FAMILY
MEDICAL
ENCYCLOPEDIA

FAMILY

MEDICAL

ENCYCLOPEDIA

An Illustrated Guide

Hamlyn

London · New York · Sydney · Toronto

Originally published under the title
Good Housekeeping Concise Medical Encyclopedia

Copyright © 1979, 1980, 1981 by the Hearst Corporation

This edition published 1982 by
The Hamlyn Publishing Group Limited
London · New York · Sydney · Toronto
Astronaut House, Feltham, Middlesex, England

Second impression 1983

ISBN 0 600 33230 6

Printed in Spain
LARSA – D. L. TF.: 1.672 – 1983
Cover design by John Miller, For Art Sake, Inc.

Acknowledgments

The publishers are grateful to the following individuals and companies for assistance in the preparation of this book:

The staff of Reference International Publishers, Ltd.: Edward R. Brace, Medical Editor; Winfred Van Atta, Associate Medical Editor; Martin Self, Editorial Director; Stephen Jones, Managing Editor; Anthony Pearce, Executive Editor; Dr. Tony Smith and Dr. Michael Hastin Bennett, Special Editorial Consultants; Dr. Andrew Brown, Picture research and captions; Julian Holland, Art director and design; Richard Bonson, Andrew Popkiewicz, Sidney Woods, Roger Twinn and George Angelini, Artists; John Cleary, Production Manager; and Robert Crocker, Production Assistant.

Robert M. Liles, Medical Editor of *Good Housekeeping* magazine, U.S.A.

Richard Bonson, who drew many of the illustrations throughout the book, and also produced all the full-color artwork.

Dr. Ian Starke and Dr. Grahame Howard for help with text for the full-color illustrations, and Sally Walters for picture research on the full-color illustrations.

Medtronic (U.K.) Ltd.
Technicon Instruments Co. Ltd.
EMI Medical Ltd.
Philips Medical Systems
GEC Medical Equipment Ltd.
for technical assistance in preparing certain illustrations.

Several illustrations in the full-color section on "The Immune System" are based on drawings in *Immunology II* by Joseph A. Bellanti; this is by kind permission of the publishers, W. B. Saunders Company, Philadelphia, PA.

The U.K. edition has been prepared with the assistance of K.E.M. Melville, L.R.C.P. and S.Ed.

Family Medical Encyclopedia is excerpted from the Good Housekeeping Family Health & Medical Guide.

Designed and produced by
Reference International Publishers, Ltd.

Common Prefixes, Suffixes and Abbreviations

The following are lists of common prefixes, suffixes and abbreviations used in medicine, together with their meanings, which the reader may find useful.

Prefixes

ab-	from
ad-	to
angio-	blood vessel
brady-	slow
card-	to do with the heart
epi-	above, upon
gast-	to do with the stomach
hyper-	excessive, above
hypo-	deficiency, below
inter-	between
intra-	within
isch-	deficiency
megalo-	abnormal enlargement
my-,	to do with muscle
myo-	
myc-	to do with fungus
myelo-	to do with spinal cord, bone marrow, myelin
orth-	normal, straight, direct
ost-	to do with bone
peri-	near, about
tachy-	abnormally rapid
trans-	across

Suffixes

-algia	pain
-cardia	to do with the heart
-cele	a body cavity
-cyte	a cell
-ectomy	surgical removal of
-itis	inflammation
-megaly	abnormal enlargement of
-odynia	pain in
-opia	defect of eye or vision
-osis	process; diseased condition
-otomy	surgical opening into
-plasia	growth, formation
-plasty	reconstruction by plastic surgery
-penia	lack of
-poiesis	formation of, production of

Abbreviations

a.c.	before food
b.d.	twice daily
I.C.D.	International Classification of Diseases
m.	in the morning
n.	at night
p.c.	after food
P.U.O.	fever of undiscovered cause (literally 'Pyrexia of undetermined origin')
Q.I.D. or Q.D.S.	four times daily
t.i.d. or t.d.s.	three times daily

Cross-Referencing System

When you start reading about one subject, you may want to learn about others that are closely related. For example, if you are reading about "agoraphobia," you may want to know about other phobias, so we suggest you look up "PHOBIA," and also compare "ACROPHOBIA" and "CLAUSTROPHOBIA." Cross-referenced subjects are set in SMALL CAPITAL LETTERS.

A Colour Atlas of the Body

The colour illustrations on the following pages show the exact location, shape, and important details of each of the body's organs and major systems, and the brief descriptions that accompany them explain the remarkable way these systems function.

To make the descriptions as clear and comprehensive as possible, the pages have been organized so that both general as well as microscopically detailed drawings of each system appear together, on facing pages. For example, on the lefthand page of colour plate IV, "Muscles," you can see how the muscles protect and interact with nerves, bones, inner organs, and the circulatory system. On the opposite page, the microanatomy of muscles is made clear in drawings that picture the incredible complexity of a single muscle fibre, the interface of muscles with the nervous system (which makes movement possible), and the detailed structure of different kinds of muscle.

Contents

The Head

The bones of the skull determine the shape of the head and also give protection to the brain and special sense organs. This view shows the intimate relationships between the various organs of the head; this compactness is one of the marvels of human evolution. The brain is by far the most complex structure in the body, and a great deal still remains to be learned about its function. With the spinal cord, it constitutes the central nervous system. The neck conveys major blood vessels, the respiratory and digestive passages and the spinal cord, and also permits extensive movement of the head around the first two cervical vertebrae.

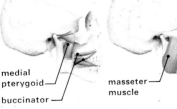

medial pterygoid
buccinator
masseter muscle
temporal muscle
temporomandibular joint

Biting and chewing muscles
Biting and chewing depend on movements at the temporomandibular joint between the lower jaw (mandible) and the rest of the skull. These movements are produced by contractions of the powerful muscles of mastication shown in the illustration above.

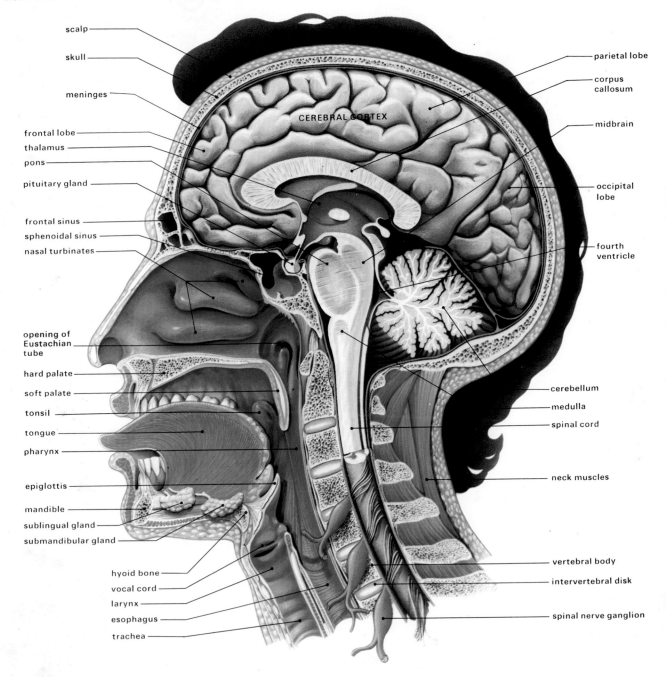

scalp
skull
meninges
frontal lobe
thalamus
pons
pituitary gland
frontal sinus
sphenoidal sinus
nasal turbinates
opening of Eustachian tube
hard palate
soft palate
tonsil
tongue
pharynx
epiglottis
mandible
sublingual gland
submandibular gland
hyoid bone
vocal cord
larynx
esophagus
trachea

CEREBRAL CORTEX

parietal lobe
corpus callosum
midbrain
occipital lobe
fourth ventricle
cerebellum
medulla
spinal cord
neck muscles
vertebral body
intervertebral disk
spinal nerve ganglion

The Bones and Joints

The skeleton gives form, support and protection to the body. It consists of about 206 bones, supplemented by pieces of cartilage. The bones, especially the long bones of the limbs, act as levers operated by the muscles (the joints forming fulcrums), thus allowing movement. Some bones (e.g., the ribs and skull) serve to protect the organs they enclose. Bones are also a reservoir of vital minerals, and some contain bone marrow, where blood cells are formed. Joints between bones are of three types: *fibrous* (allowing no movement), *cartilaginous* (limited movement) and *synovial* (freely movable).

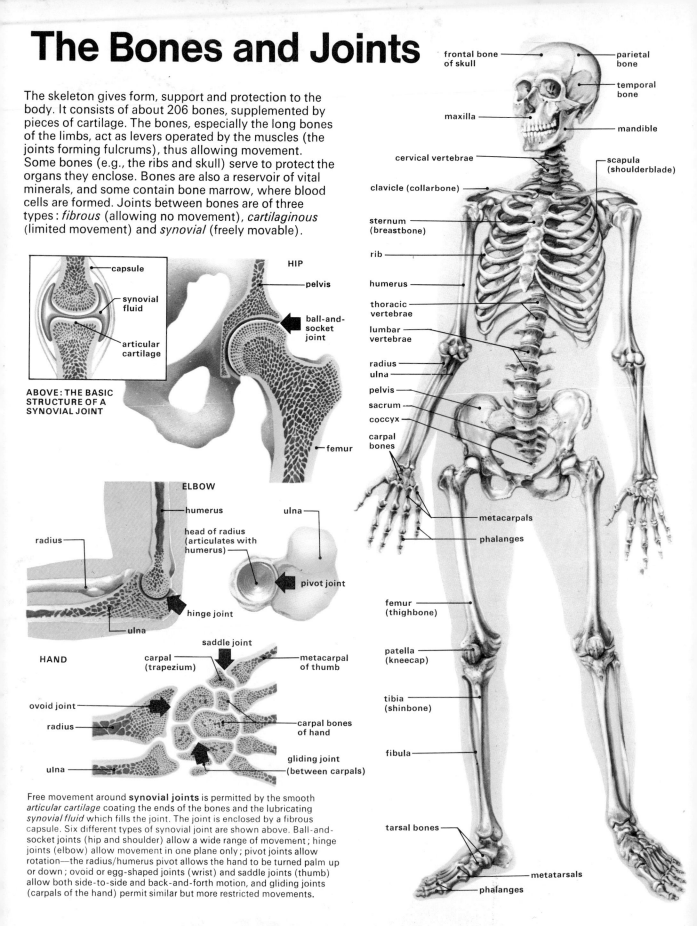

ABOVE: THE BASIC STRUCTURE OF A SYNOVIAL JOINT

Free movement around **synovial joints** is permitted by the smooth *articular cartilage* coating the ends of the bones and the lubricating *synovial fluid* which fills the joint. The joint is enclosed by a fibrous capsule. Six different types of synovial joint are shown above. Ball-and-socket joints (hip and shoulder) allow a wide range of movement; hinge joints (elbow) allow movement in one plane only; pivot joints allow rotation—the radius/humerus pivot allows the hand to be turned palm up or down; ovoid or egg-shaped joints (wrist) and saddle joints (thumb) allow both side-to-side and back-and-forth motion, and gliding joints (carpals of the hand) permit similar but more restricted movements.

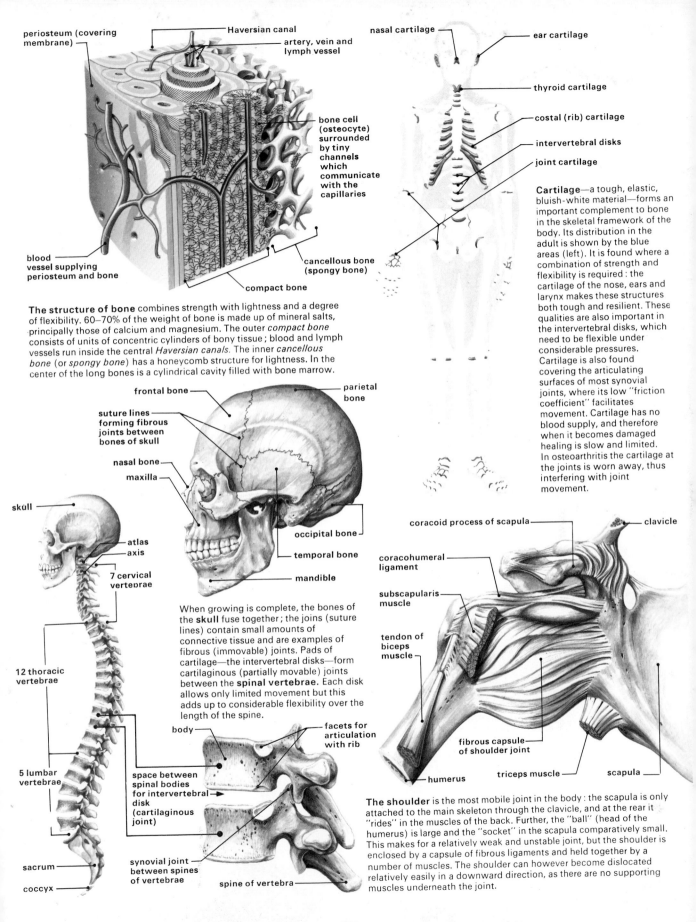

periosteum (covering membrane)

Haversian canal

artery, vein and lymph vessel

bone cell (osteocyte) surrounded by tiny channels which communicate with the capillaries

blood vessel supplying periosteum and bone

cancellous bone (spongy bone)

compact bone

The structure of bone combines strength with lightness and a degree of flexibility. 60–70% of the weight of bone is made up of mineral salts, principally those of calcium and magnesium. The outer *compact bone* consists of units of concentric cylinders of bony tissue ; blood and lymph vessels run inside the central *Haversian canals*. The inner *cancellous bone* (or *spongy bone*) has a honeycomb structure for lightness. In the center of the long bones is a cylindrical cavity filled with bone marrow.

nasal cartilage

ear cartilage

thyroid cartilage

costal (rib) cartilage

intervertebral disks

joint cartilage

Cartilage—a tough, elastic, bluish-white material—forms an important complement to bone in the skeletal framework of the body. Its distribution in the adult is shown by the blue areas (left). It is found where a combination of strength and flexibility is required : the cartilage of the nose, ears and larynx makes these structures both tough and resilient. These qualities are also important in the intervertebral disks, which need to be flexible under considerable pressures. Cartilage is also found covering the articulating surfaces of most synovial joints, where its low "friction coefficient" facilitates movement. Cartilage has no blood supply, and therefore when it becomes damaged healing is slow and limited. In osteoarthritis the cartilage at the joints is worn away, thus interfering with joint movement.

frontal bone

parietal bone

suture lines forming fibrous joints between bones of skull

nasal bone

maxilla

skull

atlas

axis

7 cervical vertebrae

occipital bone

temporal bone

mandible

When growing is complete, the bones of the **skull** fuse together ; the joins (suture lines) contain small amounts of connective tissue and are examples of fibrous (immovable) joints. Pads of cartilage—the intervertebral disks—form cartilaginous (partially movable) joints between the **spinal vertebrae**. Each disk allows only limited movement but this adds up to considerable flexibility over the length of the spine.

12 thoracic vertebrae

body

facets for articulation with rib

5 lumbar vertebrae

space between spinal bodies for intervertebral disk (cartilaginous joint)

synovial joint between spines of vertebrae

sacrum

coccyx

spine of vertebra

coracoid process of scapula

clavicle

coracohumeral ligament

subscapularis muscle

tendon of biceps muscle

fibrous capsule of shoulder joint

humerus

triceps muscle

scapula

The shoulder is the most mobile joint in the body : the scapula is only attached to the main skeleton through the clavicle, and at the rear it "rides" in the muscles of the back. Further, the "ball" (head of the humerus) is large and the "socket" in the scapula comparatively small. This makes for a relatively weak and unstable joint, but the shoulder is enclosed by a capsule of fibrous ligaments and held together by a number of muscles. The shoulder can however become dislocated relatively easily in a downward direction, as there are no supporting muscles underneath the joint.

The Muscles

Muscle is a tissue with a unique property : it can shorten (contract) when stimulated by a supplying nerve. There are three types of muscle in the body : *skeletal* or *voluntary muscle* (the "meat" of the body), *smooth* or *involuntary muscle* (found in the digestive tract, blood vessels and elsewhere) and *cardiac muscle* (found only in the heart). Skeletal muscles are attached at both ends to bones, cartilage, ligaments, skin or other muscles. When a muscle contracts, one attachment will remain static, and the other will therefore move. Muscle fibers do not increase in number with use, but each fiber becomes thicker, causing the muscles to swell and bulge.

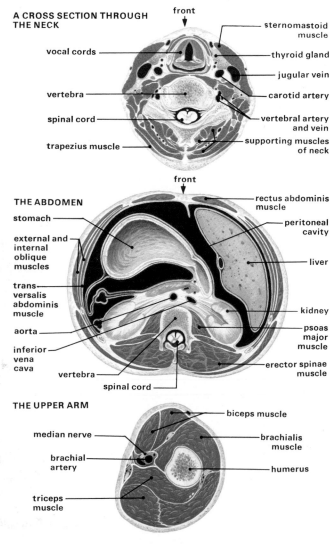

A CROSS SECTION THROUGH THE NECK

front

- sternomastoid muscle
- vocal cords
- thyroid gland
- jugular vein
- vertebra
- carotid artery
- spinal cord
- vertebral artery and vein
- trapezius muscle
- supporting muscles of neck

front

THE ABDOMEN

- stomach
- rectus abdominis muscle
- external and internal oblique muscles
- peritoneal cavity
- liver
- transversalis abdominis muscle
- aorta
- kidney
- inferior vena cava
- psoas major muscle
- vertebra
- spinal cord
- erector spinae muscle

THE UPPER ARM

- biceps muscle
- median nerve
- brachialis muscle
- brachial artery
- humerus
- triceps muscle

The arrangement of skeletal muscles in different parts of the body is shown by the cross sections above. The neck is crowded with important structures passing from the trunk to the head, including the windpipe, esophagus, spinal cord and major blood vessels supplying the brain. The many different muscles permit a wide range of head movements. The abdomen has three layers of superficial muscles giving support to the abdominal contents. Several important muscles support the spine and govern its movements, maintaining our upright posture. The section through the upper arm shows the arrangement of muscles around the humerus.

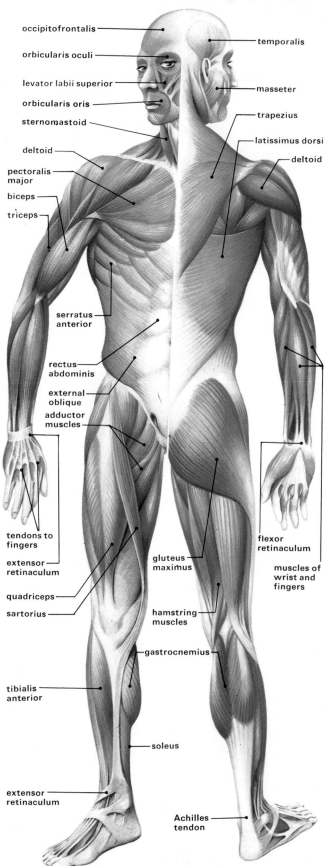

- occipitofrontalis
- temporalis
- orbicularis oculi
- levator labii superior
- masseter
- orbicularis oris
- trapezius
- sternomastoid
- latissimus dorsi
- deltoid
- deltoid
- pectoralis major
- biceps
- triceps
- serratus anterior
- rectus abdominis
- external oblique
- adductor muscles
- tendons to fingers
- flexor retinaculum
- extensor retinaculum
- gluteus maximus
- muscles of wrist and fingers
- quadriceps
- sartorius
- hamstring muscles
- gastrocnemius
- tibialis anterior
- soleus
- extensor retinaculum
- Achilles tendon

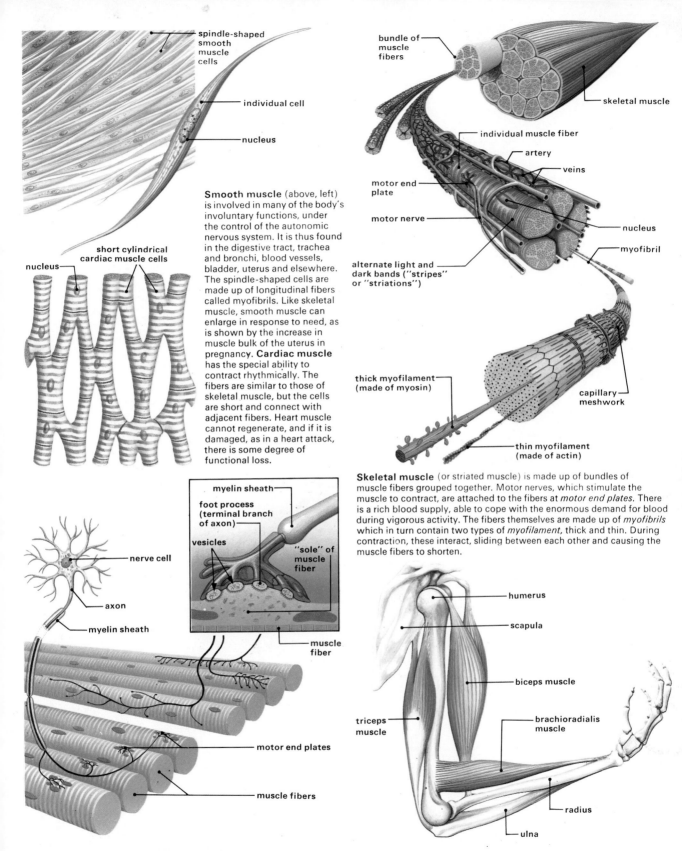

Smooth muscle (above, left) is involved in many of the body's involuntary functions, under the control of the autonomic nervous system. It is thus found in the digestive tract, trachea and bronchi, blood vessels, bladder, uterus and elsewhere. The spindle-shaped cells are made up of longitudinal fibers called myofibrils. Like skeletal muscle, smooth muscle can enlarge in response to need, as is shown by the increase in muscle bulk of the uterus in pregnancy. **Cardiac muscle** has the special ability to contract rhythmically. The fibers are similar to those of skeletal muscle, but the cells are short and connect with adjacent fibers. Heart muscle cannot regenerate, and if it is damaged, as in a heart attack, there is some degree of functional loss.

spindle-shaped smooth muscle cells

individual cell

nucleus

nucleus

short cylindrical cardiac muscle cells

bundle of muscle fibers

skeletal muscle

individual muscle fiber

artery

veins

motor end plate

motor nerve

nucleus

myofibril

alternate light and dark bands ("stripes" or "striations")

thick myofilament (made of myosin)

capillary meshwork

thin myofilament (made of actin)

Skeletal muscle (or striated muscle) is made up of bundles of muscle fibers grouped together. Motor nerves, which stimulate the muscle to contract, are attached to the fibers at *motor end plates*. There is a rich blood supply, able to cope with the enormous demand for blood during vigorous activity. The fibers themselves are made up of *myofibrils* which in turn contain two types of *myofilament*, thick and thin. During contraction, these interact, sliding between each other and causing the muscle fibers to shorten.

myelin sheath

foot process (terminal branch of axon)

vesicles

"sole" of muscle fiber

nerve cell

axon

myelin sheath

muscle fiber

motor end plates

muscle fibers

humerus

scapula

biceps muscle

brachioradialis muscle

triceps muscle

radius

ulna

A motor end plate is the junction between a motor nerve and skeletal muscle fibers. The nerve terminates in several "feet" attached to a swelling or "sole" on the muscle fiber. The nervous signal is relayed to the fibers by a biochemical "transmitter" substance, thought to be stored in vesicles near the junction.

Movement of joints usually involves contraction of some muscles and relaxation of others (skeletal muscles are generally arranged in opposing groups). Thus flexing the elbow to raise the forearm involves contraction of the biceps and brachioradialis muscles and relaxation of the triceps; to straighten the elbow, the process is reversed.

The Circulatory System

The many vital functions of the blood depend on its continuous circulation to all parts of the body. Blood is pumped by the right side of the heart through the pulmonary artery into the lungs, where it absorbs oxygen. It then returns via the pulmonary veins to the left side of the heart to be pumped through the aorta and the arterial system. It gives up oxygen — necessary for all vital bodily processes — to every tissue in the body. The deoxygenated blood returns through the veins to enter the right side of the heart once again.

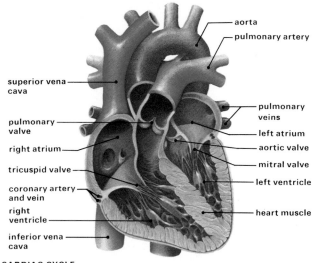

- aorta
- pulmonary artery
- superior vena cava
- pulmonary veins
- pulmonary valve
- left atrium
- right atrium
- aortic valve
- tricuspid valve
- mitral valve
- coronary artery and vein
- left ventricle
- right ventricle
- heart muscle
- inferior vena cava

CARDIAC CYCLE

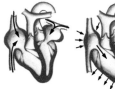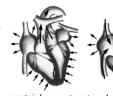

| venous blood fills atria | atria contract to fill ventricles | ventricles contract to expel blood | relaxed atria are filled again |

The heart is a double-sided pump with four chambers; valves ensure the correct flow of blood. Venous blood enters the right atrium, passes into the right ventricle and is pumped along the pulmonary artery into the lungs. Blood returns from the lungs via the pulmonary veins into the left atrium, passes into the left ventricle and is forced out through the aorta. The sequence of these events is shown in the center diagram.

ANTERIOR SURFACE OF HEART   POSTERIOR SURFACE OF HEART

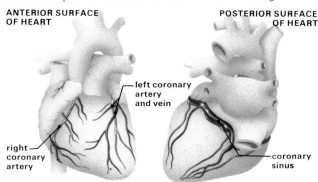

- left coronary artery and vein
- right coronary artery
- coronary sinus

The heart muscle receives its oxygen supply from the right and left **coronary arteries.** If either of these vessels becomes blocked, a "heart attack" occurs—with muscle damage, chest pain and possibly death. The **coronary veins** drain into the right atrium via the coronary sinus.

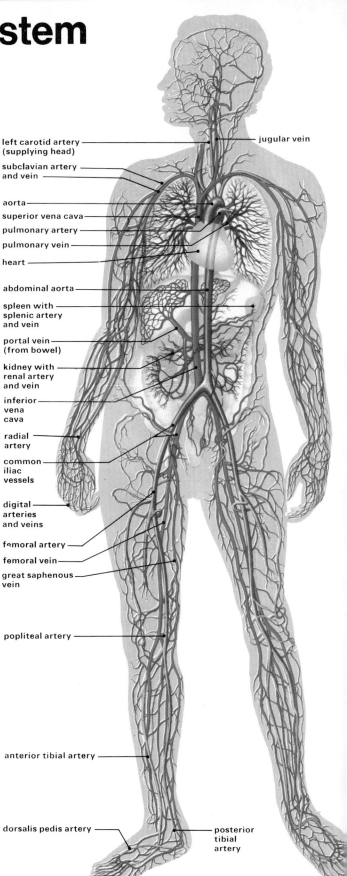

- left carotid artery (supplying head)
- jugular vein
- subclavian artery and vein
- aorta
- superior vena cava
- pulmonary artery
- pulmonary vein
- heart
- abdominal aorta
- spleen with splenic artery and vein
- portal vein (from bowel)
- kidney with renal artery and vein
- inferior vena cava
- radial artery
- common iliac vessels
- digital arteries and veins
- femoral artery
- femoral vein
- great saphenous vein
- popliteal artery
- anterior tibial artery
- dorsalis pedis artery
- posterior tibial artery

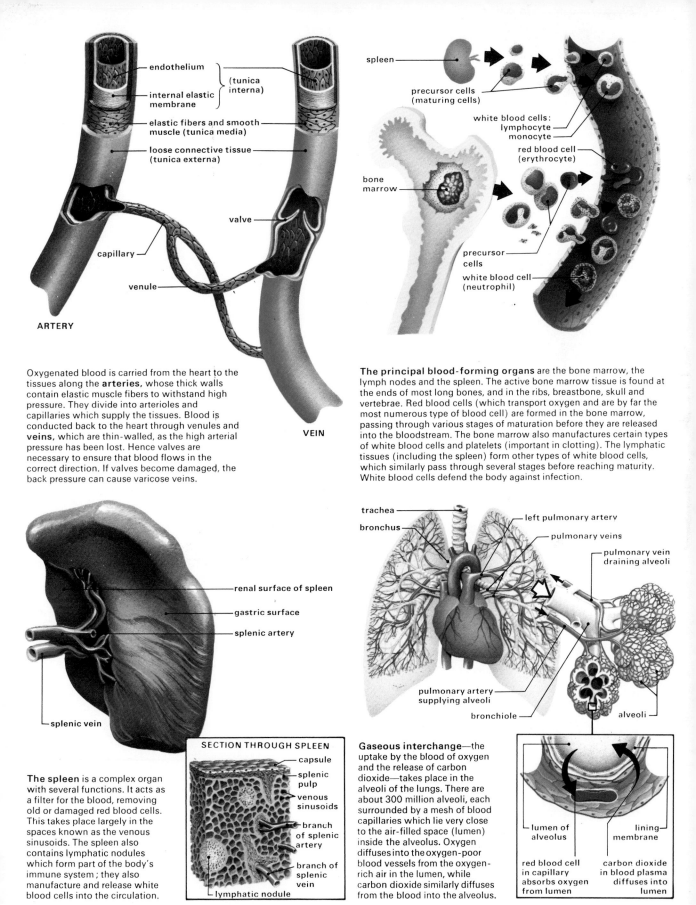

ARTERY

- endothelium
- internal elastic membrane
- (tunica interna)
- elastic fibers and smooth muscle (tunica media)
- loose connective tissue (tunica externa)
- valve
- capillary
- venule

VEIN

Oxygenated blood is carried from the heart to the tissues along the **arteries,** whose thick walls contain elastic muscle fibers to withstand high pressure. They divide into arterioles and capillaries which supply the tissues. Blood is conducted back to the heart through venules and **veins,** which are thin-walled, as the high arterial pressure has been lost. Hence valves are necessary to ensure that blood flows in the correct direction. If valves become damaged, the back pressure can cause varicose veins.

- spleen
- precursor cells (maturing cells)
- white blood cells: lymphocyte monocyte
- red blood cell (erythrocyte)
- bone marrow
- precursor cells
- white blood cell (neutrophil)

The principal blood-forming organs are the bone marrow, the lymph nodes and the spleen. The active bone marrow tissue is found at the ends of most long bones, and in the ribs, breastbone, skull and vertebrae. Red blood cells (which transport oxygen and are by far the most numerous type of blood cell) are formed in the bone marrow, passing through various stages of maturation before they are released into the bloodstream. The bone marrow also manufactures certain types of white blood cells and platelets (important in clotting). The lymphatic tissues (including the spleen) form other types of white blood cells, which similarly pass through several stages before reaching maturity. White blood cells defend the body against infection.

- renal surface of spleen
- gastric surface
- splenic artery
- splenic vein

The spleen is a complex organ with several functions. It acts as a filter for the blood, removing old or damaged red blood cells. This takes place largely in the spaces known as the venous sinusoids. The spleen also contains lymphatic nodules which form part of the body's immune system; they also manufacture and release white blood cells into the circulation.

SECTION THROUGH SPLEEN
- capsule
- splenic pulp
- venous sinusoids
- branch of splenic artery
- branch of splenic vein
- lymphatic nodule

- trachea
- bronchus
- left pulmonary artery
- pulmonary veins
- pulmonary vein draining alveoli
- pulmonary artery supplying alveoli
- bronchiole
- alveoli

Gaseous interchange—the uptake by the blood of oxygen and the release of carbon dioxide—takes place in the alveoli of the lungs. There are about 300 million alveoli, each surrounded by a mesh of blood capillaries which lie very close to the air-filled space (lumen) inside the alveolus. Oxygen diffuses into the oxygen-poor blood vessels from the oxygen-rich air in the lumen, while carbon dioxide similarly diffuses from the blood into the alveolus.

- lumen of alveolus
- lining membrane
- red blood cell in capillary absorbs oxygen from lumen
- carbon dioxide in blood plasma diffuses into lumen

The Digestive System

Digestion consists of first reducing food to its constituent parts and then absorbing the essential nutrients. Food is broken down in the stomach and duodenum by the action of enzymes released from glands in the mouth, stomach and pancreas. The absorption of nutrients into the bloodstream occurs mainly in the small intestine. In the large intestine, water is absorbed to leave semisolid waste which is passed via the rectum as feces. The liver — the largest gland in the body — is responsible for utilizing the products of digestion absorbed into the blood.

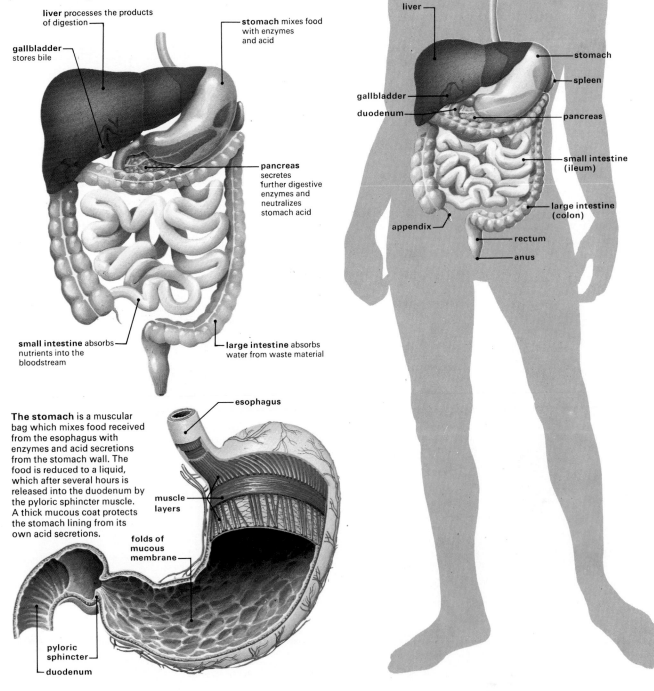

liver processes the products of digestion

gallbladder stores bile

stomach mixes food with enzymes and acid

pancreas secretes further digestive enzymes and neutralizes stomach acid

small intestine absorbs nutrients into the bloodstream

large intestine absorbs water from waste material

parotid gland

sublingual gland

submandibular gland

esophagus

liver

stomach

spleen

gallbladder

duodenum

pancreas

small intestine (ileum)

large intestine (colon)

appendix

rectum

anus

The stomach is a muscular bag which mixes food received from the esophagus with enzymes and acid secretions from the stomach wall. The food is reduced to a liquid, which after several hours is released into the duodenum by the pyloric sphincter muscle. A thick mucous coat protects the stomach lining from its own acid secretions.

esophagus

muscle layers

folds of mucous membrane

pyloric sphincter

duodenum

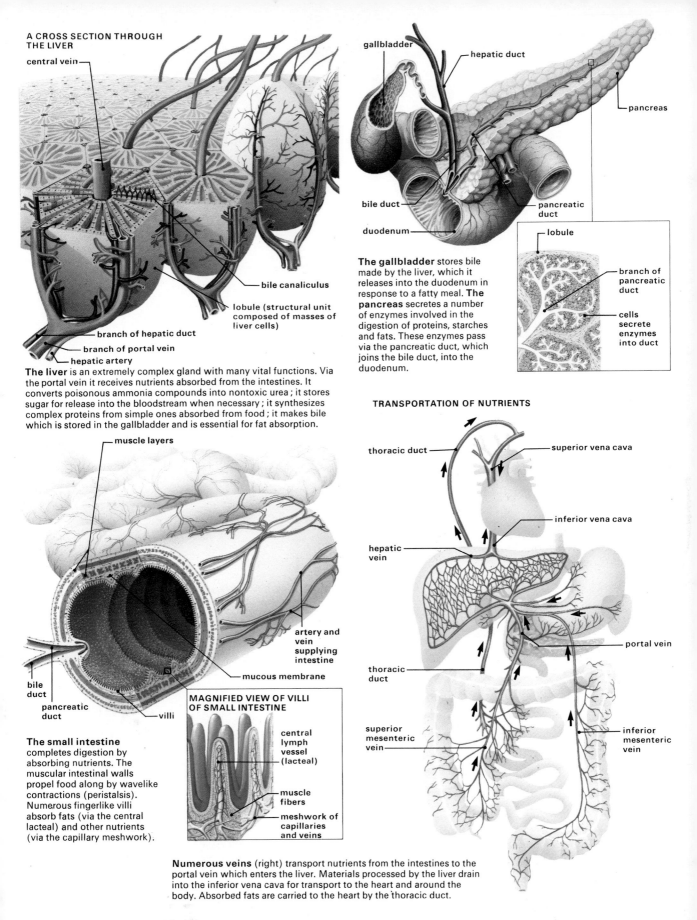

A CROSS SECTION THROUGH THE LIVER

- central vein
- bile canaliculus
- lobule (structural unit composed of masses of liver cells)
- branch of hepatic duct
- branch of portal vein
- hepatic artery

The liver is an extremely complex gland with many vital functions. Via the portal vein it receives nutrients absorbed from the intestines. It converts poisonous ammonia compounds into nontoxic urea; it stores sugar for release into the bloodstream when necessary; it synthesizes complex proteins from simple ones absorbed from food; it makes bile which is stored in the gallbladder and is essential for fat absorption.

- gallbladder
- hepatic duct
- pancreas
- bile duct
- pancreatic duct
- duodenum
- lobule
- branch of pancreatic duct
- cells secrete enzymes into duct

The gallbladder stores bile made by the liver, which it releases into the duodenum in response to a fatty meal. **The pancreas** secretes a number of enzymes involved in the digestion of proteins, starches and fats. These enzymes pass via the pancreatic duct, which joins the bile duct, into the duodenum.

- muscle layers
- artery and vein supplying intestine
- mucous membrane
- bile duct
- pancreatic duct
- villi

The small intestine completes digestion by absorbing nutrients. The muscular intestinal walls propel food along by wavelike contractions (peristalsis). Numerous fingerlike villi absorb fats (via the central lacteal) and other nutrients (via the capillary meshwork).

MAGNIFIED VIEW OF VILLI OF SMALL INTESTINE

- central lymph vessel (lacteal)
- muscle fibers
- meshwork of capillaries and veins

TRANSPORTATION OF NUTRIENTS

- thoracic duct
- superior vena cava
- inferior vena cava
- hepatic vein
- thoracic duct
- portal vein
- superior mesenteric vein
- inferior mesenteric vein

Numerous veins (right) transport nutrients from the intestines to the portal vein which enters the liver. Materials processed by the liver drain into the inferior vena cava for transport to the heart and around the body. Absorbed fats are carried to the heart by the thoracic duct.

The Nervous System

Nerves are complex fibers which conduct electrochemical impulses. Nerves to and from all parts of the body are grouped together within the spinal cord and conveyed to the brain, which controls and coordinates the nervous signals involved in any bodily function—innumerable in even the simplest activity. The nervous system can be divided into the *motor system* (muscular control), the *sensory system* (information from the senses to the brain) and the *autonomic nervous system* (bodily functions not under conscious control, e.g., digestion).

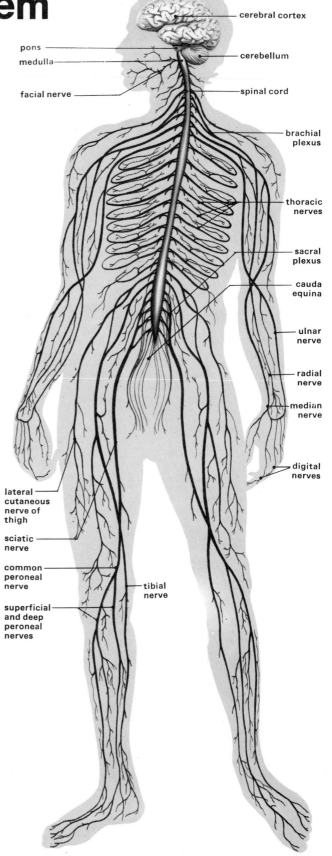

cerebral cortex

pons

medulla

facial nerve

cerebellum

spinal cord

brachial plexus

thoracic nerves

sacral plexus

cauda equina

ulnar nerve

radial nerve

median nerve

digital nerves

lateral cutaneous nerve of thigh

sciatic nerve

common peroneal nerve

superficial and deep peroneal nerves

tibial nerve

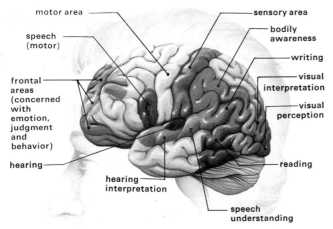

motor area

speech (motor)

frontal areas (concerned with emotion, judgment and behavior)

hearing

hearing interpretation

speech understanding

sensory area

bodily awareness

writing

visual interpretation

visual perception

reading

Each area of the **cerebral cortex** (outer layer of the brain) is concerned with a particular function. For example, voluntary movements are initiated in the motor area, while sensations of pain and touch are processed in the sensory area. Complex incoming signals may be collected together and processed in more than one area—for example, visual signals are perceived in one area and interpreted in another.

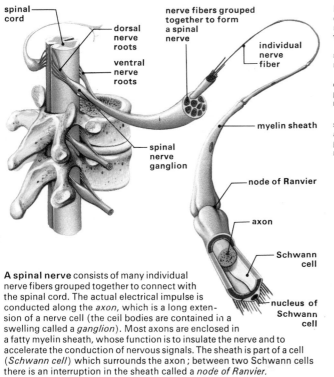

spinal cord

dorsal nerve roots

ventral nerve roots

spinal nerve ganglion

nerve fibers grouped together to form a spinal nerve

individual nerve fiber

myelin sheath

node of Ranvier

axon

Schwann cell

nucleus of Schwann cell

A spinal nerve consists of many individual nerve fibers grouped together to connect with the spinal cord. The actual electrical impulse is conducted along the *axon*, which is a long extension of a nerve cell (the cell bodies are contained in a swelling called a *ganglion*). Most axons are enclosed in a fatty myelin sheath, whose function is to insulate the nerve and to accelerate the conduction of nervous signals. The sheath is part of a cell (*Schwann cell*) which surrounds the axon; between two Schwann cells there is an interruption in the sheath called a *node of Ranvier*.

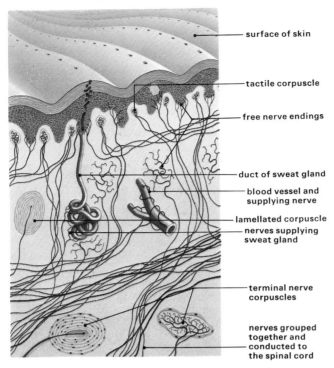

Labels (skin diagram):
- surface of skin
- tactile corpuscle
- free nerve endings
- duct of sweat gland
- blood vessel and supplying nerve
- lamellated corpuscle
- nerves supplying sweat gland
- terminal nerve corpuscles
- nerves grouped together and conducted to the spinal cord

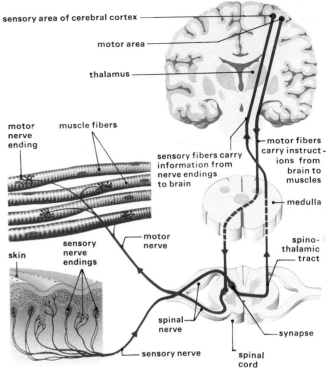

Labels (motor and sensory diagram):
- sensory area of cerebral cortex
- motor area
- thalamus
- motor nerve ending
- muscle fibers
- sensory fibers carry information from nerve endings to brain
- motor fibers carry instructions from brain to muscles
- medulla
- motor nerve
- skin
- sensory nerve endings
- spinothalamic tract
- spinal nerve
- synapse
- sensory nerve
- spinal cord

Nerve supply of the skin

Both motor and sensory nerves are to be found in and just below the skin. The autonomic nervous system supplies nerve fibers to the sweat glands and capillaries ; these control sweating and constriction or dilatation of the capillaries and thus heat loss from the body through the skin. Sensory nerve fibers supplying the skin may terminate in various types of structures called corpuscles. It is not certain whether a particular type is concerned with a particular sensation, though the lamellated corpuscle is thought to be sensitive to vibration and pressure. Other sensory nerves have free nerve endings, which may be concerned with the sensation of pain. Where there are hairs, the hair follicle is also supplied by nerves from the autonomic and sensory systems.

Motor and sensory nervous system

Sensory nerves carrying stimuli of pain, temperature, touch, etc., join the spinal cord via a spinal nerve. Those fibers carrying pain and temperature sensations (blue line) cross over to the other side of the cord ; this involves the transfer of the stimulus from one nerve cell to another at a *synapse*. (Other sensations, e.g. touch, are conducted along a different route.) The fibers then ascend the spinal cord in the spinothalamic tract to the thalamus, and from there to the sensory cortex. Here, with the aid of other parts of the brain, the stimulus is interpreted. Motor nerves carrying signals from the motor cortex to the voluntary muscles (red line) cross in the medulla of the brain stem before descending the spinal cord to leave via a spinal nerve.

THE PARASYMPATHETIC NERVOUS SYSTEM

THE SYMPATHETIC NERVOUS SYSTEM

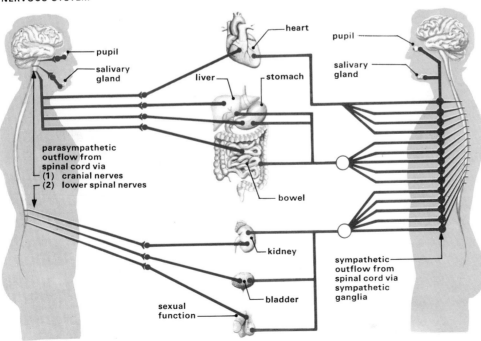

Labels:
- pupil
- salivary gland
- heart
- liver
- stomach
- parasympathetic outflow from spinal cord via (1) cranial nerves (2) lower spinal nerves
- bowel
- kidney
- bladder
- sexual function
- pupil
- salivary gland
- sympathetic outflow from spinal cord via sympathetic ganglia

The autonomic nervous system regulates the automatic functions of the body and is composed of the sympathetic and parasympathetic systems, which have opposing effects. The sympathetic system prepares the body for emergency action by reducing nonessential activities such as digestion. The sympathetic nerves are relayed from the sympathetic ganglia which form a chain along either side of the vertebral column. Stimulation of these nerves leads to increases in heart and respiration rate, blood supply to the muscles and dilatation of the pupils, while salivation, urine production and digestive activity are reduced. Ejaculation is also mediated by the sympathetic system, though penile erection is a parasympathetic function. The parasympathetic system involves the 3rd, 7th, 9th and 10th cranial nerves and the lower spinal nerves and comes into play during rest and sleep—slowing the heart and breathing, constricting the pupils and increasing digestion.

The Endocrine System

The endocrine glands (ductless glands) secrete hormones directly into the bloodstream. Hormones are complex chemical "messenger" substances; they are released in tiny amounts, yet they can produce dramatic changes in the activity of body cells. In this way they control basic body functions such as growth, metabolism and sexual development; they are also responsible for maintaining the correct levels in the blood of certain vital substances (e.g. sugar and salt).

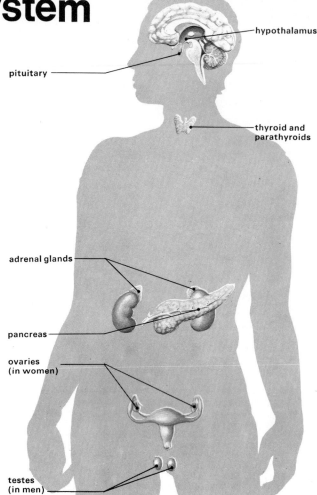

hypothalamus

pituitary

thyroid and parathyroids

adrenal glands

pancreas

ovaries (in women)

testes (in men)

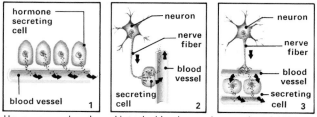

Hormones can be released into the bloodstream in a number of different ways. They may be released directly by a secreting cell (1) or when such a cell is stimulated by a nerve impulse (2). In the posterior lobe of the pituitary, nerve fibers themselves release hormones directly into the blood, which stimulate another hormone-producing cell (3).

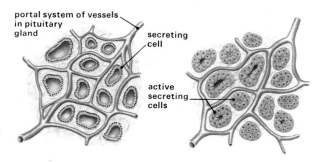

portal system of vessels in pituitary gland

secreting cell

active secreting cells

The anterior pituitary has a rich network of blood vessels connecting it to the hypothalamus. It is thought that "neurosecretions" from the hypothalamus stimulate the hormone-secreting cells.

The secretion of hormones is controlled by a complex feedback mechanism in which the nervous system is closely involved. The **hypothalamus** and **pituitary** play particularly important roles.

The pituitary gland (right) is situated at the base of the brain and is about the size of a pea; it is divided into two lobes. It is subject to the influence of the hypothalamus, to which it is connected by a slender stalk. It releases a variety of hormones which act on several "target" organs. The hormones of the anterior lobe, with the exception of somatotropin and MSH, stimulate other glands. The hypothalamus is thought to monitor the level of the hormones released by these glands and to direct the pituitary to cut off the stimulating hormone once the correct level is reached.

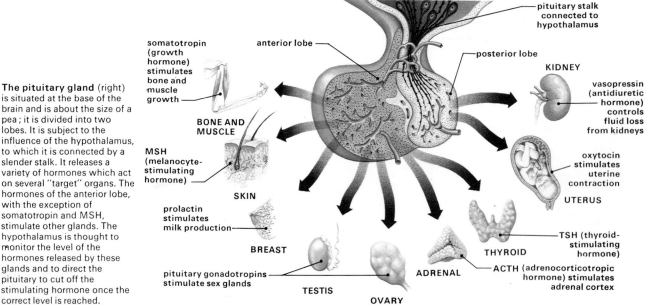

somatotropin (growth hormone) stimulates bone and muscle growth

anterior lobe

pituitary stalk connected to hypothalamus

posterior lobe

KIDNEY

vasopressin (antidiuretic hormone) controls fluid loss from kidneys

BONE AND MUSCLE

MSH (melanocyte-stimulating hormone)

SKIN

oxytocin stimulates uterine contraction

UTERUS

prolactin stimulates milk production

BREAST

pituitary gonadotropins stimulate sex glands

TESTIS

OVARY

ADRENAL

THYROID

TSH (thyroid-stimulating hormone)

ACTH (adrenocorticotropic hormone) stimulates adrenal cortex

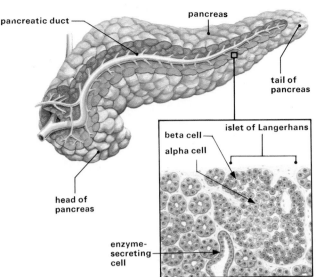

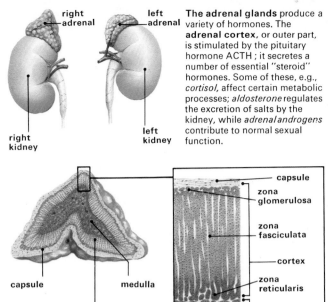

The adrenal glands produce a variety of hormones. The adrenal cortex, or outer part, is stimulated by the pituitary hormone ACTH; it secretes a number of essential "steroid" hormones. Some of these, e.g., *cortisol*, affect certain metabolic processes; *aldosterone* regulates the excretion of salts by the kidney, while *adrenal androgens* contribute to normal sexual function.

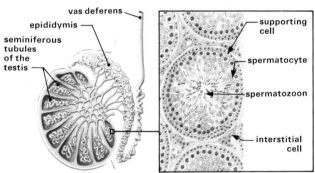

The pancreas, which lies behind and under the stomach, is a mixed-function gland; as well as containing cells which secrete digestive enzymes, it has clumps of cells known as the *islets of Langerhans* which secrete hormones. These are most numerous toward the tail or pointed end of the pancreas. The islets contain two types of cells—*alpha* and *beta* cells. The alpha cells produce the hormone glucagon which raises the level of sugar in the blood; the beta cells secrete insulin which lowers blood sugar. A lack of this hormone as the result of disease or damage to the pancreas produces diabetes.

The adrenal medulla, or inner part of the adrenal glands, is entirely separate in function from the cortex and is not influenced by the pituitary gland. It secretes the hormones epinephrine and norepinephrine (adrenaline and noradrenaline) in response to fear, anger or sexual desire; these prepare the body for instant action by increasing the heart rate and the blood supply to the muscles.

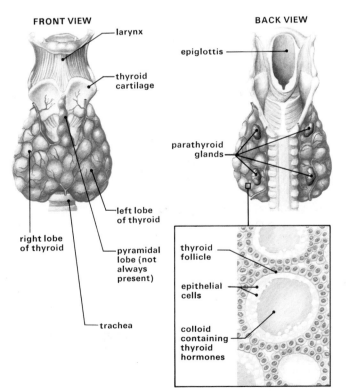

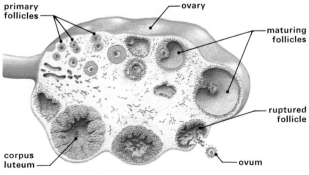

The tubules of the testes contain cells called spermatocytes which, under the influence of gonadotropic hormones, mature into spermatozoa. These are stored in the tubules and epididymis until they are conducted to the penis at ejaculation by the vas deferens. The interstitial cells between the tubules also produce the male hormone testosterone, responsible for secondary sexual characteristics.

The thyroid gland is situated at the base of the neck on either side of the trachea, just below the larynx. It is made up of follicles containing a fluid called colloid, in which the two thyroid hormones thyroxine and tri-iodothyronine (T_4 and T_3) are stored for release into the bloodstream as necessary. These hormones control the body's metabolic rate. There are four small parathyroid glands situated behind the thyroid. These secrete parathyroid hormone (or parathormone), which controls the level of calcium and phosphorus in the blood.

At birth, the ovaries contain numerous primary follicles; after puberty, these develop under complex hormonal control. At the mid-point of each menstrual cycle an ovum (egg cell) is released from a mature follicle, which then becomes a corpus luteum. If pregnancy occurs, this secretes hormones which interrupt the menstrual cycle.

The Immune System

The immune system defends the body against invasion by disease-producing organisms and against toxins they produce. It can distinguish between what belongs in the body ("self") and what does not ("non-self"), and reacts against any cells that are not recognized as "self." This reaction may be either to produce antibodies (*humoral immunity*) or to activate cells which attack the invader directly (*cell-mediated immunity*). In both cases the outcome is to make the foreign cell or invading organism subject to *phagocytosis* – destruction by certain white blood cells.

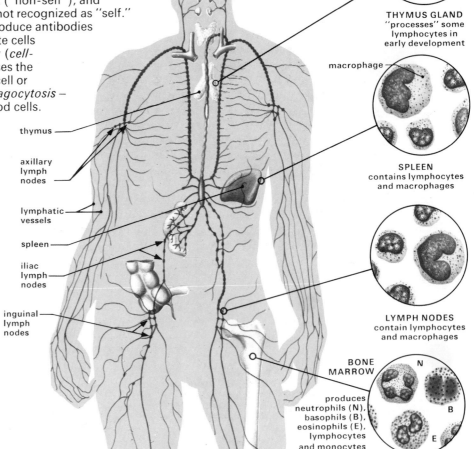

lymphocyte

THYMUS GLAND
"processes" some lymphocytes in early development

macrophage

SPLEEN
contains lymphocytes and macrophages

LYMPH NODES
contain lymphocytes and macrophages

BONE MARROW
produces neutrophils (N), basophils (B), eosinophils (E), lymphocytes and monocytes

thymus

axillary lymph nodes

lymphatic vessels

spleen

iliac lymph nodes

inguinal lymph nodes

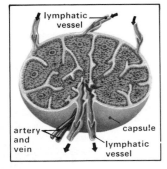

lymphatic vessel

artery and vein

capsule

lymphatic vessel

Lymph nodes (above) are pea-sized structures situated in groups at strategic points in the lymphatic vessels—the network of channels which drain the tissues and return excess fluid to the bloodstream. Foreign particles, such as bacteria, are trapped in the lymph nodes, which are inhabited by *macrophages* (white blood cells which can phagocytose, i.e. engulf and destroy, foreign particles) and *lymphocytes* (white blood cells which mount immune reactions).

The main components of the body's immune system are shown above (right). The lymphatic system and lymphoid tissues represent the basic structural framework. The magnified cells shown are all different types of white blood cell. Lymphocytes are concentrated in the lymph nodes and spleen: they are of two types—"T-lymphocytes" and "B-lymphocytes"—which inhabit different regions of the nodes and spleen and play different roles in the immune response. In early development, the thymus gland "processes" some circulating lymphocytes before they reach the lymph nodes and spleen. These become "T-cells" able to mount a cell-mediated immune response. Others, called "B-cells," are not processed in this way, but are capable of responding to antigens by producing antibodies. The bone marrow manufactures a variety of white blood cells: *monocytes,* which eventually become phagocytic macrophages; *neutrophils,* which are also mainly phagocytic, *basophils* (called Mast cells outside the bloodstream), which produce histamine, and *eosinophils,* which limit the effects of histamine release.

TWO METHODS OF ANTIBODY FUNCTION

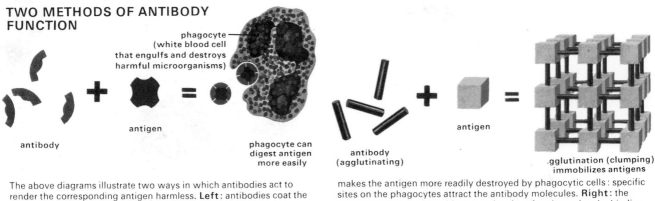

phagocyte (white blood cell that engulfs and destroys harmful microorganisms)

antibody + antigen = phagocyte can digest antigen more easily

antibody (agglutinating) + antigen = agglutination (clumping) immobilizes antigens

The above diagrams illustrate two ways in which antibodies act to render the corresponding antigen harmless. **Left:** antibodies coat the surface of the antigen. As a result of this process, certain other enzymes in the blood are activated which, if the antigen is a cell or micro-organism, damage the cell wall, killing the cell. In addition, coating makes the antigen more readily destroyed by phagocytic cells: specific sites on the phagocytes attract the antibody molecules. **Right:** the antibody can combine with two molecules of antigen, thereby binding the antigen into clumps. This process of agglutination immobilizes the antigens, which can again be ingested by the phagocytes.

PHAGOCYTOSIS AND THE INFLAMMATORY RESPONSE

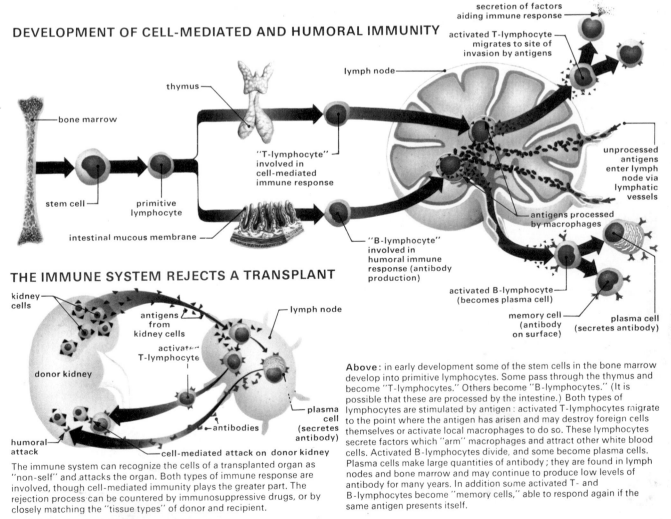

surface of skin

pathogenic bacteria

phagocytes (neutrophils)

phagocyte (macrophage)

phagocytes engulf and destroy bacteria

phagocyte attracted to area migrates from blood vessel

Mast cell releases histamine, causing dilatation of blood vessels and inflammation

blood capillary

red blood cell

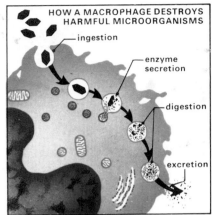

HOW A MACROPHAGE DESTROYS HARMFUL MICROORGANISMS

ingestion

enzyme secretion

digestion

excretion

Left: a rusty nail has broken the skin, carrying in with it pathogenic bacteria. Some of these are ingested by phagocytic neutrophils and by a macrophage. Antigen from the organism will reach the local lymph node, either directly or carried within the macrophage, and "antigen processing" takes place (see below). Lymphocytes are stimulated to become *plasma cells* which make the appropriate antibody; this then circulates to the tissue and combines with the antigen on the surface of the organism at the site of the wound. This reaction causes activation of enzymes in the blood, causing damage to the cell walls of the invaders. Various chemical substances are released; these attract phagocytes and cause secretion of histamine by Mast cells. Histamine causes dilatation of local blood vessels and increased migration of fluid and cells into the area, leading to the familiar features of inflammation.

DEVELOPMENT OF CELL-MEDIATED AND HUMORAL IMMUNITY

secretion of factors aiding immune response

activated T-lymphocyte migrates to site of invasion by antigens

lymph node

thymus

bone marrow

"T-lymphocyte" involved in cell-mediated immune response

stem cell

primitive lymphocyte

intestinal mucous membrane

"B-lymphocyte" involved in humoral immune response (antibody production)

unprocessed antigens enter lymph node via lymphatic vessels

antigens processed by macrophages

activated B-lymphocyte (becomes plasma cell)

memory cell (antibody on surface)

plasma cell (secretes antibody)

THE IMMUNE SYSTEM REJECTS A TRANSPLANT

kidney cells

antigens from kidney cells

activated T-lymphocyte

lymph node

donor kidney

plasma cell (secretes antibody)

antibodies

humoral attack

cell-mediated attack on donor kidney

The immune system can recognize the cells of a transplanted organ as "non-self" and attacks the organ. Both types of immune response are involved, though cell-mediated immunity plays the greater part. The rejection process can be countered by immunosuppressive drugs, or by closely matching the "tissue types" of donor and recipient.

Above: in early development some of the stem cells in the bone marrow develop into primitive lymphocytes. Some pass through the thymus and become "T-lymphocytes." Others become "B-lymphocytes." (It is possible that these are processed by the intestine.) Both types of lymphocytes are stimulated by antigen: activated T-lymphocytes migrate to the point where the antigen has arisen and may destroy foreign cells themselves or activate local macrophages to do so. These lymphocytes secrete factors which "arm" macrophages and attract other white blood cells. Activated B-lymphocytes divide, and some become plasma cells. Plasma cells make large quantities of antibody; they are found in lymph nodes and bone marrow and may continue to produce low levels of antibody for many years. In addition some activated T- and B-lymphocytes become "memory cells," able to respond again if the same antigen presents itself.

The Major Sense Organs

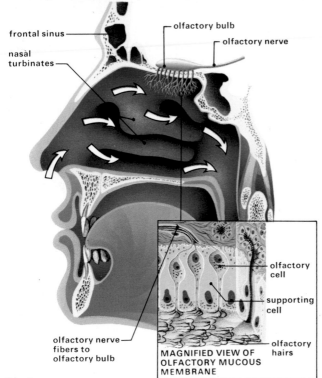

frontal sinus
nasal turbinates
olfactory bulb
olfactory nerve

olfactory cell
supporting cell

olfactory nerve fibers to olfactory bulb

olfactory hairs

MAGNIFIED VIEW OF OLFACTORY MUCOUS MEMBRANE

Smell
The olfactory mucous membrane, a small area in the nasal cavity, contains 10–20 million olfactory cells, each tipped by 10–20 tiny hairs. When air containing odorous molecules reaches the olfactory cells, certain molecules fit certain receptors on the hairs; nervous signals are then sent to the brain, where they are interpreted as odors.

Sight
Rays of light enter the eyeball through the cornea, pass through the lens and vitreous humor to the fovea centralis—the most sensitive region of the retina. This pathway is called the visual axis. By means of a complex system of muscles and nerves, the brain insures that the two visual axes remain parallel. The exception is when the eyes converge to read or study a close object.

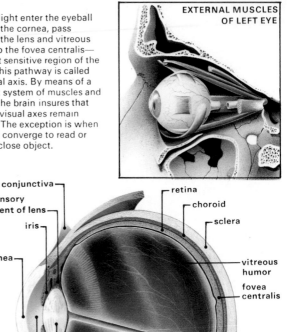

EXTERNAL MUSCLES OF LEFT EYE

conjunctiva
suspensory ligament of lens
iris
cornea

retina
choroid
sclera
vitreous humor
fovea centralis

anterior chamber
lens

hyaloid canal

CROSS SECTION THROUGH RIGHT EYEBALL

Hearing
Hearing begins when sound waves reach the eardrum; the vibrations pass through the ossicles and displace fluid within the cochlea. The fluid stimulates hair cells of the organ of Corti to send signals to the brain. The semicircular canals monitor balance by a similar mechanism.

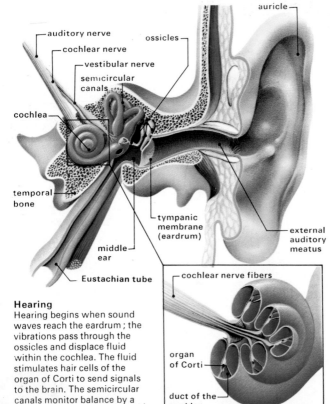

auditory nerve
cochlear nerve
vestibular nerve
semicircular canals
cochlea
temporal bone
ossicles
auricle

middle ear
Eustachian tube

tympanic membrane (eardrum)
external auditory meatus

cochlear nerve fibers
organ of Corti
duct of the cochlea

Taste
The nervous signals responsible for our sense of taste originate in the taste buds. These microscopic structures are most numerous in the grooves around the vallate papillae of the tongue. Any substance tasted must first dissolve in saliva and then percolate through tiny pores to the hair receptors of the taste bud. There are thought to be specialized receptors for each of the basic tastes : sweet, sour, salty and bitter. All flavors are made up of combinations of these four tastes.

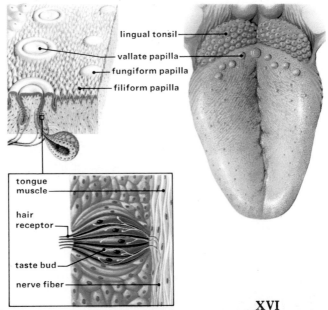

lingual tonsil
vallate papilla
fungiform papilla
filiform papilla

tongue muscle
hair receptor
taste bud
nerve fiber

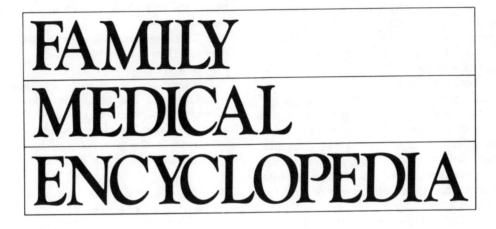

FAMILY MEDICAL ENCYCLOPEDIA

A

abdominal perforation

An acute abdominal emergency, commonly resulting from the erosion of a peptic ulcer, inflamed appendix or gall bladder, or other intestinal lesion into the abdominal cavity.

When an acute perforation occurs, there is immediate, severe pain (known as "pistol-shot") with shock and collapse. The abdominal muscles become rigid and the patient lies with his legs bent up in an attempt to ease the agonizing spasm of these muscles.

Treatment is by immediate operation, the extent of which depends on the diagnosis and on how fit the patient is. Overall mortality following operation for acute perforation is about 3% – the sooner the operation, the better the prognosis.

In cases of suspected perforation, or indeed any abdominal emergency, the competent physician will resist all pressure to administer some form of pain-relieving injection. The reason is that if he gives this, the signs and symptoms will disappear temporarily, and when the surgeon sees the patient, he is left with no option other than to perform an exploratory operation, without a firm diagnosis.

See APPENDICITIS, ULCER, ULCERATIVE COLITIS.

abduction/adduction

Two words used to describe the movements of limbs. Abduction is movement of a limb (or part of a limb) *away* from the midline of the body. Adduction is movement of a limb (or part of a limb) *toward* the midline.

When the arm is lifted away from the side and upwards toward a horizontal position, that is abduction. When it is brought down again to hang by the side, that movement is adduction. If you move your little toe outward you are abducting it; when you move it back in to lie alongside the other toes you are adducting it.

The practical importance of these terms is that they enable physicians to describe the actions of particular muscles with precision. Some body muscles are referred to as "abductors," while others are termed "adductors."

abortion

Loss of the fetus in early pregnancy.

Medically the terms "abortion" and "miscarriage" are generally synonymous, but in recent years there has been an increasing tendency for laymen to use the word "abortion" to indicate the deliberate termination of a pregnancy; "miscarriage" implies that the ending of a pregnancy has been either accidental or spontaneous.

Deliberate abortion of pregnancy has been practiced for thousands of years, but was a very dangerous procedure until quite recently. Criminal, or "back-street" abortions are still highly dangerous and may result in loss of life or serious damage to the mother's health.

Legal abortion (carried out by trained medical practitioners, surgeons or gynecologists) is a relatively safe procedure, especially if performed very early in the pregnancy. Such abortions were rarely permitted before the mid-1960s, but are now carried out on a very wide scale.

In Britain the abortion rates per 1000 women aged between 15 and 44 in 1968 were 3.46. In 1979 they had risen to 11.97.

The technique of an early abortion is relatively straightforward and usually involves aspirating the contents of the womb with a suction catheter. Later abortions (when pregnancy is advanced beyond 12 weeks) may involve more complex techniques and carry a much higher risk of side effects.

abruptio placentae

A condition of late pregnancy in which bleeding occurs within the womb as a result of partial premature separation (abruption) of the PLACENTA (afterbirth).

The cause of the placental separation is not known in most cases, although occasionally the bleeding follows an attempt at version (turning) of the fetus. Abruptio placentae is most common in women suffering from a toxic condition of pregnancy known as preeclampsia.

The features of abruptio placentae depend on whether the blood is retained within the womb ("concealed" hemorrhage) or escapes via the vagina ("revealed" hemorrhage). In the "concealed" variety, the mother suffers pain in the lower part of the abdomen and sometimes profound low blood pressure (shock). The same features are present in the "revealed" variety of the condition, but the diagnosis may be clarified by the additional presence of external bleeding.

Abruptio placentae is a danger to the mother (because of blood loss and shock) and to the baby, since severe hemorrhage may cause fetal death. Immediate admission to a hospital is thus essential. Intravenous fluid replacement and blood transfusion may be necessary. Once the condition of the mother is stabilized (and the diagnosis is differentiated from PLACENTA PREVIA) the obstetrician may attempt to deliver the baby—either by inducing labor or by carrying out a Cesarean operation.

ABSCESS

An abscess is a collection of pus in a cavity and is caused by infection with certain bacteria. Shown here are three ways in which an abscess might develop: (1) as a direct result of external infection, for example in a cut finger; (2) by local spread from a nearby site of infection, such as an alveolar abscess in the jawbone caused by a decayed tooth; (3) as a result of bacteria being transported in the bloodstream—for example, a brain abscess may follow from a lung infection.

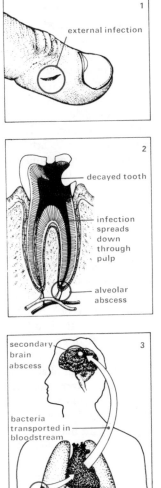

THREE ROUTES OF ABSCESS FORMATION

abscess

A collection of pus formed anywhere in the body.

Abscesses are nearly always caused by bacterial infection, although occasionally they result from the presence of an irritating foreign body such as a splinter.

The usual response of the body to the stimulus of local irritation or damage by bacteria is the concentration of a large number of white blood cells (leukocytes) in the area affected. While the overall effect is beneficial, the reaction has certain local disadvantages: the infected part becomes hot, swollen, red and painful as the blood vessels dilate to carry leukocytes to the scene of action. The leukocytes pass through the walls of the blood vessels to "mop up" invading bacteria, and the area is walled off by the formation of fibrous tissue. Eventually the area of inflammation becomes localized and the collection of dead bacteria, dead leukocytes and exuded tissue fluid liquefies to form pus under tension.

The abscess so produced tends to find the line of least resistance in the surrounding tissues and "comes to a head" on the surface. If left to itself it bursts, but if possible the doctor hastens the process by making an incision to let out the pus and so ease the pain. It is dangerous to try to open an abscess before it is ready; an injudicious incision can only spread the infection.

absorption

The process of absorbing food and other substances (including drugs) into the body.

Absorption may take place by means of a variety of routes. Medication may be given via all of them, but nutrients can be absorbed only through the gastrointestinal tract.

Food and drink are taken by mouth, pass down the esophagus, and reach the stomach. No significant absorption takes place in this organ, except in the case of alcohol and simple sugars such as glucose (which can be absorbed into the bloodstream through the stomach wall).

After a period of digestion in the stomach, nutrients move through the duodenum into the jejunum and ileum. (The duodenum, jejunum and ileum together make up the small intestine—one continuous tube about 22 ft. (6.5 meters) long.) The inside wall of the small intestine has a multitude of small finger-like projections with tiny blood vessels in them. It is in the small intestine that the absorption of food takes place: nutrients pass through the thin membrane covering the folds and enter the blood vessels lying underneath.

Many drugs are absorbed in precisely the same way, being taken by mouth and carried to the small intestine where they pass through the intestinal wall and enter the bloodstream. But drugs can also be absorbed through the skin as well as through mucous membranes of the eye, nose, mouth, vagina and rectum.

accommodation

The process that adjusts the lens of the eye for clear vision of objects either near to the eye or far from it.

If the lens of the eye were a solid immovable body (like glass and plastic lenses) it would not be able to provide a well-focused image of all objects; some would be out of focus because they were either too far away or too near. In a camera the problem is solved by moving the lens relative to the film. In the eye the distance is constant but the lens has its focal length changed. This is possible because the lens of the human eye is capable of changing its shape from moment to moment, depending on whether we are looking at objects that are near to us or far away.

When we look at a close object, the lens of the eye becomes thicker and more convex in order to focus the light from that object on the retina (the light-sensitive structure at the back of the eye). When we look at a distant object the lens becomes slimmer, so that the light from that object can be brought into focus. This alteration in the shape of the lens is the result of contraction of the *ciliary muscle*, which moves the circular ligament from which the lens is suspended and so alters its shape.

In middle age the lens loses a good deal of its elasticity, so reducing the range over which it can be focused. This loss of flexibility results in older people needing to hold a newspaper or other reading matter at arms' length or to use reading glasses. Anyone who has needed to wear glasses from childhood will probably need either two different pairs of glasses or bifocals as they grow older.

See also VISION.

achondroplasia

A congenital disorder in which the long bones of the limbs are much shorter than normal, resulting in dwarfism. The typical appearance—disproportionately short limbs and a prominent or bulging forehead—is seen in many circus dwarfs.

Achondroplasia (also known as chondrodystrophia fetalis) is an inherited form of dwarfism, although some cases occur as the result of new mutations. The disorder may affect either sex and is noted at birth.

The basic problem is retarded growth of cartilage and bone in the arms and legs (the trunk is commonly unaffected). The bones of the base of the skull also fail to develop normally, giving the appearance of a relatively large forehead. The bones that form the bridge of the nose fail to develop ("saddle nose"), giving a facial appearance that is virtually diagnostic of achondroplasia.

Muscular development is usually very good, which has helped many people with this condition to obtain employment as acrobats and tumblers over the ages. Mental ability is rarely affected and achondroplastics are sexually normal and capable of parenthood. However, achondroplastic women have abnormally small pelvises and their babies must be delivered by Cesarean section. Any person with achondroplasia should have genetic counseling before marriage.

There is no treatment. Nevertheless, the condition is compatible with a long, healthy and happy life, although it is obvious that psychological problems have to be overcome.

acidosis

An excess of acid in the body.

The human body's balance between acidity and excessive alkalinity is strictly maintained by a series of delicate control mechanisms. If this balance is disturbed the individual rapidly becomes extremely ill and, in the absence of medical treatment, may die.

The body fluids vary in their acidity. The most important fluid of all—the blood—is slightly alkaline. This mild alkalinity is due to the presence in the blood of the alkaline ion bicarbonate, which slightly outweighs the effect of the carbonic acid also present in the blood.

How then does acidosis occur? There are two principal mechanisms. The first is called respiratory acidosis and is mainly caused by respiratory disease—for instance, any disorder of the lungs that interferes with breathing. In such circumstances the carbon dioxide gas which should be exhaled in the breath tends to accumulate in the body and forms excess carbonic acid in the blood.

The second type of acidosis is called metabolic acidosis. This occurs when too many acid products accumulate in the body as a result of any metabolic or biochemical disease, such as uncontrolled DIABETES MELLITUS.

The symptoms of acidosis are ill-defined because they are usually overshadowed by those of the primary disease. Treatment is directed both toward correcting that primary disease process and (in many cases) toward correcting the body's acid-alkali balance by intravenous infusion of an alkaline solution.

acne

An extremely common inflammatory disorder of the sebaceous (oil-secreting) glands of the skin. Although several types of acne exist, described by various qualifying terms, when the term is used alone it usually refers to "common acne" (*acne vulgaris*).

Acne vulgaris can affect persons at any age, but it is especially troublesome among teenagers, where it can lead to extreme embarrassment about personal appearance or even severe emotional problems. During adolescence the sebaceous glands become particularly active and secrete large amounts of *sebum* (a fatty substance which ordinarily helps maintain the texture of the skin). This happens because of an increased production of *androgens* (sex hormones) in both males and females at the time of puberty. The sebum produced at this time is unusually thick and sticky and tends to block the sebaceous glands and their associated hair follicles. When this occurs, the follicles become dilated (stretched) with sebum and cellular debris.

If the plug of sebum extends to the skin surface,

contact with the air causes its exposed surface to turn black—thus creating a *comedone* ("blackhead"). If the blockage does not extend to the surface, a "whitehead" is formed beneath the skin. Chemical changes within the blocked follicles result in the formation of irritating substances known as *free fatty acids* (FFA); retention of the secretions encourages the growth and multiplication of bacteria. As the follicles distend they form tiny cysts, which can eventually rupture and release the free fatty acids into the immediate area—inducing an inflammatory reaction. The affected follicles are in typical instances filled with pus (papules, or "pimples") which can spread the infection if they are picked at or squeezed.

Acne vulgaris is further classified as *superficial* or *deep*, depending on the severity of the predominating lesions. The former is characterized by the formation of inflamed follicles filled with pus, which "come to a head" on the skin surface. *Deep acne*, as the term implies, affects deeper layers of the skin as well; pus-filled *cysts* may form beneath the skin, some of which discharge onto the skin surface. In the most

severe cases, as these lesions heal they may leave permanent scarring. The main site involved in acne is the face, although the neck, chest, back and upper arms may also be involved.

At one time diet was implicated as a major cause of acne; however, modern medical opinion considers this to be unlikely in most cases. It is clear that hormonal factors during puberty are mostly responsible, although some experts believe that a hereditary influence may also contribute; this is almost impossible to document, however, since acne has a worldwide incidence and is undoubtedly the most common skin disorder of adolescence.

The treatment of acne depends largely on its severity. Often the only relief is brought by time, as the lesions tend to fade as the patient reaches adulthood (in many cases they last only two years or less). In the meantime, it is wise to wash the affected areas gently at least daily with mild soap and water. This helps by mechanically removing some of the blackheads, scales and bacteria. Medicated washes have proved effective in some mild cases, as has exposure to sunlight (which tends to dry up the lesions). Antibiotic ointments are generally not used, especially since they may produce further irritation of the skin in the form of a local allergic reaction. However, in selected cases a broad-spectrum antibiotic may be prescribed to be taken orally (by mouth); one of the most effective in such cases is tetracycline. Antibiotic treatment has no effect on the underlying cause of acne, but it may help reduce the number of bacteria which are responsible for much of the associated inflammation.

Acne strikes teenages at a particularly sensitive time of life—when they are beginning to "discover" the opposite sex and are thus naturally concerned about personal appearance. Parents can be helpful in pointing out that acne is, in the normal course of events, of limited duration and that it is a nearly universal problem of those about to enter adulthood. This information may not help, of course, but there is really little else that can be done.

acromegaly

A glandular disorder which is characterized by great increase in size of hands, feet and head—producing a very typical coarse facial appearance with a large and jutting jaw.

Acromegaly is caused by excessive secretion of growth hormone in the anterior (front) part of the pituitary gland, which lies just underneath the brain. This excessive production is usually due to a tumor of the gland. (If overactivity of the pituitary gland occurs before puberty—when the bones are still

ACNE

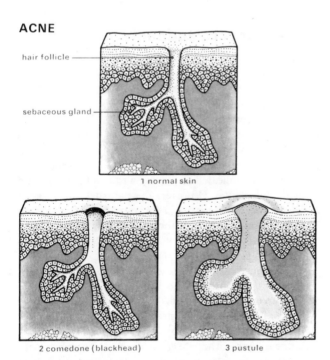

hair follicle

sebaceous gland

1 normal skin

2 comedone (blackhead)   3 pustule

Normal skin has many microscopic hair follicles opening onto its surface (1). In acne, the mouth of the follicle is blocked by a plug of oily sebum (2). The sebaceous gland continues to secrete sebum so that the follicle becomes distended and inflamed. Bacteria then multiply in the follicle, and it becomes filled with pus (3).

growing—the condition can result in GIGANTISM.)

Acromegaly is a relatively rare disease, although the fact that sufferers from it are so conspicuous has made it well known. The unusual facial appearance is illustrated in many medical textbooks, and people who are anxious about their health sometimes see such pictures and *unjustifiably* fear that they have the disease.

Early symptoms include headache or visual disturbances. The patient soon discovers that he has to take a larger size in shoes, gloves and sometimes hats. The fingers become square-ended and the tongue may enlarge. The facial features become rather coarse, with great prominence of the bony ridges above the eyes. Some patients also develop diabetes.

The disease usually runs a long course and it is not uncommon for some acromegalics to live to a great age. Treatment consists either in irradiation of the pituitary gland or surgical removal of the tumor. Unfortunately, therapy cannot reverse the changes that have already taken place in the hands, feet and skull, but it can arrest them.

acrophobia

An excessive and abnormal fear of high places. It is a natural part of human defense mechanisms to have some fear of heights because of the known danger of death or serious injury from a fall; acrophobia is merely an exaggeration of this normal fear. However, it has an element of unreason in it since the acrophobic subject will typically exhibit fear even in a room in a high building although the actual possibility of falling from it under these circumstances may be nil. It can be a very disabling condition since it may preclude the patient from going to work or attending social functions if these involve entering a building and going above the ground floor.

As with other phobias, therapy will involve analysis in an attempt to determine the possible cause of the phobia. Tranquilizing drugs may play a part and "deconditioning" the patient by teaching him to relax while in a real or imagined high place is sometimes helpful.

See also AGORAPHOBIA, CLAUSTROPHOBIA, and PHOBIA.

ACTH

ACTH is the abbreviation for adrenocorticotropic hormone, an essential hormone produced by the anterior (front) part of the pituitary gland, which lies at the base of the brain. It is also known as adrenocorticotropin or corticotropin. (The pituitary gland is the "master gland" of the endocrine system.) ACTH is of great importance because it provides the link between the pituitary and the cortex (covering) of the two tiny ADRENAL GLANDS—which lie at the back of the abdomen just above the kidneys. The cortex of the adrenal glands secretes steroid hormones such as cortisol (known pharmaceutically as hydrocortisone) and aldosterone, which are essential for maintaining the body's biochemical balance; without them we would die.

It is very important that the output of steroids is carefully controlled, since too much steroid production can be very harmful. It is the ACTH secreted by the pituitary which provides this control by means of a complex feedback mechanism.

What happens is that the pituitary secretes ACTH, which is carried in the bloodstream to the adrenal glands. There it stimulates them to produce steroids. But when the amount of steroids in the bloodstream reaches a certain level the production of ACTH by the pituitary is automatically shut off. This feedback mechanism produces a remarkably fine control of steroid production.

ACTH can be extracted from the pituitary glands of animals and given by injection in the treatment of certain diseases—such as asthma, rheumatoid arthritis and certain skin disorders.

Actinomyces/actinomycosis

Actinomyces is a genus of parasitic microorganisms formerly classified as fungi but now thought to be bacteria (some experts believe them to be intermediate between fungi and bacteria).

One species, *Actinomyces israelii*, is a common inhabitant of the mouth in persons with poor oral hygiene. The parasites cling to the teeth, gums and tonsils but rarely cause any problem—although they have been implicated as playing a role in the formation of dental plaque. However, the parasites *can* cause a severe infection if they gain entrance to the tissues, such as by means of a decayed tooth, following the extraction of a tooth, or an injury to the jaw. The resulting condition is known as *actinomycosis*.

Actinomycosis is characterized by painful, hard swellings that progress to the formation of abscesses (localized collections of pus). The sites most commonly affected are the jaws and neck, but if the parasites enter the bloodstream they may infect the lungs, intestines, kidneys and other organs. Early treatment with antibiotics, such as penicillin or tetracycline, is effective in most cases in limiting the progression of the disease.

acupuncture

The technique of producing anesthesia or attempting to treat disease by the insertion of the tips of long needles into the skin at certain special points. The needles are

ACUPUNCTURE

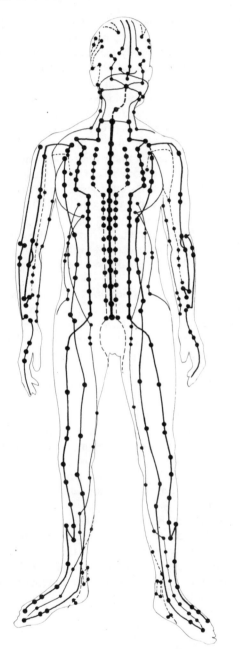

acupuncture points run along "meridians"

This is an acupuncturist's map of the body and shows the various points at which needles can be inserted through the skin in order to produce areas of anesthesia in other parts of the body. Many acupuncturists also claim that internal diseases can be cured by their skills. Contemporary Western science cannot explain how acupuncture works, and many conventional doctors are skeptical about its effectiveness.

then rotated back and forth by hand or charged with a small electric current for five minutes or so.

Acupuncture has been known in China for thousands of years, but until very recently it has been regarded by Western physicians as nothing more than one of the many forms of "quack" medicine. This view was also taken by orthodox (that is, Western-style) physicians in China itself until well into the 1950s.

However, Mao Tse-Tung's instruction to the medical profession in Communist China to "investigate the great treasure house of ancient Chinese medicine" led to a reappraisal of acupuncture. Chinese anesthesiologists were surprised to find that the technique could induce complete absence of pain during a wide range of surgical operations—although it was some years before they could convince their colleagues in the West of this.

In the 1960s Western physicians saw for themselves that operations could quite genuinely be performed under "acupuncture anesthesia" although not in all cases (some patients failed to respond to this method and continued to feel pain).

The value of acupuncture in treating disease is far less certain. Many Chinese doctors now accept the traditional oriental teaching that acupuncture can be used to treat a wide range of diseases. However, many Western physicians are very doubtful of this, pointing out that the technique has never been subjected to the careful, scientifically designed clinical trials which are essential to prove that a method of therapy is actually effective. (Almost any procedure—no matter how bizarre and useless—will have a high apparent cure rate in some medical conditions as the result of what is known as a "placebo effect.")

The value of acupuncture in anesthesiology is documented, but its effectiveness as a form of treatment is still under investigation.

Why should it work at all? No Western or Chinese doctor has come up with a truly satisfactory explanation, although some have suggested that the insertion of the needles may in some way alter the balance between two important divisions of the nervous system, known respectively as the sympathetic and the parasympathetic systems. Western-style Chinese physicians have recently theorized that the needles may affect some minute structural network of the body which has not yet been discovered by anatomists. The traditional Chinese acupuncturists maintain that the insertion of the needles along certain "meridians" affects the inter-reaction of the two life-forces, which in their philosophy are termed "Yin" and "Yang."

acute abdomen

A jargon term used by many surgeons to signify any sudden, severe and continuing abdominal pain.

The diagnosis of the acute abdomen constitutes one of the major challenges to any general surgeon. Common causes include transient and harmless conditions like "gas" or "indigestion," as well as potentially more serious ones such as appendicitis, gastric ulcer, duodenal ulcer, gallbladder disease, pancreatitis, pyelitis (a form of kidney inflammation), and diverticulitis (inflammation of abnormal pouches in the large bowel).

In women, conditions such as ectopic pregnancy (pregnancy occurring in a Fallopian tube rather than the womb), miscarriage or abortion, and a twisted ovarian cyst have to be considered as possible causes of the acute abdomen.

Adams-Stokes syndrome

A condition which mostly affects the elderly, characterized by sudden episodes of unconsciousness. It can occur at any time of the day and is not dependent on bodily position. The cause is a disturbance in the heart's rhythm, such as VENTRICULAR FIBRILLATION or a temporary interruption of the heartbeat. Absence of the heartbeat (*asystole*) for 4 to 8 seconds will cause unconsciousness in the erect position; asystole of more than 12 seconds will cause unconsciousness in the recumbent position; asystole of up to 5 minutes leads to additional signs of CYANOSIS, fixed pupils, and neurological impairment (which may be permanent, if the patient survives).

Emergency treatment usually involves the intravenous administration of isoproterenol. This may be followed by the implantation of an artificial PACEMAKER.

See also ARRHYTHMIA, BRADYCARDIA.

addiction

Physical or mental dependence on a drug. Some experts make a distinction between *addiction* (physical dependence) and *habituation* (psychological dependence); both terms have traditionally been used to describe the adverse long-term effects of certain classes of drugs on the body and mind.

The World Health Organization, however, suggests that more meaningful diagnostic terms would be *drug dependence* and *drug abuse*. The essential feature of physical dependence is the occurrence of withdrawal symptoms if regular doses are not taken. Not all drugs which are responsible for extremely serious personality disruption cause a true physical dependence of this kind. LSD (lysergic acid diethylamide) is an example of an extremely potent drug (the use of which is now illegal except in medical research) which does not cause physical addiction, but which is nevertheless potentially dangerous for the mental changes it can cause (some of

which can recur long after use of the drug has been abandoned).

The best known physically addictive drugs are the opiates or "narcotics," such as morphine and heroin. Even when prescribed legally for the relief of severe pain, prolonged treatment with opiates can lead to tolerance by the body of ever increasing doses of the drug. In these circumstances sudden withdrawal of the drug will cause cramping pains, sweating and acute mental distress. The need to relieve these symptoms by taking a further dose of the drug is the key feature of physical addiction. The fact that withdrawal symptoms occur indicates that the body's cells have themselves become dependent on regular supplies of the drug. This is why it is so difficult for a drug addict to "kick the habit"—he becomes physically ill if he does not get his regular "fix." A truly enormous amount of willpower is required over a very long period—usually with professional help—if he is to break the habit once and for all.

Other common drugs which may be addictive if abused include the amphetamines ("speed"), barbiturates and other types of sedatives ("sleeping pills"), and the major and minor tranquilizers such as chlorpromazine (Largactil), meprobamate (Miltown) and diazepam (Valium).

There is still a great deal of misunderstanding about the drugs which cause addiction. Many people do not realize that CANNABIS (marijuana or "pot") is *not* physically addictive, but that nicotine *is* (witness the very considerable withdrawal symptoms which occur in the heavy cigarette smoker when he tries to give up the habit). ALCOHOL can also be addictive, although moderate amounts do not produce addiction in the majority of people.

The treatment of addiction is often best carried out by an experienced psychiatrist working in a drug addiction program. Analysis, group therapy, and the prescription of less harmful drugs to ease the withdrawal period may all help—together with the sympathetic support of family and friends, which is essential.

See also DRUG ABUSE.

Addison's disease

A disorder in which the adrenal glands cease to function adequately, and thus do not produce normal quantities of the hormones called steroids. Also known as *adrenal cortical hypofunction* or *chronic hypoadrenocorticism*. President Kennedy is believed to have been a sufferer of the disease.

These steroids are essential to life, since they maintain the biochemical balance of the body. Without them, the classical symptoms of Addison's disease (first described by the 19th-century English physician Thomas

Addison) soon make their appearance. These symptoms include weakness, tiredness or even total collapse, vomiting, weight loss, low blood pressure, and a curious increase of dark pigmentation in the skin. This can become so marked that in some cases a European may appear to be black.

In many instances the cause of the adrenal gland malfunction is unknown. Sometimes, however, it is due to a destruction of the adrenals by tuberculosis, or by a severe generalized infection associated with meningitis. Addison's disease is less common than it was, possibly because of the fall in the number of cases of tuberculosis.

Treatment of Addison's disease is usually very successful today, since it is possible for physicians to provide replacement of the missing hormones. Steroids are given by mouth, by injection, or by implantation under the skin; this therapy may well have to be maintained for life.

adduction

See ABDUCTION/ADDUCTION.

adenitis

Inflammation of a lymph gland (lymph node). These glands are scattered through various parts of the body, some of the main concentrations being at the side of the neck, in the armpits and in the groin. Their function is to help the body's defense against infection.

Unfortunately, there are times when the infection becomes sufficiently established to produce an intense inflammatory reaction in the lymph glands. These glands then become swollen and often painful. The inflammation may rarely proceed to such a stage that pus is formed in the glands.

Typically, adenitis of the glands in the groin is caused by some infection establishing itself in the leg, or in the sex organs. Adenitis of the glands in the armpits is caused by infection somewhere in the arm, or in the breast. Adenitis in the neck glands (cervical adenitis) is caused by infection in the throat, or ear, or sometimes infection of the scalp.

The type of infection causing adenitis varies greatly. At one time tuberculosis adenitis was very common, but today most cases of adenitis are due to common bacteria such as streptococci (the organism found in many cases of sore throat) or to staphylococci (the organism found in boils). Also, adenitis of the neck glands is frequently due to viral infection—for instance, the viruses of infectious mononucleosis and German measles (rubella). Treatment of adenitis is basically treatment of the underlying infection (for instance, with the use of antibiotics).

adenocarcinoma

A type of CANCER arising in glandular tissue.

Adenocarcinomas can be distinguished under the microscope from other types of tumor, and this differentiation is of some help in assessing the likely outcome of the disease and in deciding the best method of treatment.

Adenocarcinomas mainly arise in the stomach, large intestine (colon), gallbladder, pancreas, womb (uterus) and prostate gland. They can also arise in the breast and lungs.

These tumors may spread to other parts of the body (via the blood and lymphatic systems) if they are not detected and treated early enough. When such spread occurs, the secondary tumor which is formed at another site has the same "glandular" appearance under the microscope as that of the "primary" adenocarcinoma. This may be a help in diagnosis if the site of the primary tumor is not yet known.

adenoids

Masses of lymphatic glandular tissue found behind the nose on the back wall of the nasopharynx (that part of the throat which lies an inch or two above the area that is visible when the mouth is open). Doctors can inspect the adenoids by placing a small, upward-pointing mirror in the back of the throat.

ADENOIDS

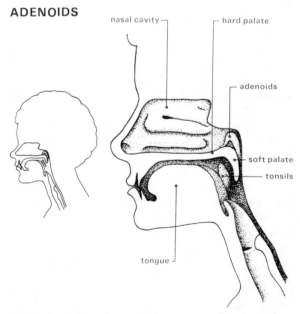

The adenoids and tonsils form part of a ring of lymphoid tissue at the entrance to the throat. Their job is to form protective antibodies against any microorganisms which attempt to enter the respiratory and digestive tracts.

These glands are often referred to as the "nasopharyngeal tonsils" because they play a similar role to the tonsils in helping to protect a child against inhaled germs. Unfortunately, they sometimes become infected and grossly enlarged—in much the same way that tonsils often do—and when this happens they may cause symptoms of nasal obstruction, since they make it difficult for air to pass in through or out of the nose.

The symptoms of grossly enlarged adenoids include inability to breathe properly through the nose, a change in the quality of the voice ("adenoidal speech") and snoring.

Adenoids usually reach their maximum size at about the age of 6, when the child is being exposed to a wide range of respiratory germs through contact with other children at school. From about the age of 9 or 10 they tend to shrink away, They usually disappear entirely by the time of adolescence and it is rare to find any trace of adenoids in adults. In view of this natural tendency to shrink, surgeons are less keen to remove enlarged adenoids than they used to be.

adenoma

A benign swelling or tumor of glandular tissue (as opposed to ADENOCARCINOMA, which is a malignant tumor of the same type of tissue).

In contrast to adenocarcinoma, adenomas are basically harmless, although their presence may cause discomfort or slight pain. They do not invade other parts of the body, nor destroy bodily tissues, and they do not spread to distant regions of the body, producing "secondary" tumors.

Adenomas chiefly occur in such organs as the breast, stomach, bowel, pancreas, liver, thyroid gland, ovary, and the adrenal glands. They are characteristically firm swellings formed of cells which resemble those of the tissues in which the adenoma has developed.

In the stomach and bowel an adenoma commonly develops a stalk, so that it grows into the cavity of the organ like a POLYP. In other situations (notably in the ovary) an adenoma may become cystic—in other words, filled with fluid. In the breast, an adenoma frequently contains a great deal of fibrous tissue and is referred to as a FIBROADENOMA; this variety is one of the most common of all adenomas.

In general, adenomas are removed surgically. Partly this is because a *definite* diagnosis of a benign adenoma cannot be made until the lump has been removed for microscopic examination. In addition, a very small proportion of adenomas do become malignant (through changing into adenocarcinomas). Surgical excision therefore not only is a wise precaution but may be essential in treating those tumors which have undergone a malignant change.

adhesion

An abnormal band of tissue developing between two internal organs, especially in the abdominal cavity.

Adhesions occur as a result of inflammation and may develop following a severe infection, such as peritonitis. Very commonly, however, adhesions form after a surgical operation, like a sort of internal scar tissue. Some people seem to be much more likely to develop postoperative adhesions than others, but the reason for this is not known.

The great importance of adhesions is that they may interfere with the function of bodily organs. In many cases a person who has had an abdominal operation may develop an intestinal obstruction a few years later. When the surgeon opens the abdomen, the cause is found to be adhesions pressing on the intestine. Cutting through the adhesive bands relieves the situation, but there is always a small risk of recurrence later.

ADHESION

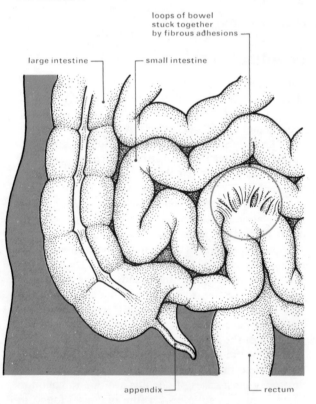

The loops of the bowel normally slide over each other freely, but occasionally become stuck together by fibrous adhesions. These may result from previous inflammation or from abdominal surgery. Adhesions may obstruct the passage of material along the bowel in which case further surgery is necessary to divide them.

adipose tissue

The layer of fat which mainly lies immediately under the skin; it acts both as an insulator and as a source of "fuel." Adipose tissue is also found in other parts of the body, but is not evenly distributed. It is quite thick in those parts most liable to sudden pressure, such as the buttocks and feet where it acts as a "shock absorber." It is also present in the bone marrow, where it supports the arteries and veins; around the heart and lungs, where it provides a cushion and support; around the intestines, to keep them warm; around the kidneys, for protection; and in the joints and muscles, where it prevents damage by sudden shock or jarring.

Excess formation of adipose tissue anywhere can be dangerous, especially around the heart—where it adds weight to that organ and impedes its movement. Heavy deposits around the lungs can restrict breathing and they can also affect the action of the heart. Excess fatty deposits can be avoided by the proper attention to diet and exercise.

adrenal glands

Two tiny glandular masses which lie immediately above the kidneys, at the back of the abdominal cavity. They are also known as the *suprarenal glands*.

The adrenal glands have two quite separate functions, and this is reflected by the fact that each of them is

ADRENAL GLANDS

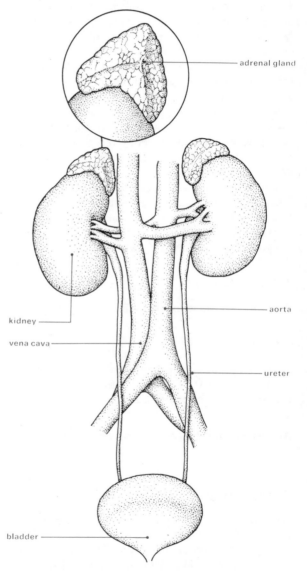

ADIPOSE TISSUE

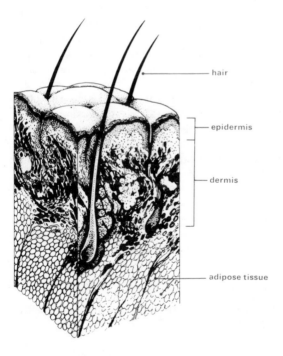

Adipose tissue is a collection of round cells full of fat; it is found throughout the body and acts as a reserve supply of energy. However, most people do not have to endure periods of starvation and tend to carry excess amounts of adipose tissue. The layer shown here beneath the skin is important for conserving body heat.

The adrenal glands sit on top of the kidneys like a pair of cocked hats. Although small, these glands are essential for life because of the hormones they produce: epinephrine and norepinephrine, which are secreted into the bloodstream when we are in stressful situations, cortisol and other stress hormones, and aldosterone, which plays an important role in regulating the blood pressure.

divided into two separate zones: an outer *cortex* and an inner *medulla*.

The cortex is absolutely essential to the body because it produces the cortisone-like hormones called "steroids," some of which play important roles in the metabolism of fats, carbohydrates, proteins, sodium and potassium, and others in sexual development and the maintenance of bodily strength. If the cortex is not functioning properly because of some serious disorder, such as tuberculosis of the adrenals, then the result may be ADDISON'S DISEASE—a condition of extreme weakness and lethargy which usually proved fatal until it became possible to provide replacement of adrenal steroid hormones by means of tablets or injections.

The medulla of the gland is entirely separate in function. It is part of the sympathetic nervous system, a division of the nerve communications network concerned with preparing the body for physical activity through release of epinephrine (adrenaline)—the chemical that prepares muscles, heart and blood vessels for instant action. It is often described as the hormone of "fight, flight, or fright." The adrenal medulla is the body's prime source of this important hormone, releasing it in bursts that are triggered off by stimuli such as excitement, fear, anger or sexual desire.

Adrenalin

A proprietary name for adrenaline (epinephrine).

adrenaline

Another word for epinephrine (a hormone secreted by the ADRENAL GLANDS). In the United States, Adrenalin is a trade name for epinephrine.

adrenocorticotropic hormone

See ACTH.

adrenogenital syndrome

A condition in which there is overactivity of part of the cortex of the ADRENAL GLANDS.

The adrenal cortex is the body's manufacturing center for the cortisone-like hormones termed "steriods," which are vitally important in maintaining the biochemical balance of our tissues. These hormones also have important effects on the sex organs, since some of them tend to promote the development of male characteristics. Overproduction of these hormones can result in the adrenogenital syndrome.

The characteristics of this condition depend on just which particular "mix" of hormones is being produced by the overactive adrenal gland. Chief symptoms,

however, tend to be masculinization in female children and adults (with excessive hairiness and enlargement of the clitoris), precocious puberty in boys (including abnormal enlargement of the penis), and sometimes high blood pressure.

The adrenogenital syndrome is fortunately rare, and the current use of hormone therapy is usually fairly effective.

African trypanosomiasis

African trypanosomiasis (also known as "African sleeping sickness") is an infection of the brain by specific protozoan parasites (*Trypanosoma gambiense* and *Trypanosoma rhodesiense*). The disease is spread by blood-sucking tsetse flies, which attack both men and animals over a broad region of central and southern Africa. In Rhodesia, Zaire, Zambia and Angola trypanosomiasis was the principal health problem until eradication campaigns controlled the numbers of tsetse flies.

The bite of the fly may pass unnoticed or it may cause a local inflammatory reaction of the skin which may develop into a characteristic hard sore. With the Rhodesian variety of the disease, symptoms develop within a week or two; elsewhere the incubation period may be months or even years. The early symptoms include a severe headache, difficulty in sleeping and a feeling of misery. If treatment is not given the disease progresses to cause weakness, apathy, increasing drowsiness and death (the mortality rate is close to 100% in untreated cases). However, drugs such as suramin and melarsoprol are capable of curing the disease in its later stages. Control of the disease depends on control of the tsetse flies; unfortunately, the political unrest and guerrilla wars in southern Africa have been followed by a huge increase in the population of flies and a resurgence of the disease.

South American trypanosomiasis (also known as CHAGAS' DISEASE) is caused by a different species of the trypanosome parasite (*Trypanosoma cruzi*).

afterbirth

The PLACENTA and associated membranes expelled after the birth of a child.

agglutination

Clumping or sticking together of numbers of small particles in a fluid. Particles or cells (for instance, red blood cells or bacteria) demonstrate this phenomenon when they are exposed to an antibody that reacts with an antigen they contain (see ANTIBODY/ANTIGEN).

The phenomenon is of considerable importance in

medical diagnosis, since it is used as the basis for many laboratory tests. For instance, if bacteria of unknown identity are obtained from a patient, they can be mixed with antibodies from laboratory animals. These antibodies are specific to a particular bacterium. If the bacteria taken from the patient clump (agglutinate) on contact with them, they can be positively identified as being the same organism and appropriate antibiotic treatment can then be prescribed.

Another variety of agglutination test uses the same principle in reverse. Serum (the amber fluid remaining after blood has clotted) of a patient who is suspected of having a particular infection is mixed with fluid containing bacteria which are known to cause that infection. If the bacteria agglutinate, this indicates that the patient has antibodies against them.

In practice, this does not mean that the patient currently has the disease but that he *has* had it at some time in the past. Often it is necessary to repeat the test after a period of time to see if the patient's titer of antibodies has risen. (The *agglutination titer* is the highest dilution of a serum which will cause clumping of the bacteria which are being tested). If it has gone up, then this is strong evidence that the infection is a recent one.

Agglutination reactions are also used in the grouping of blood for transfusion in order to ensure that the patient will not react adversely, and in the diagnosis of certain diseases (for example, rheumatoid arthritis) where there is some unusual antibody present in the blood.

See also BLOOD.

aging

The process of aging begins much earlier than most people imagine. Even in childhood there are some slight changes caused by aging—for instance, an inability to perceive the very high notes which are detectable by young infants. By the age of 18, most American males have some evidence of degeneration in their coronary arteries.

By the late 20s, most people are already showing some decline in physical prowess (many athletes have passed their prime at this age). In the 30s, the aging process continues at a gradual rate—although to some extent it can be kept in check by careful attention to diet, regular exercise and avoidance of adverse health factors such as smoking, excessive alcohol consumption and obesity.

In the 40s and 50s, the pace of aging quickens somewhat. In women it may be accelerated by the relatively rapid loss of female hormone output at the menopause. And in the 60s and 70s the classical changes of aging become apparent in most people: white hair, wrinkled skin, stiffer joints and degeneration of the arteries (leading, very often, to coronary heart disease or impaired blood circulation in the brain). The effects of aging can to some extent be moderated by leading a healthy life, with an adequate amount of exercise and well-balanced meals. In some people (and in some isolated races of mankind) the process of aging is very much slower than normal: we are all familiar with people who appear to be in their 50s, but who in fact are 75 or more.

Medical science has yet to discover why aging occurs and how the "biological clock" works, which seems to determine that it will take place. (The clock sometimes malfunctions: there are a few tragic cases of children who became prematurely aged and wizened, dying in their teens or even earlier of "old age"—a condition known as "progeria.") All we can do at the moment is to try to stave off the effects of aging by keeping as fit as possible and by treating—or better still, preventing—the various diseases which are so often associated with age.

agoraphobia

An irrational fear of open places.

Phobias are extremely common and agoraphobia is one of the most frequently encountered.

The reason why agoraphobia is so common is not known. It is the considered opinion of experts that many phobias are linked to frightening experiences that occur in early childhood, including excessively harsh or terrifying punishments inflicted by parents. It must be admitted, however, that this is still pure speculation.

The symptoms of agoraphobia are extremely distressing for the victim. When she (the disorder is much more common in women) attempts to go out into the open, there is a terrifying feeling of panic, often with racing heart, profuse sweating and trembling. The sufferer may be convinced that she is about to die, and this feeling cannot be alleviated until she gets back indoors.

In variants of agoraphobia the victim may fear only a particular type of open space—for instance, a park or even a supermarket with a high roof. Agoraphobics often have other phobias as well, such as fear of cats, insects, or of talking to other people.

It cannot be denied that treatment of agoraphobia is difficult, partly because sufferers are unable to overcome their panic in order to visit a doctor's surgery. In cases of severe agoraphobia the patient is likely to be referred to a specialist, most probably a psychologist or a psychiatrist.

Therapy may involve some form of analysis in an attempt to unravel the inner conflicts producing the panic (see DESENSITIZATION). Psychiatrists and psychologists use such techniques as desensitization (deconditioning) in which the patient is taught to relax while imagining herself in the feared situation. Tranquilizing drugs also have a small part to play in treatment, but do not solve the underlying problem.

Encouraging results have been achieved by doctors who have the knack of teaching agoraphobic patients that they have nothing to fear but fear itself—in other words, that if they can accept the symptoms of panic and not run for shelter when they occur, they will eventually triumph over the disorder.

See also PHOBIA; compare ACROPHOBIA and CLAUSTROPHOBIA.

agranulocytosis

A severe illness characterized by a gross deficiency of white blood cells. (The condition is also known as granulocytopenia.)

The white blood cells, mainly produced in the spongy center or marrow of the long bones, are of great importance in the defense of the body against infection. Unfortunately, the bone marrow is sometimes affected by disease or toxic substances (or both) and fails to produce an adequate number of white blood cells to replace those which are constantly being used up in the course of their protective work against invading microorganisms.

Failure of the bone marrow may occur as a complication of leukemia. More commonly it represents a toxic reaction to drugs such as sulfonamides, gold or arsenic preparations, phenylbutazone, chloramphenicol, or certain antiepileptic and antithyroid preparations.

Industrial poisons (e.g. benzol) may have the same effects, as may exposure to radioactive material or x-rays. Occasionally, however, the bone marrow fails to produce white blood cells for no known reason ("idiopathic" agranulocytosis).

The symptoms of agranulocytosis include those that might be expected in an individual with no real defense against infection—fever and recurrent infective ulceration of the mouth and throat, with increasing ill health, leading (if the condition is unchecked) to eventual death.

The treatment of agranulocytosis involves the administration of antibiotics to combat infection, blood transfusions to provide a temporary source of white blood cells, and steroid therapy (which is thought to encourage the bone marrow to resume its activity). In some cases the marrow will recover spontaneously once any toxic drugs have been withdrawn. Where it does not recover, it is occasionally possible to perform a bone marrow transplant, inserting marrow taken from a donor.

AID/AIH

Abbreviations used to indicate, respectively, *Artificial Insemination [by] Donor* and *Artificial Insemination [by] Husband.*

The term artificial insemination indicates the technique by means of which a man's seminal fluid is deposited in a woman's vagina or uterus under conditions other than sexual intercourse (usually with a special syringe) in the hope of achieving a pregnancy. AID and AIH, subjects of great controversy over the last few decades, have been extremely successful in providing previously childless couples with a much wanted baby.

Artificial insemination has been used by veterinary surgeons for a very long time, but it is only since World War II that the technique has been widely used in women in order to overcome a chronic failure to become pregnant.

Although some 10 to 15% of marriages in the United Kingdom are relatively infertile (in other words, the couples concerned experience difficulty in conceiving), only a minority of couples can be helped by artificial insemination.

AIH involves taking a specimen of the husband's semen and introducing it into the wife's vagina or uterus. Ordinarily the physician is responsible for the procedure but sometimes he instructs the couple how to do this for themselves at home. It is important to realize that AIH is used only in appropriate cases: where the wife has some structural or—much more commonly—emotional problem that makes successful intercourse and impregnation very difficult; where the husband is unable to achieve or maintain an erection long enough to have sexual intercourse; and finally, where the concentration of sperms in the seminal fluid is abnormally low (the physician may then use special techniques to achieve a higher concentration of sperms before introducing the semen).

Much more controversial is AID, in which the seminal fluid is provided by a male donor, whose identity should be unknown to both husband and wife. The reason for this method is the situation where the wife is fertile but the husband is not. Today many husbands are happy to approve the technique of AID if (as is so often the case) it is the only means of ensuring that their wives will have the chance to have babies. This procedure should, of course, never be carried out without the husband's permission: in most countries a legal agreement, signed by both husband and wife, is required in advance of the procedure.

'Though the artificial insemination of a married woman with the semen of a donor is not adultery, a child by AID, not being begotten by the husband, is presumably illegitimate.' (Walker, *Principles*, Vol 1).

albinism

Absence of the natural pigment from the skin, resulting in an unnaturally pale appearance.

Regardless of race, most people have a considerable amount of the dark pigment melanin in their skin; the concentration varies somewhat according to the time of year. It increases greatly after sunbathing, and this is the mechanism which is responsible for suntan. However, certain people have no melanin pigment whatever. This appears to occur as the result of an enzyme defect, which prevents the body from forming melanin from its biochemical precursor. This defect is hereditary, but is caused by a recessive gene—which means that it will appear only when two people who *both* carry the gene have children (even then it occurs in only about one in four of their children).

Albinism is very rare in Britain. It is commonest among Negroes and in people of black descent the "washed out" appearance is very striking. The hair is white and the eyes are gray or pink.

Apart from the somewhat unusual appearance, the main problem for the person with albinism (known as an *albino*) is an excessive sensitivity of the skin to sunburn. In addition the eyes may not be able to tolerate the light well.

There is no cure for the condition, although—if even a little melanin is present (as in the case with some atypical forms of albinism)—drugs can be given to stimulate melanin production. Otherwise sunscreening creams should be used to prevent sunburn. Good quality sunglasses are often helpful.

albumin

A natural protein, found in various forms in animals and plants. The best known form of albumin is egg white (the word *albumin* is derived from *albus*, the Latin for "white"). Other types of albumin are found in milk, beans and meat.

In the human body, albumin is one of the two major proteins of the blood, the other being globulin. It is formed in the liver from protein foods in the diet. Albumin has an important role in metabolism; it also maintains the osmotic pressure of the blood—that is, its water-holding capacity. If it were not present in an adequate concentration, excessive amounts of water would pass out of the blood and into the tissues, causing EDEMA. A low blood level of albumin is characteristic of protein malnutrition and is seen in certain disorders of the kidneys and liver.

There are several different kinds of laboratory tests to determine the abnormal presence of albumin in the urine—a condition known as ALBUMINURIA.

albuminuria

The presence of the protein ALBUMIN in the urine.

Albumin is one of the most important constituents of blood and is not usually found in urine. When blood passes through the kidneys, only impurities should be filtered out for excretion in the urine. When the kidney is malfunctioning, however, albumin may leak into the urine. That is why physicians make a regular practice of testing a urine specimen for albumin.

Albuminuria does not always indicate kidney disease. In women, for example, apparent albuminuria is frequently due to a small amount of vaginal secretion in the urine specimen. Other quite harmless causes of positive test results for urinary albumin include postural or orthostatic albuminuria (found in up to 5% of healthy college freshmen), in which albumin enters the urine only if the person has been standing up for some time.

Disorders which are of more significance include the various forms of nephritis (inflammation of the kidney), most types of fever, and toxemia of pregnancy.

The term PROTEINURIA (protein in the urine) is virtually synonymous with albuminuria, since albumin is the only protein ever found in significant quantities in the urine.

alcohol/alcoholism

Alcohol is the name of a type of chemical of which the most common is *ethyl alcohol*—the one obtained by the fermentation of sugar and enjoyed by man in beverages for thousands of years.

Alcoholic drinks are taken not only for their pleasant taste but because alcohol is a drug, albeit a socially acceptable one in most cultures. It is not a stimulant drug, as many people imagine, but a *selective depressant* of the central nervous system. It begins by depressing the frontal centers of the cerebrum; its effect slowly spreads back toward the cerebellum.

The effect of a small dose of alcohol is to depress the inhibitory or controlling centers of the brain, producing relaxation and a general loss of inhibitions. Larger quantities induce sedation and impair speech and muscular coordination. Very large quantities produce severe depression of the vital centers of the central nervous system and may be fatal.

Outside the central nervous system the physiologic effects of alcohol are less drastic. Small quantities increase the flow of gastric juices (thereby stimulating the appetite); larger amounts irritate the stomach lining, causing gastritis and even vomiting of blood. Alcohol also increases the flow of urine.

Unfortunately, chronic ingestion of fairly large quantities of alcohol can have highly deleterious effects on body tissues—particularly those of the liver.

CIRRHOSIS, a serious hardening and degeneration of liver tissue, kills many heavy drinkers. Cancer is especially likely to develop in a cirrhotic liver. Alcohol taken in excess over a long period may also cause a degeneration of the heart muscle (cardiomyopathy) and serious impairment of brain function. Alcoholic psychosis is one of the most common reasons for psychiatric hospitalization.

Alcoholism is a state of addiction to alcohol. Those who suffer from it are likely to develop the severe physical consequences of alcohol abuse which have been outlined above. Alcohol is not as addictive as heroin, morphine or nicotine; but research indicates that most humans (and mammals generally) can be habituated to it by prolonged, constant exposure. If a person drinks enough alcohol on a regular basis, there is a strong possibility that his body will become dependent upon it. Larger and larger doses may be required, as time goes by, to keep withdrawal symptoms at bay.

Although unhappiness and deprivation play a part in driving a man or woman to excessive drinking, it is quite untrue that only depraved and "worthless" people become alcoholics. Many Americans were astounded when the astronaut Buzz Aldrin was only one of many prominent persons to announce that he suffered from alcoholism. This brave declaration helped many people to realize that alcoholism is an *illness*, not a vice.

Treatment of alcoholism is difficult and fraught with disappointments. The alcoholic must first accept that he has the condition; he then needs caring support from his family, friends and personal physician. It may also be wise for the alcoholic to consult a psychiatrist who is thoroughly experienced in dealing with the condition.

The psychiatrist may employ analysis and may prescribe "antialcohol" drugs such as disulfiram (Antabuse), which produces a most violent and unpleasant physical reaction if alcohol is taken (including nausea and vomiting).

Other methods employed by psychiatrists include behaviorist techniques such as conditioning the patient to associate the sight and smell of alcohol with unpleasant sensations. Admission to a specialist alcoholic unit is often necessary so that the alcohol can be withdrawn completely ("drying out").

Alcoholics Anonymous is a leading organization whose supportive work in helping patients keep off alcohol has undoubtedly saved the lives of thousands of alcoholics.

alkalosis

An excess of alkali in the blood and the tissue fluids of the body.

Metabolic alkalosis ordinarily arises as the result of an excessive loss of hydrochloric acid from the stomach through prolonged vomiting. It may also arise if a person takes excessive quantities of antacids for an ulcer or an upset stomach, and as a complication of treatment with diuretic drugs, which increase the acidity of the urine formed by the kidneys. In most cases, however, the condition will resolve provided enough fluid is taken to allow the kidneys to readjust the amount of alkali (bicarbonate) in the blood. In very severe cases, treatment with ammonium chloride will speed up the return to normal.

Respiratory alkalosis is caused by an excessive excretion of carbon dioxide gas in the exhaled breath. The most common reason is hysterical overbreathing, but the normal mechanisms that control the breathing rate may be disturbed in persons on respirators and in cases of aspirin poisoning. Symptoms include a form of spasmodic muscular contraction called tetany. Treatment may be no more complex than providing a paper bag for the patient to breath into, so ensuring that the carbon dioxide breathed out is breathed back in again. When the cause is biochemical it may be necessary to give fluids intravenously to restore the blood to normal.

alkaptonuria

A rare inborn error of metabolism, which causes the excretion in the urine of a substance called homogentisic acid. This causes the urine to become dark on exposure to the air, so that urine left overnight in a pot will become almost black. (The chemical defect is the absence of an enzyme termed homogentisate oxidase, which catalyzes an important step in the metabolism of the amino acid tyrosine.)

With modern sanitation an affected individual may be unaware of the abnormality unless other symptoms develop. These include a form of arthritis and stiffness and change in color of the cartilage in the ear and elsewhere due to deposition of a pigment formed as a result of the chemical defect. The arthritis, which typically develops at about the age of 30, affects the larger joints, and especially the spine. There is no specific treatment, but life expectancy is normal.

This defect is hereditary and will not appear unless both parents carry the gene. If they do, then the disease will appear in approximately one in four of their children. Fortunately, the gene is rare; the incidence of the disease is about one in 200,000. As with other recessively inherited diseases, alkaptonuria is much more likely to appear if the parents are related to each other; thus, the disease is more common in small, inbred communities. Genetic counseling is advisable for anyone with a relative who has the disorder: the condition can be detected chemically before symptoms develop.

allergy

Allergy is the mechanism through which symptoms are caused by sensitivity to an *allergen*—an allergy-causing substance, such as pollen, feathers, fur or dust, or a chemical such as a detergent, cosmetic or drug. Allergy is the cause of hay fever and urticaria (hives) and underlies many cases of asthma and eczema.

Allergic reactions are exaggerations of the body's normal immune responses to bacteria and viruses and their toxins. Whenever an infecting organism penetrates the skin or enters the bloodstream the blood lymphocytes respond by forming antibodies. These are large protein molecules tailor-made to correspond to the chemical makeup of the bacteria or their toxins. The allergic response is essentially similar: antibodies are formed against pollen grains inhaled into the nose and lungs or against cosmetics coming into contact with the skin. However, whereas the normal immune response is designed to destroy bacteria and neutralize their toxins the allergic response causes symptoms rather than protecting against them. Characteristically, the first (sensitizing) exposure to an allergen causes no symptoms, but if the body responds by forming antibodies the stage is set for an allergic reaction on the next and subsequent exposures. Whether or not allergens such as pollen, dog hair, or strawberries provoke an allergic reaction depends on individual susceptibility. Some people are allergic to a whole range of common substances; others never develop sensitivities. Such tendencies often run in families.

The most common sites for allergic reactions are the respiratory tract and the skin. Inhaled allergens may stimulate the formation of antibodies which become fixed to the lining of the nose or lungs. Further exposure to the same allergen will cause the antibodies and antigens to react together, with the release of chemicals such as histamine from specialized immune cells (plasma cells and mast cells) in the surface membranes. It is the histamine release that causes the symptoms of hay fever such as the sneezing and eye-watering from swelling and inflammation of the conjunctiva and the nasal mucous membranes. In the lungs the predominant allergic response is spasm of the small air passages, causing asthma; in the skin the response causes swelling and irritation, though the scratching this induces may lead to secondary infection. Allergy may also affect the digestive system: allergy to gluten (wheat protein), for example, can damage the intestinal lining causing chronic diarrhea and stunted growth due to malabsorption of the food (CELIAC DISEASE).

Allergic responses may be immediate, in which exposure to the allergen causes symptoms within a few minutes, or delayed, in which there may be an interval of several days between contact with the allergen and the onset of symptoms. In delayed responses the illness may not be recognized as allergic unless careful attention is paid to the possibility.

Allergic reactions which cause troublesome symptoms may be treated either by antihistamine drugs which block the effects of histamine on the skin and blood vessels, or by drugs such as steroids or cromoglycate which suppress the formation of antibodies. Another approach is DESENSITIZATION: repeated injection of very small doses of the allergen responsible for the symptoms eventually damps down the allergic response. This form of treatment is used most frequently for persons sensitive to only one or two specific dusts or pollens.

alopecia

The technical term for BALDNESS.

alphafetoprotein

A substance that can help identify the presence of SPINA BIFIDA and similar deformities (such as ANENCEPHALY) in an unborn baby. It is also referred to as *α-fetoprotein*.

Spina bifida and other "neural tube" defects are among the most common serious abnormalities occurring in pregnancy, with a rate as high as 4 per 1,000 births in some parts of the United States. Their cause is unknown and they are difficult to treat; many affected babies are stillborn and others die in the first few weeks of infancy. Even if the child survives he may have a miserable life, with partial paralysis, incontinence, and mental handicap. For these reasons, doctors have sought a test to identify the abnormalities before birth so that the mother could be offered a clinical abortion.

A test was eventually devised, during the 1960s, by Scottish doctors. They found that if they took fluid from around the baby in the womb, by the technique known as AMNIOCENTESIS, they could estimate the level of a substance, *alphafetoprotein (AFP)*, in the fluid. High levels of AFP indicate an abnormality.

The test soon became routine in Britain for any mother known to be at special risk of producing a spina bifida baby—for example, one who had already had such a child. The test could not, however, be offered to all mothers because of its cost and its risks. Since few potential spina bifida mothers can be identified, its effect on the incidence of the condition was not great.

In 1975, however, the same Edinburgh team developed a further test for AFP in an ordinary blood sample—a much safer and easier technique. They found a good relationship between maternal blood levels of AFP and the likelihood of a deformed child, and as a result the number of affected children born in Scotland has now been dramatically reduced.

This test is now becoming more widely available and seems likely to prove to be one of the important medical advances of the 1970s.

altitude sickness

An illness occurring in persons on high mountains, or in unpressurized aircraft, as a result of the reduced quantity of oxygen in the air.

The proportion of oxygen in the atmosphere is the same at all altitudes (approximately 21%), but the atmosphere gets appreciably thinner at great heights so that less oxygen is available. At an altitude of 5,000 ft., the oxygen level is 80% of its value at sea level—a slight reduction that has little effect on a healthy person, except to make prolonged physical effort more difficult. At 10,000 ft., however, the partial pressure of oxygen falls to 69% of its value at sea level; at 15,000 ft. it is 56%, and at 20,000 ft. (say, around the summit of Mount McKinley) it is 45%. At the top of Mount Everest (29,000 ft.), it is 31%.

Man finds considerable difficulty in adapting to oxygen tensions which are 70% or less of normal—in other words, in adapting to altitudes of over 10,000 ft. The breathing rate has to be increased to permit the body to absorb the oxygen it needs, and this leads to an excessive loss of carbon dioxide from the bloodstream (see ALKALOSIS). Eventually the kidneys are able to readjust the acidity of the blood, but this process of acclimatization takes several weeks. Although small colonies of Andeans engage in quite strenuous work in their natural habitat at around 15,000 ft., it is highly doubtful if man could reside permanently at an altitude above 18,000 ft.

With careful, slow acclimatization it is possible for climbers to spend brief periods as high as the summit of Everest, even without carrying oxygen supplies. If a person does not take time to acclimatize himself, then altitude sickness is highly likely to develop at above 10,000 ft. Some people seem to be naturally much more sensitive or vulnerable than others—some cannot tolerate 7,000–8,000 ft. at all well.

Altitude sickness is best prevented by slowing the rate of ascent from sea level—the condition was rare in Everest expeditions when the climbers walked from the foothills into the Himalayas. It has become much more common now that tourists fly into mountainous regions and give their bodies no time to adjust.

Altitude sickness causes headache, shortness of breath, and coughing. In severe cases the lungs may be filled with a frothy fluid—pulmonary edema. Emergency treatment may be given with oxygen and the potent diuretic drug frusemide, but the key treatment is descent to a safe altitude.

Altitude sickness may recur on each occasion that an individual goes into the mountains: the speed of acclimatization is unpredictable and is not necessarily the same for one person on different occasions.

Alzheimer's disease

A presenile DEMENTIA

Most people suffer some degree of brain atrophy (wasting or shrinkage) as they get older, usually accompanied by a slowing of mental processes. Frequently the atrophy is so severe that the person suffers from senile dementia. Characteristically, this change takes place in some persons over the age of 70—sometimes much later.

In a small number of individuals, however, atrophy with resulting dementia occurs far earlier in life. Alzheimer's disease is caused by such an atrophy; the reasons why it occurs are not known. It tends to develop in the 30s or 40s, and the symptoms are precisely those of senile dementia: forgetfulness succeeded by irritability and then irrationality.

Unfortunately, there is no cure at present. Vasodilator drugs are prescribed in an attempt to improve the blood supply to the tissues of the brain. Psychotherapy and tranquilizers or antidepressants may be used, but "loving care" is probably the best therapy in this tragic affliction.

amaurosis

Blindness from some cause outside the eyes. Examples include the blindness sometimes associated with nephritis, toxemia of pregnancy, uremia, migraine, arteriosclerosis and Raynaud's disease.

In healthy persons, transient amaurosis sometimes occurs when standing up quickly from a prone position—caused simply by the draining of blood away from the head. There is also a hysterical variety of amaurosis. When amaurosis is of fairly short duration (as is often the case) it is referred to as *amaurosis fugax*.

The term "amaurotic family idiocy" refers to the inherited abnormality TAY-SACHS DISEASE (common in people of Jewish descent) in which blindness is a feature. The blindness, and indeed all the symptoms of the disease, are due to a lipoid degeneration of nerve ganglion cells.

amblyopia

Defective vision without any obvious disease of the eyeball. Amblyopia may be temporary or permanent and there are many possible causes; it may be partial or may progress to total blindness in the affected eye.

Poisons which may cause blindness include alcohol

and tobacco, lead, compounds that contain arsenic, and certain petroleum derivatives. *Bilateral toxic amblyopia* is common in alcoholics and is also seen in heavy smokers. Methyl alcohol ("meths") is far more dangerous than "ordinary" (ethyl) alcohol in this respect. Bilateral amblyopia may also occur as the result of poisoning with various drugs, chiefly the antimalarial agent quinine. Amblyopia can also occur as a result of damage to the region of the brain concerned with vision; some loss of vision is a common feature of strokes.

The most important preventable cause of amblyopia is strabismus ("cross-eye") in infancy. A child who develops strabismus has the eyes pointing in different directions, and his brain suppresses the image from one eye to prevent the confusion caused by double vision. If the squint is not treated the eye that is not used may become blind.

In general the treatment of amblyopia depends on the cause: cases of toxic amblyopia may improve if the source of poisoning is removed, but in cases due to brain damage or secondary to strabismus the blindness may be irreversible.

amenorrhea

Absence of menstrual periods. Amenorrhea may be primary or secondary. In primary amenorrhea, menstruation has never occurred at all; in secondary amenorrhea, a woman who has previously been menstruating ceases to do so.

Primary amenorrhea begins to give rise to some concern when a girls reaches 15 or 16 and has still not menstruated; she should then be taken to a physician for a gynecological evaluation of her condition. Primary amenorrhea at this age may be just a slight variation from normal; regular menstruation may commence shortly thereafter. But primary amenorrhea may be due to anemia, to disorders of the uterus, ovaries or pituitary gland, or to dysfunction of the thyroid or adrenal glands. Occasionally there is *false* primary amenorrhea (or cryptomenorrhea) in which a girl is menstruating but the menstrual blood is prevented from reaching the exterior by some obstacle, such as an *imperforate hymen* ("maidenhead" without an opening).

Secondary amenorrhea is common. Perhaps the most frequent causes are pregnancy and lactation. In almost any woman who has secondary amenorrhea the doctor will perform a pregnancy test. Secondary amenorrhea may also be due to anemia (often provoked by heavy menstrual blood loss in the past), by ovarian failure, by certain pituitary diseases, and by any kind of emotional disturbance or even a marked change in life style.

Amenorrhea may also occur on the contraceptive pill (or after coming off it) and in ANOREXIA NERVOSA. Treatment will depend on the underlying cause.

amnesia

Loss of MEMORY. Memories are held in the brain in short-term and long-term stores, and either or both functions may be impaired by disease or injury.

Typically, the adult has no memory for the events of infancy, but his recall of the rest of his lifetime is more or less continuous. In old age, however, the memory for recent events becomes impaired, while the events of childhood and early adult life are still well preserved. Loss of recent memory is also a feature of chronic alcoholism (in *Korsakoff's syndrome* the alcoholic invents stories to cover up his loss of memory) and some other brain diseases such as presenile DEMENTIA.

Head injuries that cause loss of consciousness—or even severe or frightening accidents that do not involve the head—may be associated with some loss of memory. Often there is a blank in the memory for some minutes or hours before the injury *(anterograde amnesia)* and for a variable period after the injury *(retrograde amnesia)*. The duration of both types of amnesia tends to diminish as the patient recovers from the injury, but often parts of memory are never recovered.

Sudden loss of memory without any injury or illness is most often due to a psychological disorder: the person who is found wandering far from home with no knowledge of his name or address is usually found to be suffering from *hysterical amnesia*, a condition provoked by emotional stress.

Despite claims to the contrary, no drug has yet been found to improve failing memory.

amniocentesis

A diagnostic test carried out in the first half of pregnancy. A needle is passed through the skin overlying the uterus to puncture the amniotic sac—the bag of membranes surrounding the developing fetus—and so to draw off into a syringe some of the amniotic fluid in which the fetus lies. The fluid can then be examined.

Amniocentesis is usually performed at about the 16th week of pregnancy under local anesthesia. When the needle is withdrawn, the tiny hole made in the amniotic sac seals itself promptly. Complications of amniocentesis are rare, although occasionally the technique may be followed by bleeding, persistent leakage of fluid or by miscarriage. It is very rare for the needle to injure the fetus accidentally, especially if the operator is guided by an ultrasound scan which enables him to locate the positions of the baby and the placenta.

Amniocentesis is one of the major diagnostic advances of recent years, since it enables the obstetrician to find out a great deal about the state of the fetus and to offer the woman termination of the pregnancy (therapeutic abortion) if a major abnormality is present.

The sample of fluid contains some cells from the fetus's skin, and these may be cultured in the laboratory. Tests on the cell culture will detect chromosomal abnormalities such as Down's syndrome (mongolism). Tests on the fluid itself will detect abnormalities such as SPINA BIFIDA and some forms of muscular dystrophy. Indeed, each year there is further growth in the number of fetal abnormalities that can be detected by amniocentesis and the related procedure of fetal blood sampling. The list includes blood abnormalities such as thalassemia, and brain disorders such as Tay-Sachs disease.

At present, however, the use of amniocentesis is restricted to cases in which there is already a higher than average risk of fetal abnormality. For instance, a woman whose last child was abnormal, or one with relatives with an inherited disease, might be referred for amniocentesis. Research is underway, however, to evaluate simple screening tests on blood samples taken early in pregnancy that can identify women at risk of an unsuspected fetal abnormality such as spina bifida and so enlarge the range of antenatal diagnosis by amniocentesis. Such diagnostic techniques require great skill in interpreting the results and the test is not available at all medical centers.

See also ALPHAFETOPROTEIN.

AMNIOCENTESIS

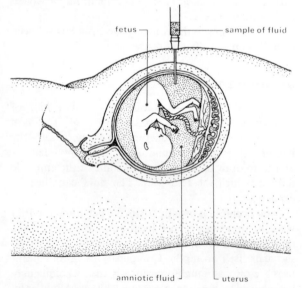

Amniocentesis is a technique for removing a small sample of amniotic fluid from the uterus of a pregnant woman. Analysis of the fluid can show whether the fetus is affected by certain serious disorders such as Down's syndrome and spina bifida. In these cases the mother can be offered a therapeutic abortion; where the result of amniocentesis is normal, she is reassured.

AMOEBA

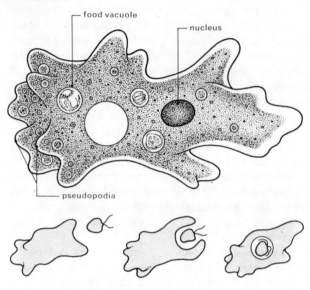

free-living amoeba ingesting a flagellate

Amoebae are single-cell microorganisms which have changeable shape and move around on temporary projections called pseudopodia. They may be free-living or parasitic: certain species can infect humans, causing disease—for example, one type is responsible for amoebic dysentery.

amoeba

A simple type of protozoon, or single-celled living organism. Many species of amoeba are found throughout the world—living chiefly in ponds and stagnant water—and are well-known to biology students.

The medical importance of the amoeba is that certain species can infect man, usually through contamination of the water supply or of food. The most important is the species *Entamoeba histolytica* which causes amoebic DYSENTERY. (This should not be confused with bacillary dysentery, which is caused by entirely different organisms.)

E. histolytica is found throughout the world, especially in the tropics. According to some estimates, 10% of all Americans and Europeans are "carriers" of the organism, although other researchers doubt this figure. The amoeba exists in the bowel in both motile and nonmotile forms; it is usually the nonmotile forms (the cysts) that spread from person to person through fecal contamination of water or food.

Only a small percentage of people infected by *E. histolytica* actually become ill with dysentery. They develop either a chronic and relatively mild diarrhea or (much less commonly) a more acute illness with abdominal pain and profuse blood-stained diarrhea.

Possible complications include amoebic liver abscess.

The diagnosis is made by identifying the amoeba in the feces. Antiamoebic drugs such as Diodoquin cure the great majority of patients.

amputation

The removal of any part of the body, especially a limb or part of a limb.

Amputation may occur accidentally, as in automobile accidents or war injuries, or may have to be performed surgically because of severe injury or disease.

Accidental amputation of toes, fingers, legs and arms is fairly common, particularly in these days of frequent traffic accidents. Other cases occur in the home through mishaps with knives, fans, air-conditioning equipment, blenders and garbage disposal units. Amputations at work are also common, particularly if safety precautions are not observed while dealing with machinery.

In all these cases, surgical treatment is required to alleviate shock, arrest bleeding and remove the damaged tissues at the edges of the wound. The surgeon will suture (stitch up) and dress the wound and take precautions to ensure that tetanus (lockjaw) and other infections do not develop. In a few cases, it is possible by very skilled surgery to stitch back the amputated part—provided it is not too damaged and there has been little delay.

Deliberate surgical amputation is one of the oldest operations. It is commonly performed in cases of great trauma where a part of the body has been irreparably damaged (so that it would be dangerous if left in place), in cases of malignancy where a cancer—most frequently of bone—has developed in a limb, and in cases of gangrene due to trauma, exposure to cold, or vascular disease.

Before the development of anesthesia, amputation was a very rapid and crude procedure; the surgeon's main intention was to remove a limb or other part in a matter of seconds so that he would spare the unanesthetized patient pain. In the last 130 years however, since the introduction of anesthesia, techniques of amputation have become much more delicate, so that a reasonably good appearance is obtained. After a limb amputation an artificial limb can usually be fitted, but the psychological adjustment required after amputation may be more difficult than the physical adjustment.

See also PHANTOM LIMB SYNDROME.

amyloidosis

The infiltration of the liver, kidneys, heart and other internal organs with a starch-like protein substance known as amyloid. (The exact composition of amyloid is not known, and probably varies.)

Amyloidosis is a late complication of chronic infectious diseases such as tuberculosis and osteomyelitis; it also occurs in some cancers of the lymphatic system, such as Hodgkin's disease, and in the bone-marrow cancer multiple myeloma. Sometimes the amyloid infiltration occurs with no predisposing cause; this *primary amyloidosis* is often a familial disorder. Despite its recognition for over 100 years, the mechanism which leads to the deposition of amyloid remains unclear. The deposit itself consists of a mixture of protein and polysaccharides (complex carbohydrates of high molecular weight) and seems to be derived in part from the proteins in the bloodstream; the high rate of antibody formation in chronic infections is probably one of the underlying factors.

The importance of amyloidosis is that the infiltration of vital organs such as the kidneys may cause their progressive failure. Vigorous treatment of the underlying infection is sometimes followed by reabsorption of the amyloid, but there is no specific treatment for the infiltration itself.

amyotonia

A rare form of progressive muscular atrophy occurring in children, often known as Oppenheim's disease or "amyotonia congenita."

It is one of the milder forms of childhood muscular atrophy, although the condition is sometimes fatal and severe disability is common.

The symptoms may be present soon after birth. The most important is a widespread lack of muscle tone, so that the limbs can be readily moved into "contortionist" positions. Because of the weakness of the muscles, the child may find difficulty in supporting his head.

There is no specific treatment for amyotonia but there is a distinct tendency for the child to improve as he gets older. Therapy is largely directed at preventing spinal deformities and lung infections, both of which may occur because of the weakness of the musculature.

anabolism

The building-up by the body of relatively simple chemical substances into fats, proteins and carbohydrates. It is part of the total metabolic process of the body (the breaking-down of food into less complex substances is known as CATABOLISM).

In certain diseases there is an excess manufacture of some chemical substances as the result of faulty anabolism. Such situations occur in PORPHYRIA, in the overproduction of *serotonin* (a potent constrictor of blood vessels), in the "carcinoid syndrome," and in CYSTINURIA (an excess of amino acids—the "building blocks" of protein—in the urine). Most errors of metabolism, including faulty anabolism, are the result of rare hereditary conditions.

See also METABOLISM.

analgesia

Loss or reduction of the sensation of pain in the conscious individual.

Drugs which produce analgesia (*analgesics*) can be divided into three main groups: (1) those which act at the site of the pain; (2) those which act centrally on the brain; and (3) those which have a specific action.

Drugs in the first group are used in cases of fairly mild pain caused by arthritis, rheumatism and various muscular discomforts. Examples include acetaminophen (Exedrin, Tylenol) and aspirin (acetylsalicylic acid). Aspirin not only is effective against mild pain (analgesic action) but also reduces the body temperature in fever (antipyretic action) and has the effect of reducing inflammation (anti-inflammatory action) in rheumatic disease (such as rheumatoid arthritis). Unfortunately, in susceptible individuals it may produce dyspepsia (stomach upset) or even bleeding from the stomach lining, as well as sensitivity reactions. Acetaminophen, which is generally less noxious, is not as effective in reducing fever or controlling the symptoms of rheumatic disease.

Examples of the second group include the opiates (such as morphine), pethidine (Demerol), methadone and codeine. These analgesics, because of their potency and potential for abuse, are used only under medical supervision (that is, available only on prescription).

The third group includes *ergotamine tartrate*, which is specific in migraine; although it relieves headache, it does not help the visual symptoms or the nausea and vomiting which may accompany an attack. It also includes *carbamazepine*, which often reduces the number and the severity of attacks of *trigeminal neuralgia* (or *tic douloureux*).

Analgesia can also result from disease of the sensory nervous system, or from overdoses of alcohol.

anaphylactic shock

Anaphylatic shock is an antibody-antigen reaction in the body which may produce a state of profound collapse. This is characterized by increasing difficulty in breathing and failure of the circulation brought about by general dilation of the small blood vessels and the escape of plasma (the fluid component of the blood) into the tissue spaces. (See ANTIBODY/ANTIGEN.)

Anaphylactic shock may be caused by the injection of certain vaccines, antisera or antibiotics, or by insect stings; it is a desperate emergency in which "half-measures" or delay may prove fatal. Hydrocortisone is given intravenously in large doses, accompanied perhaps by epinephrine or a similar drug. If respiratory distress is marked it is necessary to cut into the trachea (windpipe) to make an artificial opening (tracheostomy).

The condition is fortunately rare. Often undue sensitivity to injected substances can be demonstrated by the use of small test doses, but even a small test dose may trigger off anaphylactic shock in a "sensitized" individual.

Patients receiving injections likely to produce this condition should stay within easy distance of medical aid for half an hour after the injection. Those who feel faint or start to swell in the face after an insect bite should at once seek a doctor's help, although neither of these reactions necessarily heralds anaphylactic shock.

anemia

Anemia—literally, "lack of blood"—is a deficiency in the amount of the red pigment hemoglobin in the blood. Since men, women and children have different levels of hemoglobin, anemia must also be defined in terms of what the normal value for that group may be. Thus men have a hemoglobin level in the range of 13.5 to 18.5 g per 100 ml of blood; in men anemia is usually considered to be present when the hemoglobin value drops below 13.5 g. A corresponding figure for women would be 11.5 g and for a young child as low as 10 g. A similar lower figure would apply to a woman in the later stages of pregnancy.

Anemia has four basic causes. There may be a loss of red blood cells from the circulation through hemorrhage. There may be a deficiency of raw materials needed for the production of hemoglobin and red blood cells. The bone marrow itself may be diseased and therefore unable to produce sufficient red blood cells. Lastly, in the *hemolytic anemias*, production of red blood cells by the bone marrow is normal but the cells are destroyed unusually quickly and so do not survive for the normal period of 120 days in the circulation. Anemia may also occur as a presenting symptom of cancer, occurring for reasons that are not clearly understood and not necessarily related to any of these four causes.

Blood loss may be obvious, as in a patient with nosebleeds or a woman with heavy periods; but when it occurs internally, the patient may be unaware of it ("occult" blood loss).

The raw materials for the production of red cells include iron for hemoglobin production and vitamin B_{12} and folic acid (another B group vitamin). Deficiencies of these substances may be the result of dietary lack, failure to absorb them normally (although they are present in normal amounts in the diet), and, more rarely, an increased demand by the body (as when there is a need for more folic acid in pregnant women).

Diseases of the bone marrow causing a failure of red cell production include replacement of the marrow by cancer or leukemia cells and damage to the marrow by toxic drugs, chemicals and radiation. In many cases the marrow is depressed as an effect of a generalized disease—such as rheumatoid arthritis, tuberculosis or kidney failure (known as "secondary symptomatic anemia").

Anemia is a very common condition and in many cases goes undetected if it is not severe. For example, women, because of their menstrual blood loss, maintain their iron balance with difficulty; surveys have revealed that 5% or more of women who otherwise appear healthy are in fact anemic, while up to 30%, have no reserves of iron and are thus in danger of developing iron-deficiency anemia.

The symptoms of anemia may be minimal; but if the condition is at all severe, the patient will be pale and will complain of tiredness and shortness of breath on exertion. In addition, specific types of anemia may produce characteristic symptoms.

Blood checks for the presence of anemia and other blood abnormalities form an important part of any comprehensive medical examination. Not only may the patient's symptoms be caused by anemia, but those who are in good health usually show normal numbers of red and white blood cells and the red cell sedimentation rate will be normal (see ERYTHROCYTE SEDIMENTATION RATE). All three measurements are usually included in a "blood count" test.

If a patient is found to be anemic, the fundamental problem for the doctor to resolve is whether the anemia is the result of a specific blood disease (such as pernicious anemia or leukemia) or whether it is a symptom of blood loss or an underlying disease (such as arthritis) or infection.

The treatment of anemia may be simple, as in the administration of iron tablets in iron-deficiency anemia; in other cases it may require initial blood transfusion or other measures, or treatment may be directed toward the underlying condition of which the anemia is a symptom.

anencephaly

A congenital condition in which a developing fetus has only a rudimentary or no brain. The child is born dead or, at most, lives for only a few hours after birth. A substance called ALPHAFETOPROTEIN (which is found in abnormally large amounts in the fluid surrounding the fetus in cases of anencephaly) is today used to screen for this congenital defect, as well as other congenital abnormalities such as SPINA BIFIDA, so that the mother may be offered a clinical termination of pregnancy.

See also AMNIOCENTESIS.

anesthesia

The loss of feeling, particularly the sensations of pain and touch. It can be produced by disease or damage to the nervous system, certain psychological states, or the action of drugs. The term is usually applied to the deliberate induction of insensibility (either *general* or *local*) to make it possible to perform surgical operations.

Up to the middle of the 19th century, surgery was often a brutal business, although drugs ranging from alcohol to opium were used to diminish the pain felt by the patient. After the introduction of *general anesthesia*—induced by ether, nitrous oxide ("laughing gas") and chloroform—life became more bearable both for patients and surgeons. In 1800, Sir Humphrey Davy noted the anesthetic effect of nitrous oxide and suggested its use in surgery; the similar effect of ether was noted both in the United States and Britain in 1818.

The first practical use of general anesthetics was introduced in 1842 by Crawford Long of Jefferson, Georgia, followed in 1844 by Horace Wells of Hartford, Connecticut. Dr. William Morton demonstrated the anesthetic effects of ether in Boston in 1846; in 1847 and 1848, J. Y. Simpson of Edinburgh used ether and chloroform to relieve the pains of childbirth. Up to fairly recent times, ether, chloroform, ethyl chloride and trichloroethylene were administered by inhalation through a mask to induce general anesthesia; but nowadays intravenous injections of drugs such as *Pentothal Sodium* are used to induce general anesthesia, which send the patient quietly and agreeably to sleep.

Modern anesthetists have many drugs available. They can induce temporary unconsciousness, temporary paralysis and temporary hypotension (low blood pressure) at will. New techniques have made modern surgery possible; a complicated surgical operation depends as much for its success on the skill of the anesthetist as on the skill of the surgeon.

Anesthesia of only a part of the body (without loss of consciousness) can be produced by drugs known as *local anesthetics. Cocaine* applied to the surface of mucous membranes renders them anesthetic; but the use of cocaine has now been abandoned in favor of synthetic compounds such as *tetracaine* (also known as *amethocaine*). Other synthetic compounds, such as *procaine* and *lidocaine*, are administered by injection; if they are injected into or under the skin they produce anesthesia of the immediate area, while if they are injected into sensory nerves they produce anesthesia of the particular region of the body supplied by the nerve.

It is possible to perform some types of major operations under local anesthesia or under *spinal anesthesia*. The latter is a technique in which the local anesthetic agent is introduced into the spinal canal under strict control to bring about temporary paralysis of the motor and sensory nerve roots as they leave the spinal cord. The height up the spinal canal to which the anesthetic solution is allowed to rise determines the area of anesthesia (which is nearly always confined to the lower part of the trunk and the legs). An alternative technique involves injecting the anesthetic into the space just outside the membranes covering the spinal cord (*extradural anesthesia*), and this method is widely used during labor and childbirth.

aneurysm

Swelling at a weak point in the wall of an artery, named according to its shape *fusiform*, *saccular*, *berry* or *dissecting* and classified as *congenital*, *inflammatory*, *degenerative*, or *traumatic*.

Common sites for aneurysms are the aorta (the largest artery of the body), the arteries at the base of the brain (the "circle of Willis"), and the artery behind the knee. Although aneurysms can produce symptoms by pressure on neighboring structures—one at the base of the brain can, for example, produce double vision by

ANEURYSM

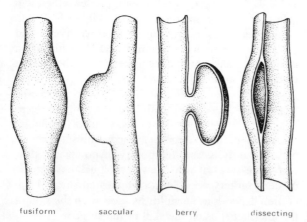

fusiform   saccular   berry   dissecting

Aneurysms form where a weak point in an artery wall is blown out by the pressure of blood. The weakness may be congenital, as with the small "berry" aneurysms in the brain which sometimes burst, causing hemorrhage. Most aneurysms, however, are due to atherosclerosis and are fusiform or saccular in shape. A dissecting aneurysm is one where blood actually runs between the layers of the arterial wall before reentering the true vessel.

interfering with nerves supplying the external muscles of the eye—the chief danger is rupture, which sets up internal bleeding with possibly fatal results.

Treatment depends on the site and nature of the aneurysm; surgery offers the only hope of cure and an operation may or may not be possible. Each case must be judged on its own merits. Saccular or berry aneurysms may have a "neck" that can be tied or clipped, and it is sometimes possible to carry out plastic reconstructions on dilated parts of the aorta.

angina pectoris

Angina pectoris (sometimes just called *angina*) is a characteristic type of chest pain caused by failure of the coronary arteries to supply enough oxygen to the heart muscle.

The pain is felt centrally in the chest but may radiate to the neck or down the left arm. It can be very severe or it may be described merely as a "tightness in the chest." A diagnostic feature is that the pain occurs during activity and will rapidly disappear if the patient stops and rests for a few minutes. Thus patients with chronic angina may come to recognize a characteristic degree or duration of exercise (walking a certain distance or exceeding a certain speed) which will bring on the pain and will learn to avoid it by keeping within their personal exercise tolerance. Emotional factors and cold may also contribute to the onset of pain.

Angina is most often caused by the narrowing of the coronary arteries by ATHEROSCLEROSIS so that the blood supply to the heart muscle is reduced. If the rate and strength of the heartbeat is increased by exercise, the blood flow required to keep the muscle adequately supplied is exceeded and the characteristic pain results. Reducing the requirement by reducing activity allows the blood flow to become adequate again. Less commonly the coronary arteries are normal but the heart muscle is "starved" of oxygen either because the blood is deficient in hemoglobin (ANEMIA) or the blood pressure is low from narrowing of the aortic valve (aortic STENOSIS). The diagnosis depends mainly on the patient's medical history, although the ECG will usually show characteristic abnormalities.

Angina is a serious disorder since its presence denotes diseased coronary arteries; all patients with angina should seek early medical advice. Under good medical care, however, many live a relatively normal life for many years with the condition.

Treatment consists of reducing the load on the heart by weight reduction, reduction of raised blood pressure, avoidance of smoking (which aggravates the condition) and possibly altering the diet to reduce blood levels of fat. Drugs which will relieve the symptoms include glyceryl trinitrate (nitroglycerin) which dilates the coronary arteries and reduces the work load of the heart, and drugs known as "beta-adrenergic blocking agents" which also reduce the work load of the heart. In severe cases, coronary BYPASS surgery may be indicated for the patient.

angiography

Radiological investigation in which a substance opaque to x rays (radiopaque material) is injected into blood vessels to make them visible on the x-ray plate or viewing screen. The process of outlining arteries is called *arteriography;* that of outlining veins is known as *phlebography* or *venography*. The technique is used not only in demonstrating abnormalities or disease of the blood vessels but also in the diagnosis of tumors, particularly in the brain. Lymph vessels can also be outlined; the technique is then known as *lymphangiography*.

ankylosing spondylitis

A disease of the spine in which there is gradual loss of mobility in the joints between the vertebrae. It occurs mainly in males between the ages of 20 and 40 and is related to RHEUMATOID ARTHRITIS.

The illness results in a progressive stiffening of the spine as the normally flexible ligaments supporting the joints gradually harden and acquire the consistency of bone. The disease begins insidiously with stiffness of the back after a period of inactivity. The ability to expand the chest diminishes and there may be pain on breathing deeply, coughing or sneezing. Later the spine may become fixed in an upright position ("poker spine") or bent sideways. The neck may be bent forward and the head may eventually become fixed so that the patient is forced to look downward when walking.

When the symptoms first appear, aspirin or similar drugs are of use to control pain. X-ray therapy has been used with some success, but in a small number of cases (about 3%) it has provoked LEUKEMIA. For this reason, many doctors prefer to control the symptoms with *phenylbutazone* (an anti-inflammatory drug), at the same time ensuring that the patient sleeps with a board under the mattress and uses a supportive pillow for the neck. The great majority (approximately 75%) of patients with this disease are able to lead relatively normal lives.

anorexia nervosa

Anorexia nervosa is a disorder which mainly affects young girls aged 14 to 17 years, although older women and occasionally men may be affected. The patient is noted to be losing weight and, when attention is drawn to this, it is usually explained as an intentional weight loss to avoid obesity or improve the figure. The dietary restriction, however, is then continued and carried to extremes, so that severe weight loss to the extent of emaciation follows. Multiple vitamin and mineral deficiencies may appear. Menstruation, if already established, usually ceases—a not uncommon effect of starvation whether voluntary or involuntary. If the condition is severe, the patient may resort to bizarre measures to increase her weight loss including self-induced vomiting, purgatives and excessive exercise. If untreated, the condition may prove fatal as the patient literally starves herself to death while continuing to assert that her food intake is adequate or even excessive.

The explanation of this curious situation is difficult to find. Physically, the patient will show only the expected findings in any case of starvation from any cause, which include changes in endocrine gland function (the pituitary, adrenal, thyroid and the sex glands).

Mentally, the patient is often depressed and hysterical; she may suffer from phobias or compulsive disorders and may be abnormally concerned about the manifestations of puberty (particularly about breast development). She may feel that any tendency to put on weight will exaggerate her breast or figure developments; it has even been suggested that the starvation is a deliberate attempt to suppress menstruation and that the patient wishes to delay puberty itself.

Treatment involves first obtaining the patient's cooperation in increasing her food intake; if this is done slowly, no problem usually arises, although she will usually also require psychiatric help to overcome her underlying psychological problems. The prognosis for restoration to normal physical health is excellent, but many patients have a subsequent relapse because the basic psychological problem remains.

anthrax

Infectious disease caused by *Bacillus anthracis*, which commonly infects cattle, goats or sheep. Humans contract the infection from the spores of the anthrax bacillus, which survive for a long time in contaminated wool, hair or hides; with increasingly hygienic methods of handling these raw materials the spread of the disease has diminished, and it is now rare in the West.

Infection can affect the skin, when it produces a severe localized reaction. The site of infection is marked by an itching "papule," which becomes surrounded by vesicles filled with blood-stained fluid. The center of the area dies as the infection spreads and becomes black, which gives the disease its name—anthrax—from the Greek word for coal.

Infection can also attack the lungs, to produce pneumonia, or it can advance to anthrax bacteremia (blood poisoning), with a high mortality rate if untreated. The old name for anthrax of the lung was "wool-sorter's disease," an illness which was usually fatal; but now anthrax of both the skin and the lungs responds to treatment with appropriate antibiotics.

antibody/antigen

When certain foreign and therefore potentially harmful substances enter the body, the body reacts to the threat of damage by producing antibodies. An antibody is a chemical compound, a protein, which has the ability to combine with and render harmless a specific foreign substance. The foreign material itself, which initiates the reaction leading to the formation of specific antibodies, is known as an *antigen*.

Most antigenic substances are protein. Proteins have a very complex and almost infinitely variable chemical composition and are constitutents of all living matter. For this reason, the antigens which cause the formation of antibodies are mostly substances derived directly or indirectly from living organisms. Common examples of antigens are the bacteria and viruses which cause human disease; "foreign" blood from an incompatible blood group, inadvertently given during a blood transfusion; and sera from other species injected into humans for the treatment or prevention of infectious diseases. Whatever the situation, the antibody formed in response to a particular antigen is unique to that antigen, reacting with no other (see illustration). The blood of an adult contains tens of thousands of individual antibodies directed against different antigens and together forming a distinct group of proteins in the serum, the *immuno-globulins*.

The basic purpose of antibody formation is defensive. One major role of antibodies is in overcoming attacks of infectious diseases and prevention of future recurrent attacks. Thus, when the patient who has never previously had an attack of whooping cough comes into contact with the whooping cough bacillus, he or she will develop symptoms of the disease. The defeat of the invading bacteria depends initially on the action of the *phagocytic blood cells* responsible for primary defense against bacterial invasion; these cells attack, kill and engulf the bacteria. As the disease runs its course, however, antibodies against the whooping cough bacilli start to appear in the blood and the final elimination of the infection is aided by their action. By the time the patient is convalescent, a good level of specific antibodies is present in the blood. In many diseases these antibodies persist at such a high level that the patient remains immune to a second attack of the disease throughout the rest of his life.

This natural phenomenon forms the basis of vaccination and inoculation against infectious diseases (see

IMMUNIZATION). Antibodies are usually produced as the result of an infection with bacteria, viruses or other microorganisms; their production can also be stimulated artificially by the introduction into the body of a special preparation of these microorganisms or their products. In whooping cough and typhoid, for example, injection of dead bacteria (of the same species that can cause the respective disease) will evoke the identical kind of antibody formation as that seen in the actual disease

ANTIBODY AND ANTIGEN – how some antibodies work

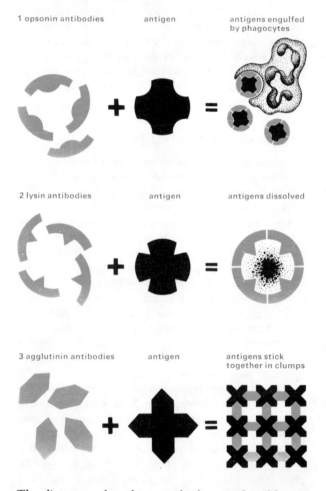

1 opsonin antibodies   antigen   antigens engulfed by phagocytes

2 lysin antibodies   antigen   antigens dissolved

3 agglutinin antibodies   antigen   antigens stick together in clumps

The diagrams show how antibodies produced by the body defend us against foreign substances (antigens). Each antibody can only combine with a specific antigen which has a complementary chemical "shape." Opsonin antibodies cling to antigens such as bacteria and make them more appetizing to certain white blood cells called phagocytes (1). Lysin antibodies kill bacteria directly by dissolving them (2). Agglutinin antibodies cause bacteria or viruses to clump together, rendering them ineffective (3).

and will confer lasting immunity. In diphtheria and tetanus, the bacteria produce their effects by means of the toxins (poisons) that they produce; injection of the toxin itself, suitably treated to render it no longer toxic though still antigenic, will enable the body to form antibodies against the toxin. Lastly, the inoculation of a specific living virus culture—which has been treated to weaken the virus to such a degree that it can no longer cause symptoms of the disease—will immunize the patient against smallpox, yellow fever, poliomyelitis and other diseases.

Most antibodies are thus acquired by contact with an antigen, but in a newborn baby some antibodies are already present that have been passively acquired from its mother and which persist for a few months after birth to provide an early protection against infections. The antibodies of the ABO blood group system are also present from birth and are not the result of antigenic stimulation.

In rare instances, antibodies may be formed against the body's own cells rather than against invading bacteria, viruses or other foreign material. In this case, damage to the tissue against which the antibodies are formed results—a condition known as an AUTOIMMUNE DISEASE.

Transplanted organs or tissues, unless they are taken from the patient's identical twin, are considered to be foreign invaders by the body and may be rejected unless immunosuppressive drugs are used (see TRANSPLANTATION).

anxiety

Anxiety is a normal response to a crisis such as an impending examination or a new job; but excessive anxiety may be socially crippling and cause physical ill health.

In *anxiety neurosis* a perfectly normal concern about cleanliness, noise or any other everyday circumstance becomes magnified to dominate the thoughts. Typically this leads to obsessional behavior, with the sufferer returning repeatedly to his house to check that the door is shut and the gas turned off, or to a preoccupation with hand washing or some other ritual. In AGORAPHOBIA, anxiety about leaving the house and meeting strangers may lead to a self-imposed imprisonment in the home. However, the anxiety may be less specific. In such cases every minor event is seen as a threat and a cause for apprehension; again, the effect is to restrict behavior to a cautious, predictable routine.

Anxiety is a common component of the *depressive illnesses* which affect a high proportion of all men and women in middle and later life (see DEPRESSION). One third or more of all middle-aged women admit to episodes of depression, often including anxiety about

their family relationships and their worth. Anxiety is also frequently provoked in middle age by an episode of illness—such as a heart attack or a head injury—that impairs self-confidence.

The symptoms of recurrent anxiety include loss of appetite and weight, palpitations, headache, excessive sweating and difficulty in sleeping. These somatic symptoms may be suppressed readily following treatment with tranquilizing drugs: such treatment is often used to control the symptoms associated with isolated life-events, such as anxiety about flying or sea voyages. More intractable anxiety warrants treatment by PSYCHOTHERAPY. Many specific phobias—such as fear of dogs—can be treated effectively by techniques such as conditioning and behavior therapy, but individuals with anxiety as a prominent feature of their personalities are unlikely to undergo any dramatic change, whatever the treatment.

apnea

Absence or cessation of breathing. In newborn babies it may be due to poor placental circulation (e.g., because of compression of the umbilical cord), birth injury or the effects of drugs administered to the mother during labor.

In later life apnea can be the result of many conditions as diverse as stroke or electric shock. A form of apnea occurs in Cheyne-Stokes respiration, when the respirations build up to a crescendo, then fade to a period of apnea, which is followed by a crescendo, and so on. It can be a terminal sign.

See also ARTIFICIAL RESPIRATION.

apoplexy

1. A sudden loss of consciousness, typically followed by paralysis, caused by bleeding from a ruptured blood vessel within the brain (CEREBRAL HEMORRHAGE) or blocking of an artery of the brain (cerebral thrombosis or CEREBRAL EMBOLISM).
See also CEREBROVASCULAR DISEASE, STROKE.
2. A condition caused by the effusion of blood into an organ, such as the lung (*pulmonary apoplexy*).

appendicitis/appendicectomy

Inflammation of the *vermiform appendix* (commonly called just the *appendix*), which is a small structure attached to the blind end of the large intestine (the *cecum*). It is about the size and shape of an earthworm.

Symptoms of acute appendicitis can vary widely and the condition is often difficult to diagnose. In the most typical case, the first symptom is diffuse discomfort felt in the area of the navel (umbilicus) with nausea and perhaps vomiting. There may be constipation or mild diarrhea. The discomfort turns into pain, and the pain settles in the lower right-hand part of the abdomen. The wall of the abdomen at first tightens when pressure is applied over the site of the pain ("guarding") and then in time becomes rigid. The patient's tongue is characteristically dry and the breath fetid. The temperature is usually only slightly raised.

Treatment is surgical removal of the appendix (*appendicectomy*). If this can be carried out within the first 24 hours or so, convalescence is usually straightforward; but if the symptoms are not recognized, the appendix may become gangrenous and burst to produce PERITONITIS. Commonly this becomes localized, and an appendix abscess forms which can be drained after it has been sealed off by natural processes.

The appendix appears to be a useless (or "vestigial") organ. The operation for its removal is usually relatively easy; surgeons are therefore inclined to perform an appendicectomy in most cases where they suspect inflammation of the organ, or remove it during the course of other scheduled abdominal surgery.

APPENDICITIS

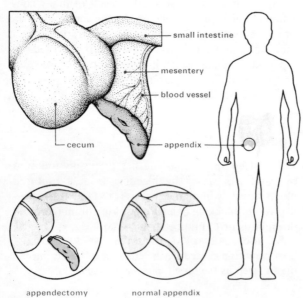

small intestine
mesentery
blood vessel
cecum
appendix

appendectomy   normal appendix

Appendicitis is the most common cause of acute abdominal pain and is a surgical emergency. In some unusual cases, accurate diagnosis may be impossible; a surgeon may then perform an appendectomy unnecessarily rather than risk leaving an inflamed appendix, which could lead to serious complications.

arrhythmia (dysrhythmia)

Any abnormality in the rhythm of the heartbeat, occurring in the normal healthy person or as a result of cardiac disease.

It can sometimes be felt as an "extra" beat of the heart, or it may only be detected by an electrocardiogram (ECG).

In the otherwise healthy person, occasional irregular beats are of no significance; many people experience extra beats, when anxious or after too much coffee or too many cigarettes. However, irregularity of the heartbeat may be a serious complication of a coronary thrombosis ("heart attack"); for that reason, patients are often admitted to a coronary care unit where the rhythm can be monitored electronically.

Dysrhythmias may also occur in diseases such as thyroid overactivity (HYPERTHYROIDISM) or as a side effect of drug treatment. Whatever the cause, the rhythm may be restored to normal either by drugs or by electric shock treatment (cardioversion); often, however, the change in rhythm is no cause for concern and no treatment may be needed.

See also BUNDLE BRANCH BLOCK; PACEMAKER; DEFIBRILLATION.

arteriosclerosis

The general term for any condition in which the walls of the arteries become thick, inelastic and hard. Popular name: *hardening of the arteries.*

The exact cause is unknown, but the condition is common and progressive from the middle years on. One particularly serious form of arteriosclerosis involves the deposition of fatty patches (atheromas) on the inner walls of the blood vessels.

See ATHEROSCLEROSIS.

arteritis

Inflammation of an artery. This may be incidental, that is, when an artery runs close to an area of infection (*nonspecific arteritis*), or it may be associated with a specific disease (of which the arterial inflammation represents only one manifestation).

In *temporal arteritis*, a serious illness which affects elderly persons, the arteries overlying the temples become swollen and painful. If the inflammation extends to the arteries supplying blood to the eyes it may cause sudden and permanent blindness. In most cases, treatment with corticosteroid drugs suppresses the inflammation and provides dramatic relief of symptoms.

Other forms of arteritis affect blood vessels in all parts of the body. These include LUPUS ERYTHEMATOSUS, POLYARTERITIS NODOSA and a number of less well defined disorders—such as POLYMYALGIA

RHEUMATICA. The importance of the occurrence of arteritis in these disorders lies in what it does, since interruption of blood flow damages the organs or muscles supplied by the affected artery or arteries.

arthritis

Joints may be affected by inflammatory or degenerative changes, which cause pain and stiffness described as arthritis. The causes of arthritis range from infection after injury to the onset of age, and include rheumatic fever, rheumatoid processes which are poorly understood, gout, osteoarthritis, psoriasis, tumors and diseases of the nervous system.

Injury impairs the efficiency of a joint by damaging the smooth articular surface; age wears out the joint surface, particularly in the joints which have borne the weight of the body for many years—the hips and knees. Gout causes the deposition of crystals of uric acid in the joints, tumors derange the anatomy of the joint, and deficiency in nervous supply can lead to insensitivity of the joint or abnormality of muscular action; this may cause bizarre movements or repeated unnoticed injuries which produce mechanical derangement of the joint.

The most common disease affecting joints in youth and maturity is RHEUMATOID ARTHRITIS, of which the cause is unknown. In Britain rheumatoid arthritis most frequently affects women in the 18–40 age group, while osteo-arthritis is most common in men over 50. The lubricating lining of the joint (synovial membrane) suffers chronic inflammatory change with consequent irreversible damage to the joint capsule and cartilage and the formation of scar tissue. Pain, swelling and deformity of the joint ensues, particularly obvious in the hands, and there is limitation of movement.

Cases of arthritis are differentiated and diagnosed with the help of blood tests and x rays. Treatment depends on the cause; there are specific drugs to treat gout, and antibiotics will be used in cases of infection. Anti-inflammatory drugs and aspirin (or similar pain-killers) are of help in cases of rheumatoid arthritis and degenerative arthritis in the elderly, but most have the drawback that they are inclined to irritate the lining of the stomach and must therefore be used with discretion. The surgical replacement of weight-bearing joints—hips in particular—has proved possible, and such operations relieve pain and restore movement. Steroids (cortisone derivatives) are used in rheumatoid disease, but their early promise has not been borne out. In nearly all cases physical therapy is invaluable.

Much research is currently in progress on these common and crippling conditions, and the patient suffering from arthritis has a much better prognosis today than in former years.

ARTHRITIS

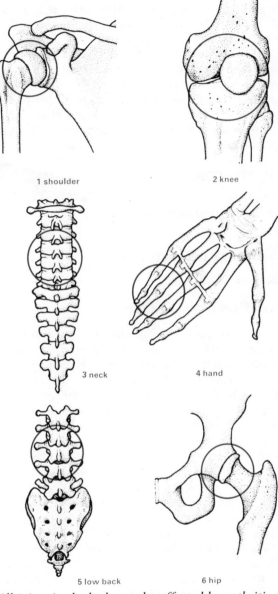

1 shoulder   2 knee

3 neck   4 hand

5 low back   6 hip

All joints in the body can be affected by arthritis. The illustration shows the joints most commonly involved, and the variety of conditions which can result. They are frozen shoulder (1); painful knee (2); pressure on spinal nerves (3); stiff fingers (4); low back pain (5); and painful hip (6).

arthroplasty

Surgical technique used to create a new joint in place of one which has become stiffened and painful through disease or injury. Arthroplasty falls into two main classes: *excision* or *replacement*.

In *excision arthroplasty*, the diseased ends of the

bones forming the joint are removed so that a gap is left. This gap can be filled with fibrous tissue as a scar forms. While such arthroplasties relieve pain and correct deformity, they leave an unstable joint unsuitable for weight-bearing.

However, in recent years it has become possible to replace diseased joints with artificial joints. Such *replacement arthroplasty* has proved very successful in treating arthritis and fractures of the hip. It is also possible to use artificial knee and elbow joints, although so far the success rate here has not been as good as it is in replacement of hip joints.

arthroscopy

The process of inspecting the interior of a joint through an optical instrument that is inserted into the joint cavity.

artificial insemination

See AID/AIH.

artificial respiration

Any emergency process by which the act of breathing is carried out on behalf of an incapacitated patient unable to perform this function for himself.

Since irreversible brain damage follows after only three minutes without oxygen and death after only a few minutes more, artificial respiration is an emergency procedure which should be started at once. Such niceties as removing dentures, ties, etc. can be performed later after the patient has received some air. For the moment, the mouth should merely be cleared of any obvious debris.

The most commonly used method is mouth to mouth, carried out as follows. The patient should be lying on his back on a hard surface and his head should be tilted as far back as possible. The operator should then place his lips over the patient's mouth (with a handkerchief in between if desired). He should pinch the patient's nostrils shut and then breathe out, using a little force with an adult, but breathing very gently if the patient is a small child or a baby. Alternatively, the patient's mouth can be left clear and breath introduced through the nostrils. In the case of small children or babies the operator's mouth must be placed over both mouth and nose.

The operator must make sure the chest rises, then remove his lips and allow the chest to deflate. This should be repeated at a rate of 12 times a minute and continued until normal spontaneous breathing resumes or until the patient is pronounced dead.

At the same time as this procedure is being carried out the patient should also be being treated for shock.

asbestosis

Asbestos is a substance made of a mixture of the silicates of iron, nickel, magnesium, aluminium and calcium; the name means "indestructible." It is used in making fire-resistant materials, brake and clutch linings, tiles and floor coverings, roofing felt, tires and many other products, including electrical insulation. Unfortunately, the lungs of workers in the asbestos industry sometimes suffer irritation from inhaled particles of asbestos and become fibrous. The patient becomes breathless, coughs, loses weight, feels tired and loses his appetite. Moreover, he is liable to contract tuberculosis and after a period (which may be as long as 20 to 40 years) to develop cancer of the lung.

Asbestos cannot easily be replaced in many of its applications, and the use of asbestos increases year by year. It is of the greatest importance that industrial processes should be rigorously controlled to prevent the inhalation of asbestos dust, for the only effective treatment of asbestosis is preventative; there is no known cure for the disease.

ascites

The accumulation of fluid, mostly water, in the abdominal cavity, contained between the layer of *peritoneum* which covers the walls of the cavity and the layer covering the organs within the abdomen. As the fluid collects the abdomen swells and becomes uncomfortable, but it is possible to draw off the fluid through a needle passed through the abdominal wall.

Ascites occurs in a number of diseases, including heart failure, abdominal cancer, and some disorders of the liver and kidneys. Treatment is directed toward the underlying condition.

aspergillosis

Disease caused by the fungus *Aspergillus fumigatus*. This microorganism is found almost everywhere and does not normally cause disease in man; indeed, it often flourishes in the mouths of healthy people. It does, however, cause disease in birds and occasionally man, where it infects the lungs and sometimes the ear or the paranasal sinuses (sinuses which drain into the nasal cavities). Infection of the lung produces cough (which may be productive of blood) and fever; parts of the fungus may break off to set up infection in the heart, brain, kidneys or spleen (carried to these sites by means of the bloodstream). Sometimes a patient with aspergillosis may develop asthma.

Treatment involves the administration of antifungal drugs (such as amphotericin B). Except in cases where the infection is widely disseminated, the outlook is good.

asphyxia

Lack of oxygen in the blood due to the cessation of breathing or an obstruction to the entry of air into the lungs. If asphyxia is prolonged for more than a very few minutes, irreversible brain damage or death may occur.

One of the most common causes of asphyxia is drowning. The entry of water into the lungs leads to loss of consciousness and breathing stops. First aid— emptying the water out of the lungs and throat and giving artificial respiration—will restore normal breathing if given quickly. Electric shock is another fairly common cause of asphyxia, which can also be reversible by prompt artificial respiration.

Asphyxia may also be due to the inhalation of air containing too little oxygen (sometimes found at the bottom of disused wells) or poisonous gases, especially carbon monoxide. Among the mechanical obstructions to breathing are ligatures around the neck, as in suicidal hanging, and choking or the accidental inhalation of lumps of food; again, prompt first aid can be life-saving. The throat may also become blocked by swelling of the tissues secondary to infections such as diphtheria and by tumors; in such cases the obstruction may be bypassed by a surgeon making an opening in the trachea below the level of the blockage (TRACHEOTOMY).

asthma

Air drawn into the lungs during breathing is conveyed to the small air sacs (alveoli) in the lungs. It is there that the exchange of oxygen and carbon dioxide (between the inspired air and the blood) takes place. To reach the alveoli, the inspired air must pass through a "tree" of air passages of ever-decreasing diameter (the *bronchi* and the *bronchioles*).

While the larger bronchi are of fixed diameter (their walls contain rigid rings of cartilage which permit no change in their "bore"), the smaller bronchioles have muscular walls and are capable of wide variation in their bore with contraction or relaxation of the muscle coat.

Changes in the bore of the bronchi are usually slight and occur in response to exercise or the secretion into the blood of certain chemically active compounds (hormones). In patients with asthma, however, the bronchioles are sensitive to stimulation by a variety of agents which produce marked contraction of the muscular wall, with narrowing of the bore to a degree that seriously obstructs the entry and exit of air in the lungs.

In an attack of asthma the breathing becomes difficult, expiration often being more affected than inspiration. The patient is short of breath and breathing may become audibly "wheezy," with coughing. The effort to draw breath increases, but despite this the movement of the chest is diminished. The patient may become agitated or confused and his skin color may change to a bluish tinge from insufficient oxygen (CYANOSIS). The attack may be short, lasting only a few minutes, or very long (*status asthmaticus*) and the patient may become exhausted by his efforts to obtain air.

There are numerous causes of the contraction of the muscular coat of the bronchioles. In some cases a frank allergy exists to a particular material; the patient responds to this by the onset of an attack of asthma, usually within minutes of exposure. Grass and tree pollens, molds and fungi, animal hair and dander, the minute "house-dust mite" (found in all areas of human habitation), and even some types of food may all provoke an asthmatic attack. In other cases a physical or chemical irritant (such as a smoky atmosphere, exhaust fumes, or acid fumes) may bring on an attack. Infections of the lungs, particularly those caused by viruses, may precipitate an attack in subjects who are susceptible. Prolonged exertion may also provoke an attack, as may a variety of emotional factors (such as stress, tension, or anxiety).

Treatment of an acute asthmatic attack involves the administration of drugs such as epinephrine or related compounds (in severe cases, injected subcutaneously), or the use of an aerosol spray (containing drugs such as isoproterenol or salbutamol). These cause relaxation of the contracted bronchioles. In most cases an impending attack can be controlled with the use of a nebulizing inhaler, which produces a fine mist of droplets that can be inhaled directly into the affected bronchioles. Regardless of whether a nebulizer or a pressurized aerosol is used, dosage must be cautiously restricted or the possibility of a dangerous overdosage may occur. Additional help may be obtained (especially if a marked allergic element is present) from the administration of a large dose of steroids (cortisone-like drugs) by mouth or injection. Oxygen may also be required for the asthmatic's treatment.

For more long-term treatment, similar drugs may be given by mouth on a regular daily basis. In addition to the administration of epinephrine-like drugs and steroids, newer drugs are proving valuable for long-term treatment.

The prognosis is usually good although in very severe untreated cases death may occur rarely, especially in status asthmaticus. When the condition first occurs in early childhood, there may be a tendency to "grow out of it," but in adults the condition has a tendency to recur.

astigmatism

A defect in the refractive surfaces of the lens and cornea

ASTIGMATISM

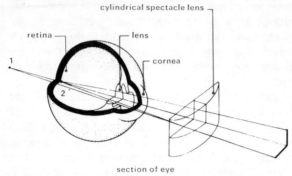

Astigmatism is incorrect curvature of the cornea or the lens of the eye with the result that the image reaching the retina is not correctly focused (1), and appears blurred or distorted. The defect can be corrected by placing a cylindrical lens in front of the eye, thereby focusing the image on the retina (2).

of the eye, which causes the image falling on the retina to be partially out of focus. In the normal eye, objects are focused sharply onto all parts of the retina. When the refractive surfaces have an incorrect curvature the focusing is distorted and parts of the image appear blurred. A spherical ball, for instance, may seem egg-shaped or only partially clear.

Astigmatism is often associated with other sight defects in children, such as short-sightedness. To correct vision, glasses are prescribed in which the lens has the shape of a slice cut off a cylinder. It thus has one curved and one flat side and is able to bend the light rays so that they come to a correct focus on the retina.

It is important that astigmatism—like any refractive error—should be corrected, since a child with such a handicap may otherwise develop permanently defective vision (see AMBLYOPIA).

See also VISION.

ataxia

Muscular incoordination, especially when attempting voluntary movements. The smoothness and precision of muscular action is impaired so that movements become unsteady, clumsy and inaccurate.

In general, ataxia is caused by lesions within the central nervous system (the brain and spinal cord). Ataxia can occur in childhood, usually as the result of congenital deficiency in the cerebellum or the nervous pathways connected with the cerebellum, although it can be caused by birth injury or subsequent disease. The child is not lacking in intelligence, but is "floppy"—when it first starts to reach out and handle objects it is

clumsy and shows a tremor (shaking). Such children are very late in starting to walk, and may be unsteady on their feet for some years. In some children ataxia is associated with the development of a spastic state of the lower limbs (spastic ataxia), a condition found in hydrocephalus and after severe meningitis or encephalitis.

In later life various diseases may affect the cerebellum to produce ataxia, which is described as "cerebellar ataxia" and is not influenced by visual guidance—unlike those forms of ataxia caused by damage to the sensory pathways of the spinal cord. Moreover, the incoordination of voluntary muscular movement results in speech disturbances so that words are slurred and produced slowly.

It is a matter of common observation that an overdose of alcohol can produce ataxia; chronic alcoholism can result in a permanent cerebellar type of ataxia. The most common causes of cerebellar ataxia, however, are the lesions of multiple sclerosis and tumors of the cerebellum. There are a number of rare conditions which involve the cerebellum and the spinal cord to produce ataxia, some of which show a family history, and various poisons such as organic mercurial salts and lead can render a patient ataxic.

Disease of the cerebellum interferes with a complicated central mechanism coordinating sensory and muscular nerve impulses to make smooth and purposeful movement possible; but ataxia will result if the sensory part of the circuit is deficient even though the central mechanism is healthy. Disease of the spinal cord may affect sensory nerve fibers running up the dorsal columns of the cord which carry impulses signaling the position of the limbs and the body. Possibly the best known example of such a disease is TABES DORSALIS (locomotor ataxia), a late manifestation of syphilis. The patient relies upon visual guidance to estimate the position of his limbs, and becomes completely ataxic when his eyes are closed or there is little or no light. Fortunately, the neurological manifestations of syphilis have become relatively rare since the introduction of penicillin.

atelectasis

Collapse of a segment or lobe of a lung (in infants, it is caused by faulty expansion of lung tissue at birth).

If an airway, large or small, in the lung is obstructed the air in the lung tissue beyond the obstruction is absorbed into the bloodstream and the lung air spaces collapse. Obstructions may be formed of sticky mucus, or brought about by the expansion of tumors or the inhalation of foreign bodies (e.g., a tooth).

Foreign bodies may often be removed through a bronchoscope; in the case of a tumor, both the tumor and the affected lung tissue must be removed by surgical operation, if possible. Bronchial secretions are excessive in conditions such as bronchitis; these tend to become dry and thick and may provoke atelectasis; to minimize the possibility of this complication, the air should be kept relatively humid.

Portions of the lung are liable to collapse after abdominal operations because the pain of the incision makes coughing (which expels bronchial secretions) an unpleasant experience to be avoided; postoperative patients thus have to be actively encouraged to clear their airways by coughing.

At birth, one of the first duties of the obstetrician is to suck any mucus plugs out of the baby's airway through a small catheter and to make sure that the lungs expand properly. Untreated areas of atelectasis may become infected and lead to the formation of a lung abscess.

atherosclerosis

Atherosclerosis (a form of ARTERIOSCLEROSIS, or "hardening of the arteries") is the condition underlying the current epidemic of coronary thrombosis ("heart attack") and STROKE. The smooth internal lining of the arteries becomes covered with yellowish fatty patches (atheromas) which narrow the caliber of the vessels. These patches (*plaques*) are often a focus for THROMBOSIS, further narrowing the arterial bore and eventually blocking the vessel completely.

Family history is probably the most important factor in the development of atherosclerosis, but the high incidence in the developed countries of the world suggests that it is also connected with some features of the Western way of life. Associated with atherosclerosis are excessive consumption of animal fats and refined

ATHEROSCLEROSIS

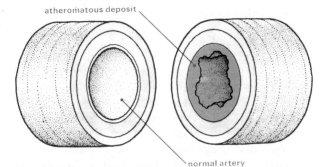

atheromatous deposit

normal artery

The illustration shows cross sections of a normal artery (left) and one in which atherosclerosis has formed. Atheroma is a fatty deposit of cholesterol which forms in the inner layer of the wall, narrowing the artery and reducing blood flow.

carbohydrates, raised blood pressure (hypertension), tobacco smoking, and lack of physical exercise; the consequences—such as coronary thrombosis—are reaching epidemic proportions in Western societies and efforts are concentrated on prevention.

The treatment of established atherosclerosis is both unsatisfactory and controversial. Apart from the treatment of the major symptoms such as stroke or ANGINA PECTORIS, other important steps are reduction of raised blood pressure and weight reduction; a low intake of animal fat is generally advised in an attempt to lower blood levels of fat. Exercise should be increased and STRESS reduced. Surgical procedures to overcome failing blood supply in certain specific sites may be helpful.

athetosis

A slow writhing movement of the limbs and facial muscles, a symptom of damage to the basal ganglia (nerve centers deep inside the brain). Most commonly athetosis is a feature of cerebral palsy or spastic paralysis, the combination of physical and mental defects caused by interference with the oxygen supply to the baby during and just after birth.

Athetosis may affect one or both sides of the body. The writhing movements are aggravated by emotion and when any voluntary action is attempted, so that they interfere with speech, eating and other daily activities. Occasionally, athetosis may develop in adult life as a symptom of tumors or infections affecting the basal ganglia.

The intensity of the movements may be reduced by treatment with drugs of the same kind used in Parkinson's disease.

athlete's foot

A fungus infection of the foot. Also known as *tinea pedis, ringworm of the foot.* See TINEA.

atresia

The abnormal closure or congenital absence of a natural opening in the body. Among the sites where atresia may be present are the anus, vagina, or in organs such as the esophagus or duodenum. These defects need to be corrected by surgery (in the first few days of life in the case of congenital atresia).

atrial fibrillation

A common consequence of ischemic and RHEUMATIC HEART DISEASE in which the normally coordinated action of the heart muscle forming the atria breaks down, allowing the muscle mass to contract and relax irregularly and rapidly. Waves of excitation pass through the muscle not at the normal rate of between 60, and 80, but at 500 to 600 a minute. Not all these waves of excitation are conducted to the ventricles, however, which beat in atrial fibrillation at about 100 to 150 a minute irregularly with much variation in force.

The patient in atrial fibrillation becomes breathless and may develop signs of HEART FAILURE. Atrial fibrillation is quite compatible with life, unlike VENTRICULAR FIBRILLATION; but as circulation ceases in the atria because the muscle is virtually paralyzed, clots are liable to form and break off as emboli.

Treatment includes the administration of digitalis to slow down the ventricular rate of contraction, and possibly of quinidine to stop the irregular contraction. DEFIBRILLATION may be effective.

atrial flutter

An abnormality of cardiac rhythm.

Atrial flutter is usually associated with coronary, hypertensive or rheumatic disease, occasionally with hyperthyroidism. In this condition the atria contract at an extremely fast rate – around 300 beats a minute—and the ventricles cannot respond to this, only to every second or third beat.

Treatment and future outlook depend upon the underlying cause of the condition.

atrophy

The wasting away or reduction in size of a part of the body as the result of disease, inactivity or disuse, or interference with its blood or nerve supply.

auscultation

The act of listening to the sounds produced within the body, especially with the aid of a STETHOSCOPE. It is a valuable part of a physician's examination routine.

The stethoscope is most often used to listen to the sounds produced by the heart and lungs. The normal heart sounds can be approximately described by the words "lubb dupp," the first sound being produced by the contraction of the heart muscle and the second by the snapping shut of the valves, which prevents a return flow of blood from the arteries at the end of the contraction. In some forms of heart disease a variety of other sounds may also be heard which are generally known as "murmurs." These are usually produced by disease of the heart valves; many murmurs, however, may have no medical significance at all. Narrowing of the valve opening (*valvular stenosis*) obstructs the blood flow and produces a harsh murmur when blood is forced through the damaged valve. Laxity of the valves causes a leakage in a reverse direction (*incompetence* of the valve)

and when the heart contraction is completed it tends to produce a softer *reflux murmur*. Disease of the *pericardium*, the membrane covering the surface of the heart, may roughen its normally smooth surface causing a "friction rub" to be heard in the stethoscope.

The entry of air into the lungs also produces characteristic sounds, transmitted through the chest wall to the stethoscope. The presence of fluid in the lungs or obstruction to the airflow will produce additional sounds (*râles* and *rhonchi*). Sounds produced in the airways, as well as voice sounds, are conducted to the chest wall and are characteristically modified by changes in the intervening lung tissue. These sounds may be blocked by the accumulation of fluid in the space between the lung and the chest wall. Diseases which roughen the smooth surface of the membrane which covers the outside of the lungs and the inside of the ribs (*pleural membrane*) may produce a "pleural friction rub" with each breath (see PLEURISY), which can be heard on auscultation.

Australia antigen

A chemical substance first detected in the blood of an Australian aborigine (thus its name) and thought originally to be characteristic of the racial group. It is now known to be a "marker" for the presence of the virus causing one type of HEPATITIS. The substance involved probably represents the virus itself and testing for it has become a valuable diagnostic aid; it is also used as one type of screening test before the transfusion of whole blood and other blood products.

autism

A psychosis in children of unknown cause, which may be related to the adult SCHIZOPHRENIA from which it differs in a number of respects.

The earliest signs are an indifference to parents and others who try to show affection and care for the child. The baby may not respond to being picked up and nursed, and may show ritualistic, repetitive play, even banging its head. It may rock to and fro. Although the child looks healthy and normal, feeding and toilet training become increasingly difficult and ineffective. The child learns to walk, but speaks late or stays mute. If it begins to speak, the words may be inappropriate, repeated and meaningless.

The afflicted children are not necessarily mentally deficient, and characteristically have an exceptional memory and high intelligence. They are upset by changes in their surroundings, for example, the rearrangement of furniture. In general, the children seem to behave as if they are alone in the world; they cannot perceive others as people, regarding them as inanimate objects, and they cannot understand that it is possible to communicate with them. Strangers will regard them as normal but very rude and ill-behaved, but it is possible to gain a little insight into their minds by imagining that they are unable to perceive the world in a normal way; somehow there is a distortion of the sensory impressions which go to make up a normal mental picture of everyday life, so that the autistic child's world is strange, incomprehensible and frightening. The natural reaction is to shut out external contacts and unfamiliar experiences, and to withdraw into surroundings which stay constant and closed.

A great deal can be done to help these children. Some suffer physical disabilities such as deafness or deficient vision which to a certain extent can be corrected; some suffer from mental deficiency; but many can be taught to communicate, although complete recovery is rare. About twice as many boys as girls are affected.

autoimmune disease

Many chronic, noninfectious diseases are due to a misdirection of the immune mechanisms which ordinarily protect the body against infections with bacteria and other microorganisms. Typically, antibodies are formed against vital structures such as the lining of the heart valves or the filtration units (glomeruli) in the kidneys, and the chronic inflammation that results causes fibrosis, scarring, and eventually failure of the organ concerned.

The body deals with microorganisms in two main ways: white blood cells engulf bacteria, destroying and digesting them and the lymphocytes and other immune cells form antibodies—protein molecules tailored to fit the organism or its toxin and so neutralize it (see ANTIBODY/ANTIGEN). Both mechanisms come into play in autoimmune diseases, although cellular infiltration is often less prominent than antibody formation. In some cases the misdirection of the immune system is easy to understand. For example, throat infections with one kind of bacterium, the streptococcus group B, are commonly followed after an interval of two or three weeks by rheumatic fever, an inflammation involving the heart valves among other parts of the body. In the individuals affected the chemical and physical makeup of the membranes lining the heart valves is very similar to the capsule of the bacterium, so that the antibodies formed against the infection also damage the heart. A similar mechanism applies to the *nephritis* (inflammation of the kidneys) that may also follow streptococcal throat infections.

However, no such bacterial infection seems to be involved in other autoimmune diseases in which antibodies are formed against structures in the liver (causing biliary cirrhosis) the thyroid (causing Hashimoto's disease, autoimmune thyroiditis), the stomach (causing impairment of absorption of vitamin B_{12}, pernicious anemia) and the joints (causing rheumatoid arthritis). What these diseases have in common is their chronic course, often marked by episodes in which the symptoms improve or become worse for no obvious reason.

Treatment of these autoimmune diseases with corticosteroid drugs (such as prednisone) is often effective in damping down symptoms, and immunosuppressive drugs (such as azathioprine) may also be useful, since they slow the formation of antibodies. More specific treatment will have to await a better understanding of the primary disease process that occurs in these disorders.

autopsy

Examination of the body by dissection to determine the cause of death. Conducted by a pathologist, an autopsy (also known as a *necropsy* or *postmortem examination*) may be undertaken with the permission of the nearest relative if death has occurred in a hospital; but if violence or neglect has been the suspected cause of death, or the cause is not precisely known, an autopsy will usually be conducted in the absence of the relative's permission on the order of a coroner or other authority.

First the pathologist (or Coroner's Medical Examiner) examines the external surface of the body and its orifices (natural openings) and notes any distinguishing marks, wounds, or evidence of disease. Then the abdomen, chest, neck and skull are opened and all the individual organs removed and examined. Specimens of tissue are taken for microscopic examination. The major blood vessels are opened to assess the state of the inner walls, and in particular the pathologist examines the arteries supplying the heart muscle (coronary arteries) and the arteries of the brain. The stomach and intestinal contents may be kept for analysis as well as specimens of blood and urine.

Where death has been caused by violence, identification of the precise cause is of the utmost importance since a criminal prosecution may rest on the proof established at autopsy. Wounds, injuries and poisons all leave particular signs that can be identified, and forensic scientists can nearly always determine with accuracy the cause of death even in bodies discovered after a considerable time has elapsed since death.

When a death has been fully investigated, the Medical Examiner will inform the appropriate authorities, who will issue a certificate for burial. However, if there is any doubt about the cause of death or there is any dispute, the body will not be available for disposal until an inquest has been held.

After the autopsy the organs are replaced in the body and the incisions sewn up to render the body presentable for the funeral.

azoospermia

Absence from the semen of living spermatozoa. In normal semen there are about 60 million sperms per milliliter, about half of which will be motile—that is, able to move about and fertilize an ovum.

Azoospermia may be caused by disease, hormonal imbalance, or inborn abnormalities of the testicles; the possibility of treatment depends on the cause. Diagnosis of the condition involves the microscopic examination of at least two ejaculates.

B

Babinski's reflex

A reflex elicited on stroking the sole of the foot.

Josef Babinski (1857–1932) was a French neurologist after whom several signs of nervous system disorders were named. The sign most commonly referred to as Babinski's reflex (or *Babinski's sign*) is an abnormal reflex (except during infancy) diagnostic of some neurological disorder of the central nervous system (in a motor nerve pathway extending from the brain to the spinal cord). When the sole of the foot of a healthy person is sharply stroked the toes turn downward. When a certain neurological disorder exists, however, the big toe turns upward instead—eliciting what is called Babinski's reflex.

In children under the age of about two, an upward movement of the toes is perfectly normal. Soon after the child learns to walk, a downward movement becomes the norm.

bacillus

Any rod-shaped bacterium.
See BACTERIA.

backache

Pain in the back may be caused by muscular strain or a "slipped" intervertebral disk, or it may also be associated with some disease of the bones and joints of the spine.

The 24 vertebrae that make up the spinal column (7 cervical, 12 thoracic and 5 lumbar) extend from the base of the skull to the sacrum, the triangular "centerpiece"

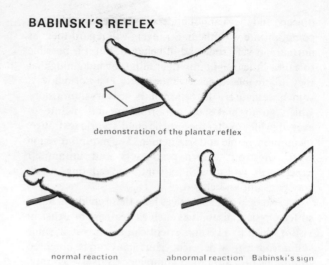

BABINSKI'S REFLEX

demonstration of the plantar reflex

normal reaction   abnormal reaction   Babinski's sign

If the sole of the foot is gently stroked with a sharp pointer in the direction shown in the upper diagram, a plantar reflex will be seen with the toes curling down. Babinski's sign, where the toes curl up, is an indication of disease in either the brain or spinal cord. A positive Babinski's sign is normal in children under 2 years of age because their central nervous systems are still maturing.

of the pelvis. They are separated by pads of tough, elastic cartilage—the intervertebral disks—which give the spine its flexibility and also act as shock absorbers. The bones are also bound together by strong ligaments and by several groups of powerful muscles which mainly run in two bands on either side of the backbone. The spine acts as the central girder of the skeleton; it also provides a protective tunnel for the spinal cord (which reaches down from the brain to the level of the second lumbar vertebra) and the nerves which branch from it.

Most commonly, backache is caused by strain of the muscles around the lower part of the spine. This may be due to unaccustomed exercise—a weekend spent shoveling snow, for example—or to sitting for prolonged periods in an unsatisfactory posture. Strains on the spine are least when the back is straight; a chair which forces the spine into a curve is likely to provoke chronic back strain.

A separate, acutely painful type of backache also originating in the muscles is LUMBAGO. Here the pain is often localized to one extremely painful spot in the muscles, usually in the lower lumbar region and slightly to one side of the midline. Lumbago is often experienced after a combination of unaccustomed exercise and cold—digging the garden in spring, for example—and may be severe enough for the victim to be unable to move out of bed. The cause is believed to be spasm of a group of muscle fibers. Even with no treatment other than rest and simple pain-relieving drugs, such as aspirin, the condition resolves within a few days; but in some cases recovery may be hastened by injection of a mixture of a local anesthetic and a steroid drug into the "trigger spot."

The second common cause of sudden severe backache is damage to one of the intervertebral disks in the lumbar region of the spine. Damage is most likely to occur from lifting a heavy weight while the back is curved. Pressure on the disk, which consists of a tough capsule and a soft, elastic center, may rupture the capsule and allow part of the central nucleus to protrude. If this protrusion extends into the spinal canal it may press upon one of the spinal nerves or even the spinal cord. Typically, this pressure causes pain extending down the main sciatic nerve which runs from the buttock to the foot. The pain (SCIATICA) is made worse by coughing, straining, or bending the back. If the symptoms persist there may also be loss of feeling in the foot or the lower part of the leg and some muscular weakness.

The basic treatment of prolapsed disk (or "slipped disk") is rest, with the patient flat on his back in bed. Rest for two weeks, sometimes more, often allows the protrusion to be reabsorbed back into the disk and the damaged capsule to heal. If the symptoms from pressure on the spinal nerves are severe, or if they do not resolve with simple rest, TRACTION may be added—with weights attached to the legs pulling the vertebrae apart and so promoting return of the disk to its normal position. The most radical treatment, which may be necessary if the prolapse does not heal or in cases of recurrent prolapse, is surgical excision of the damaged portion of the disk.

Unfortunately, anyone who has suffered a prolapsed disk is at risk of recurrence; once the acute symptoms have settled, some program of preventive treatment is important. This will include exercises to strengthen the muscles which support the spine and instruction on posture and the safe, correct way to lift weights, tie the shoes, and other simple daily activities. Sometimes a physician may advise the wearing of a protective and supporting corset.

The third common cause of sudden backache is a minor displacement of the many small joints between the vertebrae. Just how frequent this sort of problem is is a matter of dispute within the medical profession. Some physicians (and all osteopaths and chiropractors) believe that most episodes of backache can be relieved by manipulation of the spine, thus encouraging the bones to return to their normal alignment. Without doubt spinal manipulation does often relieve symptoms, but it can be dangerous if the pain is due to one of the rarer causes of backache, such as a tumor or an infection such as tuberculosis.

More chronic backache may be caused by arthritis of the spinal joints. ANKYLOSING SPONDYLITIS is a severe form of spinal arthritis, especially common in young men and related to RHEUMATOID ARTHRITIS, which may also affect the spine: both diseases cause progressive pain and stiffness of the spine. The common degenerative OSTEOARTHRITIS also affects the spine; most people over the age of 50 have some stiffness of the back from minor arthritic changes. No specific treatment is needed for this form of arthritis unless specific symptoms develop.

Among the many other causes of backache are infections (tuberculosis was especially common in the last century and is still a major problem in developing countries), tumors of the bones and of the spinal cord and nerves, and secondary deposits from the spread of cancer cells elsewhere in the body. For that reason full investigation—including x rays of the spine and blood tests—is needed before treatment is given in any case in which the cause of the pain is not obvious.

Most episodes of backache are preventable: with correct posture, care in lifting weights, and regular exercise to keep the muscles in trim, the joints in the back should remain as trouble free as those elsewhere in the body.

bacteremia

The presence in the blood of living bacteria, with or without a significant clinical response. Compare SEPTICEMIA.

bacteria

Living organisms, members of the kingdom Protista—which comprises animals and plants made up of one cell, smaller than yeasts but larger than viruses, found all over the surface of the globe in the air, soil, and water. Many live on or within larger living organisms, including man; some produce disease and are termed *pathogenic*, but not all are harmful. Some are actively useful—for example, the bacteria that produce nitrogen in the soil for plant growth.

Bacteria may be classified by their shape: round (*cocci*), straight rods (*bacilli*), curved (*vibrios*) and wavy (*spirilla*). Most are unable to move, but a few are motile by virtue of their flagellae (tails). Cocci are very often found in typical groups: *staphylococci* are gathered in bunches like grapes, *streptococci* form chains and *diplococci* are paired. All bacteria given the right circumstances can multiply very quickly, some doubling their numbers every half hour. In an unfavorable environment most die, but some can form spores—thick walled cells resistant to heat and drying out (dessication)—which lie dormant until conditions become favorable again.

BACTERIA

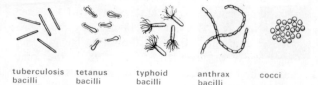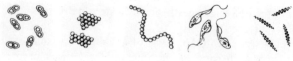

| tuberculosis bacilli | tetanus bacilli | typhoid bacilli | anthrax bacilli | cocci | diplococci (pneumonia) | staphylococci (boils) | streptococci (rheumatic fever) | trypanosomes (sleeping sickness) | spirochete (syphilis) |

Bacteria are single-cell microorganisms, classified according to their shapes into bacilli, cocci, spirilla and vibrios. Most are harmless—indeed many types are beneficial to us—but certain types of bacteria are responsible for infectious diseases, which were notorious killers before antibiotics were discovered.

Pathogenic bacteria cause disease in two basic ways. They may gain access to the tissues and there multiply to damage their surroundings, or they may release substances called *toxins* which poison remote parts of the body. *Endotoxins* are contained inside the bacteria to be released when they die, and *exotoxins* are produced by living bacteria. Usually the signs and symptoms of disease are produced by exotoxins—e.g., in tetanus, where the bacteria multiply in a dirty wound and produce an exotoxin which damages the nervous system.

Dangerous organisms are usually transmitted from man to man by direct contact, by breathing air exhaled from diseased air passages, by contact with contaminated excreta, or by insects. In most cases the body is able to deal with harmful bacteria, but if they gain a foothold and produce disease the defensive processes of inflammation and antibody formation can be aided by the use of drugs designed to kill pathogenic organisms or prevent their multiplication. These drugs, antibiotics, are called *bactericidal* if they kill bacteria or *bacteriostatic* if they inhibit their multiplication.

Antibiotics must not be used indiscriminately, because continued exposure to a particular antibiotic may result in the development of resistant strains of bacteria.

Methods of controlling bacteria in the environment include the use of chemical disinfectants, the application of heat (either dry or steam heat) and, sometimes, irradiation.

bagassosis

A lung disease caused by the inhalation of the moldy fibrous waste (bagasse) of sugar cane.

Baker's cyst

A painless soft cyst at the back of the knee, commonly occurring when the knee joint is damaged by OSTEOARTHRITIS. The condition is named after William Morrant Baker (1839–1896), a 19th-century British surgeon.

The synovium (joint lining) produces an excessive amount of joint fluid, which escapes from the joint either by rupturing through the synovium or by pushing the synovium out ahead of it.

The size of the cyst may be reduced by drawing out the fluid with a needle and syringe, followed by an injection of hydrocortisone (a drug which reduces inflammation) into the affected area. Alternatively the whole cyst may be removed surgically.

balanitis

Inflammation of the tip of the penis. Balanitis is generally associated with PHIMOSIS—narrowing of the opening of the foreskin so that it cannot be pulled back.

In infancy the condition is usually of the type called *ammoniacal* balanitis. In such cases the inflammation is due to irritation caused by ammonia produced by the action of bacteria on the urine. It can usually be prevented by promptly changing wet diapers.

When balanitis occurs in older children and adults, it may be related to sugar in the urine and it may therefore be a warning sign of DIABETES MELLITUS. Other possible causes in adults are an underlying syphilitic sore (a chancre) or cancer of the penis.

Because the tip of the penis and the foreskin are in close contact, inflammation of one seldom occurs without inflammation of the other. Inflammation of both structures is called balanoposthitis.

In addition to the administration of an appropriate antibiotic (if required to control bacterial infection), treatment is directed at the primary or underlying cause.

baldness (alopecia)

The loss of hair on the head.

Hair grows from the base (bulb) of hair follicles, tiny tube-like structures in the skin. Although some hair is constantly being shed (as an actively growing hair expels an older one from its follicle), baldness does not usually occur.

Hair loss resulting in baldness may occur in disease or

in the normal individual as a hereditary phenomenon.

Skin infections which reach deep enough to affect the base of the hair follicles may cause temporary or permanent bald patches. Other skin diseases, burns, radiation injury, chemical injury, or any injury which causes scarring can lead to permanent bald patches. Some drugs cause an increased rate of shedding of the hair.

Increased shedding may also accompany several illnesses—such as prolonged fevers, certain malignancies, uncontrolled diabetes mellitus, or diseases of the thyroid, pituitary and adrenal glands. There is no special treatment for this type of baldness, which is often reversed as the underlying disease is treated.

Some women experience a temporarily increased rate of hair loss after pregnancy.

By far the most common type of baldness is *male-pattern baldness*—which starts around the temples and spreads to the crown, leaving behind a rim of hair at the sides and back. As in other types of baldness, the bald areas are seldom completely hairless but covered with a downy type of hair which is barely perceptible.

The tendency to male-pattern baldness is hereditary and nothing can prevent it. It usually occurs in middle

PATTERNS OF BALDNESS

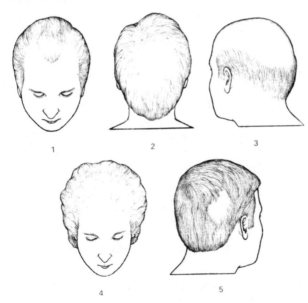

Male-pattern baldness is an inherited condition which usually starts in middle age around the temples (1) and the crown (2). In severe cases only a rim of hair remains around the back of the head (3). Baldness in women is uncommon but sometimes occurs after pregnancy (4). Patchy loss of hair (5) can either result from a skin infection (for example, ringworm of the scalp) or from a condition called alopecia areata.

age, although it may start as early as the late teens. It is irreversible and no successful form of treatment exists. In selected cases, however, a course of hair transplantation may improve appearance.

Hair loss of the male-pattern type may also occur in women, but usually results in severe thinning rather than actual baldness.

One type of baldness that can be very upsetting is *alopecia areata*—a patchy baldness which comes on suddenly. The bald patch may increase in size or new bald areas may form on the scalp, in the eyebrows, or in the beard region. Occasionally there is extensive loss of hair on both scalp and body.

The cause of alopecia areata is not known. Recovery usually occurs without treatment, especially if only a few areas are affected. The only treatment that may be of value is the injection of a corticosteroid drug.

Banti's syndrome

A condition (also known as *Banti's disease*) characterized by an enlarged spleen, anemia, leukopenia (an abnormal reduction in the number of circulating white blood cells), gastrointestinal bleeding and cirrhosis of the liver.

It was first described in 1898 by Guido Banti (1852–1925), an Italian pathologist. He thought that the disorder originated in the spleen, which produced a toxin causing cirrhosis of the liver. Doctors now know, however, that the primary disorder is obstruction of the blood circulation between the intestines and the liver (the "portal system"). The result is a condition known as portal hypertension (see LIVER DISEASE), leading to venous congestion in organs such as the spleen and stomach.

Blood cells are normally destroyed by the spleen, and the anemia and leukopenia are a consequence of a large and overactive spleen.

There are many causes of obstruction of the portal system, but cirrhosis of the liver accounts for about 70% of all cases.

barium meal/barium enema

X-ray studies of the digestive tract. In a barium meal, barium sulfate is swallowed before x rays are taken; in a barium enema, barium sulfate is introduced into the rectum through a tube under gentle pressure.

X rays do not pass through barium sulfate, so the barium sulfate shows up as an opaque mass on the x-ray picture. Like any liquid, the barium sulfate conforms to the shape of its container; a clear outline of the stomach and intestines can thus be obtained by taking x rays as the barium sulfate passes along them.

A barium meal is used to diagnose abnormalities of

BARIUM MEAL/ENEMA

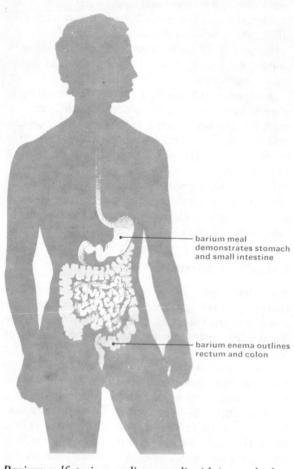

barium meal demonstrates stomach and small intestine

barium enema outlines rectum and colon

Barium sulfate is a radiopaque liquid (one which x rays cannot pass through) and is extensively used by radiologists to outline the digestive tract. The barium is either swallowed as a meal or injected through the anus as an enema. Using these techniques the radiologist can diagnose peptic ulcers, cancers, pockets in the bowel wall, and other diseases of the bowel.

the upper gastrointestinal tract down to the small intestine, while a barium enema is used to study the large intestine.

battered-child syndrome

A condition in which young children, usually under the age of three, are deliberately injured (often repeatedly) by someone in a position of trust such as a parent or guardian.

The violence is totally inexcusable and occurs on the most trivial provocation. It results in bruising, fractures, injury to internal organs, burns and even death.

Besides being physically injured, the child may be deprived of food, care and affection; but battering can also occur in children who are otherwise well cared for.

It has been said that every parent is a potential child batterer; but no matter how exasperating a child's behavior may be, most parents fortunately do not resort to violence.

Child batterers come from all social classes and all levels of intelligence; some may be difficult to detect because they appear concerned over the child's injuries and extremely willing to cooperate with the doctor in every way. However, there are certain typical characteristics of child battering.

There may be a few hours' delay before the child is brought to a doctor. The explanation given is one of an accident, such as falling down the stairs or bumping into a crib or table. But examination reveals injuries incompatible with the history and may also reveal past injuries. Often there are similar injuries on opposite sides of the body, such as bruises on both legs or on both sides of the neck. The parent may try to explain away bruising by saying the child bleeds easily.

The child is very often an unplanned or unwanted child.

A greater proportion of child batterers come from the lower socioeconomic classes; there is usually a history of social, financial, or emotional problems within the family. Batterers are often in their twenties. In some cases the father is unemployed or may have a criminal record, and the mother may be pregnant or in the premenstrual period. Although generally one parent is the batterer, the other is usually aware that the battering is going on.

There may be no evidence of a psychopathic personality in batterers, but violence toward their children is considered to be a temporary psychosis resulting from emotional immaturity. In such cases treatment must be directed at both the child and the parents, who need all the help they can get for social rehabilitation. Otherwise, in more than half the cases, the child will be injured again.

BCG (bacille Calmette-Guérin)

A vaccine used in the control of tuberculosis.

The vaccine was developed by two French bacteriologists, Albert Léon Charles Calmette (1863–1933) and Camille Guérin (1872–1961). Their work began in 1906, with a painstaking series of culturing and subculturing of the causative organism of tuberculosis (the tubercle bacillus) until a stable and safe form of the vaccine was achieved. It was first used in the prevention of tuberculosis in 1921 (in a newborn baby whose mother had died of the disease). Culturing the organism in a succession of artificial media removes its virulence, so that while the vaccine can confer immunity or partial immunity against tuberculosis it does not produce the disease in the person vaccinated.

BCG both reduces the incidence of tuberculosis and results in a less progressive form of the disease when it occurs.

BCG is now being used experimentally to treat cancer. The rationale behind this is that the vaccine stimulates the production of antibodies which are thought to increase the body's general defense system. These antibodies may attack cancer cells and destroy them in the same way that they destroy the tubercle bacilli.

See also ANTIBODY/ANTIGEN, IMMUNIZATION.

bedsores

Sores caused by lying immobile in bed for long periods. They are also known as *pressure sores* or *decubitus ulcers*.

The skin and the tissues beneath it receive their nourishment from very small blood vessels. When these blood vessels are compressed for a sufficient length of time—for example, when the patient is lying down in bed—the skin becomes deprived of its nutrition and becomes vulnerable to death of cells in the area (necrosis). Continuing pressure is likely to progress to a large area of tissue destruction and the formation of an ulcer.

Healthy people do not get bedsores because they move about during sleep and because they shift position when pressure areas become uncomfortable. Pressure sores develop either because the person concerned is semiconscious and so does not feel the discomfort caused by pressure, or because weakness makes them unable to move. Anyone who is unconscious for more than a few hours may develop pressure sores if left unattended.

Bedsores usually begin as a reddening of the skin, which later assumes a bluish tinge. Once an ulcer forms, healing is difficult. It may become infected and so severe that the underlying bone becomes exposed. Treatment, like prevention, depends on relief of pressure: nursing the patient on an air bed or in a net hammock will allow the damaged skin to heal.

Prevention is the best method for coping with bedsores. People confined to bed should be helped to turn every two or three hours. Their skin should be washed regularly. Sheets should be clean and smooth, because movement against a crumpled sheet can hasten damage to the skin. The heels and elbows most frequently become sore from friction caused by constant contact with the bedding. Pressure points may be supported against soft cushions or pads, or on an air ring. Special air and water beds are now available to reduce the risk of pressure sores developing.

bedwetting (enuresis)

There is no precise age at which bedwetting becomes abnormal. Most children are dry at night by the age of two or three, but others not until five or seven.

Even after good control is achieved, occasional bedwetting may occur up to the age of nine or ten or even older. These lapses of night-time control are usually associated with fatigue or emotional upset and should not be a cause for concern.

Most cases of bedwetting persist from infancy although sometimes regular bedwetting starts after a period of good control. There is usually a family pattern for the age at which control is achieved. As a rule, bedwetting does not require investigation until after the age of three or four.

Bedwetting is very rarely associated with nocturnal epilepsy, a disorder of the spinal cord, abnormality of the urinary tract, uncontrolled diabetes mellitus, or diabetes insipidus. But in most cases there is no obvious cause and the condition is thought to be a sign of a temporary emotional or psychological disorder.

The most common cause of persistent bedwetting extending from infancy is too vigorous and too early attempts at toilet training. In general children are not able to achieve voluntary daytime control before the age of 15 to 18 months.

Bedwetting may represent a desire for more parental attention. In contrast, some psychologists attribute the condition to unconscious resentment of the parents, while another proposed explanation is anxiety caused by an unconscious fear of injury to the genitals (associated with feelings of guilt due to sexual fantasies or activities such as masturbation).

Treatment is essentially training based on encouragement. Shaming, nagging, scolding or punishment should be avoided as they may only aggravate the problem. The parents' attitude is extremely important. They should not be overanxious about the bedwetting and should not make an undue fuss when carrying out measures aimed at preventing bedwetting.

These measures include restricting fluids for about two hours before bedtime and waking the child up so that he may empty his bladder before he wets the bed. Drugs are of doubtful value but a bell and pad may be helpful. This is a conditioning type of treatment in which a bell rings and wakens the child when the urine passed completes an electrical circuit in a pad placed beneath the child.

Another measure that may be worth a trial is based on the assumption that bedwetting is the result of a smaller than average bladder capacity. Some doctors believe that the bladder capacity can be increased by giving plenty of drinks during the day and encouraging the child to suppress the urge to go to the bathroom.

If a strong psychological disorder is the underlying cause of bedwetting, none of these measures will work and the help of a psychotherapist may be required.

Bell's palsy

A paralysis of the facial nerves resulting in a characteristic lopsided appearance of the face, due mainly to drooping of the angle of the mouth on the affected side.

There are several causes of facial nerve paralysis. Bell's palsy refers to cases of unknown cause, although exposure to cold has been implicated. The condition was first described in 1828 by Sir Charles Bell, a Scottish surgeon.

It has a rapid onset and mainly affects people aged 20 to 50. Recovery is usually spontaneous and begins within a week. About 75% of patients fully recover in several weeks. Occasionally, especially if the disease persists for a long time, the eventual recovery may be only partial. In such cases, facial spasms may accompany voluntary facial movement. It has been suggested that cortisone-like steroid drugs may help if prescribed early in the course of the disease.

bends

Pains experienced by deep-sea divers and compressed-air tunnel workers when they move too rapidly from areas of high pressure to areas of lower pressure. Bends are symptoms of decompression sickness (caisson disease).

Nitrogen, present in the air we breathe, can dissolve in the blood. As a person moves into areas of increasingly higher pressure, more nitrogen in the lungs dissolves in the blood and enters the circulation. However, the reverse process—when nitrogen moves from the blood to the lungs—takes longer. So if a diver surfaces too rapidly, nitrogen bubbles remain in the circulation where they form air locks and block the blood supply to various tissues.

The pain of bends is felt mainly in the muscles, bones and joints. It can range in severity from an ache to a severe cramp and may occur while the person is moving from high to low pressures, or within a few hours afterwards. Bends are relieved almost immediately if the person returns to high pressures again; a diver could go back into the deep sea or into a special recompression chamber.

Decompression—that is, moving from high to low pressure—should always be gradual because severe decompression sickness can cause immediate collapse, permanent brain damage or death. Repeated attacks of even mild decompression sickness can result in bone damage many years later. Modern diving procedures and special equipment minimize the risk of the bends.

beriberi

A disease caused by the dietary deficiency of vitamin B_1 (thiamine), seen especially in those parts of the world where the diet consists primarily of polished rice. It affects both the circulation and the nervous system and leads to heart failure and swollen limbs from EDEMA, a loss of sensation in the limbs and paralysis.

berylliosis

A disease caused by poisoning from inhalation of the fumes or dust of beryllium or its compounds. (Beryllium is a white metallic element, formerly used in combination with other substances to coat the inner lining of fluorescent lamps and still widely used in industry in the form of beryllium-copper alloys because of its hardening qualities.)

Acute beryllium poisoning causes symptoms a few weeks after exposure, resembling those of bronchitis or pneumonia. Most cases are relatively mild and the patients usually recover within one to six months; corticosteroid drugs may be prescribed in moderate to severe cases.

Chronic berylliosis (also known as *beryllium granulomatosis*) mainly affects the lungs. It occurs after several months of exposure, although some cases have been reported decades later. In addition to progressive damage to the lungs, the disease may involve the heart and present a direct threat to life. The chronic form of the disease is characterized by the formation of small masses or nodules (known as granulomas) in the liver, kidneys, spleen and skin (often leading to ulceration of the skin).

Treatment and control of berylliosis involves the prescription of corticosteroids, which can be very effective if begun early during the course of the disease.

Up to 30 years ago, when beryllium was used to make fluorescent powders, excessive exposure to beryllium was quite common. Now it is used largely for making alloys or heat-resistant ceramics and there are strict controls on the amount that can be found in the factory environment.

bilharziasis

Another name for SCHISTOSOMIASIS.

biopsy

Removal of a small specimen of tissue from the living body for diagnostic purposes. Diagnosis is made by examining thin slices of the tissue under a microscope.

Since only very small pieces are required, tissues can be obtained from within the body by means of special instruments without a major surgical operation. To obtain tissue from the bronchi, intestines or bladder (all of which have natural openings onto the body surface) slender illuminated instruments are used known as *fiberoptic endoscopes:* bronchoscopes, gastroscopes, and cystoscopes—for viewing the bronchi, stomach and bladder, respectively. These are flexible tubes with special attachments which can be introduced into the appropriate body opening to the point at which a tissue specimen is to be taken. A gastroscope, for example, is passed via the mouth and esophagus into the stomach where the gastric lining can be viewed and a biopsy taken.

Biopsies of internal organs such as the liver and kidney are performed by means of a long hollow needle, which is passed through the skin and into the organ concerned.

Most biopsies are sent to the laboratory for processing before being examined under the microscope. This may take a day or two. But sometimes a biopsy is taken during an operation and an immediate result is required for the surgeon to decide how to proceed. In such cases a "frozen-section biopsy" is performed. This is a quick but less satisfactory means of processing the tissue by freezing before slices are made.

A diagnosis made on biopsy findings is generally a firm one. However, a disease may affect organs in a patchy manner; since only extremely tiny pieces are removed, these bits may not have come from the affected parts. To reduce the chance of missing affected parts, where possible several "bites" are taken at biopsy.

bird breeder's lung

An allergy to substances contained in the excreta ("droppings") of birds. The condition is also known as *pigeon breeder's disease*—although it can be caused by other species of birds, such as parakeets.

The allergic reaction results in chills, fever, cough and shortness of breath. The attacks usually occur a few hours after handling or being otherwise closely associated with birds. Some patients experience only the breathlessness without fever and chills; others may have substantial weight loss as well. The chronic inflammation of the lungs (alveolitis) may cause progressive breathlessness as well as permanent lung damage.

Bird breeder's lung due to regular contact with pet parakeets (or other cage birds) is now recognized as an important cause of chronic respiratory disease. Removal of the birds will relieve symptoms. The allergic reaction may also be suppressed by desensitization or by the administration of antihistamines or steroid drugs.

birth injury

Damage to a baby at birth whether avoidable or unavoidable. Birth injuries may be either mechanical or due to a lack of oxygen at birth (anoxia).

Premature babies and those who lie in awkward positions in the uterus are most likely to suffer mechanical injuries, which include bruises, fractures and nerve injuries.

The most common life-threatening birth injury is hemorrhage into the brain. If the injury is severe, death may occur at birth or within a few days. Those who survive may recover fully, although they sometimes suffer permanent brain damage. It is often difficult to predict the effect the brain damage will have in later years.

The liver is another internal organ occasionally injured during birth. Injury may occur during delivery or as a result of external heart massage during attempts at resuscitation. The prognosis depends on the degree of injury.

Sufficient oxygen is essential because the brain can withstand only a few minutes of anoxia. Anoxia may result when the placental circulation has been inadequate during pregnancy, for example in conditions such as PREECLAMPSIA (toxemia of pregnancy), multiple pregnancy or hemorrhage before the onset of labor.

Anoxia may also occur when the baby fails to breathe spontaneously at birth. Failure of spontaneous breathing (APNEA) is more likely following some complication of pregnancy such as premature birth, multiple pregnancy, toxemia or maternal diabetes mellitus. When these complications are present, however, apnea can be anticipated and skilled staff and specialized equipment for resuscitation can be prepared.

Sometimes, however, apnea is totally unexpected. As with brain hemorrhage, it is often difficult to predict how much and what kind of permanent brain damage, if any, will result.

birthmark

A skin blemish present at birth.
See NEVUS.

birth weight

The average weight of a baby at birth is approximately 7 lb. (3.2 kg) with boys being slightly heavier than girls. There is obviously great variation between newborn infants but 95%, weigh between 5 lb. (2.3 kg) and 9.5 lb (4.3 kg).

The baby is often heavier than average if one of the

parents is unusually large or if the mother is diabetic or prediabetic. Large size is not necessarily dependent on late delivery (that is, after a pregnancy lasting for more than 42 weeks).

In the United Kingdom a premature birth is held to be one in which the birth weight is less than 5½ lb. (2.5 kg). A birth weight of 3.3 lb. (1.5 kg) or less can be associated with ill health and a risk to life. Responsible factors can include a diminished length of pregnancy (less than 37 weeks from the first day of the last menstrual period, making them "premature") or the rate of intrauterine growth may be less than expected ("small-for-date"), although the baby is born perfectly healthy.

Premature birth resulting in a low birth weight is associated with several factors: disease in the mother during pregnancy, such as toxemia or nephritis; maternal age below 20 or above 35; and low social and economic status.

blackheads

Dried plugs of fatty material in the ducts of the sebaceous (oil-secreting) glands. Also known as *comedones*. The black color at the surface of the plugs is not dirt, as people often believe. In fact albinos (who lack the pigment melanin) have light-colored "blackheads."

The blackhead is produced by faulty functioning of the sebaceous follicle, which does not release the *sebum* (fatty secretion of the sebaceous glands) in a correct manner. The consequent obstruction to the gland leads to enlargement of the opening of the follicle. Infection by bacteria living on the skin may lead to inflammation and so to the characteristic papules, or "pimples," of ACNE.

Blackheads should never be squeezed; this increases the risk of infection. Gentle bathing with warm water and soap should release most of them.

blackout

A momentary loss of consciousness or vision, which is caused by an interruption of the blood supply to the brain.

bladder problems

Bladder problems can be separated into those arising from infection within the bladder, those due to growths within the bladder and those associated with loss of bladder control.

Inflammation of the bladder (CYSTITIS) is common and is most often due to bacterial infection. The symptoms of burning pain on passing urine and increased frequency or urination may, however, also occur without any evidence of infection; this non-bacterial inflammation is especially common in women. Pregnancy and sexual intercourse both increase the likelihood of cystitis, which in women is often a consequence of infection spreading to the bladder from the genital organs. Treatment includes the drinking of large quantities of fluid and the administration of appropriate antibacterial drugs. Women who develop symptoms of cystitis in association with sexual intercourse need to pay special attention to regular washing of the genital region.

The bladder is occasionally the site of a growth. The most common is a benign wartlike tumor (papilloma), but only specialist investigation can distinguish these from malignant tumors. In either case the first sign is blood in the urine, occasionally rather than constantly, without associated pain. Later the symptoms may resemble those of cystitis. Small bladder tumors can be removed through a tube passed into the bladder (cystoscope), but regular medical follow-up is needed to keep a lookout for any recurrence.

Urinary INCONTINENCE is involuntary urination; it may be caused by a defect in the nervous control of the bladder or a mechanical problem. Children often have episodes of urinary incontinence, especially during sleep (see BEDWETTING).

Stress incontinence—the leakage of a few drops of urine during coughing or straining—is common in women and is most often due to damage in childbirth to the muscles around the neck of the bladder. Surgical repair may be necessary in such cases. (Pregnant women may sometimes experience stress incontinence merely as a result of the growing fetus pressing against the bladder.)

Inability to pass urine (retention) may be caused by an obstruction at the opening of the bladder from a tumor or a bladder stone; but in men the most common cause is enlargement of the prostate gland. The early symptoms of prostatic enlargement include increased frequency of urination, and slowness and hesitancy of the urinary stream. These symptoms can be relieved by a surgical operation to remove all or part of the prostate gland (PROSTATECTOMY). Inability to pass urine may also be due to an injury or disease of the spinal cord, such as MULTIPLE SCLEROSIS. In such cases the bladder may need to be emptied by passing a narrow tube (catheter) up through the urethra to the bladder.

See also URINARY TRACT INFECTION for further information.

blepharitis

Inflammation of the margins of the eyelids, where the

skin joins the conjunctiva of the eye.

The symptoms are usually mild, but there may be heat, itching and grittiness resulting in considerable pain. The eyes may seem tired, unduly sensitive and intolerant to light, dust, or heat. Causes include allergies, bacterial infection, external irritants (such as foreign particles and wind) and eyestrain. The nature of the skin itself (pale-skinned people are generally more susceptible) may also influence the condition. (In addition, seborrhea of the scalp may also cause blepharitis.)

Squamous blepharitis is a superficial dermatitis in which the area is congested, swollen, inflamed and accompanied by scaling of the skin. The lid looks bleary and swollen as the result of congestion; the scaling skin forms yellow crusts as it adheres to the secretion produced. Later the margins become permanently swollen, thickened and disturbed in position.

The result is wetting of the lids; this induces rubbing, followed by eczema and eversion of the lid margin. Dirty handkerchiefs and fingers aggravate the infection.

If the condition is chronic the lashes become damaged and may be lost (usually temporarily, but sometimes permanently).

Follicular blepharitis is a less common but more serious form. The inflammation is deeper, pus is produced, and the inflammation may extend outside the hair follicles and form abscesses (resulting in destruction of tissue and ulceration). The lid margins are red and inflamed and the lashes matted. Healing eventually occurs with scarring.

The complications of blepharitis are chronic conjunctivitis, permanently red lids, loss of lashes and eversion of the lid (exposing its inner surface).

Treatment must include attention to general health and scrupulous cleanliness of the face. Antiseptics and soothing lotions may help. Where required, the doctor may prescribe antibiotics (to control any associated bacterial infection that occurs) or ophthalmic steroid preparations.

blindness

In the literal sense, blindness is the state or condition of being sightless. But in a legal or practical sense it also includes serious impairment of vision to the extent that certain types of activity or employment may be extremely difficult or impossible. Blindness may be permanent or transient and affect only one or both eyes. It may arise suddenly or develop gradually over months or years and may affect the entire field of vision or only part of it.

Blindness has many possible causes, but in each case one or more of four basic areas are affected: (1) the eye itself; (2) the blood supply which nourishes the *retina* (the light-sensitive structure at the back of the eye); (3) the *optic nerve* (a bundle of over one million separate nerve fibers which conveys impulses from the retina to the brain); and (4) the *visual cortex* (an area toward the back of the brain which is primarily concerned with interpreting impulses from the retina as visual images).

Sudden loss of vision may affect only part of the visual field of one or both eyes. An unobservant person may at first remain unaware of visual loss in one eye until the other is inadvertently covered up. Total loss of vision that occurs suddenly may be caused by blockage of the artery or vein supplying the retina or by hemorrhage within the eye. Sudden loss of part of the visual field may occur when a part of the retina becomes detached from its normal position (see DETACHED RETINA) or when a blood clot forms in the blood vessels which supply the nerve tracts from the eye to the brain.

Several conditions may affect the arteries which supply blood to the eyes. These include: spasm of the vessels (which can cause temporary visual impairment); thickening of the arterial walls from the deposit of fatty material on their inner linings (ATHEROSCLEROSIS), which may seriously impede or block the flow of blood to the eye and cause a wasting away (atrophy) of the tissues of the retina and the optic nerve; and hemorrhage into the retina sometimes associated with high blood pressure (particularly as a complication of KIDNEY DISEASE or DIABETES MELLITUS).

Blindness can be caused by a congenital defect of the eye, optic nerve, or the visual cortex of the brain. Other causes include injuries or wounds affecting these areas, tumors of the eye or brain, meningitis (inflammation of the membranes which cover the brain), complications that occur as the result of chronic inflammation of the eye, CATARACT (an opacity of the crystalline lens of the eye), and GLAUCOMA (abnormally raised pressure within the eye, which can exert damaging pressure upon the optic nerve). The three major causes of a gradual loss of vision, mainly affecting the elderly, are cataract, glaucoma and senile macular degeneration (discussed below).

Cataract may be hereditary or a complication of German measles (rubella) in the mother during pregnancy. It may also follow injury (with or without rupture of the lens capsule) or inflammation within the eye.

Glaucoma is a disease of obscure cause, characterized by increased fluid pressure within the eye. It may arise suddenly or over a long period and is thought to be the result of an aging process in the vessels and tissues of the eye. The raised pressure of the internal watery fluid (aqueous humor) impairs the vision indirectly. Sight is gradually destroyed, beginning as a blind patch and gradually extending. Treatment involves controlling the pressure with drops or by surgical decompression.

Senile macular degeneration is the third main cause of blindness (after cataract and glaucoma). It is caused by degenerative changes in the retina associated with the general process of aging and is irreversible. Visual loss is gradual but progressive; older persons afflicted with this condition probably adapt better to a simple magnifying glass for reading than to elaborate aids such as telescopic glasses.

Blindness can occur as a complication of certain infectious diseases, including SYPHILIS, TUBERCULOSIS, MEASLES, DIPHTHERIA, SCARLET FEVER and the afore-mentioned German measles. At one time, babies born to mothers who harbored the microorganisms of GONORRHEA were frequently in danger of acquiring the infection—which often led to blindness. The practice of putting drops of silver nitrate or an antibiotic in the eyes of newborn babies has made this complication ex-tremely rare today, in addition to the fact that gonorrhea—because of its symptoms arising from acute inflammation of the Fallopian tubes—is commonly diagnosed and treated before a pregnant woman gives birth.

Some forms of blindness or severely impaired vision (such as cataract) can be corrected with prompt medical or surgical attention. Early treatment of other causes of defective eyesight (such as glaucoma and detached retina) can frequently limit or arrest the progress of impaired vision before blindness occurs.

Permanent blindness, whether present at birth or occurring later in life, is a condition which most sightless persons have learned to cope with successfully. It is important for sighted persons to realize that *the blind generally take great pride in being able to function with a minimum of outside assistance*. For example, even in such an apparently simple matter as offering to assist a blind person to cross a busy street it is important that the sighted person not "force" his help, but merely ask if he *may* help and then offer his arm as a guide. No one—sighted or not—likes being *dragged* across a road! A condescending manner always should be rigorously avoided.

Various institutions and societies exist which offer valuable training and assistance for the blind, including those which provide guide dogs and others which teach the reading and printing of Braille (a system of raised dots, felt with the fingertips, used to represent letters and other characters).

blisters

Outpouring of fluid under the outer layer of the skin as a result of local damage produces a blister. Blistering may be caused by repeated friction on tender skin (parti-cularly of the hands or feet), by heat (as in the case of burns and scalds), or by irritating chemicals.

Blisters caused by the friction of unaccustomed physical work on the hands or by ill-fitting shoes on the feet will heal easily if the source of friction is removed and the blister kept clean so that it cannot become infected. The extensive blistering and broken skin caused by burning or scalding needs careful treatment under medical supervision if infection and subsequent scarring are to be avoided.

blood

There are approximately $10\frac{1}{2}$ pints (5 liters) of blood in the circulation. Two-fifths of this volume consists of *erythrocytes* (red blood cells). The other cellular components, the *leukocytes* (white blood cells) and *platelets*, though equally important, are a thousand-fold less numerous and therefore occupy a relatively small proportion. The remaining three-fifths consists of *plasma*, a watery solution of proteins and salts in which the blood cells are suspended.

The basic concept of the blood as a vital body fluid is familiar enough to most people, and we know its appearance and consistency. We also know that it is pumped around the body by the heart, that it is under pressure in the arteries and that a cut artery bleeds profusely and possibly dangerously. It is also not difficult to imagine the failure of the pumping system if the bleeding leads to too great a reduction in the volume of blood in the circulation. We know that death follows because our "life blood" is gone.

The functions of the blood which make it so vital to life are less well known to the average person. These functions may be described under three main headings: (1) transport, (2) the maintenance of a stable internal environment and body temperature and (3) defense against infection and uncontrolled hemorrhage.

The fact that it is in constant movement around the body suggests that a principal function of the blood is as a *transport medium*. All the body's vital processes depend on a supply of oxygen to "burn" sugar and fat to produce energy. This oxygen is obtained from the air in the lungs and carried by the HEMOGLOBIN pigment in the red blood cells to all parts of the body; the unique properties of the pigment allow uptake of oxygen in the lungs and its subsequent release of the tissues. The principal waste product of energy production, carbon dioxide gas, is also carried in the blood—in both the red cells and the plasma—and is released in the lungs to be expelled in the expired air.

The food we eat, after digestion has reduced it to simpler chemical compounds, is absorbed mainly through the walls of the small intestine into the bloodstream. A variety of special transport mechanisms for individual compounds exists. Iron, for example, has its own "transporter protein" to which it is bound on entry into the circulation, to be "unloaded" when it reaches the red blood cells where it is needed for hemoglobin production. All the proteins, fats, sugars, vitamins and minerals required by the body tissues are similarly carried in the blood—either in simple solution, or attached to a transporter protein. This may involve the movement of absorbed food materials from the small intestine direct to the site where they are required or, if not immediately required for use, to storage in the liver or the "fat depots."

The processing of food materials and the replacement and repair of tissues produce waste products, which if allowed to accumulate would be harmful. These are transported either to the liver for further processing to render them less toxic or directly to the kidneys for excretion from the body.

Control of the body's functions depends to an important degree on "chemical messengers" (hormones) carried in the blood. These indispensable chemicals, which are produced by the endocrine glands (such as the pituitary and thyroid), are carried by the bloodstream to all parts of the body, thereby providing rapid and efficient control of its physical and chemical activities.

The tissues of the body can function efficiently only if their physical and chemical environment remains constant within fairly narrow limits. The enzymes (ferments), which drive the chemical processes of the body, function optimally at 98.6°F (37°C) and the blood plays a vital role in maintaining all parts of the body reasonably close to this temperature. Heat produced from chemical processes occurring deep in the body is carried by the blood to warm the extremities. In hot conditions, excessive heat production by the body is controlled by increasing the flow of blood to these exposed parts; heat is dissipated through the skin (which is cooled by sweating). In cold conditions, however, the body prevents excessive heat loss by reducing the blood flow to the extremities.

The salt concentrations at which the body cells can function properly are similarly limited. The blood circulation ensures an even distribution of salts throughout the body, with excretion of any overall excess via the kidneys. This allows the tissues to maintain the correct balance of water and salts within their cells—without which the cells would collapse, or swell up and rupture or die.

In defense, the leukocytes (white blood cells), mostly produced together with the red cells and platelets in the bone marrow, are vital in combating infection. The *neutrophil leukocytes* directly attack bacteria invading the body and remove the debris of dead bacteria and damaged cells resulting from infection. The *lymphocytes* produce antibodies which act as specific chemical "antidotes" to invading bacteria and viruses and their

BLOOD FILM

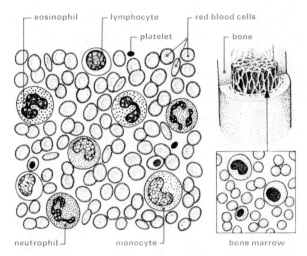

This drawing of a blood film gives an idea of the various cells a hematologist might see when he looks at blood under a microscope. In fact, not all the different types shown here would be present in any one sample. All these blood cells are derived from large primitive cells in the bone marrow.

products, helping to overcome their initial attack and to provide a lasting immunity to further attacks.

Finally, when body tissues are damaged and bleeding occurs, the blood flow through the tissues ensures a continuing supply of platelets and blood clotting factors carried in the plasma which will allow blood clotting to occur and thus control the bleeding.

See also AGGLUTINATION, AGRANULOCYTOSIS, ANEMIA, ANTIBODY, BLOOD CLOTTING, BLOOD GROUPS, BLOOD PRESSURE, BLOOD TRANSFUSION, CELL, CYANOSIS, ERYTHROCYTE SEDIMENTATION RATE, HEMORRHAGE, ISCHEMIA, LEUKEMIA, PHAGOCYTOSIS, PLATELETS, POLYCYTHEMIA, PULSE, RH FACTOR, SEPTICEMIA.

blood clotting

When a blood vessel is damaged, control of the resulting hemorrhage involves first the spontaneous contraction of the muscular wall of the vessel to reduce the flow and then clotting of the blood in the vessel and the wound.

The end result of clotting is the conversion of liquid blood to the familiar gelatinous, red material of a blood clot. This takes place by the conversion of a soluble protein material in the blood, *fibrinogen*, to insoluble *fibrin*—which is deposited in fine strands in which the red and white cells become enmeshed to form a clot.

The first step toward this end result is taken when the continuity of the wall of a blood vessel is interrupted by an injury (or when a blood sample removed from a vein is placed in a laboratory test tube). The lining membrane of the blood vessels allows blood to remain in close contact with it without change in its cells or chemical constituents. As soon as a vessel is damaged, however, contact is established between the blood and other tissues and blood clotting is initiated.

Platelets (cellular components of the blood which play an essential role in clotting) adhere to the damaged area and liberate chemical substances which set in motion a complex chain reaction involving a dozen or more protein constituents of the blood. (There are more than 15 million platelets in a single drop of blood.) Each of these constituents exists in two forms, an inactive precursor and an active material derived from it. The chain reaction is thus seen as a "cascade" or "domino" phenomenon in which activation of one factor by a chemical derived from damaged platelets leads to its conversion to its active form. This in turn will activate the next chemical in the chain, and so on, until the reaction is complete.

The final stages involve the conversion of the protein *prothrombin* to *thrombin;* this substance can convert fibrinogen to fibrin, leading to the formation of a blood clot as described above.

THROMBOSIS is a condition in which blood clots within an intact blood vessel. This may be associated with an abnormal slowing of the circulation (as in a patient restricted to bed following major surgery) or with various changes in the clotting factors or platelets. (See also EMBOLUS.)

The normal mechanism of blood clotting is disturbed in certain disorders (mostly notably HEMOPHILIA, an inherited defect of the clotting mechanism), which exposes the patient to the danger of uncontrolled bleeding—even after what in most people would be a relatively minor injury. Various diseases or disorders that affect the bone marrow (where blood cells are produced) may lead to an underproduction of platelets or an abnormally low quantity in the circulation (a condition known as THROMBOCYTOPENIA).

blood groups

The first human blood groups were discovered in 1900 by Karl Landsteiner (1868–1943). He described the separation of human blood cells into four classes, A, B, AB and O—which we now know as the *ABO blood groups.*

Characterization of these ABO blood groups depends not only on the detection of specific characteristics on the surface of the red cells of each group (*antigens*) but on the presence in the plasma (the liquid portion of the blood) of characteristic *antibodies* which are capable of clumping together (agglutinating) red cells of a specific group. Thus, persons of group A have in their plasma an antibody (agglutinin) which agglutinates cells of group B (anti-B), while those of group B have the complementary agglutinin (anti-A) which reacts with A cells. Those of group O have both anti-A and anti-B in the plasma, but their cells are agglutinated by neither of these agglutinins. Those of group AB have no agglutinins in the plasma but their cells will obviously be agglutinated by both anti-A and anti-B agglutinins. In general, there will be no agglutinin in the plasma acting against the subject's own cells since the agglutination in circulation which would result from such a situation would be incompatible with life.

For many years it was thought that the ABO groups were the only groups that existed; but when, during World War I, some steps were taken to use Landsteiner's discovery to provide BLOOD TRANSFUSION to combat blood loss, it soon became apparent that the situation was more complex. While the ABO system remains the most important for transfusion purposes, many more blood group factors have now been demonstrated—including rare subgroups of the ABO system, the important "Rhesus groups" and others (such as the "MNS system"). The last two systems differ from the ABO system in that no corresponding agglutinins occur naturally in the blood but only appear as a result of blood transfusion or pregnancy involving a blood group differing from the patient's own group. Progress in understanding various blood group factors was initially slow; the Rhesus groups, for example, were not discovered until 1940. (See RH FACTOR.)

The blood groups are inheritable characteristics, passed from parents to their children and following the Mendelian laws of inheritance.

Today, the blood groups are of importance not only in blood transfusion work but also in the establishment of paternity and in forensic pathology. Lastly, since different blood groups have widely different frequencies in different races, they are of great interest to the anthropologist.

blood poisoning

See SEPTICEMIA.

blood pressure

Blood pressure is normally defined in terms of the *systolic* pressure, which is the maximum pressure produced in the larger arteries by each heartbeat (see SYSTOLE), and the *diastolic* pressure, which is the constant pressure maintained in the arteries between heartbeats (see DIASTOLE). The blood pressure, measured by means of a SPHYGMOMANOMETER, is expressed in millimeters of mercury. The "textbook normal" figure for the systolic pressure is 120 millimeters and for the diastolic 80 millimeters, usually expressed in abbreviated form as 120/80 ("one-twenty over eighty").

Many people have a blood pressure reading that is slightly below the average. This is normally no cause for concern.

It is important to realize that no fixed value exists for the blood pressure and that the "standard" figure of 120/80 is really the average of a fairly wide range. In a group of normal individuals, few will have a blood pressure of exactly 120/80. In a single individual, considerable fluctuations in blood pressure will occur from minute to minute, from hour to hour, and from day to day. The figure may be affected by rest, exercise, emotion or anxiety; the normal range typically widens with increasing age.

When a physician measures your blood pressure, he is unlikely to accept the first figure he obtains if it is at all raised, since anxiety about your visit to him may have considerably affected the reading. He may ask you to wait a few minutes (either sitting down or lying down) before taking it again, or may ask you to return on another day for a check. Only when he has decided that your blood pressure is constantly raised above an acceptable figure for your age, and that this is causing or is likely to cause symptoms, will he decide that you suffer from high blood pressure (hypertension) and initiate the appropriate treatment.

High blood pressure may be a primary disease entity (*essential hypertension*) or a symptom of a number of disorders affecting the kidneys (*renovascular hypertension*), blood vessels, or the adrenal glands. It may also be an unwanted side effect of drug treatment for other diseases.

Whatever the cause, the symptoms are extremely variable. In some cases, the pressure may be appreciably raised for many years without any notable symptoms. Headache, particularly in the early morning, may occur as well as giddiness—especially on a sudden change of posture. There may be palpitations and shortness of breath on exertion and changes in eyesight, with blurring of vision in one or both eyes. The patient may need to get up with increasing frequency during the night to pass urine. If the raised blood pressure is the result of another disease, such as kidney failure, the symptoms may be predominantly those of the underlying disease rather than a direct effect of the raised blood pressure.

The main effects of raised blood pressure involve the heart and blood vessels. High blood pressure is one of the major risk factors in the development of *coronary thrombosis* (also known as *myocardial infarction* or "heart attack") and coronary artery disease. It is also an important factor in the development of a STROKE, whether caused by brain hemorrhage or blood clots in the blood vessels of the brain. Taking the blood pressure is therefore an important part of any medical examination.

If treatment is necessary, the first step will involve tests to ensure that the disorder is not a symptom of kidney damage or some other disease. (If such a disease is found, obviously it will be treated.) Attention will then be given to other risk factors for the development of coronary artery disease, such as cigarette smoking, obesity or a high intake of animal fat in the diet (see CHOLESTEROL). Reduction in weight alone will often produce a fall in blood pressure and also a fall in blood levels of fat. If stress or anxiety is present, a change in life style or the use of tranquilizing drugs may be sufficient to control the disorder in mild cases.

If these measures fail to bring the blood pressure within normal limits for the individual, specific treatment will be required. Before any is given, it will be important to decide whether the patient has recently had a rise in blood pressure which is now causing symptoms or whether the blood pressure, particularly in elderly patients, has been raised for many years. In this latter group of patients there is frequently hardening and narrowing of the arteries (ARTERIOSCLEROSIS), particularly those supplying the brain, and the circulation is maintained at adequate levels only by the increased blood pressure. A sudden reduction in blood pressure may actually be harmful and the patient may become confused, unsteady and even mildly demented as the result of a poor blood supply to the brain.

The first line of treatment involves a simple reduction of the volume of circulating blood, which will in turn lower the blood pressure. This is achieved by giving a *diuretic* drug, which causes the kidneys to pass more urine. In some cases this, together with other measures (such as weight reduction), may be all that is required. If these measures are not effective, specific drugs that act to lower the blood pressure will be required. Many such drugs are now available and their action exerts a direct effect on the heart and blood vessels. They can often be usefully combined with a diuretic drug. The best choice of drugs is sometimes difficult, however, and the physician may have to try several before he is satisfied that he has selected the one most suitable for an individual patient.

Unfortunately, these drugs are not always free from unwanted side effects. They may be responsible for producing giddiness on sudden changes of posture (postural hypotension), diarrhea, depression and (occasionally, in men) impotence. For this reason the decision to initiate treatment may be difficult; it is important for the doctor to ensure that the side effects caused by the drug have not been added to the patient's other symptoms without significant benefit in other ways.

blood transfusion

The discovery at the beginning of the 20th century of the ABO BLOOD GROUPS made possible for the first time the safe transfusion of blood to patients who would otherwise have died of hemorrhage. Previous attempts to give randomly selected blood had usually led to disastrous consequences, although occasional success had been achieved by chance.

Blood for transfusion is today provided by national blood transfusion organizations and by the blood banks of large hospitals, where it is collected from donors and stored. Blood is drawn from donors into sterile bottles or plastic bags containing chemicals to prevent clotting (anticoagulants). A maximum of 500 milliliters every six months is usually considered safe for donors.

Blood is administered through a special plastic bag (drip set) connected to a needle or plastic cannula placed in a vein in the arm. The rate of administration varies with the needs of the recipient, but in routine cases 500 milliliters will be given over two or three hours.

All blood for transfusion is ABO and Rhesus (RH) typed. Except in grave emergencies, blood of the patient's own ABO and Rhesus type is always used and direct compatibility tests performed between the blood of the donor and that of the recipient. See also RH FACTOR.

Modern transfusion practice involves much more than the routine provision of "whole" blood for transfusion. This is basically a wasteful procedure since whole blood contains many valuable components, only some of which are required by the individual patient. Thus a severely anemic patient may need red blood cells but not the plasma in which the cells are suspended and this can be separated before the blood is used, leaving "packed red cells." Other patients specifically require platelets or clotting factors from the plasma or specific protein fractions containing antibodies against infectious diseases (or whole plasma in the case of severe burns).

It is increasingly likely that the individual patient will receive packed cells, platelet concentrates, plasma or clotting factor concentrates rather than whole donor blood. This results in a great economy in the use of this scarce and expensive material.

In some cases (as in the treatment of "hemolytic disease of the newborn") whole blood will be used in a procedure known as an *exchange transfusion*—in which all or most of the patient's blood is periodically replaced with donor blood.

boil

A painful red swelling in the skin (also known as a *furuncle*) caused by bacterial infection of a hair follicle

BLOOD TRANSFUSION

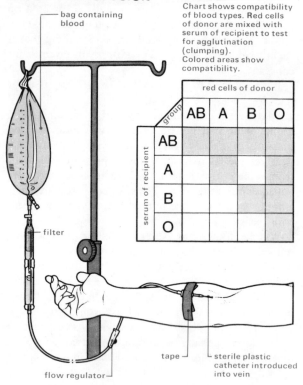

Chart shows compatibility of blood types. Red cells of donor are mixed with serum of recipient to test for agglutination (clumping). Colored areas show compatibility.

Blood transfusion can be lifesaving, but stringent checks are necessary before it is performed. The first step is to determine the patient's major blood group (AB, A, B, or O) and Rh (Rhesus) type so that possible donor blood can be selected. Before every transfusion, the blood is "cross matched" as an extra precaution—a sample of the recipient's serum is mixed with the donor's red blood cells to check that they do not agglutinate.

or sweat gland. Infection is usually caused by staphylococci, bacteria which are normally found on the skin. Boils are unusual unless there is some additional factor to provoke infection. This may be an underlying disease (such as diabetes) or it can be simple friction, which is why boils occur around the neck, on the forearms and on the seat.

The first sign of a boil is a red swelling which may be painful and cause itching. In some cases the boil will go no further and will subside after two or three days. But the more usual course is that after about six or seven days the swollen boil bursts and releases pus.

It is important to treat boils because an untreated one can lead to the development of further boils or to generalized septicemia (blood poisoning).

The new synthetic penicillins are the drugs of choice against staphylococcal infection.

bone

The substance of which the skeleton is made—a mixture of calcium carbonate, calcium phosphate and fibrous tissue. There are more than 200 bones in the human skeleton, made up of "compact" and "cancellous" bone. Compact bone, found in the shafts of the limb bones, consists of a hard tube surrounded by a membrane (*periosteum*) and enclosing a fatty substance (*bone marrow*). Cancellous bone forms the short bones and the ends of the long bones and has a fine lacework structure (it is also called "spongy" bone).

Bone is a living tissue and even the most dense is "tunneled" by fine canals in which there are small blood vessels, nerves and lymphatics, by which the bones are maintained and repaired. In children the bones include a plate of cartilage in which growth occurs; in the long bones (such as the femur and humerus) this plate is at one end only, the "growing end." At the end of puberty bone replaces the cartilage, the long bones cease growing, and the skeleton no longer increases in size.

Bone is repaired by cells of microscopic size. One type, the *osteoblast*, lays down strands of fibrous tissue between which calcium salts are deposited from the blood. The other, the *osteoclast*, dissolves and breaks

BONE

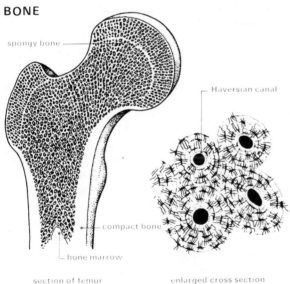

spongy bone

Haversian canal

compact bone

bone marrow

section of femur

enlarged cross section of compact bone

Bone is a combination of mineral salts and fibrous material which is very resistant to mechanical stresses. The upper end of the femur, or thighbone, has a strongly developed meshwork of "spongy" bone designed to transmit the weight of the body. The shaft of the femur consists of "compact" bone, able to resist bending because of its structure—concentric rings of bony tissue.

down dead or damaged bone. These processes occur when a bone is broken. The skeletal bones not only determine the body's "architecture," but are also vital because it is in the marrow of cancellous bone that new red blood cells are constantly formed.

botulism

A dramatic, life-threatening illness caused by the bacterium *Clostridium botulinum*. This microbe produces a toxin which is absorbed from the intestine.

Clostridium botulinum occurs in soil, in watery environments such as the sea bed, and in fish and many other animals. The disease is acquired from contaminated food which has not been heated to at least 250°F (121°C), the temperature at which the organism is killed. Thus, smoked or lightly cooked or raw food may be responsible. Faulty preparation of home-preserved foods (e.g., inadequate boiling) is one of the commonest causes of botulism.

Outside the body, the organism is in spore form, which does not cause disease even when it contaminates fresh food; the spores must have germinated and actually produced toxin. The toxin is quickly absorbed from the intestine. Within 36 hours there are gastrointestinal symptoms of nausea, vomiting and abdominal pain, as well as weakness and unsteadiness. The nervous system is then attacked by the toxin resulting in blurred vision, difficulty in swallowing, muscular weakness of the arms and legs and—potentially much more serious—paralysis of the muscles used in breathing.

Treatment of botulism is mainly directed toward preservation of lung function by use of a respirator, if necessary. Antitoxin is also given and a drug called guanidine has proved of some value. In spite of this, the disease is fatal in up to 65% of cases.

bowel and bowel movements

The intestinal tract—the basically hollow tube which extends from the stomach to the anus—has a total length of approximately 25 ft., although its length in life varies considerably with the contraction or relaxation of the muscle fibers in its wall. The main sections are the *small intestine*—comprising, from above downwards, the *duodenum*, *jejunum* and *ileum* (together, approximately 20 ft. in length) —and the *large intestine* or *colon* (about 5ft. in length).

The duodenum, the shortest section, is only 12 in. or so long; it is slightly wider in diameter (1½ in.) than the remainder of the small intestine. The jejunum forms about two-fifths of the small intestine (about 5 ft.) while the ileum is the longest segment (about 14 ft.); both are approximately 1 in. in diameter.

The colon ("large bowel") is the part of the intestinal

BOWEL

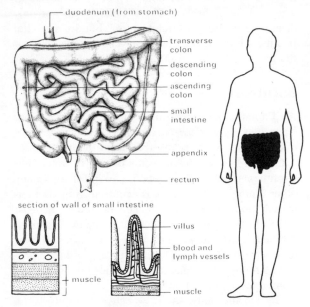

duodenum (from stomach)

transverse colon

descending colon

ascending colon

small intestine

appendix

rectum

section of wall of small intestine

villus

blood and lymph vessels

muscle

muscle

The bowel, or intestine, is a long muscular tube where food is digested and absorbed, and waste material travels to the rectum to be excreted as feces. The magnified sections of small intestine show the folds, or villi, which are important for absorption of nutrients into the blood.

tract usually referred to when the term "bowel" alone is used. It varies in diameter from about 1 to 3 in.

The whole of the small intestine and the greater part of the colon is supported in the abdomen by a membrane (*mesentery*), which is attached to the back wall of the abdominal cavity and carries in it the blood vessels and nerves which supply the intestines.

The function of the intestinal tract is to digest food particles introduced into it from the stomach, to allow the essential nutrients broken down into simpler compounds by the act of digestion to be absorbed into the bloodstream (this occurs mainly in the small intestine), and to excrete the unwanted residue from the body. Waste products are largely deprived of their water content in the large intestine (the water is reabsorbed into the body—and then formed into the semisolid mass known as feces (or "stools").

The intestinal tract has three coats: (1) the *mucosal membrane*, which lines it throughout; (2) the *muscular coat*, which surrounds the mucosa; and (3) the outer *serosal coat*, which is in fact part of the *peritoneum* (the smooth, moist membrane which lines the entire abdominal cavity).

The mucosal membrane both secretes digestive juices and allows absorption of the products of digestion to take place. Its surface area is greatly increased by its

being thrown into innumerable folds running around the bowel wall. In the small intestine, its surface can be seen under a microscope to be densely covered with minute "finger-like" processes (the *villi*), which measure about half a millimeter in length. The presence of these villi produces a further enormous increase in the surface area available for absorption—as is well seen when, as a result of disease, they are destroyed and absorption becomes severely impaired (see CELIAC DISEASE, a disease in which the small intestine fails to absorb fats, vitamins, and other nutrients, and MALABSORPTION, a term applied to a number of conditions in which normal absorption of nutrient is impaired). The mucosal cells also secrete digestive juices which act in combination with those produced by the salivary glands, stomach, liver and pancreas.

The muscular coat of the bowel consists of two layers—one of circular fibers, the other of longitudinal fibers. This allows it to contract both in diameter and in length. The essential wavelike movement of the bowel is called *peristalsis*; it moves food material down the bowel as digestion proceeds. A ring of contraction appears at one point in the bowel, producing a narrowing; this contraction ring then passes down the length of the bowel, literally squeezing the fluid contents along before it, while the muscle wall relaxes again after the wave of contraction has passed. For the most part, we are not aware of this process; however, if there is gas as well as fluid in the bowel, we may be aware of gurgling noises or sensations of intestinal activity as peristalsis occurs. If the bowel is irritated or inflamed, the contractions become more vigorous and may be painful.

The contents of the small intestine are fluid; but on entering the colon, water is progressively absorbed until by the time the rectum is reached they are converted to semisolid (though normally soft) feces. These accumulate in the rectum until increasing distension produces a desire to open the bowels (defecation). The ring of muscle which controls the anus (anal sphincter) relaxes and contraction of the muscular walls of the rectum causes the feces to be passed.

In most persons a bowel movement occurs once or sometimes even twice daily, but there are wide variations that are dependent on diet and other factors. There is absolutely nothing abnormal about having a bowel movement only once every two or three days, providing the pattern is regular and relief is achieved without difficulty.

For further information, see also DIGESTION, CONSTIPATION and DIARRHEA.

bowleg

Bowleg is an outward bending of the legs. It is common during infancy and requires no treatment or undue concern unless the condition persists. A normal posture occurs after the child has been walking for about one year. But abnormal bowleg may arise in various conditions where growth is disturbed, such as rickets or OSTEOGENESIS IMPERFECTA.

If the bowlegged state of infancy does not improve spontaneously or if other disease is clearly evident, or if the infant is not developing normally, then further investigation is necessary.

There is a rare condition, the result of intrauterine deformity, in which congenital dislocation of the knee is present at birth. The resulting bowleg deformity is avoided by immediate treatment.

Another condition that causes severe bowing of the legs is known as *tibia vara*. It occurs mainly in infants but is sometimes seen in adolescents, particularly those from the West Indies and West Africa. The bone deformity, which is present at the upper end of the tibia (shinbone), may be due to the laxity of the ligaments in these races and their custom to walk earlier. The condition cannot be confused with the normal bowleg of infancy because it fails to improve and requires surgical correction.

See also KNOCK-KNEE.

BOWLEG AND KNOCK-KNEE

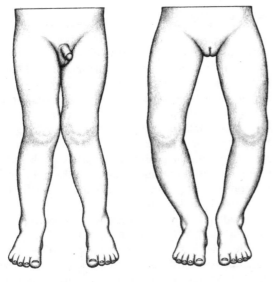

knock-knee   bowleg

Most young babies have bowleg but the condition corrects itself when they begin to walk. Very rarely, if the deformity persists, it may be necessary for the child to wear corrective splints at night. A mild degree of knock-knee is also very common in children under 6 years of age and only needs active treatment if it is severe. Either of these deformities in adults can result from trauma, rickets, and Paget's disease.

bradycardia

A slowing of the heart rate below 60 beats per minute. It can be a normal occurrence in fit young people at rest or during sleep (especially among well-trained athletes) and results from the inhibitory action of the vagus nerve (the Xth cranial nerve). In other circumstances bradycardia may be a sign of acute myocardial infarction ("heart attack"), depressant drug action (from the administration of drugs such as digitalis, morphine, reserpine, propranolol or prostigmine), low blood volume (as the result of internal bleeding or severe fluid depletion), heart block, or the ADAMS-STOKES SYNDROME.

In most cases bradycardia requires no treatment. However, in patients who have persistent symptoms of lightheadedness, fainting, angina pectoris, or congestive heart failure as the consequence of an abnormally low heart rate or insufficient acceleration of the heart under conditions of stress, an artificial PACEMAKER may be required. Compare TACHYCARDIA.

brain

The control center of the central nervous system, enclosed and protected by the skull.

More than 10 billion cells in the brain receive and transmit messages to and from all parts of the body; they filter, store and form associations between information received through the senses. The brain is often compared with a computer, but is thousands of times more complex than any existing electronic circuitry.

During fetal development the top end of the spinal cord thickens and expands to form distinct areas within the brain. Broadly speaking, the "higher" the center in the brain the more complex its function, culminating in intelligent or "cerebral" behavior.

A diffuse network of cells and fibers called the *reticular activating system* (RAS) extends through the core of the brain stem from the top of the spinal cord up into the hypothalamus. The RAS is the seat of consciousness and governs the states of sleep, arousal and attention. The RAS and the higher centers of the cerebral cortex have extensive two-way connections so that their levels of activity are mutually controlled.

At the back of the skull is the *cerebellum*, which coordinates reflex actions that control posture, balance and muscular activity. Deep within the brain, where the brain mass seems to tip forward, is the center for basic or "uncritical" appreciation of pain, temperature and crude touch—the *thalamus*. It is the main relay center for incoming sensory impulses (except those of smell), which it transmits to other parts of the brain, including those concerned with consciousness. Vital automatic functions, such as blood pressure, blood circulation, heartbeat, and hormone secretion are in part regulated by the *hypothalamus*, which is situated just below the thalamus (as its name implies). It also plays an important role in the experiencing of basic drives, such as hunger, thirst and sex.

Above and billowing out to fill the skull are the convoluted *cerebral hemispheres*, where the nerve centers exist that are responsible for conscious thought and action. In man, this part of the brain (the cerebrum) is larger in relation to total body weight than in any other animal. A dense layer of nerve cells—the *gray matter* of the cerebral cortex—forms the active "roof" of the brain. Deeper within the cerebrum are insulated nerve fibers of these cells, which intermingle to form the *white matter*.

Distinct areas have been mapped out for many voluntary movements and for sensations from most parts of the body. But the brain's "computer" activity, which is responsible for functions such as reason and memory, is basically a mystery. Indeed, experts still understand little about the phenomenon of consciousness itself.

BRAIN

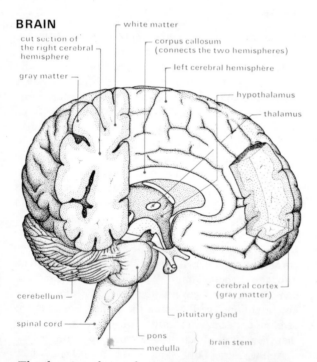

The drawing shows the important structures of the human brain. Centers in the brain stem control the heart and breathing. The cerebellum smooths out our movements. The thalamus relays signals to and from the cerebral cortex, the thin layer of gray matter. The hypothalamus is concerned with "instinctive drives" and with emotions: it has intimate connections with the pituitary gland, controlling the body's hormones.

brain death

Brain death is a relatively new concept. It occurs when there is: (1) a prolonged failure of the brain to show any evidence of electrical activity (as indicated by electroencephalography); (2) absence of general neurological activity (manifested by fixed pupils, absence of spontaneous breathing, absence of any response to painful stimuli, etc.); (3) a prolonged state of deep unconsciousness. Head injury and brain hemorrhage are the most likely causes.

There has been deep public concern over brain death, especially accompanying controversial cases of patients in prolonged comas where relatives have wished to switch off life-support machines.

One view is that to switch off is to "allow" a patient to die, not that he has already died. Another is that indecision over death deprives people of dying with dignity, as when intensive care supports a vegetable-like body with an irreversibly damaged brain.

The informed consensus which now governs much of medical practice (although there are still controversial cases) is that if two or more doctors are convinced that brain death has occurred then the respirator (and other life-support equipment) should be switched off.

brain tumor

An abnormal growth in any part of the brain.

Brain tumors may be benign or malignant (cancerous). Unfortunately many are malignant, and these may be primary or secondary—that is, originating in the brain or caused by the spread of cancer cells from another part of the body.

The tumors may appear at any age. As they grow within the enclosed space of the skull they have little room for expansion against the delicate brain cells. Therefore, even quite small tumors in the brain may have serious consequences. As with many growths, the cause is usually unknown.

The gradually increasing pressure in the brain tissue causes many general symptoms. A dull nagging headache and vomiting are common. With some tumors, convulsions may sometimes precede other symptoms. Mental changes may occur, such as drowsiness, lethargy and possibly a change in the personality. Other symptoms depend on the part of the brain affected—for example, partial paralysis, dimming of vision or possibly speech problems.

Diagnosis involves specialized x rays, lumbar puncture, and EEG tests. In recent years the advent of computerized x-ray scanning of the brain has improved diagnosis. It gives earlier diagnosis and a more accurate picture of the tumor than was possible in the past.

Treatment is mainly surgical; for benign tumors this

may be quite successful. In cases of malignant tumors, however, a permanent cure is difficult to achieve, although surgery may relieve the symptoms. Radiotherapy and drugs may play a subordinate therapeutic role.

breast

The mammary, or milk-secreting, gland.

It was originally a sweat gland but has developed during evolution. It is also a potent sexual symbol with an important erotic function.

The breasts develop slowly under the influence of hormones during puberty. Each breast consists chiefly of fibrous tissue radiating from the nipple and dividing it into 15 to 20 lobes. Under hormonal control, these lobes produce milk following delivery of a baby. Each lobe has many small ducts draining into a main duct, which finally emerges as a tiny opening on the surface of the nipple. Just under the nipple these ducts dilate, forming reservoirs of milk during feeding. Pressure by the infant's mouth on the areola, the distinct circle of dark skin surrounding the nipple, causes milk to be ejected from the 15 to 20 ducts.

Surrounding the glandular tissue is a large pad of fat cells which give the breast its shape. The entire breast mass extends over a large area, reaching up into the armpit. (Thus, the importance of thorough feeling during self-examination of the breasts for early signs of cancer.)

There are no muscles in the breasts; if they lose their youthful firmness, exercise is unlikely to restore it. Despite the vagaries of fashion and the women's liberation movement, many women find that they do prefer to wear a brassiere—both for the sake of comfort and, hopefully, to ward off stretching and sagging. Support is especially important during a woman's pregnancy.

Throughout pregnancy the breasts become fuller. This and tingling nipples are, for many women, among the first indications of pregnancy. The areola itself may further darken, especially in dark-haired women.

Although boyish figures are promoted as fashionable, many women worry if their breasts are very small. Little can be done to enlarge breasts without expensive plastic surgery. Expensive creams and massage are virtually worthless. But size tends to increase after the age of 35 or so, chiefly due to fat being deposited in the breast.

Ideal size and shape of the breasts vary among different cultures as well as among individuals. Polynesians are said to admire small conical breasts, while North American Indians admire elongated drooping breasts.

See also BREAST CANCER, BREAST FEEDING, MAMMOPLASTY and MASTECTOMY.

breast cancer

Most of the great variety of tumors or growths which may occur in the female breast are not cancerous. Nevertheless, it is essential to seek immediate medical attention at the first sign of any suspicious changes or abnormalities in the breast since early diagnosis and treatment of breast cancer can be life-saving. Breast cancer continues to be the most common form of cancer in women—especially in those between the ages of about 40 to 45—and claims approximately 8,000 lives annually in the United Kingdom alone.

Despite massive worldwide research efforts to discover the possible causes of breast cancer in women and to evaluate the best methods of medical and surgical treatment, little significant progress has been made within the past 30 years. Indeed, great controversy still exists within the medical profession regarding the best method of treating various forms of breast cancer.

Experts are aware that the risk of breast cancer is highest among unmarried women with no pregnancies and who began their menstrual cycles at a relatively early age. But the obvious suggestion that this is definitely linked to prolonged exposure to high levels of ESTROGENS during menstrual cycles over many years (unrelieved by becoming pregnant) has not been substantiated scientifically. Objective evidence still does not exist that the female hormones contained in oral contraceptives (the "Pill") increase the incidence of breast cancer; indeed what evidence there is suggests that the Pill may even protect against breast cancer. Likewise, women receiving estrogen therapy have not been definitely proved to be more susceptible to cancer of the breast. In both cases, however, these possibilities are still being investigated in long-term research studies.

What *has* been shown to be true—even though the reasons are unclear—is that breast cancer is more common (1) in women in the higher socioeconomic classes; (2) in those with a family history of the disease; (3) in those with previous disease of the breast (regardless of the cause); (4) in single women who have not been pregnant; and (5) in those whose first menstrual cycles started at or before the age of 12. For some unexplained reason, breast cancer is also more common among Jewish women than among non-Jewish women. It is also more common in Western women than in Asiatics such as the Japanese. It is relatively rare in women below the age of 25, reaching its highest incidence just before, during, or after the MENOPAUSE (the "change of life").

Among the possible causes of breast cancer which have been extensively investigated is some form of viral infection. (Experiments have clearly demonstrated that certain viruses can cause mammary cancer in mice—animals which provide an important "model" of the

BREAST SELF-EXAMINATION

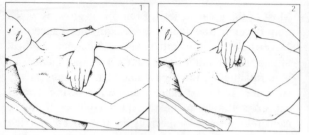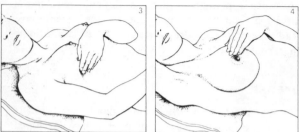

Most breast lumps are not cancerous, but any woman discovering a lump should consult a doctor. The correct method of self-examination is shown above. Feel with the flats of the fingers, not the tips (1). Start with the upper outer quadrant of the breast and remember it extends up into the armpit (2). Then examine the remainder of the outer half and underside of the breast (3). Feel around the nipple and gently roll the inner half of the breast over the ribs (4). Self-examination should be performed monthly because treatment is more successful in the early stages of breast cancer.

human form of the disease.) Another possibility under current investigation is the part played by diet. A popular belief exists among many women that a blow to the chest may be responsible for the subsequent development of breast cancer; this has never been substantiated, however, and it is generally thought that such a cause is most unlikely. (Breast cancer in men is an extremely rare disease.)

Warning signs. Among the warning signs of breast cancer are: (1) the appearance of any unusual lump or nodule in either breast (which may or may not be a harmless cyst or other benign growth); (2) changes in the nipple, either by alterations in position or by retraction ("inverted nipples"); (3) puckering of the skin on the breast; (4) bleeding or other discharges from the nipple; (5) an unusual rash on the breast or nipple; and (6) an unusual prominence of veins over the breast (however, in pregnant women this is fairly common). Many women may have one or more of these symptoms without having cancer. But because of the rapid growth of many breast cancers, medical attention must be obtained immediately—especially if any unusual lump is evident.

Self-examination. Many experts recommend monthly self-examination of the breasts. This can be performed while standing or sitting in front of a mirror or even while taking a shower. However, it is desirable to observe the shape of the breasts in a mirror in addition to feeling for any abnormal changes in the consistency of the breast tissues. The visual examination should be

made first with the arms raised and then with the arms hanging loosely by the sides. The light should fall evenly on the chest from the front, which will aid in recognizing any dimpling of the skin or changes in the size or shape of the breasts. About 95% of all women with breast cancer seek medical attention after discovering some abnormality or suspicious change as the result of self-examination. It is best to conduct this examination on or about the same day each month, preferably when the breasts are softest (after the menstrual period).

Note any changes of the shape with the arms upstretched, then feel every part of the breasts and up into the armpits for any lumps or changes (see illustration). Lumps may well be painless but should not be ignored.

Breast cancer may also be diagnosed at an early stage—before any lump can be detected—by regular screening using x rays (MAMMOGRAPHY) or infrared imaging (THERMOGRAPHY). At present this form of SCREENING is recommended for women in high-risk groups and for all women aged over 50.

Treatment. Treatment of breast cancer may involve a combination of surgery (see MASTECTOMY), irradiation and drug therapy. The choice of therapy will depend largely on the extent of invasion of the breast and surrounding tissues with cancer cells. In some cases it may be possible to remove a small lump or nodule of cancerous tissue without removing the entire breast (a procedure known as a *lumpectomy*). In other cases, where the cancer cells have spread to involve the lymph nodes of the armpit and surrounding areas, it may be necessary to remove the breast and the underlying muscles, as well as tissues nearby which have become invaded by cancer cells (*radical mastectomy*). Between these two extremes, it may only be necessary to remove all or most of the affected breast without recourse to removing other tissues (*simple mastectomy*).

There is no general agreement regarding the best combination of therapy for the treatment of breast cancer. Some experts believe that the possible spread of cancer cells can be controlled following mastectomy by exposure of the tissues to x rays (*irradiation therapy*). Other experts at treating breast cancers believe that the use of anticancer ("cytotoxic") drugs may be a possible alternative to radical mastectomy, although the research studies designed to answer that question are not yet complete. The aim of this *adjuvant chemotherapy* is the destruction of any small "satellites" of cancer cells in the bones, the liver or other organs that are remote from the breast.

Alternative means of treating breast cancer are currently being investigated, such as the administration of a vaccine ordinarily used for the prevention of tuberculosis. This vaccine, known as *BCG* (bacille Calmette-Guérin), stimulates the production of antibodies that in some cases are thought to destroy cancer cells. At present, however, such attempts to stimulate the body's immunological defense system (*immunotherapy*) in the control of breast cancer remains only a possibility.

The outlook for treatment of breast cancer remains guarded but there are some hopeful trends. Publicity and the growth of screening programs have encouraged women to seek treatment earlier, and the breast tumors removed by surgeons are now on average substantially smaller than ten years ago. The combination of early treatment and adjuvant chemotherapy should improve the cure rate in the next decade.

breast feeding

The natural way to feed small babies.

In this century breast feeding has largely been abandoned in affluent countries in favor of bottles. The use of a special formula of cow's milk, in bottles, is becoming widespread in developing nations. Pediatricians are trying to reverse this worrying trend. They are encouraging mothers to give their babies the advantages of breast milk for some time, even if only for a few weeks.

A chief advantage is that, not only does it give the baby some digestible milk proteins, but breast milk protects against infections such as gastroenteritis and pneumonia during the first few months of life when the baby's own immune system is immature. Immunity is passed from mother to baby through the milk. Breast-fed babies are also thought less likely to become overweight. There is some speculation that breast feeding may also protect against heart disease in later life. And it is also theorized that babies who have nonhuman milk early in life are more liable to develop allergies.

Suckling helps to develop close emotional links between mother and baby, demonstrated by the fact that a baby's cry a few rooms away will cause a "let down" of the mother's milk. Nursing also stimulates release of a hormone from the hypothalamus in the brain which aids the shrinking of the uterus back to normal size following childbirth.

Breast size is immaterial to successful feeding. Even quite flat-chested women may manage to feed twins. During pregnancy, the glandular tissue of the breast proliferates in readiness for lactation. When the baby suckles, the hormone oxytocin is released from the pituitary gland and stimulates milk production.

During the first few days, the breasts secrete small amounts of a thick yellow fluid known as colostrum— a substance quite adequate for the baby, which has its own initial reserves of food—after which the milk "comes in."

The modern trend is to feed babies "on demand" and allow them to establish their own feeding pattern. A continued flow of milk depends upon the demands made by the baby. When the baby is weaned, the falloff in the sucking stimulus means that less milk is produced; eventually, the flow ceases.

Most women who want to feed successfully can do so. Worry, emotional upset and illness are major reasons why milk may fail. However, it is no failure if a woman is unable to feed her baby. Hundreds of thousands of happy adults were bottle fed.

Bright's disease

A somewhat vague or imprecise term for chronic inflammation of the kidney (nephritis), accompanied by proteinuria (the abnormal presence of protein in the urine). In modern medical terminology it is basically equivalent to GLOMERULONEPHRITIS.

The disease was named after the English physician Richard Bright (1789–1858), who described it in 1827.

bronchiectasis

A chronic condition in which one or more of the main airways in the lungs (bronchi) lose their elasticity and become permanently dilated. Mucus secretions collect in the damaged section of lung and secondary bacterial infection is a common complication. The disease is characterized by severe bouts of coughing that occur early in the day as the sufferer tries to bring up the infected sputum.

Bronchiectasis may be associated with a congenital defect in the lung. More usually it occurs after pneumonia or some other infection, especially whooping cough. Bronchiectasis is also common in the genetic disorder CYSTIC FIBROSIS (mucoviscidosis), in which the mucus secreted by the lungs is excessively thick and sticky.

However, with antibiotic treatment readily available for prompt treatment of respiratory conditions, damage is less likely to occur than it once was. In very severe cases, but where damage is confined, an affected lobe of the lung may be removed surgically.

bronchitis

Inflammation of the air passages of the lung. Bronchitis may be acute or chronic.

Acute bronchitis very often follows a cold or an attack of influenza, for bacterial infection is facilitated by viral inflammation.

First the windpipe (trachea) becomes inflamed; then infection spreads through the bronchial tree to reach the larger air passages (bronchi) and so into the smaller bronchioles. In a severe or untreated case, inflammation may spread into the lung tissue itself to give rise to bronchopneumonia. There is no hard and fast line between these states.

Initially there is a hard and unproductive cough (i.e., no sputum is coughed up) with mild fever, malaise (a general feeling of being unwell), aching muscles and depression. After a day or two the patient begins to bring up sputum, and the cough is less painful. Treatment includes bed rest, warmth, steam inhalations and hot drinks; if necessary, antibiotics are given to cut short the duration of the illness and to prevent the development of bronchopneumonia, especially in the aged.

Chronic bronchitis is a different disease, the result of repeated irritation of the lining of the air passages by smoke, dust, fumes and general atmospheric pollution. It occurs in all industrial communities, and members of the managerial and professional classes are affected less than unskilled and semi-skilled workers. Men are more commonly affected than women.

The patient may be said to have chronic bronchitis when he continues to cough up sputum for at least three months in two years. Usually he becomes out of breath, because the disease is accompanied by EMPHYSEMA— enlargement of the bronchioles, the small terminal air passages, with dilation and destruction of the alveoli (air sacs) where gaseous exchange takes place during respiration. The basic process in chronic bronchitis is excessive secretion of mucus, which interferes with the proper drainage of the respiratory tract and aids the development of recurrent infection. Eventually the lung tissue loses is normal elasticity, the air spaces become disrupted, and there is interference with the blood circulation in the lung which may lead to increased pressure in the right side of the heart and its consequent failure.

Symptoms of chronic bronchitis include chronic productive cough, increasing breathlessness, wheezing and sometimes depression. The patient should stop smoking; usually it is impossible for him to change employment or to move into a more favorable climate without gross pollution of the air, but by doing so he may lengthen his life and diminish his discomfort. Acute flare-ups of the disease are treated with antibiotics, as they are typically caused by the addition of bacterial infection.

Breathing exercises may help, and in very severe cases the administration of oxygen and the use of bronchodilator drugs under medical supervision may improve the condition.

bronchopneumonia

Inflammation of the lungs, usually beginning in the terminal air passages (bronchioles).

See PNEUMONIA.

brucellosis

A bacterial infection (also known as *undulent fever*) transmitted to man from cattle, hogs, and goats. It is mainly an occupational disease of those in contact with animals or meat, but it can also be contracted from unpasteurized milk.

The bacteria (of the genus *Brucella*) can enter the body through the nose, mouth or broken skin. The first symptoms usually appear within two weeks of infection, but the incubation period varies from about five days to several months. Symptoms include fever, headache, chills, fatigue and depression. Often there are no physical abnormalities except the high temperature and brucellosis can easily be mistaken for influenza. The fever sometimes recurs in repeated waves (or undulations) with intervening periods of several days without symptoms.

Even without therapy, the symptoms of acute brucellosis usually disappear within one year. However, nonspecific symptoms of chronic brucellosis may persist for many years. Treatment of acute brucellosis with tetracycline antibiotics reduces the chances of a relapse; once established, chronic brucellosis is difficult to cure and causes great personal misery.

bubonic plague

The most common variety of plague which—as the "Black Death"—killed an estimated 25 million people in Europe during the 14th century. Today it is more prevalent in insanitary areas of tropical countries, but limited outbreaks do occur occasionally in the western parts of the United States.

The infecting bacteria, *Pasteurella pestis*, are transmitted to humans from the bite of infected rat fleas, which abandon rats dying of plague in favor of domestic animals such as cats and dogs.

The characteristic features of the disease are fever and swellings—buboes—of lymph glands in the armpits and groin. Bleeding into the skin results in dark blotches, which give rise to the historical name "Black Death."

The onset of the disease is very sudden. After a few sporadic cases, the disease may suddenly spread and reach epidemic proportions.

However, modern drugs have dramatically changed the outlook for plague victims. Treatment once used to consist of careful nursing and administration of antibubonic serum. Today a combination of sulfonamides and antibiotics is used with great success. Prevention of the disease involves the use of insect repellants to ward off the infective fleas and attempts to control the rodent population.

(*Pneumonic plague*, the other common form of plague, involves a severe infection of the lungs. In the absence of appropriate medical treatment it can prove fatal within two to five days of the onset of symptoms.)

Buerger's disease

Another name for THROMBOANGIITIS OBLITERANS.

bundle branch block

A defect in the electrical conduction system of the heart. There is a delay or block of the wave of electrical impulses that spreads out from the region of the heart's atrial chambers (responsible for controlling the heartbeat).

This causes one ventricle to contract before the other, resulting in an abnormal pattern of heart rhythm. The electrical impulses are conducted through a network of fibers known as the *bundle of His*. This bundle forms two branches: a block in the left branch usually means that heart disease is present, whereas a block in the right bundle (although linked with disorders of the heart) may occur in people with no evidence of abnormality.

Bundle branch block may occur in people suffering from arteriosclerosis, rheumatic heart disorders, or congenital heart disease.

Diagnosis is usually made with the help of electro-cardiograph recordings. The outlook depends on the severity of the underlying disorder.

bunion

An unsightly deformity of the joint at the base of the big toe. It looks as if the joint has been pushed out of place and is the result of undue pressure on the joint over long periods.

Although injury which has not been treated satisfactorily may cause a bunion, badly fitting shoes are the most common cause. Pointed shoes which compress the feet push out the joint, as do shoes which throw the weight of the body onto the ball of the foot. As a result of pressure on the joint, the sac or bursa alongside the bones may also become inflamed and tender. Pus may be

BUNION

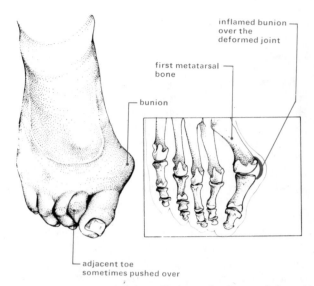

inflamed bunion over the deformed joint

first metatarsal bone

bunion

adjacent toe sometimes pushed over

A bunion is a painful swelling at the base of the big toe which results from tight shoes rubbing over a deformed joint. The primary cause is that the first metatarsal bone deviates away from the rest of the foot resulting in a prominent joint. A sac of fluid develops over this joint as a result of friction, and this sac may become inflamed and tender or even go septic (produce pus).

present.

Strapping, splinting and attention to wearing comfortable shoes may improve matters by reducing pressure. Once the damage is done, the only really effective treatment is surgical removal of the deformity. This operation is usually very successful.

Burkitt's lymphoma

A malignant tumor of the lymphatic tissue mainly affecting young children in certain parts of Africa, although it also occurs sporadically throughout the world.

It is named after Denis P. Burkitt, a 20th-century British surgeon who drew attention to the disease while working in Uganda. The characteristic feature is gross rapid swelling of the jaw. Many other bones and organs may be affected, and without treatment the disease is fatal in a few months.

Following Dr. Burkitt's interest in the disease, the tumor proved very amenable to powerful anticancer drugs. In Africa there are now many cases of complete cure. In other parts of the world, however, treatment has not been quite so successful.

There is very strong evidence to suggest that Burkitt's lymphoma is caused by the *Epstein-Barr virus* (the same microorganism which causes infectious mononucleosis). It is one of the very few human cancers in which a particular virus is so strongly implicated.

burns

Damage caused to the skin by either dry or wet heat (scalds). The biological properties of skin are destroyed just as when egg white is heated. Anything bringing about this change is said to cause burning—fire, boiling liquid, electricity, acids, alkalis and other corrosive fluids, or even excessive cold.

The severity of burns is assessed by considering the depth to which the skin is damaged and the surface area affected. A 1% burn would cover an area equivalent to that of the hand.

Fluid loss is a serious consequence of extensive burns. Plasma leaks out from blood vessels near the burned area. Small burns cause only a little leakage with local blisters, but very large burns (where skin is severely damaged) may interfere with the circulation to such an extent that large volumes of fluid are lost. There is a danger of a severe drop in blood pressure (shock) and the fluid loss requires prompt replacement with the transfusion of plasma, which may be immediately more important than treatment of the damaged tissue.

A 15% to 20% burn may well require transfusions. Burns over 25% of the body are virtually certain to require them; burns over 75% of the body are nearly always fatal. Children and the elderly are particularly at risk.

Burns are often divided roughly into three categories: first, second and third degree.

First degree burns involve superficial reddening of the skin with no blistering. This layer of the skin is usually shed and replaced naturally and healing is uncomplicated. Major treatment is unlikely to be necessary, although the patient may suffer some degree of shock.

In *second degree burns* the skin is actually destroyed and there may be extensive blistering as fluid seeps out of the blood vessels. But enough tissue is left for the surface layer to be fully replaced in time. The chief threat is from infection when the blisters burst.

In *third degree burns* the entire thickness of the skin is involved and cannot be renewed naturally. New skin will grow at the edges of the wound but destroyed skin must be replaced by skin grafts. These thin layers of skin—taken from other parts of the body—speed up the healing process, help prevent infection and reduce deformity. Grafts of pigskin are sometimes used to speed recovery when large areas are affected. Infection is the chief danger and badly burned patients are usually nursed in germ-free isolation units; they may be uncovered in the early stages. Devices such as air beds are used to prevent pressure on the damaged areas.

Although there is still some dispute over the first-aid treatment of burns, most experts advise cooling burns immediately. This certainly applies to minor household burns and scalds: the area should be cooled in running cold water for at least 10 minutes. Heat is retained in the skin following removal from the source of the burn and continues to "cook" unless cooled. Cooling also helps to relieve and prevent pain. However, concern with this should not prevent rapid removal to the hospital of more severely burned victims. Smoldering clothing should be peeled off but clothes adhering to damaged skin must be left.

Burns with acids or alkalis or other corrosive liquids should always be flushed with water. Acids should not be used to neutralize alkalis, or vice versa. Corrosive liquids in the eye should be flushed with water for some time and the patient should be encouraged to blink. Pain caused by chemicals in the eye may induce the patient to keep the eyelids tightly shut. They have to be gently opened to let the water flow under them and over the eyeball.

Blisters must be left strictly alone. Pricking them gives bacteria entry to a perfect breeding ground. Small trivial wounds may be covered with a sterile dressing, but larger burns should only be covered lightly if at all. A clean laundered sheet or handkerchief may be more suitable than gauze, which tends to stick. Ointments, creams or butter should *not* be applied.

Medical attention should be sought where there is any doubt. Burns caused by an electric current may be more serious than they look, as tissue below the surface can be damaged.

bursitis

A painful condition affecting certain joints, caused by inflammation of a bursa.

A bursa is a closed sac which helps muscles and tendons to move smoothly across places where bones are prominent, such as in the knee, shoulder, hip and bottom. Bursitis can be extremely painful; often the pain starts suddenly, especially in the shoulder—the most common joint to be affected.

The cause of bursitis in most cases is unknown, but it can be caused by injury, inflammatory arthritis, gout, rheumatoid arthritis, infection, or repeated friction. One popular name for bursitis involving the bursa in front of the kneecap is "housemaid's knee."

Acute bursitis often responds to injection into the affected bursa of hydrocortisone, following infiltration of 1% procaine. An anti-inflammatory drug such as phenylbutazone or indomethacin may also be helpful.

Once the worst is over, exercise of the joint will help to get it moving once more. This physical therapy, under proper supervision, is important to prevent any permanent loss of joint movement.

BURSITIS

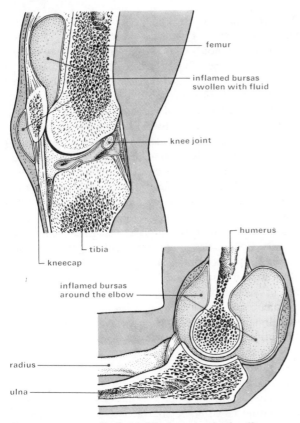

- femur
- inflamed bursas swollen with fluid
- knee joint
- humerus
- tibia
- kneecap
- inflamed bursas around the elbow
- radius
- ulna

Bursas are small, fluid-filled sacs which allow tendons and skin to move freely over prominent bones. Repeated trauma to these areas leads to bursitis—painful, inflammatory swellings of the bursa. This is particularly likely to occur in bursas around the knee ("Housemaid's Knee") and at the elbow ("Tennis Elbow.")

bypass

When an artery becomes narrowed as a result of ATHEROSCLEROSIS or other disease causing hardening of the arteries, there may be harmful effects on the organ or tissue supplied by the vessel. In addition, a narrowed vessel is likely to become the site of a blood clot, which may then completely stop the flow of blood. Narrowing of the coronary arteries (which nourish the heart muscle) may lead to ANGINA PECTORIS or to CORONARY THROMBOSIS (myocardial infarction, or a "heart attack"). In the limbs, a narrowed artery may produce INTERMITTENT CLAUDICATION with pain developing in the limb on exercise. In the brain, narrowing of the blood vessels may cause mental deterioration or confusion.

In certain sites, the problem may now be overcome by the use of grafts to replace the narrowed portion of the vessel or to bypass it. In the heart, narrowed coronary arteries producing angina pectoris can be bypassed by using a graft of a vein taken from the leg. Once the graft has "taken," the vein soon assumes the structure of the artery it replaces. In the leg and in the major blood vessels at the lower end of the abdominal aorta (the main artery from the heart carrying blood to the lower part of the body), narrowed or obstructed vessels may be replaced by a variety of plastic grafts, usually of woven nylon or Teflon to give flexibility. Other bypass procedures may shunt blood from the portal vein to the vena cava in the abdomen, or may be done to provide additional blood to the brain when a carotid artery is obstructed. All these procedures demand a high level of specialized surgical skill, but the results can be extremely successful.

CORONARY BYPASS

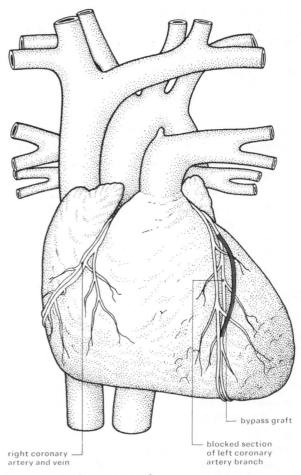

- bypass graft
- blocked section of left coronary artery branch
- right coronary artery and vein

In principle the coronary bypass operation is simple and involves bypassing the blocked section of coronary artery with a length of vein taken from the patient's leg. In practice, it calls for a formidable surgical team and expensive equipment.

byssinosis

A lung disease caused by the inhalation of dust and foreign substances (including mold, fungi and bacteria) contained in cotton, flax and hemp. It primarily affects workers in industries where these materials are processed. Retention of dust in the lungs does not invariably lead to disease, but it may cause suspicious shadows on a lung x ray if the dust is sufficiently dense.

C

cachexia

A severe wasting (atrophy) of the body produced as the consequence of disease. Wasting occurs, of course, in any patient who is starved for any reason; but the term *cachexia* is usually reserved for those in whom an underlying illness exists and in whom merely providing a well-balanced diet is usually ineffective in restoring normal health.

Simple starvation plays some part in many cases of true cachexia. For example, a patient with cancer of the esophagus ("gullet") or stomach may be quite unable, for purely mechanical reasons, to take in enough food to maintain health. In starvation, however, body fat is first lost; only when this has been consumed for energy production will essential tissue, such as muscles, be broken down. In some debilitating diseases, loss of body fat and muscle wasting often occur simultaneously as a relatively early sign of the disease and cannot always be easily explained by a loss of appetite or diminished food intake. This is particularly true of patients with cancer (*malignant cachexia*).

When a physician takes a patient's medical history he will often inquire about any recent loss of weight. He will sometimes be inclined to take a more serious view of the problem if there has been any significant weight loss over the preceding weeks or months. On the other hand, weight loss may simply be associated with a reduction in food intake as a result of anxiety or depression, without any underlying disease. Lastly, certain glandular disorders—including overactivity of the thyroid gland (HYPERTHYROIDISM) and a rare disorder of the pituitary gland (known as *pituitary cachexia* or *Simmond's disease*)—may cause severe weight loss and wasting of the tissues, which can usually be corrected by appropriate treatment of the glandular disorder.

caisson disease

A technical name (together with *decompression sickness*) for the BENDS.

calculus

An accumulation of solid material (a "stone") in any of the hollow organs or passages of the body.

Calculi commonly cause symptoms when they occur anywhere in the urinary tract—the kidney, ureter, bladder, prostate gland or urethra—or the biliary tract (GALLSTONES). The next most common sites for stone formation are the ducts of the salivary glands.

Urinary calculi usually form as a result of abnormally high blood levels of calcium or other metabolic abnormalities. Stasis of urine, infection and inadequate fluid intake are sometimes contributing factors.

Most *gallstones* are caused by an imbalance in the concentrations of cholesterol, phospholipid and bile salts in the bile; but infection may contribute and a few cases are due to other diseases, such as hemolytic anemia. For reasons not yet understood, gallstones are becoming more common in Western societies; the most likely explanation is that the modern diet is especially rich in fats and proteins.

Calculi may cause no symptoms and their presence may first be recognized only on x-ray films taken during a routine health check. However, if symptoms do develop they may be severe. If a stone blocks the bile duct (leading from the liver to the duodenum) or the ureter (leading from the kidney to the bladder) the result is severe abdominal pain. The muscles of the blocked duct go into spasmodic contractions in an attempt to overcome the obstruction, causing repeated bouts of intense pain (colic).

Often an attack of colic will be short-lived as the calculus is passed into the bladder or the intestine. Sometimes, however, the obstruction may persist. In the case of a gallstone this will cause JAUNDICE. If the ureter is blocked the kidney cannot function and may be permanently damaged. Even if they do not cause obstruction, the presence of stones in the kidney or the gallbladder encourages inflammation.

When the cause of stone formation is known, as in some types of kidney stone associated with inborn biochemical defects (such as the presence of excessive quantities of uric acid in the circulating blood, which can lead to GOUT), treatment may be given with drugs such as allopurinol (Zyloprim) or with dietary modifications to reduce the chances of further stones being formed. Treatment with the drug *chenodeoxycholic acid* can cause the gradual dissolution of some types of gallstone. However, in most cases in which stones cause repeated symptoms the treatment is primarily surgical. Removal of the gallbladder (cholecystectomy) can provide a permanent cure of ill health from gallstones in many cases. Removal of kidney stones does not give a guarantee of cure either, but it is usually combined with dietary advice to reduce the risks of recurrence.

CALCULI

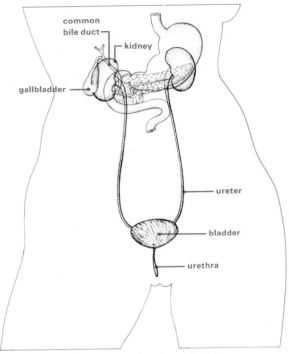

COMMON SITES FOR CALCULI (STONES)

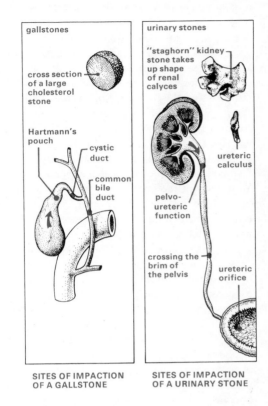

SITES OF IMPACTION
OF A GALLSTONE

SITES OF IMPACTION
OF A URINARY STONE

Calculi or stones form in concentrated bile or urine. Multiple gallstones are often found in the gallbladder. Urinary stones can form anywhere in the urinary system. Large "staghorn" calculi in the kidney may be unnoticed, but tiny stones passing along the ureter cause excruciating pain and blood in the urine.

callus

1. A local hard growth of the outer layer of the skin. Also known as a *callosity*.

Calluses are a normal reaction of the skin to friction or pressure. For example, many people have a callus on the side of the middle finger of their writing hand, caused by pressure from a pencil or pen.

Calluses rarely require treatment because they are painless and protective. They are occasionally removed for cosmetic reasons; this is pointless, however, unless the provoking factor is also removed, for they tend to recur. In contrast, corns may need treatment by a chiropodist.

Calluses rarely require treatment because they are painless and protective. They are occasionally removed for cosmetic reasons; this is pointless, however, unless the provoking factor is also removed, for they tend to recur. In contrast, corns may need treatment by a podiatrist (an expert on care and treatment of the feet).

2. The lump of soft, unorganized new bone which forms

at the site of a healing fracture and ultimately is transformed into organized bone that fixes the fractured bone ends firmly together.

cancer

Cancer is most easily understood as the development and later spread throughout the body of cells from a malignant tumor. With the exception of the leukemias, cancers almost always originate in a single isolated growth; at that early state removal of the solitary tumor will cure the disease. Once the cancer cells spread (metastasize) to the bones, liver or other major organs, however, the disease is controllable only by drug treatment or by radiotherapy.

The unique feature of cancer cells is, then, their readiness to multiply outside their organ of origin. Carried in the bloodstream or in the network of lymphatic channels to distant parts of the body, cells from the primary tumor "seed" themselves and grow, infiltrating and eventually destroying the healthy tissues around them. It is these secondary, "metastatic islets" of cancer which cause most of the serious and fatal complications of the disease.

Cancers are divided into four main categories on the basis of the site and nature of the primary tumor. Tumors of glandular organs—such as the breast, stomach, pancreas, lung, skin and intestines—are termed *carcinomas.* Tumors of muscle, bone and the other fibrous and supporting tissues of the body are termed *sarcomas:* these are often slower growing than carcinomas. Thirdly, the *lymphomas* (such as HODGKIN'S DISEASE) are tumors of the lymphatic system, affecting the lymph nodes in the neck, groin, armpits, and the liver and spleen; and similar in their symptoms and their response to treatment are the *leukemias,* the cancers of the blood-forming bone marrow.

The fundamental change in a cancer cell that distinguishes it from normal is in its *nuclear protein.* Seen beneath the microscope, cancer cells have large, often misshapen nuclei, and they often have two or three times the normal number of chromosomes. As the cells multiply those characteristics are passed on to each generation, perpetuating the abnormality in their growth pattern. What is not yet clearly understood is the nature of the event that changes a cell so that it becomes cancerous (malignant). It is clear, however, that most cancers originate as a response by the body to external factors. Some of these have been identified: nuclear radiation from substances such as radium, from atomic weapons, and from x rays and radioactive isotopes used in medicine or industry; alcohol and tobacco smoke; industrial minerals and chemicals such as asbestos and polyvinyl chloride; and hormone drugs such as estrogens. Others are only suspected: viruses in particular are believed to play a part. There also seems to be an association between intestinal tumors and a diet rich in meats and animal fats, but the constituent responsible has yet to be identified. Another equally important factor is the genetic and constitutional makeup of each individual: some cancers are found more commonly in racial groups such as the Japanese, and in other cases a tendency to one form of cancer may be found in successive generations of a family. Furthermore, while, for example, heavy cigarette smokers have a high risk of lung cancer, most of them (90%) do not develop the disease. This may be due to variations in the biochemical makeup of the individuals concerned, and much current cancer research is concerned with the identification of high-risk groups.

In their early stages cancerous tumors may be indistinguishable from other, benign growths such as warts, moles or cysts. Indeed, most lumps in the breast (for example) are not cancerous. Treatment is more likely to be curative, however, if it is given before the cancer has begun to spread, so that any lump or swelling in or beneath the skin in any part of the body, whether or not it is painful, must be suspected as potentially cancerous until proved to be benign. (See BREAST CANCER.) Warning signs of the possible presence of a malignant tumor in an internal organ include: the presence of blood in the urine or feces; abnormal bleeding from the vagina; change in the regularity of menstrual periods; change in the frequency of bowel movements or in the passing of urine; change in the voice; unexplained loss of weight; pain in the chest; coughing up blood; sudden onset of shortness of breath; or a persistent cough.

All of these symptoms may be associated with a disease other than cancer, but all may also be signs of an early cancer. Medical examination is needed for accurate diagnosis and effective treatment.

Treatment of cancer
Many cancers are now curable. Surgical removal of an isolated tumor in the breast or the intestine is successful in 60% or more of cases—in that there is no recurrence of the disease within a ten-year period. Radiotherapy is the best treatment for most early lymphomas; in Hodgkin's disease, for example, the cure rate is about 80% in such cases. Drug treatment for leukemia has made dramatic advances in the past decade; the cure rate in the most common childhood leukemia is now close to 50%, whereas a generation ago the disease was uniformly fatal.

It is still true, however, that all forms of cancer are most susceptible to treatment in their early stages and that in some cases the disease is widely spread before symptoms occur. Even in those circumstances a combination of drugs, radiotherapy and surgery may achieve a remission of symptoms for several years. One current research interest is the stimulation of the body's own defenses against cancer—*immunotherapy*—by injecting killed cancer cells or bacteria into the bloodstream; this and the development of new drugs are extending the survival—in reasonable health—of patients with widespread cancer.

Prevention
As more of the external causes of cancer are discovered, prevention of the disease becomes possible by protecting people from exposure to these "carcinogens" at work, in food and drink, and by education about the dangers of smoking.

The second branch of the preventive approach to cancer is the promotion of early diagnosis. Screening tests have been proved effective in a number of common cancers: the best known example is cancer of the cervix (neck of the womb), detected by a "Pap smear," and screening by mammography (x rays of the breast) has been shown to achieve earlier diagnosis of breast cancer in women aged below 50.

Screening is also valuable for people exposed to carcinogens at work and for those with a family history of the cancer. For the rest of us, however, the key to early diagnosis lies in alertness to the warning symptoms listed earlier.

Candida (Monilia)

A genus of yeastlike fungi (formerly known as *Monilia*), often harmlessly present in the mouths of healthy people. In some circumstances, however, the micro-organisms may proliferate to produce a symptomatic infection of the mouth, intestines, vagina, skin, or (rarely) the entire body. The species most often involved is *Candida albicans* and the infection is known as *candidiasis* (or, formerly, *moniliasis*). When the infection involves the mouth or the vagina the condition is commonly referred to as "thrush."

Thrush occurs particularly in babies, but it may also occur in debilitated adults or those with dentures. It usually forms a white curdlike deposit on the tongue, cheeks and palate which may cause severe discomfort.

Vaginal candidiasis is one of the most common causes of inflammation and itching of the vagina and vulva, typically producing a white, curdlike discharge. Vaginal candidiasis is becoming increasingly common, perhaps partly because of changes in vaginal acidity brought about by oral contraceptives. It is often seen in pregnant women and diabetics. The condition is not usually acquired during sexual intercourse but sometimes may cause a symptomatic infection in the male partner.

Candida albicans may occasionally infect the entire intestinal tract, causing anal itching and forming a reservoir for repeated accidental infection of the vagina.

The fungi may also infect the skin—particularly in moist areas, such as beneath the breasts of large women and in the finger webs of those working with water.

Infections with *Candida* are usually effectively treated with an antifungal drug such as nystatin—in the form of a mouthwash, lozenge, pessary, or a cream; intestinal infection is treated with nystatin tablets to prevent reinfection elsewhere.

Vaginal candidiasis tends to recur; avoidance of sexual intercourse during treatment reduces the recurrence rate.

Patients with reduced immune defenses (for example, those with any severe illness and those on drugs that suppress immunity) may get a generalized *Candida* infection involving most organs. This is a life-threatening condition that requires the intravenous administration of amphotericin B, a powerful (but quite toxic) antifungal agent used especially in the treatment of persistent deep-seated infections.

See also VAGINITIS.

cannabis

A drug derived from the flowering tips and shoots of *Cannabis sativa*, a plant which grows wild or cultivated all over the world.

The active substances in the drug are chemicals called

INDIAN HEMP (Cannabis Sativa)

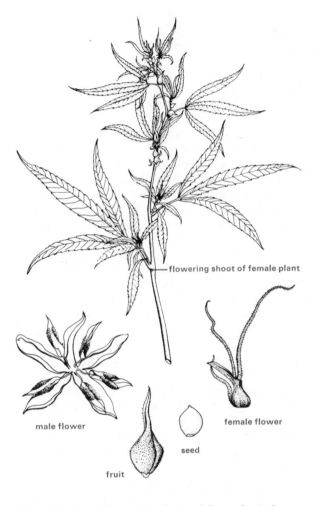

flowering shoot of female plant

male flower

female flower

seed

fruit

Cannabis (marijuana) is obtained from the Indian hemp plant pictured above; it can be taken either by mouth (mixed with food or drink), or smoked in a pipe or cigarette. It is not considered to be an addictive drug, although heavy users may become psychologically dependent.

tetrahydrocannabinols. Cannabis is also known as hashish, Indian hemp, marijuana, grass, pot, tea, weed, ganja and many other names.

It is one of the oldest known drugs and was used in early surgery to produce drowsiness and euphoria. It has few legitimate medical uses today, but is widely consumed throughout the world—illegally, in most Western countries. The plant and its flowers are dried, ground up, and smoked in a cigarette (a "joint") (It has been used experimentally in the treatment of glaucoma and in the relief of symptoms in patients with terminal cancer.)

In the West, cannabis resin is smoked in a small pipe

("hash pipe"); in some parts of the world (e.g., the U.K.) it is mixed with tobacco and the smoke inhaled from a cigarette. It can also be drunk as an infusion (bhang), as in India, or eaten in food.

Cannabis has been widely used in the U.S. since the 1930s, when it was probably introduced from Mexico or from the Caribbean (perhaps into New Orleans). Originally its use was largely confined to urban minority groups, but since the 1960s it has spread to many millions of middle-class Americans. Its popularity is also growing in other Western countries.

The effects of cannabis vary with the individual. Mild intoxication is characterized by cheerfulness, giggling and easygoing extrovert behavior. With more severe intoxication there may be irritable outbursts, feelings of unreality, auditory and visual hallucinations, and even frank psychosis. The effect usually wears off within 12 hours or less.

Long-term use of cannabis has not been shown to have major dangers—but neither has it been shown to be safe. Chronic users often appear to be generally apathetic ("a motivational syndrome"), but this could be a reason for the long-term use rather than the result of it. Suggestions of brain damage due to prolonged use have not been confirmed, but decreased sexual function and potency seem to be a real, if slight, hazard.

Physical dependence on cannabis does not occur but psychological dependence may be severe. Cannabis does not directly lead the user toward "hard" drugs or crime, but the drug subculture in which it is often used may expose him to greater dangers, and its hallucinogenic activity may tempt him to seek the stronger effects of LSD or other drugs.

Cannabis is probably no more harmful than alcohol (many experts believe that it is much less so), but it is debatable whether this is a sufficient argument for its legalization.

carbohydrates

Natural compounds, relatively high in caloric value, of which sugars and starches are the best known examples. They are capable of producing energy or heat and form one of the three classes of nutrients (the others being protein and fat).

Carbohydrates make up the bulk of the organic matter on earth, occurring predominantly in plants—particularly, as the structural carbohydrate cellulose. In animals, including man, the principal structural material is protein; but carbohydrate (in the form of mucopolysaccharide) is an important part of skeletal and other connective tissue.

Carbohydrates provide energy for synthetic processes and other work undertaken by the cells; they also provide many of the simple starting materials required for the synthesis of complex substances. The liver is an organ of particular importance in carbohydrate metabolism.

Carbohydrates may be classified into: (1) *monosaccharides*, simple sugars such as glucose and fructose; (2) *oligosaccharides*, compound sugars of two to ten monosaccharide units, such as sucrose and lactose; (3) *polysaccharides*, complex polymers of ten or more units, such as starch, glycogen, cellulose, dextran and mucopolysaccharides.

Carbohydrate yields four calories per gram; in developing countries it supplies up to 75% of the energy in the diet, mainly as unrefined cereal. In the United States 55% of dietary energy comes from carbohydrate, largely in the form of the refined carbohydrate sucrose (i.e. ordinary sugar). Sucrose contains none of the other nutrients found in unrefined carbohydrate sources and is thus a source of "empty calories." Most Westerners eat too many calories, and sucrose intake should be reduced.

The carbohydrate cellulose is indigestible by man, but is of great importance in providing dietary fiber ("roughage"), which is important in the maintenance of good health.

Excessive carbohydrate intake is the cause of obesity and dental caries. Carbohydrate intake must also be controlled in diabetes and in other more rare conditions where its metabolism is disturbed.

carbuncle

A large boil with multiple openings.

Carbuncles may reach the size of an apple. They cause severe throbbing pain, associated with fever and a general feeling of being unwell (malaise).

Carbuncles usually occur where the skin is thick, especially on the back of the neck: extension beneath the skin is probably favored by its thickness, when elsewhere the infection would "come to a head." The infecting bacteria are usually *Staphylococcus aureus*. Carbuncles are particularly common in patients with reduced defense to infection due to other debilitating illness.

Treatment of carbuncles involves the administration of appropriate antibiotics. The application of local heat may relieve pain. Surgical drainage is sometimes performed, but is often ineffective since there is no single collection of pus.

Before antibiotic therapy was available carbuncles were potentially dangerous, often leading to septicemia (blood poisoning) and even death. With appropriate antibiotic therapy they are now usually cured, although in some cases the infecting microorganisms become resistant to one or more of the antibiotics, making successful treatment more difficult.

carcinoma

Any of various types of malignant cancerous growths composed of epithelial cells—the cells which line the body's organs and ducts.

See CANCER and the major article on **Oncology.**

cardiac massage

A technique used in the attempt to restore function to a heart which has stopped suddenly.

Direct cardiac massage is massage of the heart itself; it is only performed by doctors, usually after heart surgery.

External cardiac massage or compression is performed by means of pressure applied over the chest wall; this technique can save life when performed correctly by a fully trained person.

Cardiac massage should not be given to a patient dying of a general illness such as cancer, since it is ineffective and distressing for all concerned. Its main use is for otherwise healthy people whose hearts stop suddenly, usually following a heart attack (myocardial infarction), or after drug overdoses, electric shock, drowning, or other accidents.

Cardiac massage is appropriate *only* when the heart has stopped. It is unhelpful and dangerous in someone who has simply fainted, where a slow pulse can still be lightly felt.

The technique can lead to complications. Rib fractures are quite common, especially in the elderly. Although this is sometimes inevitable, such fractures are usually the result of excessive pressure and may allow air to enter the chest cavity. Excessive pressure may also rupture the liver, spleen, or the heart itself and cause death. It is thus considered best not to attempt external cardiac massage without the proper training.

What to do:
1. Note the time. Call for help and an ambulance. Act quickly—you have about three minutes only before brain death starts.
2. Confirm that the heart has stopped by feeling for the neck (carotid) or groin (femoral) pulse. If either is present cardiac massage is inappropriate.
3. Lay the patient on his back on a hard surface—usually the floor—and kneel beside him.
4. Thump the lower end of the sternum (breastbone) hard once with your fist; this is sometimes sufficient to restart the heart.
5. If not, put the heel of one hand on the lower end of the sternum, put the other hand on top of it, and compress the chest with all your weight. Effective massage produces a femoral pulse which can be felt by an assistant. Repeat 60 times a minute.

6. Most patients with cardiac arrest also stop breathing and need artificial respiration. This is best performed by an assistant at one forced breath for every five to eight cardiac massages, but the two procedures can be performed by the same person if essential.
7. Keep going. Recovery may occur after an hour or more of cardiac massage, although this is uncommon.
8. Other measures are urgently required but must await medical assistance.

When resuscitating children, whose rate of respiration is different than that of adults, care must be taken not to use excessive force.

caries

Decay and death of calcified tissue. Originally the term was applied to the death of bone, but it now always means *dental caries.*

CARIES

STRUCTURE OF TEETH

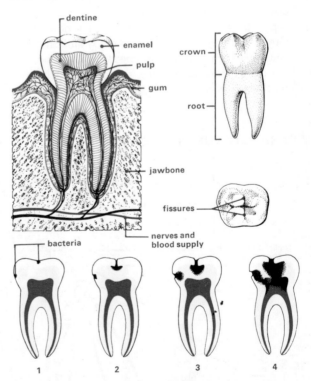

Caries or dental decay is the most common disease of Western man. Bacteria collect in the pits and fissures of the teeth and produce acid from refined sugar (1). The acid eats into the enamel (2). Decay then spreads more rapidly through the softer dentine (3). When the pulp becomes infected, irritation of the nerve leads to toothache (4).

Dental caries is the decalcification of a portion of a tooth, accompanied or followed by the disintegration of the living part of the tooth—resulting in the formation of "cavities."

Dental caries causes no symptoms during the early stages of decay, but when the living zones of the tooth are affected toothache results. The affected teeth eventually become visibly decayed and discolored.

Dental caries is a disease of modern Western man; the major cause is dietary. There are many relevant differences between a primitive unrefined diet and what most people eat today. But the most important is the consumption of refined sugar (sucrose), which adheres to the surface of teeth and encourages the growth of the bacteria which damage the teeth. The combination of sucrose, food debris and bacteria is known as *dental plaque*, which covers the area where caries develops. Sticky sweet foods are more likely to adhere to the teeth than granular ones; the more frequently the food is eaten, the worse the effects.

Almost all Westerners have some caries, but their frequency and severity can be reduced by avoiding sweet foods, by regular use of a toothbrush and dental floss to remove plaque, by fluoridation of the water supply, by the direct application of fluoride to the teeth as paints or in toothpaste, and by more modern techniques such as *fissure sealing*. Regular inspection by a dentist and the use of *disclosing tablets* help to reveal areas of plaque.

The development of caries can be arrested but not reversed; thus, preventive care as well as proper treatment of the resulting cavities are essential. If left untreated dental caries destroy teeth completely, with the added risk of serious infection (osteomyelitis) of the jawbones.

carpal tunnel syndrome

The symptoms resulting from compression of a large nerve (the *median nerve*) as it passes through the tendinous "tunnel" in the wrist.

The carpal tunnel syndrome is fairly common. Symptoms include numbness, tingling and burning pain in the part of the hand supplied by the median nerve—that is, the thumb, index finger, middle finger and part of the ring finger. The symptoms typically first occur at night, often waking the patient; later they may also be experienced during the day and interfere with normal use of the hand. In advanced cases the thumb becomes quite weak.

The condition is seen in women more than men and is often a problem in pregnancy, although it disappears after delivery in nearly all cases. Sometimes there may be a demonstrable cause, such as acromegaly, myxedema, or arthritis; symptoms are often made worse by activities such as gardening, knitting, or typing. The common factor is *pressure on the median nerve* as it passes beneath a bridge of tough, tendinous tissue

CARPAL TUNNEL SYNDROME

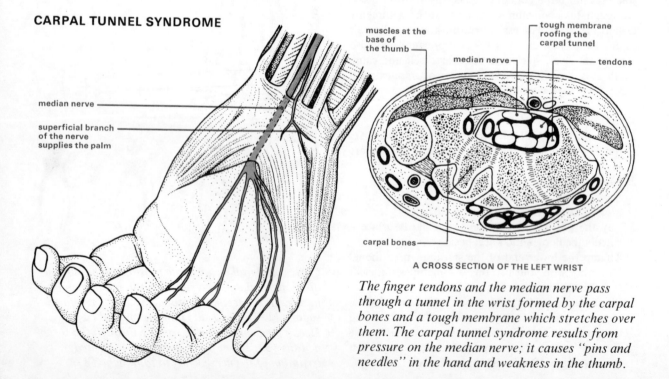

median nerve

superficial branch
of the nerve
supplies the palm

muscles at the
base of
the thumb

median nerve

tough membrane
roofing the
carpal tunnel

tendons

carpal bones

A CROSS SECTION OF THE LEFT WRIST

The finger tendons and the median nerve pass through a tunnel in the wrist formed by the carpal bones and a tough membrane which stretches over them. The carpal tunnel syndrome results from pressure on the median nerve; it causes "pins and needles" in the hand and weakness in the thumb.

underlying the skin creases at the wrist. Swelling of any of the other structures that pass through this "carpal tunnel" will compress the nerve.

The diagnosis is usually obvious, but if necessary it can be confirmed by special nerve conduction studies. Mild cases are relieved by rest or by splinting the wrist at night. Sometimes local injections of cortisone-type steroid drugs into the wrist will cure the condition; as a rule they at least produce some relief of the pain. The most effective and permanent treatment, however, is a minor surgical operation to reduce pressure in the carpal tunnel by dividing the wrist ligaments which lie above it.

cartilage

A tough, dense, elastic tissue which—together with bone—constitutes one of two main skeletal tissues of the body. Mature cartilage contains no blood supply of its own, but obtains nutrients for its living cells from the surrounding tissue fluids. (In meat, it is called "gristle.")

In the developing human embryo, the skeleton is formed of cartilage which is eventually transformed into bone by the process of *ossification* (the deposition of calcium within the cartilage). At this stage the cartilage is penetrated by small branching canals containing blood vessels. Cartilage persists until adolescence in the rapidly growing regions of the skeleton, and in particular at the ends of long bones (as *epiphyseal plates*). In adults, cartilage is restricted mainly to the frontal ends of the ribs (*costal cartilage*), the surfaces of joints, and certain areas outside of the skeletal system— such as the rim of the ear, in the nose, and in the respiratory passages (especially in the trachea and larynx).

The cartilage on the surfaces of most joints (articular cartilage) acts to reduce friction. The low "friction coefficient" of cartilage (three times more slippery than one ice cube moving across another) aids joint movement; it also has a cushioning effect.

Pads of cartilage mixed with tough fibrous tissue (fibrocartilage) are found as intervertebral disks between the bones of the spine. Fibrocartilage pads are also found in the knee, called "semilunar cartilages" because of their half-moon shape. These are sometimes injured in contact sports and have to be surgically removed (see MENISECTOMY).

Cartilage is occasionally the site of a benign tumor (CHONDROMA) or a malignant tumor (chondrosarcoma).

See also CHONDROCALCINOSIS and CHONDROMALACIA.

catabolism

The breaking down of complex chemical substances into

CARTILAGE OF THE KNEE

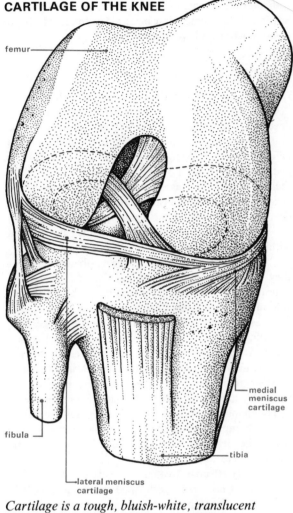

femur

medial meniscus cartilage

fibula

tibia

lateral meniscus cartilage

Cartilage is a tough, bluish-white, translucent material. Its perfect smoothness facilitates movement at joints. Thus at the knee, the contacting ends of the femur and tibia are covered with a thin layer of cartilage. In addition two crescent-shaped plates of cartilage, the menisci, help the bones to fit together snugly.

simpler ones by the living cells of the body, with the release of energy.

Catabolism occurs in all living cells, side by side with ANABOLISM (building up processes). The two processes in combination are known as METABOLISM.

The energy released in catabolism is used in maintaining body temperature, movement and other functions, as well as in the synthetic (anabolic) processes involved in energy storage, growth and repair.

The normal adult has a net equilibrium of catabolism and anabolism and is said to be in "metabolic balance." In severe illnesses, such as SEPTICEMIA, the patient may enter a "hypercatabolic state" in which catabolism predominates and the body tissues are broken down with a resulting rapid loss of weight. Unless this process is stopped with appropriate medical treatment it leads to severe wasting and eventually death.

cataract

An opacity in the lens of the eye causing defective vision.

Cataracts may be present in one or both eyes and may develop at any age. Fully developed cataracts cause BLINDNESS, but initially the symptoms include spots before the eyes (which do not move and can thus be distinguished from normal "floaters"), short sight (helped at first by glasses) and gradually diminishing vision. Cataracts do not cause pain or discomfort. Fully developed cataracts at birth may prevent the normal development of visual ability unless they are treated within a few months.

Cataracts in childhood may have no obvious cause or they may be caused by syphilis, German measles or abnormally low levels of calcium in the blood (hypocalcemia) in the mother during pregnancy.

Cataracts may also result from injury to the lens, including injury by heat or ionizing radiation. In adult life, cataracts occur in patients with diabetes but they are most common in the elderly (senile cataracts)—where they are considered to be an extreme case of the inevitable hardening of the lens that occurs with age.

The change that occurs in the lens in cases of cataract can be compared with the change that occurs in egg white when it is cooked. (Its protein is "denatured" and the opacity cannot be reversed.)

The only effective treatment is surgical. Operations for cataract have been performed as long ago as 1000 B.C. The modern operation for cataract extraction is a direct development of one first described in 1752.

The opaque lens is removed through the front of the eye under local or general anesthesia. Complications are

CATARACT

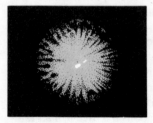
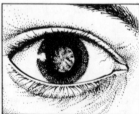

early cataract seen with an ophthalmoscope

mature senile cataract

A cataract is any opacity in the lens of the eye. Most cataracts are associated with aging ("senile cataract") and are present in both eyes, leading to progressively blurred vision and eventual blindness. However, surgical removal of the lens improves sight in over 90% of cases.

fairly uncommon and it is no longer necessary to wait until the patient is nearly blind before operating. It is safe to operate on both eyes at the same time, when necessary. Modern anesthesia has made the operation safe in many elderly patients who previously would have been considered unsuitable.

There is no possibility of recurrence in the same eye after the operation, but the patient needs an aid to vision in the absence of his own lens. Special glasses are commonly used but they may produce confusing visual images. Contact lenses—especially modern soft lenses worn permanently—give better results. Another alternative is the implantation of an artificial lens within the eye (an intraocular lens implant), but this is not always possible.

catarrh

A popular (not strictly medical) term for inflammation of the air passages of the nose and throat.

The symptoms under the general heading "catarrh" vary according to what the patient means by the word, but they usually include one or more of the following: a blocked nose, a runny nose, facial discomfort due to sinusitis, hearing difficulty due to obstruction, sore throat and a cough.

This range of symptoms may be caused by a number of nose and throat diseases, the most common of which is infection—especially the common cold and sinusitis. Allergy is also a common cause, while rarer possibilities are a deviated septum or nasal polyps.

Treatment depends on the exact cause. There is no cure for the common cold, although nasal symptoms may be relieved by the vasoconstrictor drugs (such as ephedrine) contained in many "cold cures" and nose drops. While these proprietary drugs are useful for short periods of symptomatic relief, they should not be used for long because they can damage the lining of the nose.

Sinusitis may need antibiotic treatment and sometimes surgical drainage of the affected sinuses.

Allergic causes of catarrh may sometimes be overcome by DESENSITIZATION or by removal of the allergen. Alternatively. drug treatment with vasoconstrictors or cortisone-like steriods may help in the short term.

A deviated nasal septum (wrong positioning of the cartilage that separates the nostrils) and nasal polyps can be treated surgically if necessary.

In general, however, what people describe as catarrh is a simple and harmless infection which disappears rapidly without any treatment. The term "catarrh" is becoming obsolete, although the signs and symptoms represented are generally referred to under the medical phrase *chronic rhinitis*.

catatonia

A combination of mute withdrawal and abnormalities of movement and posture, found in some forms of schizophrenia.

The patient may be completely immobile and remain in any position in which his body is placed (a state known as *flexibilitas cerea*). For example, if his arm is lifted above his head he may leave it there until it is again moved for him. He may also obey verbal orders to move his body to an uncomfortable posture or he may precisely imitate the movements of another person.

Long-continued repetition of a meaningless word or phrase or the same movement (*perseveration*) is also common—for example, repeated eating motions with a knife and fork long after the food is finished. In extreme forms of catatonia the stupor may be extreme enough for there to be complete unresponsiveness, with failure to eat and drink (often necessitating tube feeding) and incontinence or retention of urine and feces. Such a phase may last from a few hours to several days.

The cause of catatonia—like that of schizophrenia—is unknown. Treatment is directed at the underlying schizophrenia and may include drugs, electroconvulsive therapy (see ECT), or psychotherapy.

catheter

A tube used to introduce fluids into or withdraw them from any of the body cavities or passages.

Early catheters were rigid and usually made of metal. The development of rubber and plastic catheters over the past few decades has greatly extended their uses.

Many catheters with special uses are now available—there is at least one specially made catheter for every space in the body. Some of the more common ones are as follows:

Urethral catheters are inserted through the urethra into the bladder to drain urine in cases of urethral obstruction (for example, when caused by an enlarged prostate gland). They are also needed in certain other medical and surgical situations, such as kidney failure or following gynecological surgery. Most patients require urethral catheters for only a short period, but patients with a paralyzed bladder may need permanent catheterization.

Intravenous catheters (or "cannulas") are inserted into a vein to take blood or administer fluids and drugs.

Cardiac catheters are passed via arteries and veins to the heart to measure cardiac function. Cardiac catheterization is often a routine preliminary to HEART SURGERY.

Vascular catheters of other kinds may be used—for example, to remove blood clots from the femoral and pelvic veins.

A *peritoneal dialysis catheter* is inserted through the abdominal wall into the peritoneal cavity to allow exchanges of fluid necessary for peritoneal DIALYSIS.

A *nasogastric tube* is a catheter passed via the nose to the stomach for the administration or removal of fluid.

An *epidural catheter* is used for the administration of anesthetics into the subarachnoid space surrounding the spinal cord during childbirth.

caudal anesthesia

An anesthetic injection into the lower back, especially used during CHILDBIRTH to produce painfree labor. (It is distinguished from *spinal anesthesia* in that the injection is made not into the dura, the outermost of the three membranes that surround the spinal cord, but into the "epidural space.")

Sensory nerves carrying pain impulses run from the uterus, vagina and perineal area (between the vagina and anus) to the spinal cord. Fortunately these nerves are much more sensitive to local anesthetic drugs than are the motor nerves which control movement in the same area. It is therefore possible to deaden the pain of childbirth while at the same time allowing muscle contraction and movement.

The spinal cord, which runs through the bony hole in the center of the vertebrae, is surrounded by a white membranous coat called the *dura*. The space between this coat and the vertebral bone (the *epidural space*) contains nerves running to and from the spinal cord, together with fatty tissues and blood vessels. An anesthetic injected into this space numbs pain sensations.

The injection is sometimes given near the beginning of labor at the stage when contractions start to become very painful. The woman usually lies on her side with her knees drawn up to her chin. The injection may be given by an anesthesiologist or by the obstetrician. With great care he inserts a needle between two vertebrae into the epidural space. He then pushes a fine tube, or catheter, through the needle into the space and withdraws the needle. The anesthetic drug is then injected through the tube. Its effect lasts for about two hours, after which it may be reinjected if necessary.

With some patients the injection may fail or may not be completely effective, sometimes for technical reasons. However, it is completely effective for about 90% of patients. The chief complications are a fall in blood pressure in about 5%, but this is easily corrected. Some women experience temporary sensations of heaviness or weakness in the legs after the anesthetic has worn off.

Epidural injections are expensive and time-consuming. Although many women can manage quite well without them, for difficult or prolonged labor they have been welcomed.

causalgia

A chronic, severe, burning pain of the skin that may occur after partial injury to a nerve. It occurs most often in the palm of the hand (after damage to the median nerve) or the foot (after sciatic nerve injury), although it may affect any part of the body. The pain is usually continuous and is often aggravated by pressure on the affected skin, which is typically shiny, thin and hairless. There may be excessive sweating, and the affected hand or foot is often abnormally cool. Ultimately, the muscles and bones in the area may waste away (atrophy) from lack of use.

The condition is common after gunshot wounds, traffic accidents and industrial injuries. It may also occur in patients with peripheral neuropathy (disease of the outlying nerves). Relief may be given by the application of local ice packs and by analgesics (pain-killers) and sedatives. The symptoms often improve without treatment, but in longstanding cases they may be suppressed by surgical division of the nerve fibers concerned.

cautery

The use of an agent to burn or destroy tissue. The term may also mean the agent used.

The main use of cautery is to prevent unwanted bleeding during surgical operations. Bleeding from small cut vessels can usually be stopped by cautery, thus obviating the need to tie off many vessels (which would delay the operation).

The most simple form of cautery is heat applied by a hot piece of metal, but this is seldom used in modern medicine. In surgery, cautery is usually achieved by an electric current which heats the tissues and produces hemostasis (localized arrest of blood flow). Electrocautery is also used for *surgical diathermy*, a common technique in which a heated blade is used to cut tissue, ensuring hemostasis as it cuts.

Extreme cold may also be used for cautery. Electrically cooled probes are used routinely in delicate operations (for example, in the eye) to destroy tissue by freezing. Cryocautery (cold cautery) may also be achieved by liquid nitrogen or solid carbon dioxide, as in the destruction of skin warts.

Chemocautery involves the use of caustic chemicals and is another technique used to destroy skin lesions.

celiac disease

A disease in which the small intestine fails to absorb fats, vitamins and other nutrients.

Although the condition was originally described in children, it is now clear that there is an adult counterpart ("nontropical sprue") which is probably common, though sometimes mild.

In the childhood form of the disease a previously healthy child loses weight, passes foul-smelling loose stools, and becomes irritable—usually at the age of six to nine months and always after solid feeding has started. Later the child's abdomen protrudes, his limbs waste, and ANEMIA and RICKETS may develop as the result of iron and vitamin deficiencies.

Adult celiac disease may develop at any age. Foul-smelling stools which are difficult to flush away (because they are frothy and light) are a prominent symptom; in addition weight loss, wasting and anemia often occur.

Celiac disease is caused by sensitivity to *gluten*, a protein found in wheat, rye and other grain. This was discovered during World War II, when it was noted that Dutch children with celiac disease improved when bread was unavailable. In some unknown way gluten leads to damage (fortunately reversible) in the lining of the small intestine, which results in the malabsorption of food.

Diagnosis usually involves BIOPSY of the lining of the small intestine by swallowing a small capsule on the end of a flexible tube. The treatment is to avoid all foods containing gluten. Special gluten-free flour, pasta and other foods are available. The restricted diet should probably be continued for life, but this is not yet certain. Vitamin supplements are required until the intestine has recovered.

Untreated celiac disease may lead to total wasting and eventual death, although milder forms of the disease are common. Treatment restores normal health. There is an increased risk of intestinal cancer in patients with this disease, but this is not great and the overall prognosis following the initiation of treatment is good.

cell

The functional unit of which all animals and plants are composed.

The human body contains an astronomical number of cells. The brain alone has billions of cells, and the total number of red cells in the blood is around 30 trillion (an average of 5 million in every cubic millimeter). Cells are quite variable in their size and shape. The average cell is around 7 microns (millionths of a meter) in diameter, but some are much smaller. Nerve cells are characteristically long and thin; in fact, some single nerve fibers stretch from the spinal cord to the tips of the toes.

A typical cell is composed of a *nucleus* (containing the genetic material DNA) and *cytoplasm* (which contains the enzymes necessary to translate the genetic information stored in the DNA into chemical action).

The cytoplasm contains a number of "organelles" in which the various metabolic processes are organized.

CELL

A GENERALIZED CELL

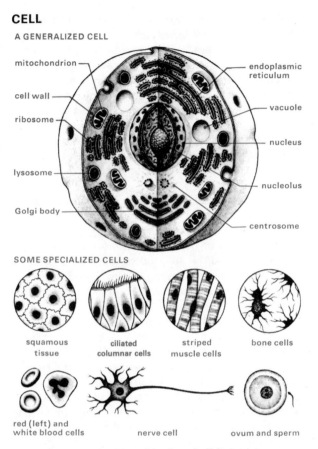

mitochondrion

cell wall

ribosome

lysosome

Golgi body

endoplasmic reticulum

vacuole

nucleus

nucleolus

centrosome

SOME SPECIALIZED CELLS

squamous tissue

ciliated columnar cells

striped muscle cells

bone cells

red (left) and white blood cells

nerve cell

ovum and sperm

Cells form the building blocks of all living tissue. Essentially, they consist of a sac of fluid enclosed by a membrane. Floating in the cell are smaller membranous sacs, or organelles, such as mitochondria and ribosomes, which are the sites of specialized activity. The varied shapes of the cells in the lower part of the drawing show how they adapt to perform many different jobs.

These can be clearly identified with the electron microscope and include the ribosomes, endoplasmic reticulum, mitochondria and lysosomes. The cytoplasm is surrounded by the cell membrane.

The internal environment of the cell is remarkably constant and differs greatly from the surrounding tissue fluid. This difference is maintained by active processes in the cell membrane. These processes, together with the other metabolic activities necessary for life, require a continuing supply of energy in the form of oxygen and nutrients.

All the cells in the body are derived by division from the original fertilized ovum. As the embryo develops, cells take on specialized functions; most remain capable of division in the event of injury. Nerve cells have no such potential, and mature red blood cells have lost their nuclei and are simply envelopes of cytoplasm. Most cells

are capable of regeneration if they are partially injured.

The study of individual types of cells has contributed to medical understanding of abnormalities in many diseases, including cancer and metabolic disorders.

cellulitis

A severe inflammation of the tissues just beneath the skin or certain deeper structures (such as the connective tissue that surrounds the uterus). The inflammation, usually caused by bacterial infection, typically spreads through the tissues producing sheets of pus.

In addition to the local pain and discomfort, toxins (poisons) released by the infection produce high fever and a general feeling of being unwell (malaise). The infecting bacteria probably enter the skin through a small scratch or wound.

ERYSIPELAS, in which there is little pus but the skin is raw, red, and painful, is a form of cellulitis caused by a specific streptococcus (*Streptococcus pyogenes*). It is usually cured by penicillin or similar antibiotics.

The bacteria that cause cellulitis are spread by the small lymph vessels. Patients with lymphatics blocked by disease or with congenital blockage of the lymph system are at particular risk of recurrent cellulitis.

cephalohematoma

A swelling on the head of a newborn baby, caused by bleeding under the membrane (pericranium) covering the bones of the skull. It is usually on one side of the head, but it may appear on both sides over the forehead or at the back of the head.

A cephalohematoma becomes obvious on the second or third day of life, when the normal molding of the head produced by birth disappears. It is soft and fluid-filled, and its borders are fixed to the edges of the affected bone. In about a week the rim of the swelling hardens and the softer center becomes depressed. At that stage it appears like a skull fracture, which may at first confuse the diagnosis.

A cephalohematoma needs no treatment, since it disappears completely within weeks or months. Attempts to aspirate it carry the risk of infection.

cerebral embolism

Embolism occurs when part of a blood clot, formed in a major artery or in the heart itself, separates and is carried by the circulation to a smaller artery. It lodges there, closing off the blood supply to the tissues beyond. Cerebral embolism—embolism in a blood vessel of the brain—can occur in patients whose cerebral blood vessels are otherwise normal.

When it happens in people aged under 50 years, there

is usually some heart disorder such as RHEUMATIC HEART DISEASE, or a "dead" segment of heart wall (myocardial infarction) following a heart attack.

In older patients, cerebral embolism may be a consequence of the breakup of areas of severe fatty degeneration of the aorta (the main artery leading from the heart) or its branches to the brain.

Emboli may be large, causing the catastrophic and irreversible changes of STROKE in which the brain tissue dies through lack of oxygen and nutrients. Small emboli, which pass briefly through the circulation, may cause transient symptoms such as dizziness or lapses of consciousness, without leaving permanent damage. These small emboli, collections of blood platelets or cholesterol crystals, may sometimes be seen during a medical examination passing along the blood vessels in the eyes of patients with such attacks.

Infected cerebral emboli may arise in patients with lung or heart infections, such as pneumonia and endocarditis, resulting in brain abscess and localized encephalitis.

The onset of illness in cerebral embolism is sudden. There is often a headache for a few hours before the signs of neurologic damage arise, such as paralysis or loss of feeling. Sometimes the illness starts with convulsions, which may be localized to a particular group of muscles before becoming generalized. About one quarter of patients become unconscious for some minutes, then return to consciousness in a confused state.

How much damage remains depends upon the site and size of the embolus. Embolism can occur in any major artery in the brain, so that residual damage varies from patient to patient.

Cerebral embolism is a minor cause of stroke. In a review of 873 stroke patients without cerebral hemorrhage in a large hospital, 8% were ascribed to cerebral embolism. The others were caused by blood clotting in the cerebral arteries themselves.

See also EMBOLISM/EMBOLUS.

cerebral hemorrhage

Leakage of blood inside the brain.

Cerebral hemorrhage is very serious, carrying a high death rate, and is the cause of about one in ten of all sudden circulatory disorders in the brain. Although its causes vary, the symptoms always follow the same pattern, arising from increased pressure within the skull and death of brain cells.

Cerebral hemorrhage starts with a sudden, very severe headache—much more intense than other headaches—which often extends to the neck and back. For a short initial period the patient may be able to feel the pain in one particular place, such as the front, back, or one side

of the head. This localization can be helpful in detecting the site of the lesion, as the pain quickly spreads throughout the head. Next, to add to the headache, come dizziness, vomiting, sweating and shivering, then progression from drowsiness to stupor and unconsciousness. In mild cases the patient recovers consciousness, but for many days or even weeks afterwards there is lethargy, clouding of intellect, confusion or delirium.

In the first 72 hours after the cerebral hemorrhage, the accumulation of blood around the surfaces of the brain and spinal cord leads to irritation of nerves and stiffness of the neck muscles.

At the same time, the brain damage causes various disturbances: unequal pupils, squint, paralysis, and loss of sensation. Fever lasts for several days.

Examination of the CEREBROSPINAL FLUID reveals traces of blood in 80% of patients with cerebral hemorrhage. The discovery of this blood rules out cerebral embolism or thrombosis as the cause of symptoms.

Most cerebral hemorrhages arise from a ruptured artery. In younger patients the most common cause is "berry" aneurysms—small balloonings of thinned arterial walls—usually on the system of arteries lying at the base of the brain. The aneurysms appear to form at points of weakness in the arterial wall which develop after infancy. Other causes of arterial rupture include high blood pressure, congenital abnormalities of the arteries and tumors involving the blood vessels.

cerebral palsy

Any disturbance of function of the muscular system associated with a congenital defect of the brain or birth injury. The term covers a wide range of disabilities, including paralysis of the muscles, inability to coordinate their movements and the occurrence of involuntary movements in an otherwise normal person.

Cerebral palsy affects two children in every thousand. Most cases are due to birth injury, either from instrumental or obstructed delivery or from lack of oxygen during labor or birth. Other causes include developmental defects of the brain, maternal infection during pregnancy, RHEUMATIC HEART DISEASE and JAUNDICE in the first few days of life. A quarter of all cases start in infancy, after a brain infection, thrombosis, embolus or injury. The condition is more common in first babies, particularly boys.

Patients may be hemiplegic—that is, with spastic paralysis (muscular rigidity accompanying partial paralysis) and poor growth of one side of the body. Arms are more severely affected than legs and the children walk with a "scissors" gait. Mental impairment sometimes occurs.

Forms of cerebral palsy with ATAXIA (awkwardness

of movement) vary from minor clumsiness to severe difficulties with coordination and balance. Such children may be of normal or even high intelligence. "Dyskinetic" patients are affected by involuntary muscle movements and changing muscle tone, which disappear only during sleep.

The outlook for the child with cerebral palsy depends on his reponse to help in overcoming the disability.

Physiotherapy, speech and behavior therapy, and mechanical aids may be useful.

cerebrospinal fluid

The clear, colorless fluid surrounding the brain and spinal cord and filling the spaces and channels (ventricles and aqueducts) within them. It is examined in the diagnosis of certain diseases.

Most of the cerebrospinal fluid (CSF) is formed in the ventricles of the brain from tufts of tiny blood vessels in their walls, called *choroid plexuses*. The CSF flows out over the surface of the brain through openings just above the base of the skull, and is later reabsorbed into the venous system by tongue-like processes. Some CSF flows downwards, within and around the spinal cord, and out into the nerve lymphatics. The CSF acts as a "water cushion" between the brain and skull and between the spinal cord and vertebrae.

CSF has a similar density to water. In a healthy person it is alkaline, almost protein-free, totally free of red blood cells, and with very few white blood cells. Its content of salts (such as sodium, chloride, bicarbonate and potassium) is similar to that of the blood.

Examination of CSF taken by needle from the lower back (*lumbar puncture*) or neck (*cysternal puncture*), helps in the diagnosis of neurologic disease. CSF pressure and protein levels may be raised in cancer; blood may be present in cerebrovascular disorders; white cells and bacteria are found in meningitis.

cerebrovascular disease

Any disorder of the circulation of blood in the brain. The most common is disease of the blood vessel wall or clotting of the blood within the vessels.

Cerebrovascular disease is responsible for over 80,000 deaths in Great Britain each year and many more people suffer from some of the effects of the disease. Attacks are likely to recur and those who survive are often permanently disabled and dependent on others.

The symptoms of paralysis, numbness, apathy and loss of intellect or memory arise from a reduction of the oxygen supply to the brain cells.

See also APOPLEXY, CEREBRAL HEMORRHAGE, CEREBRAL EMBOLISM, STROKE.

CEREBROSPINAL FLUID (CSF)

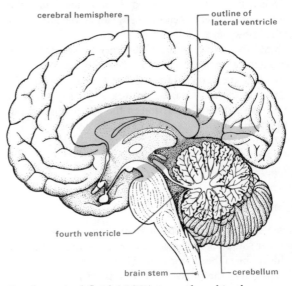

Cerebrospinal fluid (CSF) is produced in the ventricles of the brain. It escapes through openings in the roof of the fourth ventricle to bathe the surface of the brain and spinal cord. If the flow of CSF through the ventricles is blocked, pressure builds up leading to the condition of hydrocephalus. The composition of CSF changes in meningitis and certain other diseases.

cerumen

The technical name for EARWAX.

cervical smear

A test in which the cells on the surface of the neck of the womb (cervix) are gently removed and examined microscopically. It was pioneered by Dr. George Papanicolaou (1883–1962) and is sometimes called a "Pap smear" or "Pap test."

Smear tests were originally aimed at early identification of cancer of the cervix—the second most common cancer in women after breast cancer—and this is still the main use of the technique. But its value has spread to include assessments of hormone imbalance in menstrual and menopausal disorders, infections and other nonmalignant changes in the tissues.

The technique is simple and painless and can be performed quickly without sedation or anesthesia. It has been adopted for mass screening of populations in developed countries, where experts in analyzing the smears are readily available. The tissues may be sucked into a round nozzled glass pipette (the original Papanicolaou method) or scraped away with a smooth wooden spatula. The latter is more likely to detect cancer cells, but is less useful for hormone studies.

When the material obtained is examined under the microscope, potential cancer cells can be detected by a skilled observer.

Since its first use in the 1940s, cervical smear testing has enabled doctors to prevent the onset and spread of cancer of the cervix. Detection and treatment of the disease in the early stages, before symptoms arise, has led to a significant reduction in the death rate among apparently healthy women. The test is advised for women entering their late twenties or early thirties, and for younger women whose family or personal history puts them at special risk.

Cesarean section

The delivery of a child through an incision made in the mother's abdomen, named after Julius Caesar who was said to have been born in this manner. For a full discussion of the subject see CHILDBIRTH.

Chagas' disease

An infectious disease caused by a species of parasitic protozoa (*Trypanosoma cruzi*). The disease (also known as *South American trypanosomiasis*) affects more than seven million people in Central and South America.

The infecting protozoa are transmitted to man by the bite of certain species of blood-sucking bugs known as *reduviids*, which are often found in the cracked walls of mud houses or in the thatch on the roofs. They deposit their contaminated feces on the skin of their victims, who then scratch the area and permit the protozoa to gain entrance to the body through the resulting abrasion.

The parasites eventually enter the blood circulation. Many of them are carried to the heart, where they invade the heart muscle (myocardium). As they undergo developmental changes they can cause inflammation of the heart muscle (MYOCARDITIS). In this stage of the disease there may be enlargement of the heart and eventual HEART FAILURE. Severe damage can also be caused if the parasites migrate to the digestive system, with consequent dilation of the esophagus, stomach and small and large intestine.

There is no specific treatment as yet for Chagas' disease, although research is being conducted into the possibility of developing an effective vaccine. Drugs are not available which can remove the parasites from the heart muscle and other tissues, but some drugs are effective in eliminating them from the blood circulation. Preventive measures involve control of the bugs that spread the disease (by means of insecticides) and improved domestic hygiene.

Compare AFRICAN TRYPANOSOMIASIS.

chalazion (meibomian cyst)

A cyst of the eyelid.

Chalazion is caused by blockage of an oil-secreting (sebaceous) gland in the eyelid (also known as a *meibomian gland*). The gland slowly enlarges, producing a lump in the eyelid which is more of a nuisance and a disfigurement than a source of pain or discomfort. Small chalazia are often not noticed until the finger is run over the eyelid. Everting the eyelid reveals a purple or red discoloration over the surface of the chalazion in the early stages, which later turns gray.

Pressure building up within the cyst may force the extrusion of the contents through the inner surface of the eyelid, giving rise to a chronic irritating discharge from the eye. If the gland becomes infected the swelling may be red and painful with a yellowish discharge. In *marginal chalazion* the inflammation affects only the duct of the gland.

The treatment is surgical removal of the cyst. There is no need for dressings or stitches.

chancroid

A sexually transmitted disease caused by infection with a bacterium called *Hemophilus ducreyi*. This germ is thought to enter the genitalia through a minor abrasion during sexual intercourse.

The first sign of chancroid, often not noticed by the patient, is a small pustule appearing on the external genital organs a few days after the contact. The pustule enlarges and erodes deeply into the tissues; it then bursts, leaving a shallow, painful purulent (pus-filled) ulcer with an irregular edge.

The center of the ulcer usually remains soft, a characteristic which distinguishes it from the firmly based chancre of syphilis. The ulcer is usually about 2 cm (less than an inch) in diameter and its base commonly settles to a clean granular appearance. But neglect and further infection with other bacteria may lead to destruction of the tissues and even gangrene.

Chancroid in women may lead to ulcers covering the genitalia, perineum and anus. (The perineum is the area between the opening of the vagina and the anus.) In men the ulcer is usually confined to the shaft of the penis rather than the tip. The disease may be caught from people who have no sign of it themselves but are "carriers" of the bacteria.

A common complication of chancroid, particularly in men, is painful swollen lymph glands in the groin. These may become greatly enlarged, rupture, and discharge foul pus (which may infect other areas of skin by contact).

A 10- to 20-day course of antibiotics such as tetracycline or sulfonamides usually cures chancroid.

cheilitis

Inflammation of the lips.

The lips, being particularly sensitive and often in contact with various irritants, are subject to inflammation—even when there is no inflammation in other organs.

In acute cheilitis the lips become swollen, tender and painful. In chronic cheilitis they are dry, cracked and peel easily. Patients with chronic cheilitis often pull or bite pieces of inflamed skin, thereby increasing the irritation and inflammation. As the lips become dry, cracked and sore, many patients resort to frequent licking in an attempt to ease the discomfort. Some cases of cheilitis are of nervous origin.

Cheilitis can be caused by allergy to chemicals in lipsticks, dentifrices, perfumes, and—particularly in young children—food. Deep fissures from chronic cheilitis may be persistent and annoying. "Splints" of gauze treated with collodion may be applied to them.

People with protruding lower lips constantly exposed to sunlight may develop "actinic" cheilitis, a condition which may later develop into cancer.

"Cold sore," or herpes simplex infection of the lip, is a common form of cheilitis. Repeated herpes attacks occur in the same places on the lip, suggesting that there may be a dormant virus which is reactivated at intervals, leaving minimal scarring. Such attacks are often precipitated by sunburn or fever. Nibbling at warts on the fingers may transfer the virus to the lips in warty cheilitis.

chest pain

Pain in the chest is a common complaint—so common, in fact, that it is mostly disregarded. Often only persistent or severe pains bring a patient to the doctor.

The pain may be a symptom of a potentially serious heart disease, or it may represent a relatively minor condition such as "heartburn" (pyrosis) brought on by the overindulgence in food or alcohol. In other cases a person may be unduly concerned about his or her heart and develop an anxiety state in which chest pains are experienced, or said to be experienced, without any physical cause (a condition known as *cardiac neurosis*).

Chest pain may arise from any of the organs in the chest or the upper part of the abdomen, or it may be "referred" from disease of the spine. A thorough physical examination, plus certain tests (which may include an electrocardiogram—a tracing of the electrical activity of the heart) will help in the diagnosis.

Most people when they suffer severe pain in the chest fear heart disease, and most physicians will first try to exclude the possibility of heart disease before they consider an alternative diagnosis. Pain that actually arises from the heart is produced by *ischemia* of the heart muscle—that is, a deficiency of the heart's blood supply brought about by disease of the coronary arteries (see ANGINA PECTORIS).

Peptic ulcers and gallbladder disease may both produce pain referred to the lower part of the chest, often associated with mealtimes. HIATUS HERNIA can cause pain or discomfort behind the sternum (breastbone).

In the process of making his diagnosis, the physician may wish to keep the patient at rest until his investigations are complete, rather than find too late that he is dealing with a condition that should have been treated with rest from the start.

Pain from the respiratory apparatus may be central, arising from the trachea ("windpipe") as a result of infection by viruses or bacteria, or it may be on the side—arising, for example, from inflammation of the membranes that cover the lungs (PLEURISY). Chest pain may be a consequence of lung inflammation secondary to pneumonia or it may be associated with a tumor of the lung; in such cases the pain is made worse during breathing in.

Occasionally, pain in the chest is caused by PNEUMOTHORAX or PULMONARY EMBOLISM, both conditions being accompanied by breathlessness. The skin of the chest may be affected by HERPES ZOSTER (shingles), a painful inflammation of the sensory nerves—characterized by blistering of the skin along the line of the nerve (in the case of the chest, one of the *intercostal nerves* which run around the body below each rib). In a number of cases no cause for chest pain can be found, and the physician may attribute it to "psychogenic tension."

In all cases, treatment of chest pain is directed at the underlying condition. Symptomatic relief can be given with analgesics such as aspirin or other drugs.

chickenpox

A highly infectious but rarely serious disease of childhood caused by the herpes virus. Also called *varicella*.

Chickenpox most commonly affects children during the early school years (between the ages of 5 and 10) and usually occurs in limited outbreaks in the winter and spring. It rarely attacks infants in the first six months of life, or adults. One attack virtually ensures permanent protection against future infections.

Chickenpox is passed on by close contact with a patient in the first week of the rash. The incubation period of 14 to 21 days is followed by a short period when the child feels generally unwell, perhaps with a mild fever and headache. Crops of spots appear during the next five days. They are thickest on the trunk and face and relatively sparse on the limbs. Some may appear inside the mouth and throat.

The rash develops from pink, flat spots into tiny single blisters which become dry and encrusted within two to four days. During the blister, or "vesicle," stage the patient is highly infectious, although he may not appear to be particularly unwell.

The rash often itches severely and younger children are strongly tempted to scratch. Scratching should always be discouraged because it can lead to bacterial infection of the skin and the subsequent formation of scars ("pockmarks"). Hygienic measures—such as close cutting and frequent cleaning of fingernails, and daily baths—are also useful in preventing infection.

Crusts may be removed from the skin by compresses or the use of carbolized oil. Once the last crop of blisters has become dry and encrusted, the patient is no longer a source of infection. There is no specific treatment for the disease. As a rule it is self-limiting and resolves completely with no adverse effects. Exceptions to that rule are children with leukemia or who are taking cortisone-like steroid drugs, who may develop pneumonia or liver problems. Chickenpox pneumonia may occur in adults, leaving many small lung scars which are seen on chest x rays after the illness has cleared up.

The virus that causes chickenpox is the same as the one that causes HERPES ZOSTER (shingles). In fact, shingles—a disease mainly of adults—is thought to arise from reactivation of the virus which has remained dormant in the body since an attack of chickenpox during childhood.

chilblain

Hot, red, swollen patches of intensely itchy skin on the toes, feet, fingers and hands caused by exposure to cold and moisture.

Chilblain affects women and children more than men, especially those who are not well protected from exposure to the cold.

Acute chilblain usually disappears after a few days, but it can become chronic, with dull violet discoloration of the skin and the appearance of painful blisters containing blood-stained fluid. Ulceration may follow. Repeated exposure to cold may produce several areas of chronic chilblain which leave scars on healing.

The disease is much less common in the Northern United States than in parts of Europe with similar cold climates; the more widespread use of central heating in North America helps prevent it.

Prevention of chilblain is easier than cure; the condition hardly ever occurs in people provided with enough warm dry clothing (including gloves and footwear) in the colder seasons. High doses of various vitamins and vasodilators (drugs that dilate blood vessels) have been used in the management of chilblain, but their benefit has not been established.

childbed fever

Another name for PUERPERAL FEVER.

childbirth

The birth of a child, either by way of the vagina (vaginal birth) or by surgical means (*Cesarean section*).

Some 280 days after the beginning of the last menstrual period before conception, the term of pregnancy normally culminates in the birth of a child. While the child is developing in the uterus, the mother can prepare herself for the birth mentally as well as physically. In nearly every community, classes are available for prospective mothers—and fathers—where the mechanism of pregnancy and labor is fully described and discussed. The value of such classes is inestimable, for the knowledge that enables the mother to understand the changes in her body and the events that bring a child into the world can transform an event traditionally associated with anxiety and pain into one of complete fulfillment.

It is possible by using the methods of *psychoprophylaxis*—which teach the physiology and anatomy of childbirth and show the mother how to achieve good muscular relaxation by controlled respiration—to shorten labor, control pain and reduce muscular tension during labor to such an extent that a minimum of medication is needed—or in some cases no medication at all.

The individual mother's needs in the time of pregnancy will vary. Some are more affected emotionally than others, finding relaxation and confidence more difficult to attain. Some find themselves pregnant for the first time; others already have a family, so that preparation for the new birth will include particular attention to the siblings to help them accept the new baby with pleasure rather than jealousy. Increasing attention is now being paid to the manner in which the new arrival is welcomed into the world, for it is recognized that birth can be a traumatic experience to the baby as well as to the mother. The labor ward should ideally be a quiet place, without the glaring lights and sudden noises which contrast so alarmingly with the peace of the womb.

In a normal labor there are three stages. The first stage consists of a series of contractions of the muscles of the uterus to allow the cervix (neck of the uterus) to open. The baby starts to descend through the pelvis during the second stage when its presenting part, usually the back of the head, has passed through the fully opened cervix. At some time during this process the "bag of waters"

CHILDBIRTH

THE THREE STAGES OF LABOR

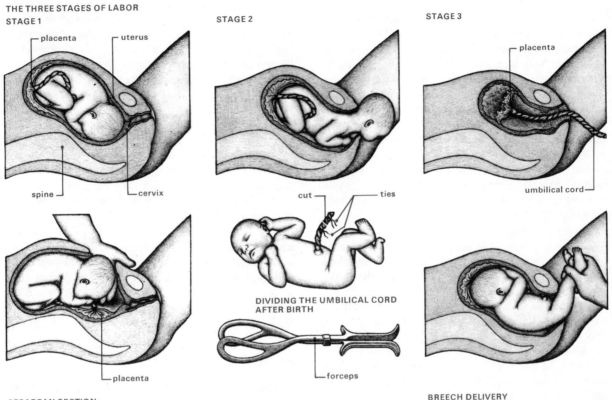

STAGE 1

placenta · uterus

spine · cervix

STAGE 2

cut · ties

DIVIDING THE UMBILICAL CORD
AFTER BIRTH

forceps

STAGE 3

placenta

umbilical cord

placenta

CESAREAN SECTION
(delivery through a
lower abdominal incision)

BREECH DELIVERY
(bottom or feet first)

During Stage 1 of labor, which often lasts as long as 12–16 hours, the cervix or exit from the uterus widens so that the baby can pass through. Stage 2, begins when the cervix is fully open and ends, in under an hour, with the delivery of the baby. Stage 3, expulsion of the placenta and umbilical cord, takes only five minutes. Cesarean section or forceps are sometimes necessary to assist childbirth.

within which the baby lies bursts and the fluid escapes.

After the beginning of the second stage of labor the mother is able to aid the delivery by pushing with her abdominal muscles in time with the frequent pains or contractions of the muscles of the uterus. As the baby's head descends through the pelvis it may press upon nerves, causing pain in the back and legs. Pressure of the head on the vaginal outlet gives a sensation of fullness in the anus and a flattening of the outlet. The appearance of the baby's head at the outlet is called "crowning."

In normal childbirth the nape of the baby's neck rests behind the mother's pubis. With the final push the head is expelled, the neck extending as it does so in order that the narrowest diameter of the skull will pass through the pelvic outlet. The back of the skull is delivered first, then the forehead, face and chin.

During a brief period of rest, the baby's head slowly rotates, to face one thigh. This allows an easy delivery of the shoulders with the next contraction, and the rest of the baby quickly follows. With the baby comes the remainder of the amniotic fluid and a little blood. The womb is now contracted and can be felt through the stomach wall as a firm, ball-shaped mass.

The umbilical cord is tied, clamped and cut. The baby should have gasped and cried on being born. It will be briefly checked by the obstetrician, nurse, or pediatrician, then passed to the cradling arms of the mother (if she is conscious).

When the baby is born it may at first appear quite ugly, with a swollen head, flattened nose and greasy skin. It may be partially covered by the remnants of the *amnion,* the membranous bag of waters which contains the fetus in the womb. But the swelling of the head usually begins to disappear in a matter of hours, and the greasy matter, or *vernix,* which covers the skin—composed of secretions from the sebaceous glands and cells shed from the surface of the skin—if left goes in a day.

Childbirth is not complete until the PLACENTA, or "afterbirth," is delivered, usually 10 to 15 minutes after the baby.

Normal childbirth depends on the infant's head being completely bent down, so that the chin rests on its chest. The blunt apex of the skull, pressing down into the pelvis, helps to open the cervix effectively. The shape of the mother's pelvis guides the head into the position in which the baby is born—facing the mother's back. Approximately one birth in ten occurs with the baby facing forward. Labor in such cases is usually slower, the stronger contractions are needed to bring the head into the lower part of the pelvis. The baby's position is much less flexible and the head is strikingly molded during delivery. Face-to-pubis deliveries are more exhausting for the mother, and the baby is at greater than normal risk of oxygen starvation. However, most infants entering the pelvis in this position rotate spontaneously to the safer backward position.

During a normal labor it is possible for the perineal tissues to be torn as the head passes through the vaginal outlet; the obstetrician often prevents the uncontrolled rupture of tissues by making an incision (EPISIOTOMY) through the stretched perineum extending backward and to the side, for by doing so he can ensure that the tissues part in the line which will make subsequent repair easy and efficient.

The use of obstetrical forceps—instruments designed to enable the obstetrician to guide and help the birth of the baby's head—is sometimes necessary in cases where the second stage of labor has been long, and the mother needs assistance in the birth of the head because she is becoming over-tired or the baby is showing signs of distress. The application of forceps is not as common as it once was, for the modern conduct of maternity cases is planned to avoid the occurrence of complications at birth. When applied properly, forceps do not injure the baby or the mother, and the obstetrician has the choice of a number of different types which are used for different purposes—some to rotate the head and some to apply gentle traction.

The relief of pain and anxiety in childbirth by drugs must be tempered by their effect on the fetus, for drugs administered to the mother will pass into the fetal circulation. Each obstetrician has his own well-tried favorite preparations and techniques. The risks of general anesthesia, particularly for the infant, have led to the use of regional local anesthesia. In the widely used CAUDAL ANESTHESIA, the anesthetic agent is injected into the lower part of the spinal canal outside the membrane (dura mater) which contains the spinal cord and the nerve roots descending from it (cauda equina), so that it anesthetizes the nerve roots as they emerge. Continuous caudal anesthesia ensures analgesia in 90% of patients, who remain alert and cooperative throughout delivery.

In a number of cases the obstetrician will consider that it is dangerous for the baby to be born through the natural birth passages, and will advise delivery by Cesarean section. In such cases an incision is made through the lower part of the abdomen and the lower part of the uterus, through which the child is delivered. Indications for the operation include the following: disproportion between the size of the fetal head and the mother's pelvic outlet; malpresentation of the fetus, the most common of which is the breech presentation (although it is possible for a breech presentation to be delivered naturaly); signs of fetal distress; and PLACENTA PREVIA, in which the placenta is implanted in such a position that it covers the internal opening of the cervix of the uterus.

Indications in the mother for Cesarean section include diabetes (where section is best undertaken in the 37th week of pregnancy), heart disease, and a bad obstetric history. Tumors in the pelvis may preclude normal delivery, and a failed induction of labor may make Cesarean section advisable. Many obstetricians will consider performing a section on the older mother who is having her first child. A mother who has been delivered by Cesarean section will almost always be advised to have further children in the same way.

chill

The popular name for an attack of shivering, accompanied by the sensation of being cold, resulting from a disturbance of the nerve centers in the brain which regulate body temperature. Despite feeling cold, the patient may have a fever. Typically, the chill occurs as the fever rises; when the fever breaks, the chill stops and the patient perspires profusely.

Most "chills" are due to minor virus infections of the nose, throat or chest; but an unexplained fever may be due, for example, to bacterial blood poisoning (septicemia), to infection of the kidneys or bladder, or to a protozoal infection such as malaria.

Whatever the cause of a fever, treatment should include plenty of fluids to replace those lost in sweat. If the temperature rises above 104°F the patient may be cooled by sponging the chest and forehead with cool but not ice cold water. Persistence of a fever for more than 48 hours or the development of further symptoms provides grounds for seeking medical advice.

chiropody

See PODIATRY

chiropractic

A method of treatment which assumes that anatomical faults cause functional disturbances in the body and that, therefore, illnesses can be treated by "manipulation"—particularly of the spine. The specialty of chiropractic began (as did osteopathy) with the ancient techniques of "bonesetting." Eventually, chiropractors began to treat all types of strains, sprains and dislocations. Well before the end of World War II, the practitioners of spinal or skeletal manipulation considered themselves far more than mere bonesetters; they firmly believed that they had helped to develop a new system of medicine.

Since its foundation nearly 100 years ago by Daniel David Palmer in the U.S. chiropractic has become probably the most successful form of alternative medicine (about 40,000 practitioners in the U.S. alone) despite fierce opposition from the American Medical Association (AMA). In Britain, where there are about 150 qualified practitioners, some 50,000 new patients are treated each year.

Palmer believed that minor displacements of bones in the spine lead to nerve irritation and that this, in turn, leads to illness. The theory is that if the chiropractor then manipulates the spine to correct the anatomical faults, the pressure on the involved nerves is relieved. This is said to be beneficial on the course of the illness. In its basic philosophy it differs little from osteopathy, but some practitioners make medically unjustified claims for it (including the ability to treat organic diseases such as cancer). This is one of the main reasons for the AMA's opposition; but, in virtually all U.S. states chiropractic is recognized by insurance companies as a legitimate form of medical treatment. In Britain many insurance companies will accept reports from a chiropractor.

In addition to manipulation, chiropractors employ such orthopedic techniques as immobilization and traction. They also use a wide range of special electrical or mechanical devices in therapy.

chloasma

A localized brown coloration in the skin associated with pregnancy or the MENOPAUSE.

Chloasma is most obvious on the face, where the areas affected are known as "liver spots," but it also occurs on the nipples and around the genitals. The cause is thought to be a disturbance in hormone production which leads to a rise in the amount of melanin (brown pigment) formed in the deeper layers of the skin. Although chloasma is sometimes disfiguring, it usually disappears at the end of pregnancy or after the menopause.

In severe or persistent cases, some success in reducing the pigment has been achieved with hydroquinone drugs. Surgical "planing" of the affected area is also sometimes performed in order to remove the discoloration.

Very rarely, chloasma is a sign of an ovarian tumor.

cholecystectomy

Surgical removal of the gallbladder.

The gallbladder is a reservoir for bile produced by the liver and destined for the small intestine. It can give rise to symptoms caused by inflammation, the formation of gallstones, or a tumor. Stones are usually associated with inflammation, although they may occur "silently." Cholecystectomy is performed when the illness has caused recurrent fever, pain or jaundice.

The risk of gallbladder disease increases with age. As the number of elderly people in the general population has increased, cholecystectomy has become a very common operation. Gallbladder problems are most common in overweight, middle-aged women, but they can affect both sexes of all ages and weights.

The symptoms of gallbladder disorders may be acute or chronic. In acute inflammation there is severe abdominal pain, usually under the border of the right ribs. It starts suddenly and persists for some hours; relief can usually be obtained only with the injection of a potent painkiller. The patient may appear pale, vomit bile, and have a rapid pulse and damp hands. The abdomen is often rigid and very tender; the pain can also radiate to the back and right shoulder. Cholecystectomy is performed only after the acute symptoms have subsided under special medical treatment. In the elderly, surgery may be considered earlier if the symptoms persist.

Chronic cholecystitis occurs as repeated attacks of indigestion with discomfort in the upper right part of the abdomen. Other features of the illness include intolerance to fatty foods, heartburn and flatulence. Repeated attacks of inflammation can reduce the gallbladder to a shriveled nonfunctioning sac contracted around gallstones. Treatment of chronic cholecystitis includes a low-fat diet and in obese patients may require weight reduction. Cholecystectomy is generally recommended if symptoms persist or if gallstones are a problem.

Disagreement exists among medical experts regarding the most appropriate treatment for patients with gallstones but no symptoms. Some surgeons leave things alone; others remove the stones to prevent future problems. Research continues toward the development of drugs that will dissolve some forms of gallstones. At the present time, however, surgical removal of the gallbladder is the only available effective treatment in severe cases.

Tumors of the gallbladder are rare. They typically develop only in the presence of stones—perhaps because of chemical or mechanical irritation of the gallbladder wall. Unfortunately, such tumors have a tendency to spread to the liver, at which stage cholecystectomy is seldom successful.

cholecystitis

Inflammation of the gallbladder, usually associated with the presence of gallstones.

Acute cholecystitis is the most common form of the disease and may appear merely as "indigestion" along with tenderness and pain on the right side of the abdomen. More severe cases include spasm of the abdominal muscles. When gentle pressure on the spot is released, a flash of pain is experienced—a phenomenon called "rebound tenderness."

The body temperature is usually raised to over 102°F and nausea and vomiting are very common. Jaundice occurs in about 25% of patients.

The diagnosis can initially be confused with peptic ulcer or acute appendicitis, but is confirmed by the estimation of several enzymes in the blood and by ECG and x-ray investigations.

Treatment of acute cases is surgical removal of the gallbladder. Most surgeons prefer early operation; others like to wait a few days, during which time they administer intravenous fluids and antibiotics. Tube feeding may be given to rest the intestines.

Chronic cholecystitis is much less common. It is characterized by some tenderness and upper abdominal pain, but the symptoms are so general as to make the disease hard to diagnose. X-ray studies are essential for accurate diagnosis. Treatment commonly requires surgical removal of the gallbladder.

cholera

Cholera is caused by infection with comma-shaped bacteria known as *Vibrio cholerae* (or *Vibrio comma*). It occurs most often in India and other parts of Southeast Asia.

The usual picture is a sudden outbreak of a large number of cases in a particular locality. These epidemics arise when people come into contact with water or food contaminated by the feces of infected persons. Cholera epidemics are therefore a reflection of poor sanitation and living conditions. The severity of the disease can vary widely. On occasions it is fairly mild, but in some outbreaks up to 50% or more of those infected have died.

The symptomless incubation period may be as long as six days, but once the illness starts it is dramatic. The most prominent symptom is watery diarrhea, in which gray "rice water" stools are passed almost nonstop. Fluid loss may be as much as 20 quarts in a day. The liquid stools are flecked with mucus and there is little or no sign of fecal matter. There may also be vomiting, and the catastrophic loss of body fluid causes cramps and collapse. There is little or no output of urine and without prompt medical treatment death can occur within 48 hours. In the mild case, however, complete recovery typically occurs within one to three weeks.

The key to the treatment of cholera is replacement of the water and salts lost in the diarrhea. If treatment is given early the fluid may be taken by mouth, but in severe cases the fluid has to be given by direct infusion into a vein. Once the "drip" has been set up, an antibiotic such as tetracycline is given to overcome the bacteria. Vaccination every six months offers some protection for those who must remain in affected regions.

Control or prevention of cholera involves measures to purify public water supplies and the establishment of modern methods of sewage disposal. Also important is abandonment of the practice of fertilizing crops with human waste. Outbreaks in Western countries are rare and are usually confined to travelers returning from the Middle East, Central and South America.

cholesterol

A substance (technically known as a sterol) found in animal oils and fat, nervous tissue, bile, blood and egg yolks.

It has been found that those who suffer from arterial disease have a higher than average concentration of plasma cholesterol, and it has therefore been thought that a high level of cholesterol in the blood increases the risk of developing ATHEROSCLEROSIS. It has been shown that if animal fat in the diet is replaced by vegetable oil containing polyunsaturated fatty acids, the plasma cholesterol falls and remains low as long as animal fats are omitted from the diet. The relevance of a low cholesterol level, however, is still in doubt.

It is interesting to consider that man has been an omnivorous hunting animal for about two million years, during which time his natural diet must have been rich in animal fat. In fact the reasons behind the development of atherosclerosis remain obscure, although it is sensible for those who in middle age have any suspicion that they may have atherosclerosis to give up tobacco, take exercise and reduce their intake of fatty meat, butter, cream, salt and sugar. There are a number of drugs, such as clofibrate, which can reduce the concentration of cholesterol in the plasma.

The steroids, which include the sex hormones and the hormones of the adrenal glands, are derived from cholesterol—which is thus essential in limited amounts.

chondrocalcinosis

A disease, affecting the middle aged and elderly, which produces pain and swelling of one of the larger joints (for example, the knee). It is also known as *pseudo-gout*, for there are recurrent attacks of acute inflammation of one joint followed by chronic arthritis.

During the acute phase, crystals of calcium pyrophosphate are present in the synovial fluid of the affected joint and x rays of the joints show calcification in cartilages and joint capsules.

Treatment includes aspiration of fluid from the joint, and perhaps the injection of steroids; pain is relieved with the use of phenylbutazone or large doses of aspirin.

chondroma

A benign tumor composed of cartilage.

chondromalacia

A rare disease of connective tissue especially involving cartilage, the white gristlelike substance that cushions the joints and plays a structural role (for example, in the nose and ear). Inflammation causes the cartilage to soften and produces deformities such as saddle nose and floppy ear. The windpipe, lungs and joint cartilages can all be affected.

Chondromalacia can occur in men and women of all ages. It is a chronic disease which from time to time flares up to produce pain, reddening of the overlying skin, and swelling of the affected cartilage. Fever and a raised white blood cell count are usually present. The softening effect mentioned above is the aftermath of acute attacks of this kind.

Regular administration of corticosteroid drugs may keep inflammatory episodes to a minimum.

chorditis

Inflammation of the vocal cords. Small inflamed fibrous nodules are found on the surface of one or both cords, and inflammation may extend to the membranes of the larynx in which the vocal cords are housed.

Chorditis is especially common in people such as professional singers and clergymen, who repeatedly subject their voices to considerable strain (a popular name for chorditis is "clergyman's throat"). Heavy smokers and drinkers are also at special risk.

Symptoms vary from slight huskiness or hoarseness of the voice to complete loss, together with pain on swallowing and difficulty in breathing. Diagnosis is helped by the use of the laryngoscope, which enables the doctor to obtain a direct view of the inflamed parts.

The first essential treatment is total rest of the voice; any attempt at its continued use makes things worse. Some doctors apply astringent solutions such as lactic acid and silver nitrate to the affected area, and the patient may be directed to inhale iodine or eucalyptus vapors. Alcohol, tobacco and spicy foods must be avoided. If necessary, thickened sections of the chords can be removed by a minor but delicate operation.

In singers and public speakers there may be the underlying problems of incorrect voice production, in which case speech therapy may be required.

chorea

Disordered movements of the body due to lack of muscular control. In chorea normal movements are interrupted unpredictably: walking may suddenly be replaced by disorganized lurching, while the face may grimace and the eyes screw up. Interference with other muscles may affect breathing and speaking and the sufferer is unable to sit still. The power of the muscles cannot be sustained so that the grip squeezes and relaxes intermittently producing "milkmaid's grasp."

Huntington's chorea was first described in 1872 among families in Long Island by an American physician, George Huntington (1851–1916). It is a tragic condition which occurs worldwide with an incidence of between four and seven per 100,000 people. Since the condition is inherited and is genetically dominant, the incidence can rise to 50% in closed communities. The symptoms are those of chorea with progressive mental deterioration. They do not usually begin until the 30s or 40s but the disease is unsparingly progressive, terminating in death five to twenty years following onset.

To diagnose Huntington's chorea with certainty doctors need an honest family history, but concealment is common. Opinion in the medical profession is divided on the question of how much counseling affected parents should be given, but it is agreed that children at risk must be informed of the hazards ahead. At birth the child of a parent with Huntington's chorea has a 50% risk of developing the disease; by the age of 40 the risk has dropped to 33%—still a depressing statistic.

There are variations from this typical picture. When the onset is delayed until old age the condition is often not associated with mental impairment and in some cases there is muscle rigidity rather than the typical symptoms of chorea, although this presentation occurs in only about 6% of adult cases. Conversely, rigidity is found in half of the rare juvenile cases.

There is no cure and very little that can be done to relieve the symptoms.

Sydenham's chorea (also known as *St. Vitus' dance*) is a disease of childhood. It has become very rare since rheumatic fever, with which it is usually associated, has declined in incidence since World War II. Sydenham's chorea is one of the complications of previous infection with bacteria of the type known as group A hemolytic streptococcus.

The onset of the disease is usually insidious and progressive over a period of months, although about 20% of cases show acute dramatic symptoms. In half of the cases abnormal movements are restricted to one half of the body only. The age group most commonly affected is between 5 and 20 years. Psychological changes are common and the child typically becomes emotionally volatile, irritable and disobedient.

About a third of patients also show evidence of heart involvement at the same time, although this usually subsides within six months.

Treatment consists of rest and sedation. Penicillin may be given regularly until about the age of 20, to prevent further streptococcal infection. The chorea resolves within about six months; recurrences occur in about a third of cases but eventually the disease is self-limiting.

It is worth noting that women who have had Sydenham's chorea in childhood have been known to have a recurrence if they take the contraceptive pill. (It must be emphasized that this condition is not hereditary, does *not* involve mental deterioration and bears no relation whatsoever to Huntington's chorea.)

chorionepithelioma

A malignant tumor usually arising in the membranes surrounding the fetus in the womb, or occasionally in the testes, the ovary (where it is associated with a teratoma), or the pineal gland.

About half of the tumors follow the development of a HYDATIDIFORM MOLE in the uterus, another quarter follow abortions, and there have been some after an ECTOPIC PREGNANCY. About one third of these tumors occurs in women after the age of 40. The tumor appears a few months after pregnancy and induces vaginal bleeding. There may be abdominal pain and discomfort; the tumor may spread to produce secondary growths in the lungs or brain.

Diagnosis mainly depends on recognizing the possibility of chorionepithelioma. All cases of hydatidiform mole are watched very carefully. A firm decision is reached on the basis of repeated hormone measurements.

Today chorionepithelioma is treated with methotrexate and actinomycin D—a pairing of drugs which, most unusual for cancer, can have a devastating effect on this particular growth: in one study, only 2 out of 87 patients failed to show substantial regression of the tumor if not complete recovery. Surgery tends to take a back seat, but may be tried in the occasional patient who fails to respond fully to drugs.

chromosomes

The blocks of genetic material in the nuclei of all cells in the body. They carry the *genes*—the units responsible for the transmission of parental characteristics to the offspring and also for passing on essential information with each cell division during the development of the embryo, during the growth of a baby to an adult, and throughout life. The material that makes up the chromosomes is *deoxyribonucleic acid (DNA)*, and it is this long-chain molecule which provides the "templates" for the formation of the protein building blocks of the cells of every tissue and organ in the body.

Human cells contain 23 pairs of chromosomes; 22 are identical pairs, but the 23rd pair, the sex chromosomes, are identical only in females, who have two X chromosomes. In males the 23rd pair contains only one X chromosome and a smaller Y chromosome. The sex cells themselves (the spermatozoa and ova) contain only half the normal number of chromosomes—one of each of the 23 pairs—so that when fertilization takes place the full complement of 46 is restored. All ova contain an X chromosome, but sperm may contain *either* an X or a Y; the sex of a child is thus determined by whether or not the sperm cell which fertilized the ovum carried an X chromosome (giving a girl) or a Y chromosome (giving a boy).

In the process of cell division in the sex organs which leads to a reduction of the 46 chromosomes to 23, the chromosomes are split and reformed so that each sperm or ovum contains a slightly different selection of the genetic characteristics of the parent. It is this "shuffling of the DNA pack" which insures that children are not carbon copies of each other or of their parents. However, the process is also susceptible to errors, and the resulting change or mutation may be either beneficial or harmful. Many congenital defects, such as DOWN'S SYNDROME (mongolism), are due to chromosomal abnormalities. Less obvious mutations are also responsible for disorders such as hemophilia and muscular dystrophy, which may then be passed on from one generation to the next.

To determine an individual's chromosome pattern, doctors take a cell sample from anywhere in the body—usually inside the mouth—and treat it so that the cells divide. On division the chromosomes become visible under the microscope: they are then photographed to be counted carefully later. The technique can be used for prenatal diagnosis of chromosomal abnormality by the examination of fetal cells taken from the womb by AMNIOCENTESIS.

circadian rhythm

Circadian rhythm describes an observed daily pattern in the behavior of body processes. Temperature, blood pressure, pulse, blood sugar levels, etc., change, rising and falling about every 24 hours. For example, body temperature drops at night by a degree or two and climbs during the morning to a plateau near which it

CHROMOSOMES

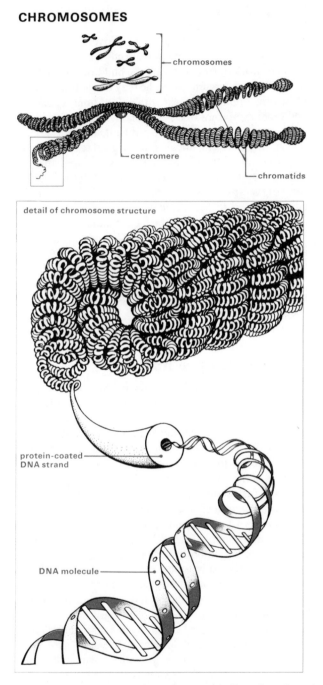

The chromosomes present in every cell nucleus in the body contain DNA and protein. Each DNA molecule consists of two long chains wound in a double helix. Genes, the units of inheritance derived from both parents, consist of long lengths of DNA chains. By controlling manufacture of the body's proteins, genes are ultimately responsible for each person's characteristics. Except for sex cells (spermatozoa and ova), all human cells contain 46 chromosomes (23 pairs).

remains throughout the rest of the day.

This "internal clock" usually continues to operate when people are kept in isolation. Individuals deprived of their wristwatches and natural sunlight have often continued to live a roughly 25-hour day. Studies of circadian rhythms in animals have led some enthusiasts to suggest that surgery, for instance, should be carried out when the body is at a physiological peak. The disabling effects of JET LAG have also been blamed on disruption of circadian rhythms.

circumcision

The minor surgical procedure of removing all or part of the foreskin (prepuce) of the penis. The historical basis of this practice is unknown, but it can be traced back to ancient times. When circumcision is performed for non-medical reasons—i.e., as a religious rite or as a routine hygienic measure—the operation is best done in the first one or two weeks of life.

In some ethnic groups circumcision is performed as a traditional religious rite—notably, among male Jewish babies on the eighth day after birth. But it is also practiced among Ethiopians, Muslims and some Christians for religious reasons. The Old Testament of the Bible refers to this practice as Abraham's Covenant with God (the "Law of Moses").

The main nonreligious reason for circumcision is the belief that it improves cleanliness. It would also appear to provide a significant degree of protection against cancer of the penis, as this is extremely rare in Jewish and other circumcised men. Cancer of the cervix (neck of the womb) is also said to be less common in women who are married to circumcised men. However in uncircumcised men, proper hygiene—by daily retracting the foreskin and washing the tip of the penis, to clean out the secretions which may have become trapped beneath it—is generally considered sufficient to minimize any health risks. Circumcision for specific medical rather than ritual reasons is performed in cases such as abnormal tightness of the foreskin which causes painful or difficult urination (see PHIMOSIS).

Some tribes (mostly African) ritually "circumcise" their women on reaching puberty. Varying amounts of genital tissues are removed, usually including the clitoris. This practice is becoming increasingly rare.

cirrhosis

A condition induced in the liver by scarring secondary to destruction of liver cells by infection, poisoning, or any other cause. The term was originally coined to describe the tawny color of the cirrhotic liver as seen after death. The essential feature of cirrhosis, however, is that much of the liver is replaced with a thick fibrous tissue; the relatively few remaining normal liver cells are left to cope with the vast biochemical functions of the organ.

Cirrhosis may follow virus hepatitis (infectious jaundice) and it is also commonly seen in association with alcoholism (*alcoholic cirrhosis*). Cirrhosis may also develop as a complication of heart failure (*cardiac cirrhosis*). Whatever the cause, the features of the disorder are due partly to the failure of the liver cells to carry out their normal functions and partly to *portal hypertension*—a raised pressure in the veins draining into the fibrotic liver from the intestinal tract.

In an attempt to compensate for the deficiency of normal liver cells the organ often initially increases in size; enlargement of the liver (hepatomegaly) is one of the early signs of the disease.

The liver cell failure leads to a whole range of biochemical defects. Accumulation of breakdown products causes the yellow discoloration of the skin (JAUNDICE). The amount of protein in the blood is reduced, leading to retention of fluid and swelling of the abdomen (ascites). Blood clotting may be slower than normal. In the later stages of the disorder the breath may have a characteristic sweet smell and an increase in the ammonia content of the blood may cause mental disturbances and eventually coma.

The portal hypertension causes the spleen to enlarge (splenomegaly), and the raised pressure may lead to bleeding into the stomach from engorged varicose veins at the lower end of the esophagus.

When cirrhosis is due to alcoholic poisoning the condition may be halted if drinking is stopped. In some other forms of cirrhosis the progress of the disease may be slowed by treatment with corticosteroid drugs. The symptoms may be relieved by a diet containing little protein; and fluid retention may be reduced by diuretic drugs. The complication of portal hypertension may require surgical treatment. In some cases the pressure in the portal vein may be lowered by diverting the blood flow into an alternative pathway, a surgical procedure known as a portocaval shunt.

claudication

The technical name for *limping*.

See INTERMITTENT CLAUDICATION.

claustrophobia

Fear of closed spaces or of being shut in. It is natural for us all to feel some fear of confined spaces, since there are circumstances in which one might be trapped in a narrow cave passage, a wrecked automobile, or a closet or small room where the door has swung shut and can be opened only from the outside. For the claustrophobic patient, however, even a closed room or the inside of a building will prove unbearable, even though he has only to open the door and walk out.

Such a phobic condition may prove severely disabling, preventing the patient from entering a vehicle to travel to work or from entering the building in which he works. In such circumstances he may develop shortness of breath, a rapid heartbeat with palpitations, sweating and other symptoms of a panic that he cannot control.

Treatment of all phobias is difficult. Psychotherapy may be useful if it can uncover the original reason for the development of the phobia, and it may be possible to relieve it by further analytical therapy. Another useful form of therapy is *desensitization*, in which the patient is either exposed to the feared situation or instructed to imagine himself in it while being continually reassured and encouraged by the therapist. This process may be assisted by the use of tranquilizing drugs. A cooperative and sympathetic relative may also help a great deal.

The prognosis, however, remains uncertain as many patients will subsequently relapse despite initially successful therapy.

See also ACROPHOBIA, AGORAPHOBIA, PHOBIA.

cleft palate/hare lip

Cleft palate and hare lip are developmental deformities present at birth. Besides the physical disfigurement, there are often feeding problems as well as difficulties with speech and hearing. However, modern plastic surgery can usually provide remarkable repair of even the most severe deformities.

Clefts of the lip and palate arise because the processes of tissue fusion that normally take place early in the development of the fetus either fail or break down. Defects may vary from minor nasal and lip notching to deep splits running the full length of the roof of the mouth to the lip on both sides of the mouth.

Cleft palate and hare lip occur in two to three live-born babies in every thousand, with males affected more than females. Japanese have a higher incidence than white Americans (black Americans have a lower incidence). There may be a family history of deformity.

The treatment of a child with cleft palate involves a team of surgical and other specialists, who follow his progress into adult life. Normally the lip is repaired at the age of 3 months and the palate at 12 to 15 months; major surgery involving the hard palate is usually postponed until late adolescence. In addition to correcting the deformity of the hard palate (which forms the roof of the mouth), the surgeon also examines the soft palate at the back for less obvious defects.

The child should return to the clinic for regular checkups and correction of any minor defects that may arise with growth. Speech, hearing, and dental problems require special attention and help.

CLEFT LIP/CLEFT PALATE

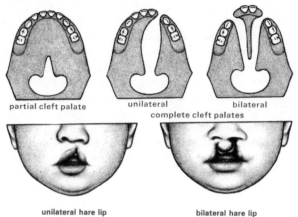

partial cleft palate

unilateral   bilateral
complete cleft palates

unilateral hare lip   bilateral hare lip

The face, lips, and palate normally form in the embryo by the fusion of many different components. About one baby in every 500 is born with a cleft deformity caused by failure of this fusion process. There is a wide spectrum of cleft defects ranging from minor lip notching to bilateral complete clefts of the lip and palate.

clonus

A rhythmic muscular spasm characterized by alternate contraction and relaxation. It is to be contrasted with *tonus*, in which the muscle is held in a partial but steady contraction.

Clonus of the ankle or foot is encountered in patients with spastic diseases such as paraplegia and paralytic hemiplegia. When the foot is forcibly flexed (tipped up) with the knee extended, rhythmic clonic movements occur at the ankle joint. This is one of the tests used in the examination of such patients.

Clonic facial spasm is nearly always confined to elderly people, usually women. Almost without exception it is restricted to one side of the face and the patient suffers from the embarrassing problem of involuntary winking. The only treatment in troublesome cases is surgical division of the upper fibers of the facial nerve.

Clonus is one of the possible signs of cramp, experienced as jerky painful muscular contractions. Cramp is usually brought on by poor blood circulation, as in cases of varicose veins, but may arise in healthy people engaged in strenuous physical activity. Treatment of the condition involves stretching the contracted muscles.

Clonus is sometimes found in people who are anxious, and it often affects healthy people who are under stress; they may notice rhythmic contractions of the calf muscles when the foot is pressed on the ground so as to stretch the Achilles tendon. In these cases clonus is of no significance.

clubbing

Clubbing of the fingers and sometimes the toes refers to an overgrowth of hard tissue in the region of the nailbed. It was first described by Hippocrates in the 5th century B.C. in patients with tuberculosis of the lung. Finger clubbing is present in approximately one third of patients with lung cancer but is also seen in an enormous variety of respiratory and other diseases.

The first stage in clubbing involves a filling in of the angle between the nail and the surrounding skin. The nailbed thickens and the top joint of the finger expands so that it resembles a drumstick. Rarely the nose may also thicken.

Besides the link with lung cancer, finger clubbing may be a sign of fungal infection of the nailbed or diseases of the heart, liver and thyroid gland; in some cases it may be an inherited trait and represent no cause for concern. Clubbing can arise in *pulmonary osteoarthropathy*, a condition which produces severe joint pain and in about 80% of cases is associated with lung cancer.

One theory about clubbing suggests that the tissue overgrowth is caused by an overly rich supply of oxygen through tumor-induced activation of the numerous short circuits between the arterial and venous circulations that are found in the finger. But this idea, like others, does not explain how clubbing can arise in such a diversity of diseases.

The treatment of clubbing necessarily involves treatment of the underlying disorder.

clubfoot

A deformity present at birth which prevents the foot being placed flat on the ground. Boys are affected twice as often as girls. Clubfoot may also be acquired as a result of paralytic disease such as poliomyelitis, or it may be associated with a hidden or obvious spinal abnormality.

The main defect is usually in the heel, which is pulled inward and upward so that the patient walks on his toes. Alternatively, the toes are pulled back and he walks on his heel. The foot itself may be twisted so that only either the outer or inner edge of the sole touches the ground. The foot arch is often abnormally high. Both feet are usually affected.

The structural faults in uncorrected clubfoot are due to defects in the shape and alignment of the bones of the foot. However, there may be secondary contractures in the soft tissues and shortening and tightening of the Achilles tendon and ligaments. Children with clubfoot can be divided into two main groups: (1) those with flexible clubfoot and less severe deformity and contracture, and (2) those with rigid clubfoot and poorly developed muscles, a small heel and deformed forefoot.

VARIETIES OF CLUBFOOT

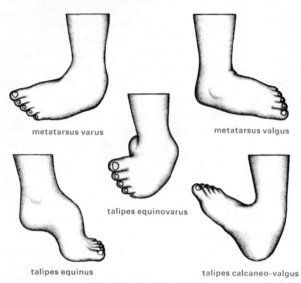

metatarsus varus

metatarsus valgus

talipes equinovarus

talipes equinus

talipes calcaneo-valgus

"Clubfoot" usually refers to talipes equinovarus *(center, above)—a relatively common congenital deformity of unknown cause. The other varieties are much less common. The deformity can be corrected if treated immediately after birth.*

The key to successful reversion of clubfoot is early treatment, particularly in cases of flexible clubfoot where the outlook is good. Manual manipulation of the deformed soft tissue should begin immediately after birth so that the various parts of the foot can be coaxed into proper alignment. If this is not done the rapidly developing bones of the foot may be irreversibly distorted. It is common for the surgeon to teach the various manipulative techniques to the parents so that therapy can continue at home. Correction is maintained by strapping and splinting the foot.

If manipulation is not completely successful, surgical correction of clubfoot is usually performed when the child is three months old. The foot is then kept in a plaster cast for about six weeks. Special boots are worn for at least two years thereafter.

Surgery in adolescence is usually reserved for the occasional patient with crippling painful deformity. Today such interventions are being carried out with decreasing frequency. This is evidence of the value of early manipulative treatment.

coccidioidomycosis

A fungal infection that first attacks the lungs and can spread to the skin, bones and brain. It consistently arises in people living in desert areas of the United States and Central America. The disease is picked up by breathing in dust from soil contaminated with microscopic spores of the fungus *Coccidioides immitis*. For this reason laborers are often affected.

Coccidioidomycosis usually produces a mild influenzalike illness (sometimes known as *valley fever* because of its prevalence in the San Joaquin Valley in California), which with adequate bed rest soon passes. In about 10% of cases the infection spreads and abscesses and deep-seated weeping wounds (sinuses) may result. It can also cause MENINGITIS (inflammation of the membranes which cover the brain and spinal cord). In such severe instances large doses of *amphotericin B* are necessary. The overall mortality rate is less than one in a thousand.

cold

1. See COMMON COLD.
2. See CHILBLAIN, FROSTBITE, HYPOTHERMIA.

cold sore

A blister on the lips caused by infection with a virus.
See HERPES SIMPLEX.

colic

Any severe abdominal pain of a spasmodic nature, caused by contractions of the smooth muscle in the walls of a hollow organ under tension.

Biliary colic is the chief symptom of gallstones, caused by the gallbladder and bile duct dilating and contracting after a stone has lodged in the cystic duct. Attacks of pain usually begin abruptly several hours after a heavy meal. The pain is felt in short sharp bursts just below the rib cage. Each attack can last up to 30 minutes but may take up to a few hours before subsiding. The victim may be so distressed that he writhes and doubles up. Treatment involves the administration of powerful painkillers; surgical removal of the gallbladder may be necessary.

Renal colic is caused by a stone in the ureter, the tube linking the kidney to the urinary bladder. The excruciating pain of renal colic begins in the loin or flank and fans out downward to the inner surface of the thigh or the genitals. The urine commonly contains traces of blood. If the stone is small it may pass spontaneously, otherwise it may have to be removed surgically.

Intestinal colic produces widespread cramps, which are often worse just below the level of the navel. This type of pain may be caused by blockage or intestinal inflammation. If it is due to blockage the pain is accompanied by vomiting, swelling of the abdomen, and high-pitched gurgling sounds in the intestine.

Other forms of colic may be caused by lead poisoning, appendicitis, and difficulties in menstruation.

colitis

Inflammation of the lining of the large intestine (colon). It affects roughly 1 person in 2,000, begins most often in people in their 30s, and is a chronic condition characterized by sudden repeated attacks interspersed with periods of remission. Colitis should not be confused with the far less serious complaint of *spastic colon*, which is caused by emotional factors.

Among the possible causes of colitis are bacterial infection of the intestine, food allergies (especially milk) and genetic factors. In most cases, however, the cause is unknown or at least not documented.

Colitis may begin insidiously or suddenly. In about half the patients the first indications are malaise (a general feeling of being unwell), vague abdominal discomfort, and mild diarrhea or constipation. As more severe signs and symptoms appear, such as lower abdominal pain or bleeding from the rectum (indicative of a condition known as ULCERATIVE COLITIS), the patient is driven to seek medical advice. If the disease strikes abruptly there is worsening fever, bloody diarrhea, loss of appetite and weight loss. This happens in about a third of cases.

The first step in the diagnosis of colitis is direct visual inspection of the walls of the intestine with an endoscope (sigmoidoscope). A small sample of the diseased tissue is removed for further examination and to test for the presence of infection. X rays of the intestine are also taken. Further tests may be needed to rule out diseases such as colonic cancer, diverticulitis and infectious enteritis which can coexist with colitis or produce similar symptoms.

Patients are classified on the basis of the severity of their symptoms. Those with mild disease can be treated at home and allowed a normal diet. A second "moderate" group are usually cared for in the hospital; in addition to the appropriate drug therapy they usually receive a high-protein diet with replacement of salts and fluids lost during bouts of diarrhea and bleeding. Seriously ill patients may require blood transfusions and surgical removal of all or part of the intestine and a COLOSTOMY.

collagen diseases

A group of poorly understood disorders affecting connective tissue, which is largely made up of collagen, a protein of exceptional strength. These diseases are thought to be due to some impairment of the IMMUNE SYSTEM, by means of which the body defends itelf against the introduction of foreign proteins.

There is evidence that the immune reaction can turn against the tissues it normally should protect, and that there are a number of diseases associated with this state (see AUTOIMMUNE DISEASES). Those affecting connective tissue include systemic lupus erythematosus (SLE), polyarteritis nodosa (PAN), rheumatoid arthritis (RA), and dermatomyositis.

Systemic lupus erythematosus occurs mainly in women between the age of 20 and 50, and is associated with complex disorders of the immune mechanism. It may start with symptoms of arthritis and pain in the muscles, pleurisy and pneumonia, the passage of protein in the urine, myocarditis (inflammation of the heart muscle), anemia, enlargement of the spleen, skin rashes, hepatitis or a combination of these. The diagnosis is made by specific tests on the blood. Treatment includes rest, analgesics, the administration of corticosteroids and chloroquine, and avoidance of exposure to strong sunlight. The patient should take as few drugs as possible.

In *polyarteritis nodosa* the lesion is thought to be due to hypersensitivity to an unknown antigen with a consequent reaction involving the arteries. The signs and symptoms are varied; they include loss of weight, fever, a high pulse rate, chronic bronchitis, recurrent pneumonia, abdominal pain, acute diarrhea, passage of protein in the urine, arthritis and pain in the muscles. The treatment resembles that used for SLE.

Women are affected more frequently than men by *rheumatoid arthritis;* the usual age at onset is between 20 and 50. It is fairly common, but the incidence is lower in the tropics than in temperate climates. Some studies put the incidence as high as 3% of the adult population, with a slight familial tendency. There is usually a preliminary illness lasting a number of weeks with raised pulse rate, fatigue, loss of weight, sweating and discomfort in the limbs. This is followed by the development of arthritis in the hands, which spreads to affect the wrists and elbows; the feet, ankles and knees may also be affected. The joints are hot and swollen and painful, and the muscles acting on the joints waste. There may be anemia, and nodules may be found in the skin. The most common complication in the lungs is pleurisy, with an effusion; patients with a long history of the disease develop an atrophied skin and ridged nails as well.

Treatment includes rest, with physical therapy directed at joints and muscles. The diet must be good. Salicylates and other anti-inflammatory drugs are usually prescribed; corticosteroids are of limited use, but may be introduced directly into affected joints. Gold salts by injection may be used under strict medical supervision, and the drug penicillamine is also useful, although research remains to be carried out in order to define its precise place in treatment. In chronic disease, orthopedic surgery may have much to offer; for example, hip joints that have been crippled by chronic rheumatoid arthritis may be restored by HIP REPLACEMENT.

Colles' fracture

This fracture of the wrist is named after the Irish surgeon Abraham Colles (1773–1843) who described it in 1814, long before x rays were available. It is quite common at all ages, but especially in women over 40. Colles' fracture is usually caused by a heavy fall on the outstretched hand.

The fractured bone is the *radius*, which runs from elbow to wrist and which "carries" the hand at the wrist. It is usually broken across, within one inch of the wrist. The force of the blow displaces the separated end a little sideways, toward the thumb side and backwards, taking the hand with it. This gives the typical "dinner fork deformity"—the forearm being the "handle" of the fork with a depression just before the wrist and the hand forming the curve of the "prongs" of the fork. Very often the other bone of the forearm (the *ulna*) is also involved, its lower and outer tip (the *styloid process*) being detached; the cartilage of the wrist joint may also be damaged.

Treatment generally demands an anesthetic, under which the bones are manipulated back to their correct

COLLES' FRACTURE

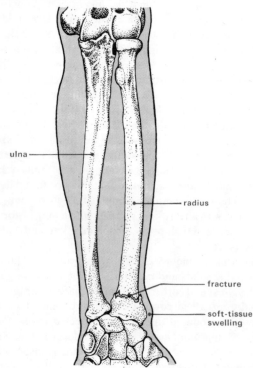

Colles' fractures of the lower end of the radius result from falling onto the outstretched hand and are very common in the elderly. This is partly because the elderly tend to fall heavily, but also because their bones are brittle.

positions. The wrist and the forearm to above the elbow are then immediately immobilized in a plaster cast. The fingers and the further end of the palm are left free so that the fingers can move fully. It is often necessary to take another x ray soon after immobilization to make sure that correction has been maintained.

The cast has to be worn for up to six weeks, after which light work can be undertaken; heavy work should not be resumed for about another six weeks. While the wrist is "out of action" the patient is encouraged to exercise fingers and shoulder—with disuse they may stiffen up, especially in the elderly. Many housewives (common victims of Colles' fracture) find that they are able to continue their usual everyday tasks.

Once the cast is removed, strengthening and mobilizing exercises may be given for the wrist itself.

colonic cancer

Cancer of the large intestine (colon) accounts for about one sixth of all malignant tumors in the Western countries. It is extremely rare in Japan and Africa. Some 70% of the cancers occur in the rectum; if these are excluded, then 50% of cancers of the large intestine are found in the sigmoid, or pelvic, colon on the left of the abdomen—25% in the cecum or the ascending colon on the right side of the abdomen, and the other 25% in the transverse colon, descending colon and the flexures.

Predisposing factors include ulcerative colitis and papillomatous conditions of the intestine. There may be a hereditary factor, and diet is thought to play a large part in the development of colonic tumors. It is interesting to note that the incidence of these tumors is four times as high in Japanese born and brought up in the United States as those born and brought up in Japan. In Britain in 1979, 4,324 men and 6,057 women died of cancer of the colon.

The most common warning symptom is an alteration in bowel habits. Growths occurring on the right do not often cause intestinal obstruction, but they do cause discomfort, loss of weight, anemia and fever. Those on the left frequently obstruct the passage of intestinal contents; there may be marked abdominal distension and pain. The tumor may sometimes be felt through the abdominal wall. Investigations include endoscopy and contrast radiography.

The aim of the treatment is to remove the tumor completely with as many of the regional lymph glands as possible, and to restore the continuity of the bowel. It may be necessary during surgical treatment to use a temporary COLOSTOMY, but the end result of surgery is designed to avoid the necessity of permanent colostomy. Overall results are much better than those of surgery for cancer of the lung or the stomach, and about four out of every five patients make a good recovery.

colostomy

An artificial opening in the large intestine so that it can discharge its contents through the abdominal wall. Colostomies can be temporary or permanent.

A *temporary colostomy* may be performed when cancer has attacked the bottom end of the intestine and the surgeon wishes to divert the bowel contents to facilitate treatment. Patients suffering from severe inflammation of the intestinal wall may also require a temporary colostomy. If the disease is so severe that the rectum must be removed, a permanent colostomy is unavoidable.

In the operation to form a temporary colostomy, the surgeon makes an opening in the abdomen and connects to it the tip of a loop of the transverse colon (the middle portion of the large bowel). Once the disease responsible for the temporary colostomy has been successfully treated, the opening is closed. It is usual to wait about three months before closure.

COLOSTOMY

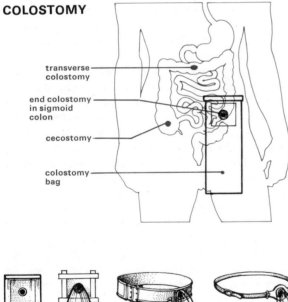

transverse colostomy

end colostomy in sigmoid colon

cecostomy

colostomy bag

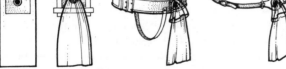

colostomy bags can be held in place by magnets, adhesive tapes or belts

A colostomy is an opening (stoma) made into the large intestine in order to relieve an obstruction. It may either be temporary or permanent depending on the site. Cecostomies and transverse colostomies are both temporary diversions. End colostomies are permanent openings in the sigmoid colon.

In a *permanent colostomy* the lowest section of healthy intestine is fastened to the skin of the abdomen. The opening is positioned to one side of the midline so that the colostomy appliance (collection bag) is in a comfortable site.

In the first few days after the operation the effluent is fluid and is collected in a transparent disposable bag attached to the opening (stoma) by an adhesive seal. The bag is changed at least once daily. Later, when the feces become more solid, many patients switch to bags attached by a plastic flange. They need to be changed less often and problems of skin irritation are less common. Cosmetic factors are of great importance and "stoma therapists" advise on the use of medicaments to improve security of adhesion and reduce odor.

Once the immediate postoperative period is over, most patients find that their colostomy empties only two or three times a day. Often the timing is so regular that the bag can be emptied before the patient leaves home in the morning. Careful attention to diet can minimize problems with excess gas production or diarrhea, and a permanent colostomy need hardly restrict normal physical and social activities.

color blindness

An abnormality of the eye in which a person cannot distinguish colors. The most common forms are inability to distinguish between red, green and yellow or blue, green and yellow. Total blindness (monochromatism) is extremely rare.

About one man in eight suffers from some degree of red-green confusion, but the condition is far less common in women—only about one in 200 being affected. Overall, perhaps one person in 50 is afflicted to an appreciable extent.

Color blindness is usually present from birth and persists throughout life. It is believed to be inherited from the mother, who nearly always has normal color vision despite carrying a defective "color gene." Such congenital color blindness cannot be corrected. There have been reports of color blindness being acquired by people who drink or smoke heavily; cutting back on smoking has been known to restore normal color vision.

Color blindness is thought to be caused by deficiencies or defects of the color-sensitive cells (cones) in the retina. There are three kinds of cone, one for each of the primary colors: red, green and blue. All other colors are made up of combinations of these. Every color corresponds to light of a particular wavelength. Color confusion arises because cones that are tuned into one wavelength (or color) have some sensitivity to light of neighboring wavelengths. For instance, if someone has defective cones for green he may see this color as blue. The degree of color blindness in affected persons varies between a slight loss of brilliance at a distance to an inability to choose between vividly contrasting colors. Usually those with red-green blindness see these two colors as shades of gray or yellow.

The *Ishihara color test* (named after the Japanese ophthalmologist Shinobu Ishihara, b. 1879) is used to detect color blindness. This involves presenting the subject with a mosaic of colored dots in which there is a partly hidden symbol such as a number or letter. The color-blind person is unable to distinguish this symbol.

Color blindness may keep an affected person from holding certain jobs where color perception is essential (such as soldering color-coded wires), but it may not always be the handicap it appears. At a major scientific conference held in England in 1977, it was suggested that John Constable (1776–1837), one of the greatest landscape painters who ever lived, might have been color blind.

For further information, see also BLINDNESS and VISION.

coma

A state of unconsciousness so deep that the reflexes are lost and the eyeball can be touched without making the eye blink, while the most painful stimuli fail to have any effect.

Coma can be caused in a number of ways, all of which affect the higher functions of the brain while leaving the lower "vegetative" centers of the nervous system working (such as those which control breathing and the heartbeat). Direct damage to the brain sustained in head injuries or produced by intracranial bleeding, tumor or infection can result in coma. If part of the blood supply to the brain is cut off by a clot in one of the cerebral arteries (cerebral thrombosis), or if the blood pressure falls so that the blood flow to the brain becomes grossly impaired—as a result of surgical shock, massive loss of blood or a heart attack—the patient can become comatose.

Unconsciousness after an epileptic attack can be deep enough to be called coma. Other causes include electric shock and profound HYPOTHERMIA; biochemical changes in the blood may so interfere with the proper metabolism of the brain cells that coma ensues. The most common causes of such biochemical changes are diabetes, uremia and liver failure. Poisons can produce coma, perhaps the most common being the excessive ingestion of alcohol.

Treatment of coma is directed toward the underlying cause; but in all cases it is imperative that the airways be kept clear.

A patient who is comatose will require artificial feeding by means of an intravenous infusion of nutrients.

common cold

The common cold is a viral infection of the upper respiratory passages. It differs from other respiratory infections in that fever is most often absent and the symptoms are generally milder. Modern research has revealed that any one (or a combination) of over 100 different viruses can cause a cold. Colds are spread by direct person-to-person contact, although some people can become infected and spread the cold viruses without having any symptoms.

Colds tend to occur most frequently in the young. The preschool child has an average of six to twelve colds per year, parents with young children have about six colds a year, and older adults usually escape with two or three colds per year. (Some people, of course, have very few or none at all.) Colds are more widespread in the winter: about half the population picks up a cold during the winter quarter. This figure drops to around 20% in the summer. The cold has a significant economic impact: among the American working population of 60 million, colds account for the loss of 1 million man years or roughly six days per person per year. This represents one quarter of the total time lost from work.

Contrary to popular belief, cold weather does not actually appear to *cause* colds. The results of studies in the Arctic and among volunteers exposed to cold weather have not shown any increase in the number of colds. The observed link between wintry conditions and colds remain unexplained. Colds tend to come in waves. The first outbreak is usually in the autumn a few weeks after the schools have opened, the second in midwinter; and the third in the spring.

The precise symptoms of the common cold vary from one individual to the next. Some people always seem to get "head" colds while others suffer from pharyngitis or cough. The first signs of a cold are usually sneezing, headache and a general feeling of ill health (malaise). Then come chilly sensations, a sore throat and heavy nasal discharge. Often, after a brief respite, the patient progresses to the classic symptoms of the common cold—chief of which is nasal congestion as the mucus changes from being clear and thin to become thick, tenacious and yellow-green in color. By this stage the sore throat has normally disappeared, but cough may become an increasing problem and last until the cold has completely resolved (generally one to two weeks).

Because so many viruses can cause a cold, and because the illness is short and readily dealt with by the body's natural defenses against infection, doctors usually recommend only supportive treatment. This means bed rest and warm clothing to make the patient feel more comfortable. If breathing difficulties occur drugs such as expectorants and nasal decongestants may be used. Aspirin is effective in relieving headache and malaise. Physicians tend to frown on the exotic "cocktails" of vitamins, multiple painkillers, antihistamines, tranquilizers, and so on, that are widely advertised as the remedy for colds. Antibiotic drugs are helpful only when a secondary bacterial infection follows "on the heels" of a cold—a relatively common event.

complex

An organized collection of emotions and ideas of which the individual may not be fully aware but which strongly influence attitudes and behavior.

The OEDIPUS COMPLEX is one of the main planks of PSYCHOANALYSIS, a method of psychiatric treatment originated by Sigmund Freud. It refers to a distinct group of linked ideas, instincts and fears which are most commonly observed in male children between three to six years and form a normal part of development. During this period a boy's sexuality is at a peak and is primarily directed toward his mother, accompanied by feelings of hostility toward his father. Baby girls go through a similar phase, but this time sexual interest is centered on the father and aggression on the mother. This is referred to as the *Electra complex*. At the age of five or six, sexuality wanes and the Oedipus complex normally passes.

In our society it is typical for parents to discourage overly intense expression of infant sexuality. This in itself is not wrong provided that it does not become an excuse for rigorous repression. With firm but loving direction, sexual and aggressive impulses can be channeled into constructive activities such as learning and play. Parents must certainly guard against viewing infant sexuality as abnormal or wicked.

A number of complexes relate to adolescent or adult life. One of the most widely known is the *inferiority complex*, in which the sufferer experiences an acute sense of inadequacy; this shows up as extreme shyness or compensatory aggressiveness. The *Cain complex* refers to excessive jealousy of a brother and the *Diana complex* to ideas leading to the adoption of masculine behavior by a female.

In everyday language the word "complex" is often used to describe feelings of apprehension or fear directed toward some particular object, person, or social situation. To some extent such tensions are normal, but if they become severe can cripple an individual's behavior. They are then more properly described as *anxiety states, phobias,* or *obsessions*—depending on their exact nature. Patients with these disorders usually need psychiatric help.

For a description of these conditions, see ANXIETY, OBSESSION and PHOBIA.

concussion

Cerebral concussion means a loss of consciousness immediately following a blow on the head. It is nearly always followed by loss of memory for the blow and the incidents leading up to it (retrograde amnesia). The extent of the amnesia is roughly related to the severity of the injury and the period of unconsciousness.

The mechanism is not properly understood, but it is thought that at the time of injury there is a wave of very high pressure inside the skull which is transmitted to the brain. This may produce many small pinpoint hemorrhages; the concussion is assumed to stop the higher centers of the brain from working for a while, although the lower centers continue to function. It is probable that the injury suffered by the brain in concussion differs in degree rather than in kind from the more severe injuries that result in coma.

Recovery from unconsciousness in concussion is followed by a period of minor confusion and headache; there should be no lasting effects other than the retrograde amnesia, which shortens in time and may eventually recover completely. A person who loses consciousness after a blow on the head should be put to bed under observation for 24 hours. Such a period of observation not only guards against insidious development of more severe complications to the injury but lessens the likelihood of postconcussion headaches and dizziness.

The presence or absence of scalp wounds or fractures of the skull has no influence on the state of concussion, although they may allow the surgeon to estimate the degree of violence involved in producing the concussion.

condyloma

A flat moist skin lesion raised from the surface like a wart. It usually affects the genital area of the body and can occur in both sexes at any age.

Condylomata are of two main types: those caused by a virus that is similar to that responsible for common warts (*condylomata acuminata*) and those that appear during the secondary stage of syphilis (*condylomata lata*).

Over the last few years viral condylomata have become increasingly common, possibly as a result of greater sexual freedom. They are moderately infectious and are transmitted by direct contact. They begin as tiny pinpoint spots which rapidly enlarge to form soft clusters of red or yellow warts. Condylomata thrive in moist regions of the body, which is why they tend to infect the penis and the vulva. Small condylomata can be treated with applications such as podophyllin, but larger lesions may require surgical removal. Sometimes they recur.

The condylomata of secondary syphilis are usually about half an inch or less in diameter and often appear in large numbers grouped closely together on the vulva and around the anus. The have a pink or violet color and may cause the skin surface to break down to form a shallow gray-pink ulcer which exudes a sticky puslike fluid. Examination of a sample of this fluid under a microscope reveals the presence of the highly mobile *Treponema* spirochete and enables the doctor to distinguish between these and viral condylomata. The lesions are highly infectious.

congenital dislocation of the hip

The hip is a ball and socket joint; if the socket (acetabulum) in the pelvis is abnormally shallow and the ball (the head of the femur) is small, the joint is unstable and easily dislocated.

Some babies, particularly those of Central European and North Italian descent, are found to have hips dislocated at birth; the deformity tends to run in families. Routine examination at birth includes examination of the hips for dislocation. If found, flexible metal splints are used to hold the legs abducted so that the head of the femur rests properly in the acetabulum.

The sooner treatment is started the better the results. If the deformity becomes apparent as the child starts to walk, a plaster cast is fitted to hold the joint in the right place, and it may be needed for six to nine months. Older children may need operative treatment to reduce the dislocation.

If the deformity persists untreated into adult life, it is usually left alone unless the joint is affected by severe osteoarthritis, in which case suitable surgical treatment may be indicated.

conjunctivitis

Inflammation of the conjunctival membrane covering the outer aspect of the eyeball and the inner aspect of the eyelids. It is commonly the result of invasion by various microorganisms or allergies.

Acute conjunctivitis is often caused by *Staphylococcus aureus*, sometimes by *Streptococcus pneumoniae* or an adenovirus; classical epidemic "pinkeye" is caused by the *Koch-Weeks bacillus, (Haemophilus aegyptius)*, or the *Morax-Axenfeld bacillus (Moraxella lacunata). Gonococcus (Neisseria gonorrhoeae)* may produce conjunctivitis, as may *Corynebacterium diphtheriae*. Chemicals splashed into the eye can produce severe inflammation, as can the irritating presence of an eyelash or other foreign body.

The affected eye feels gritty and burning, the discomfort being worse on movement and blinking. Both eyes soon become inflamed in most cases, and the discharge may become yellow and sticky. Antibiotic eyedrops are usually prescribed when bacterial infection is thought to be the cause of the inflammation. The patient is warned that the infection can be spread easily through contaminated towels, washcloths, etc., so that he or she must be very careful not to share toilet articles.

In some cases treatment is not immediately successful and the condition becomes chronic. This is sometimes the case in viral infections; or it may be that there is an allergic cause, for the conjunctiva can become sensitive to a number of cosmetics and drugs, including penicillin and atropine. A particular type of chronic conjunctivitis of great importance is TRACHOMA, which is due to a large virus-like organism. It occurs in all dry parts of the tropics and subtropics in communities that are afflicted by poverty; about 400 million people are affected. Trachoma is the chief cause of blindness in the world.

constipation

The frequency with which bowel movements occur varies greatly (see BOWEL AND BOWEL MOVEMENTS). It is not necessary to have a bowel movement every day; some quite healthy people have bowel movements every two or three days or twice or more during the day. However, when emptying of the rectum is delayed there is increasing reabsorption of water from its contents so that the stools become excessively hard and dry. This in turn may lead to difficulty in passing them at all. The patient who has a bowel movement without difficulty every third day has no problem, but if difficulty results he suffers from constipation. In severe cases, the hard feces cannot be passed; but "paradoxical diarrhea" may occur with fluid feces from the large bowel being passed around the hardened mass of stool.

The causes of constipation include diseases of the bowel itself, an unsuitable diet containing too little roughage or dietary fiber (low-residue diet) and certain neurological disorders resulting in paralysis of the muscular walls of the bowel. Of much greater importance, however, is a failure by the patient to adhere to a regular bowel-opening habit. This may be due to inadequate toilet training as a child, to an unwillingness to open the bowels because of pain from piles or other anal conditions or, most important, a willful neglect of the urge to open the bowels because of lack of time, laziness or other factors.

Treatment of constipation depends on its cause. Any painful condition such as piles must be relieved. A diet containing plenty of dietary fiber should be taken and breakfast should be a meal of adequate bulk. If laxatives have been previously taken, they should be replaced by one of the bulk-producing preparations such as agar or mineral oil In severe cases, the bowel may have to be initially emptied by means of enemas or even by manual removal of the dry feces by the doctor or nurse.

Laxatives fall into three main categories. These are bulk-forming laxatives, stool softeners, and bowel stimulants or irritants. It is important to note that prolonged or excessive use of chemical laxatives can lead to potassium depletion, muscle weakness and chronic diarrhea.

contact lenses

Contact lenses are molded to fit snugly over the cornea and sometimes the conjunctival surface of the eye. Over 99% are intended solely to correct refractive errors while allowing the wearer to dispense with the use of glasses; in other words, their function is normally purely cosmetic.

The lenses are made of various plastics, most commonly an acrylic resin which is reliable and cheap, and are molded (unlike glass lenses, which must be ground). Softer plastics have also been introduced, which are permeable and therefore cause less irritation. In time they will doubtless replace the older type, but at present are considerably more expensive and have a relatively short life of about two to three years due to the fragility associated with their softness.

The period for which contact lenses can be worn without interruption depends on the individual; but, if they are fitted correctly, most people can wear them all day and need only remove them at night. Soft lenses can often be left in position longer.

Fitting lenses is liable to be uncomfortable, but the optometrist applies local anesthetic drops before beginning his assessment. In ordinary use no such preparation is necessary.

It should be remembered that about 15% of refractive errors (especially high degrees of astigmatism) are not suitable for correction by contact lenses because the corneal surface is too irregular. Certain medical conditions are greatly helped by contact lenses. One of these is congenital absence of the lens of the eye. Contact lenses are also beneficial in some cases following cataract removal. Rarer disorders, particularly those affecting the cornea, often benefit enormously from the use of contact lenses; but in these abnormal circumstances there can be hazards associated with their application. Very specialized medical advice is thus required.

Finally, it should not be forgotten how useful contact lenses are to some sportsmen and members of the armed forces—even though there have been occasional reports of injury from the lens itself.

Use of colored contact lenses for movie and television work is only worth mentioning to remind us that passport entries about eye color now seem pointless.

CONTACT LENS

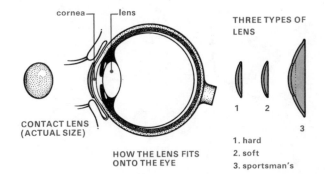

cornea — lens

THREE TYPES OF LENS

CONTACT LENS (ACTUAL SIZE)

HOW THE LENS FITS ONTO THE EYE

1
2
3

1. hard
2. soft
3. sportsman's

Most of the focusing of light rays takes place at the cornea in the front of the eye, with the lens making further adjustments. Contact lenses, which are placed directly onto the cornea, perform exactly the same function as glasses and are only preferred for reasons of appearance.

contagion

The spread of disease by direct contact.

contraception

Men and women have sought out ways to control conception since they began to understand the mechanism of reproduction, and measures such as douching, coitus interruptus and the use of tampons are very ancient. Curious objects and materials have been inserted into the vagina with varying results. The Egyptians put their faith in crocodile dung, and Casanova recommended the juice of half a lemon—the lemon skin being used as a Dutch cap (placed over the cervix).

In 1916, Margaret Sanger started the world's first birth control clinic in Brooklyn; in 1921 Marie Stopes opened a clinic in Britain. In the ensuing years the problems of population control, together with a more liberal outlook on the individual's needs, have brought the matter well into the open.

The simplest, but perhaps the least reliable, method of contraception is the observance of the "safe period." It is based on the belief that ovulation takes place midway in the menstrual cycle, and that the period during which fertilization of the ovum is possible is limited to the 10th to 17th days inclusive of a normal 28-day menstrual cycle. The method is allowable for Catholics, but while it decreases the risk of pregnancy it by no means precludes it. More effective is *coitus interruptus*, the technique of premature withdrawal of the penis from the vagina; but it is still unreliable and in some cases psychologically unsettling.

CONTRACEPTION

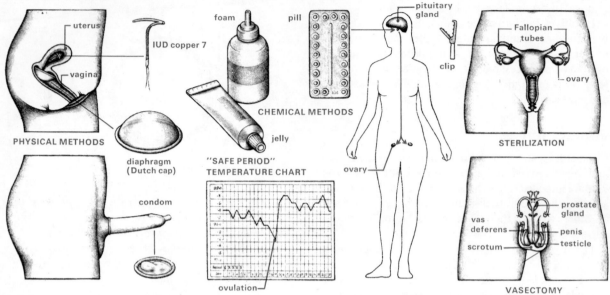

PHYSICAL METHODS — uterus — IUD copper 7 — vagina — diaphragm (Dutch cap) — condom

CHEMICAL METHODS — foam — pill — jelly — "SAFE PERIOD" TEMPERATURE CHART — ovulation — ovary

pituitary gland — clip — STERILIZATION — Fallopian tubes — ovary

VASECTOMY — prostate gland — penis — testicle — vas deferens — scrotum

Most contraceptives are either physical devices such as the condom and diaphragm, which act as barriers to the sperm, or chemical methods which either kill the sperm (foam or jelly) or prevent ovulation (the pill). The intrauterine device (IUD) occupies an intermediate position in that it probably works both by having a spermicidal coating of copper and by preventing implantation of a fertilized egg in the womb. Sterilization by dividing the Fallopian tubes or a vasectomy, in which the vasa deferentia are cut, provides permanent contraception.

Condoms ("safes," "prophylactics," or "rubbers") have been known since the 16th century. They were at first crude; but the invention of vulcanizing rubber in the 19th century made possible their manufacture on a large scale, and they were further improved by the use of latex about 50 years ago. Some are now made of plastic material. Their safety depends on their integrity, and many authorities recommend the use of chemical methods in addition to the condom. Nevertheless they form the most widely used method of birth control in the West, and are made and used in astronomical numbers.

Cervical occlusive devices for use by women have been known for many years. The modern vaginal *diaphragm* was introduced in Germany towards the end of the 19th century, and was enthusiastically promoted by Malthusians in Holland; it therefore became known as the Dutch cap. The vaginal diaphragm is made of thin rubber in the shape of a shallow dome, with a flat circular spring contained within the rim. When in place, it covers the uterine cervix, sloping from the vault of the vagina toward the pubic bone. It is effective if it is

combined with a chemical contraceptive, and is quite harmless.

Chemical contraceptives in the form of gels, pessaries, foam and creams containing spermicidal compounds are not entirely reliable if used on their own, but form a strong reinforcement to the use of occlusive diaphragms and condoms.

The permanent intrauterine contraceptive device (IUD or IUCD) has been known for over a hundred years, but early devices were liable to introduce infection into the genital tract and therefore became unpopular. The introduction of plastic devices to a great extent prevented septic complications; at present there are a large number of designs available, some of which are covered by copper (which is said to increase the efficacy). Some authorities consider that they should not be used by women who have had no children, in cases with a history of pelvic infection, or in women who have painful or excessive periods. IUCDs are acceptable to about 75% of women; 25% tend to expel them. They are not completely effective, and rarely pregnancies can occur with the device in position. The precise mode of action is not understood.

The most effective method of contraception is the use of sex hormones—the oral contraceptive pill. The pill contains a combination of estrogen and a progestogen and is taken by mouth for 21 days with a gap of 7 days between courses, during which time there is withdrawal bleeding (which simulates the woman's menstrual period). There are a large number of preparations on the market; the choice is wide, but may be influenced by the observation that the incidence of thromboembolism may be related to the total amount of estrogen. It is therefore wise to use the lowest effective dose.

Disadvantages of the use of hormones are that some women tend to put on weight; some complain of headaches, nausea and a general feeling of being unwell (malaise); some may have discomfort in the breasts, and some become agitated and nervous. The greatest hazard to health is the risk of venous thrombosis, which is higher in those taking the contraceptive pill (but it should be remembered that there is also a risk of developing thromboembolism after childbirth).

Some evidence exists to suggest that there is an increased risk of developing hormone-dependent cancer after many years of taking the sex hormones, and it would seem that older women should be wary of the contraceptive pill. In any case, women taking the pill should be sure to have regular medical checkups, and as they pass the age of 30 they may care to discuss alternative methods of contraception with their family physician.

See also STERILIZATION and VASECTOMY.

contracture

Abnormal shortening of the muscles or soft tissues surrounding a joint.

Most muscle contractures affect the hand, where they produce a clawlike deformity. Causes include nerve paralysis and scarring from burns. One of the most common contractures affects the fingers, the ring finger in particular. Named *Dupuytren's contracture*, it develops with age in some persons of European origin, a little more commonly in men than women. It may be inherited but is also associated with epilepsy and alcoholic cirrhosis of the liver. Often it progresses so slowly that it causes little disability. In several cases surgical treatment is possible.

Joint contracture usually affects the hips, knees and shoulders of elderly people. It is caused by lack of use of the joint, which the patient is eventually unable to flex freely.

convulsion

A sudden involuntary twitching or contraction of the body caused by an abnormal discharge of electrical activity in the brain. Convulsions are commonly associated with EPILEPSY, being the most disturbing feature of the major epileptic seizure or fit. But they can be brought on by many other disorders, such as stroke, meningitis, kidney disease, and heatstroke. In young children convulsions may be caused by high fever.

In the typical convulsive attack, as in the major form of epilepsy, the patient first loses consciousness and falls heavily to the ground, his muscles locked. For a brief period breathing may be impaired, which accounts for a temporary bluish discoloration of the skin. Next comes a series of rapid, jerky and uncontrolled movements in the trunk and limbs. The jaw and tongue may also be affected, so that sometimes the patient lathers his saliva into a foam and appears to froth at the mouth. The tongue may be badly bitten. This period of frenzied activity usually lasts between two and three minutes. After a further few minutes of unconsciousness the patient generally regains consciousness, often to complain of a severe headache. He may remain in a state of confusion for several hours after an attack.

corneal grafting

This simple transplant technique is used to preserve the sight of people who are threatened with blindness when the cornea (the transparent area on the front of the eyeball) turns opaque.

With the exception of blood transfusions, corneal grafting is the most successful of all surgical operations involving the transfer of tissue from one person to another. The cornea can be removed from the eye of the donor up to six hours after death.

There are two main types of corneal graft: partial or full thickness. Some surgeons prefer not to replace the whole thickness of the cornea when only the outer layers of the recipient's cornea have turned opaque. Whole-thickness grafts are better optically than *lamella* or partial grafts. Partial grafts are sometimes performed, however, because of special circumstances in individual cases.

About three quarters of corneal transplants are successful, but the failure of one operation does not necessarily doom the patient to blindness. In a few cases it has taken as many as six operations to restore vision.

It can take a month or so for a transplanted graft to "knit" naturally, during which time it is held in place by sutures or special disks. These have to withstand considerable pressure, since the pressure behind the cornea exceeds that of the atmosphere.

A major reason for the high success rate of corneal grafting is that the cornea contains no blood vessels, so that the body's defense system of rejection antibodies cannot get into it; these antibodies account for failure in many other transplant operations, in spite of the use of immunosuppressant drugs. (See ANTIBODY/ANTIGEN, IMMUNE SYSTEM.)

Few people are aware of the long history of corneal grafting. The first operation was performed in 1817 by Reisinger, a European surgeon, although the first successful graft was not performed until 1905. Inconsistent results thereafter underlined the need for better techniques, which were to emerge with better instruments and finer suture material. Even today there is a degree of mystery as to why corneal grafts sometimes fail.

corns

A painful localized thickening of the skin of the foot. It is shaped like a cone, the point of which is directed inward, known as the eye or root of the corn. A CALLUS or callosity is a thickening over a wider area.

Corns on the upper part of the toes are caused by wearing tight or badly fitting shoes. Those on the underside of the foot are due to unevenness in the sole of the shoe. Where the skin is pinched or continually rubbed it grows more rapidly and, under the effect of pressure, gradually hardens. Corns between the toes are moist and are referred to as *soft corns*.

The first essential of treatment (despite the demands of fashion) is to start to wear sufficiently large and properly shaped shoes. These should not be pointed; the width of the sole at the level of the little toe should equal that of the bare foot when supporting the full weight of the body.

Corn plasters are circular pieces of felt which, when applied over a corn, give relief by spreading the unwelcome pressure of the shoe over a larger area.

Corns can be removed by soaking the foot in hot soapy water and then carefully cutting away the upper part of the softened corn. The affected area is dried and painted with a salicylic acid solution (included in many corn-removing lotions) to soften the corn even more and break it down. These lotions can damage healthy tissue surrounding the corn and should be used with great care. Finally, the eye of the corn may be picked out or rubbed away with a nail file, emery board or pumice stone. After complete removal of the corn, the foot should be washed or soaked in salt water every day to help return the skin to normal.

If foot problems continue, your physician may be able to recommend a foot specialist in your area.

coronary artery disease

See HEART DISEASE.

coronary bypass

See BYPASS.

coronary care unit

See INTENSIVE CARE UNIT.

coronary thrombosis

Blockage of one of the arteries that supplies the heart muscle (coronary artery) with a thrombus. Common name: *heart attack*.

See HEART DISEASE, THROMBOSIS.

CORN

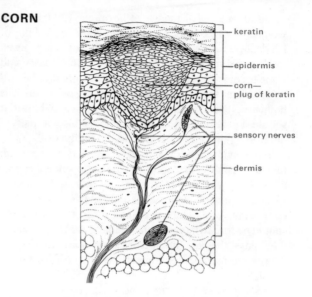

keratin
epidermis
corn—plug of keratin
sensory nerves
dermis

A corn is a horny thickening in the skin, and may occur at any point of continued pressure. It consists of a compressed mass of keratin (dead skin cells), and usually has a conical shape with a broad base on the skin surface and a point extending down into the dermis. Pain is caused by pressure of the horny plug on nerve endings.

cor pulmonale

A heart condition that can afflict people suffering from lung diseases such as chronic bronchitis, emphysema and chronic asthma.

It is often brought on by a chest infection. This worsens an already poor respiratory performance and leads to a lack of oxygen in the capillary vessels of the lung. These constrict so that the right chamber of the heart has to pump harder to keep the blood moving. The overall result is an enlarged heart working under considerable strain—rather like a domestic water pump faced with clogged pipes.

The typical signs of cor pulmonale include a bluish discoloration of the skin, especially in the hands and feet (which are often warm to the touch). The pulse is usually full and easily detected and there may be swelling of the limbs and ankles.

Stethoscopic examination of the chest can reveal abnormal heart sounds. The electrocardiogram (ECG), which provides a graphic record of the heart rhythm, typically contains various abnormalities.

The main danger in cor pulmonale is failure of the overworked heart (see HEART FAILURE). Treatment is aimed at improving lung performance, and antibiotics such as tetracycline and ampicillin may be administered to overcome the chest infection. Patients with severe breathing difficulties frequently receive oxygen therapy.

cosmetic surgery

The stigma formerly attached to this small and highly specialized branch of surgery is gradually disappearing. It has become increasingly popular during the last 20 years and about a million Americans a year now have "image-enhancing" operations.

Disfiguring facial deformities sustained during World War I provided a great impetus to the development of *plastic surgery*, from which cosmetic, or "beauty," surgery has evolved. The public still tends to identify plastic surgery only with elective cosmetic surgery, but the subspecialty also deals with cosmetic repair following injuries like burns and removal of tumors. However, in this entry we will discuss only those operations designed to "beautify" or otherwise improve outward appearance and sought by the patient.

The work falls broadly into three categories: (1) removal of blemishes and scars; (2) repair of congenital defects; and (3) improvements in contour. Most cosmetic operations are designed to eliminate wrinkles and pouches of baggy tissue to provide a firmer skin and a more youthful appearance, although one procedure—breast enlargement through silicone implantation—*adds* rather than removes for its enhancing effect.

Theoretically, there is no limit to the amount of cosmetic surgery any one person can have. The effects of a procedure like a face lift usually last about seven years.

Many patients are afraid that cosmetic surgery will scar them. Scars are inevitable, but they can be hidden beyond the scrutiny of the eye. Any reputable surgeon will advise about treatment and the likelihood of noticeable postoperative scars.

The following are some of the more commonly performed cosmetic operations.

Rhytidectomy (standard face lift). The surgeon separates the facial skin and part of the skin of the neck through an incision just beyond the hairline. He then pulls the skin up to the temples and back toward the ear, cuts away all the excess and closes the incision. People such as film stars, to whom a youthful appearance is often particularly important, may have several operations over the years.

Rhinoplasty (alteration of the nose). One of the most common surgical procedures. A large nose can be reshaped with the removal of cartilage or bone. Conversely, a sunken or flat nose can be remodeled by implantation of a carved piece of bone or cartilage. No scars are visible, since incisions are made within the nasal cavity.

Blepharoplasty (eyelid correction). A basically simple technique to improve a tired-looking pair of eyes by removing excess skin from the upper and lower creases of the eyelids. Scars can be concealed in the remaining skin folds.

Supraorbital rhytidoplasty (eyebrow correction). Drooping eyebrows can give a tired look to the eyes. The incision is made above the brow, which is raised with the removal of an ellipse of skin. The suture line can be hidden within the upper hairline of the brow.

Mammoplasty (cosmetic breast surgery). Silicone implants can be used to restore the shape of the breasts after mastectomy; this is an extremely valuable procedure in making necessary mastectomy operations a more tolerable prospect to many women. Other operations can be performed to enhance or reduce the size of the breasts.

Many people have unrealistic expectations about what a change of looks will do for them; thus, any responsible plastic surgeon will subject a potential patient to searching questions about her motives. Some women seek cosmetic surgery fearing that their husbands are losing interest in them and are attracted to younger, more beautiful women. It must be fully understood that cosmetic surgery cannot perform miracles and cannot be used as a means of solving some deep-seated emotional problem that has been wrongly blamed on external appearance. Not all beautiful people have happy lives, by any stretch of the imagination!

cot death

The sudden and unexpected death of an infant who was either well, or almost well, prior to death and whose death remains unexplained even after autopsy. The medical term is *sudden infant death syndrome*.

About 800 cot deaths occur every year in England and Wales. Throughout the world the incidence is consistently between 1 and 2 per 1,000 live births, with the highest frequency occurring in urban areas. Most cases involve infants of two to four months of age who die at home, in the night and unobserved.

More males than females are affected, and the children of minority groups and lower socioeconomic backgrounds experience a higher rate of cot death than others. The rate among siblings of victims is four times higher than usual. The mother is often young, with a large family, and inexperienced. The homes where cot deaths occur are frequently overcrowded. They are more common in winter.

The mechanism of cot death is unknown, although commonly a minor virus infection of the upper respiratory tract was present beforehand. Since cot death invariably occurs in sleep, one theory links depression of respiration during sleep with the viral infection and perhaps a reduced immune response.

Sometimes autopsy reveals a severe virus infection, in which case it is not strictly a "cot death." There is no evidence to suggest that sleeping position is responsible, nor neglect on the part of the parents. It may be that an immature respiratory control center is responsible and prevention is difficult where this cannot be recognized.

The rate of cot deaths has been reduced somewhat by improvement in urban housing, education of the vulnerable parents by special classes and instruction on the subject of baby care. Even so, cot deaths do occur in well-educated, affluent families.

The parents suffer a desperate feeling of loss made worse by a sense of guilt, which is invariably unjustified. Parent groups have done much to alleviate this suffering through contact and useful literature.

cough

Sudden noisy explosive discharge of air from the lungs and air passages, which clears them of excessive mucus or irritating foreign matter.

Coughing depends on the integrity of a complicated reflex action during which (1) the chest first expands; (2) the glottis then closes; (3) the muscles of the chest contract, so that pressure builds up in the lungs; and (4) the glottis opens suddenly to release the air in a rush.

Any condition which increases the secretion of mucus in the lungs will produce a cough, for example, inflammation or a tumor; a dry, irritating cough typically follows infection of the upper air passages. Excessive secretions from the nose of the paranasal sinuses (which drain into the nasal cavities) may drip down the back of the throat, and set up attacks of coughing ("postnasal drip"). The only cure for a cough is the cure of the condition which causes it. But coughing can be suppressed by drugs acting centrally on the cough reflex (codeine, pholcodine) or alleviated by drinking soothing liquids, one of the most effective being lemon juice and honey in warm water. Various compounds are said to loosen thick sputum, but none is unfailingly effective.

Persistent cough is rarely an early sign of a potentially serious underlying disease. Cough which produces blood, however, should receive immediate medical attention.

Coxsackie virus

Coxsackie viruses belong to the *enterovirus* group, which also includes the ECHO viruses and polioviruses. They are common infecting agents in humans and produce a wide variety of diseases. Thus, they may produce a condition resembling either the common cold or influenza, with a sore throat and painful neck glands. The sore throat may be accompanied by small blisterlike lesions in the back of the throat (a condition known as *herpangina*); a similar condition may involve the feet and hands as well (*hand, foot and mouth disease*). The pleura (the membrane lining the chest cavity and covering the outer surface of the lungs) may be affected to give a painful chest condition known as EPIDEMIC PLEURODYNIA or *Bornholm disease*. In both children and adults, the heart muscle may be affected (MYOCARDITIS) and the membranes surrounding the brain and spinal cord (MENINGITIS).

Infections produced by this group of viruses are usually not serious though they may be painful and distressing to the patient. Death is unusual except in young children.

cramp

A sudden, involuntary and prolonged spasm of the muscles causing severe pain.

It can occur in the abdominal muscles due to immersion in cold water (*swimmer's cramp*) or in groups of muscles used continually (e.g. *writer's cramp*). Hard physical labor in the heat leads to excessive salt losses by sweating and causes *heat cramps*. The elderly and the young, especially, also get cramps in the leg muscles while sleeping. This is brought about by impaired circulation that results from lying in one position too long.

The treatment of muscle cramp is to relax the spasm and improve the local circulation: keep the limb warm, rub and massage it, and avoid excessive fatigue. Heat cramps should be treated by drinking plenty of water with a little salt in it.

craniopharyngioma

A very rare tumor of the brain occurring only in children.

It is a congenital "leftover" piece of tissue at the base of the brain that should have evolved in the embryo into part of the mouth. As the child grows, this tissue grows and presses on the pituitary gland or the optic nerve. The result may be dwarfism, a rise in pressure in the skull, or progressive blindness. Craniopharyngioma is diagnosed by skull x rays when any of the symptoms arise, usually in late childhood.

The only treatment is surgical removal of the tumor.

cretinism

A congenital condition characterized by retarded physical and mental development caused by a deficiency of thyroid hormone.

Inadequate or absent secretion of hormones by the THYROID GLAND in fetal or early neonatal life retards growth of the skeleton and the brain. This underactivity of the thyroid gland can be the result of inadequate nutrition and particularly the lack of iodine in the diet; it may occur when the mother has been taking antithyroid drugs before or during pregnancy; or it may be due to a biochemical abnormality in the thyroid (sporadic cretinism).

In the first months of life a cretin fails to feed properly and has a protruding tongue, thick dry skin, slow reflexes and poor muscle tone. These signs in a baby may lead to an early diagnosis. If not, then later, delayed dentition (development of the teeth), constipation, yellow scaling skin and retarded growth indicate the need for biochemical investigations. The tests will show depressed thyroid function and will clearly establish the diagnosis.

It is important to diagnose cretinism early before permanent brain damage occurs. Treatment with thyroid hormone has to be continued with increasing dosage as the child grows. Early treatment and good control can produce normal development and a complete cure.

Cretinism occurs endemically in areas of the world where the dietary intake of iodine is inadequate, especially in mountainous limestone districts, where rainfall has washed the iodine out of the soil. In such regions GOITER occurs in the adult population. Both conditions can be prevented by the dietary use of "iodized" salt.

Crohn's disease

A disorder of the intestines. It is characterized by recurrent episodes of abdominal pain (usually on the right lower side), diarrhea, fever, weight loss and appetite depression.

The disease was first described by the American gastroenterologist B. B. Crohn in 1932. It is also called *regional ileitis* and *regional enteritis*.

Crohn's disease mainly affects young adults and in the early acute attacks it is often misdiagnosed as appendicitis. The stools are loose, watery and continual. If the disease is not treated, serious complications such as peritonitis and abscesses may occur. It attacks both males and females and most ethnic groups, although it is unusually common among Jewish people.

The cause is unknown. Diet, infection and allergy have all been implicated, but without precise identification of the actual mechanism involved. Emotional stress undoubtedly leads to exacerbations and recurrences are seen at times of psychological disturbance.

The initial symptoms in most patients are nonspecific for this disease and include a low-grade fever with recurrent bouts of diarrhea over a period of months. Weakness and loss of weight become obvious and in former times tuberculosis of the intestines would be considered as a diagnosis. (It is now known that TB is not a cause of Crohn's disease.) As the attacks get worse

and more frequent, diagnosis requires investigation by x rays (a barium enema—see BARIUM MEAL/BARIUM ENEMA) and biochemical analysis. The typical x-ray picture confirms the diagnosis.

In approximately a third of the cases the disease eventually resolves by itself and subsides. In the remainder it has to be treated by a high-calorie, high-protein diet and special drugs to relieve the stress and diarrhea. Cortisone-like steroid drugs help in overcoming the acute phase and bring about a remission; however, they are not a cure and the problems of continual medication with such powerful agents is considerable because of the side effects.

Surgery is usually necessary for severe cases and for patients over the age of about 50. Excision of the affected area of the intestine can bring short-term relief in all cases and long-term cure for some. The disease can recur after surgery, however; such patients are then treated with a combination of dietary care, medication and support.

croup

An inflammation of the larynx ("voice-box") leading to difficulty in breathing accompanied by a harsh croaking noise. The condition is virtually confined to small children.

Croup is usually a complication of a virus or bacterial infection of the upper respiratory tract. Inflammation in the larynx leads to the gap between the vocal cords being narrowed, so obstructing the breathing. The attack usually appears at night, when the child is lying down; the breathing becomes strident and difficult and the child will usually be frightened. Croup can be dangerous if the gap between the vocal cords is completely closed, and urgent treatment may be needed to overcome the obstruction either by passing a tube down the windpipe (intubation) or by making an opening through the neck into the windpipe (TRACHEOSTOMY).

Once a child has had an attack of croup it is liable to recur, so he should be guarded against cold and damp conditions which tend to encourage respiratory disorders. If a child suffers from an attack of croup and is having difficulty in breathing, a doctor should always be called. In the meantime, opening the window in a centrally heated house can bring relief, since hot dry air seems to encourage croup. For the same reason, a vaporizer or cold mist nebulizer should be placed in the bedroom. In the home, humidity may also be increased by running hot water from the shower and faucets. However, is it potentially dangerous to increase the humidity of the child's bedroom by means of a boiling kettle or pan, as scalding accidents are not uncommon. The parent should not panic, but be reassuring and assume a relaxed attitude.

crush syndrome

A serious condition that can develop following a massive crushing injury to large groups of muscles, as in being trapped under heavy debris in a mining or industrial accident or being the victim of a traffic accident where part of the body (especially an arm or leg) is pinned. It has also occurred as the result of leaving a tourniquet on a limb for prolonged periods without relief.

The condition was first described by German physicians during World War I and was further investigated by British and American physicians during World War II (the falling debris from air strikes resulted in hundreds of military and civilian personnel being the victims of the crush syndrome). Even so, the underlying mechanisms are still unclear. Probably the kidneys are damaged by the complicated breakdown products of the injured and dead muscle cells that enter the circulation; the low blood pressure associated with SHOCK (circulatory collapse) is another factor.

Trouble typically starts two or three days after the injury, when the patient appears to have recovered reasonably well from the shock and the surgical treatment of the injuries. Urine production becomes scanty and eventually kidney function stops. The patient becomes apathetic, restless and delirious with the rise in blood concentrations of urea (the major nitrogenous waste product of metabolism) and other poisonous substances (toxins). (See UREMIA.)

Death was common before the invention of hemodialysis (the "artificial kidney") in people who had been severely crushed and trapped for prolonged periods. Despite modern surgical and medical advances, however, the condition still proves fatal in some cases. Early amputation of the crushed limb seems to be an important factor in reversing the kidney failure. The administration of intravenous fluids containing *mannitol* in the period immediately after the injury can also help to reduce the incidence of the crush syndrome. For those patients who experience the signs and symptoms of the condition, however, hemodialysis may be needed for a week or ten days before the kidneys begin to recover.

Cushing's syndrome

A disease with many symptoms, caused by excessive secretion of cortisone-like hormones by the adrenal glands. It was first recognized in 1932 by the Boston neurosurgeon Harvey Cushing (1869–1939).

Among the signs and symptoms of Cushing's syndrome are protein depletion causing muscle wasting and weakness, fragility of the blood vessels causing increased susceptibility to bruising, decalcification of the bones causing spinal curvature, occasional biochemical disorders such as diabetes, and—most obvious of all—the "moon face" and "buffalo hump" caused by facial obesity and redistribution of body fat. Women also suffer masculinization: excessive hair grows on the body, the voice deepens, and menstruation ceases.

Cushing's syndrome is relatively rare, more common in females than males, and most frequently develops in women over 30, particularly after a pregnancy.

The complicated disorders of the body seen in Cushing's syndrome—all due to an excess of cortisone-like hormones—are nowadays more commonly seen as a result of long-term or excessive treatment with cortisone or similar steroid drugs. People who depend on steroids to control such conditions as asthma, rheumatoid arthritis or colitis develop the characteristic "moon face" of Cushing's syndrome as an early sign of chronic overdosage.

Apart from excessive steroid treatment, the cause of Cushing's syndrome is usually a small tumor of one of the adrenal glands (which lie just above the kidneys). If the tumor cannot easily be identified and surgically removed, treatment consists of irradiation of the pituitary gland at the base of the brain—which controls many of the other hormone-producing glands.

The diagnosis is made by careful biochemical assessment of hormone output, and in particular measurement of the urinary excretion of cortisone breakdown products over a given period. Skull x-rays (to reveal a possible tumor of the pituitary gland) and complicated blood tests are also necessary. Once the diagnosis is made, drugs are necessary to compensate for the chemical, mineral and other hormonal deficiencies.

Then the diseased adrenal gland is removed surgically along with the tumor, the remaining gland is often found to be shrunken. Thus, supplements of the correct amount of cortisone-like hormone are necessary until the other gland recovers function, and they may also be necessary for life.

cyanosis

Blue coloration of the skin due to lack of oxygen in the blood. Normally most of the pigment (HEMOGLOBIN) in the blood is combined with oxygen, giving it a bright red color. If for any reason the blood lacks oxygen a substantial proportion of the pigment is in its "reduced" form, giving the blood a dusky blue color. This is most noticeable in the patient's lips, face, fingernails, hands and feet.

Babies born with heart defects such as HOLE IN THE HEART, children and adults with diseases causing respiratory or cardiac failure, and the elderly with circulatory or cardiac inefficiency all show signs of cyanosis due to inadequate oxygenation of the blood. Poor circulation in the limbs may also cause cyanosis—for example, in RAYNAUD'S DISEASE, VARICOSE VEINS, or exposure to cold.

The condition is a *sign*—not a disease in itself—and may appear whenever an extra demand is made on a circulatory or respiratory system that cannot cope with more than its normal work. A "blue baby" is cyanosed because some of its blood bypasses the lungs and so is not oxygenated. A cardiac invalid may become cyanosed when he sustains a respiratory infection.

Treatment depends on the underlying cause, but if cyanosis appears during an illness, hospitalization and the provision of oxygen are usually necessary. Cardiac surgery may be required for the baby with congenital heart disease.

cyst

An abnormal sac or pouch within the body, usually filled with fluid, semifluid, or solid material (gas-filled cysts occasionally occur).

A common example is a SEBACEOUS CYST. Sebaceous glands in the skin secrete an oily material (sebum) essential to the maintenance of normal skin texture. Blockage of the opening of the gland leads to an accumulation of sebum in the duct of the gland. As it becomes greatly dilated, a rounded mass develops immediately beneath the skin, with its walls formed by the original lining of the duct. Such cysts are commonly half an inch in diameter but may occasionally be much larger.

Cysts may occur in any organ which produces a secretion if the duct becomes blocked while secretion continues. Cysts of this type may occur in the breast, mouth, genital tract, in the specialized sebaceous glands in the eyelid (CHALAZION) and in many of the internal organs, such as the ovaries, pancreas and kidneys. Other types of cyst may occur as the result of imperfect development of glands before birth, with the gland forming but its duct being absent. A *dermoid cyst* occurs when a portion of skin becomes buried in the tissues, either as a result of a penetrating injury or at the junction of two developing skin folds before birth. Occasionally, a tumor may develop a cystic area within itself and eventually come to resemble a cyst.

Cysts may also develop as a result of infection with parasitic worms, which form cystic structures in the tissues at certain stages of their life cycles (*hydatid cyst*).

Treatment of cysts may be unnecessary if they cause no symptoms. If they are unsightly, cause pressure on surrounding structures, or are suspected of originating in a tumor, surgical removal will be usually required. In some cases, simple aspiration of the cyst contents is performed to establish its nature.

cystadenoma

An ADENOMA containing cysts.

cystic fibrosis

An inherited disorder which primarily affects the PANCREAS (an organ in the abdominal cavity responsible for producing insulin and some enzymes essential for digestion).

The disease, also known as fibrocystic disease of the pancreas, causes obstruction of the gland's ducts and thus a deficiency or total absence of its secretions. In severe cases childhood development is severely retarded.

The pancreatic deficiency means that the patient cannot digest fats. This inability causes the bulky, offensive smelling stools consistently produced, and leads to malnutrition with shortened stature if the diagnosis is not made early and treatment started promptly.

Cystic fibrosis also effects the mucus-producing glands of the respiratory system. Chronic severe chest disease and proneness to chest infection are characteristic of cystic fibrosis.

Tests show that one in four of the immediate relatives of a child born with this disease has a partial tendency toward it. The test used is the "sweat-test," which indicates abnormality in the body's chemistry. The incidence of cystic fibrosis is one in a thousand Caucasian live births, while it is rare in blacks and never reported in Mongolian races.

Cystic fibrosis is diagnosed by measuring how well the patient digests fat from "test" meals. The fat content of the stool is analyzed. An increase of salt excretion in the sweat and a history of chronic lung disease are also diagnostic signs. Blood tests may confirm the diagnosis of the disease.

It is possible today to reduce fat intake through careful dietary control, to give pancreatic enzymes as a medication taken by mouth, and to replace the vitamin deficiencies. As a result, the outlook for patients has improved in recent years. The pancreas still produces insulin so diabetes does not occur. Control of the chest symptoms remains a problem: every minor infection presents the risk of bronchitis and chronic blockage of the air passages by excess mucus leads to permanent chest damage. Treatment involves the administration of antibiotics, physiotherapy to encourage the drainage of mucus, and nebulizers to promote the breakup of thickened secretions.

Survival used to be rare, but modern medical care and dietary control make the outlook for children born with cystic fibrosis more promising.

cystinuria

A rare inherited, or congenital, disorder of the kidneys in which the urine contains excessive amounts of an amino acid called cystine and related substances. This occurs because of an inability of the tubules of the kidneys to reabsorb these substances.

Cystine excretion poses no threat to life. The excess in the urine, however, may lead to stone formation in the kidneys or bladder and surgical treatment may then be necessary. Prevention of stones depends on the regular and frequent drinking of water as a lifetime habit for those who inherit cystinuria.

cystitis

Inflammation of the membrane lining the urinary bladder.

Urine is normally sterile and this freedom from infection is dependent on a number of factors. Firstly, the bladder lies wholly within the body and is connected with the exterior only by means of the narrow lower urinary passage (urethra). The external sites, in both male and female, at which the urethra opens teem with bacteria but their ascent up the urethra to reach the bladder is normally prevented by the constant downward flow of urine. Complete emptying of the bladder is important and obstruction to the outflow of urine, as by enlargement of the prostate gland in the male, or paralysis of the bladder, greatly increases the likelihood of ascending infection. The urine itself has antibacterial properties and the bladder membrane is resistant to the establishment of infection.

Infection of the bladder is much more common in women than in men since the urethra is much shorter in a woman and the infecting bacteria have less far to travel. The passage of instruments (*cystoscopy* or *catheters*) into the bladder will also tend to carry infection up the urethra. "Honeymoon cystitis" is a common condition in women following frequent sexual intercourse; both bruising of the urethra and bladder wall and a tendency to force infected material up the urethra play a part in its cause.

The symptoms of cystitis include pain in the lower part of the abdomen, a desire to pass urine frequently, pain on urination, and the passage of cloudy, blood-stained or foul-smelling urine. There may be more generalized symptoms with fever and lassitude. Examination of a urine sample in the laboratory will reveal the presence of pus cells and bacteria can be cultured from the urine. It may also contain protein and blood.

Treatment involves giving plenty of fluids to increase the urine flow and the administration of appropriate antibiotics for all but the mildest attacks. Recurrence of bladder infection in a woman (or, in a man, the occurrence of even a single attack) may indicate the need for further investigation to seek a local cause, such as an obstruction to urine flow.

Recurrent bladder infections may, in some patients, give rise to more serious infections of the ureters (the passages from the kidneys to the bladder) or of the kidneys themselves (*pyelitis*, *pyelonephritis*) and the patient should always seek medical advice.

cystocele

A herniation of the urinary bladder into the vagina sometimes occurring as a complication of multiple childbirth or as a complication of PROLAPSE of the uterus. In the latter case, weakening of the muscles which support the floor of the pelvis allows the uterus to descend from its normal position high in the pelvis so that it presses on the vagina from above, telescoping its walls and allowing the cervix (neck of the womb) to lie low in the vagina near its opening.

The uterus lies in the pelvis close to the bladder in front of it and the rectum behind. The distortion of the normal anatomy which occurs in prolapse of the uterus frequently causes the wall of the bladder to be forced downward as well so that it forms a pouch bulging down into the front wall of the vagina (cystocele). A similar situation may occur if the rectum herniates into the vagina (RECTOCELE).

In addition to the symptoms of a prolapse (vaginal discomfort, a dragging sensation in the pelvis and backache), a cystocele can produce its own specific symptoms. These include difficulty in emptying the bladder completely, with a resulting increase in the frequency of passing urine, a tendency to recurrent bladder infections and (most commonly) difficulty in preventing escape of urine when the bladder is full, especially on coughing or straining ("stress incontinence").

Treatment usually involves a surgical procedure known as *colporrhaphy*. The ligaments supporting the pelvic floor are tightened, the muscle layers repaired and the normal anatomic relationships of the bladder, uterus, vagina and rectum restored. In older women the procedure may be combined with surgical removal of the uterus (HYSTERECTOMY).

cytomegalovirus disease

A disease that attacks the salivary glands, liver, spleen and lungs. It was first recognized in the late 1950s; the name literally means "a large cell with a large virus inside."

In babies the unidentified virus—visible on microscopic study of tissue from the affected gland—causes pneumonia and a severe blood disorder which leads to hemorrhage in the tissues and death. Newborn babies are thought to be infected before birth via the placenta and they have insufficient immunity to fight the disease. Most adults have antibodies against the virus, suggesting that infection in a minor form has been encountered and overcome—perhaps as a misdiagnosed attack of a "mumps-like" disease. It is the occasional nonimmune mother who is infected by the virus in late pregnancy who will pass it to the fetus.

Cytomegalovirus disease of the newborn is thought to be responsible for a small proportion of CRIB DEATHS. In nonimmune adults some cases of virus pneumonia are due to infection with the cytomegalovirus, but they usually recover unless leukemic-type complications occur as a result of damage to the tissues that produce blood cells.

No treatment for the disease is known (immunity cannot yet be produced by vaccination) but the presence of antibodies in most of the adult population suggests that many attacks are relatively harmless.

D

dandruff

A dry scaly eruption of the scalp; it may also less commonly occur as thick greasy scales. It is thought to affect about 60% of people to some degree; the condition, although unsightly, is of little consequence except that those who suffer to a marked extent may develop skin disorders such as common ACNE and ROSACEA. They also incline to react more sharply than normal to contact with chemicals, developing sensitivity states, and are prone to superficial bacterial infection of the skin by *Staphylococcus aureus* and *Streptococcus pyogenes*.

There are a large number of preparations on the market designed to relieve this common condition. Among the most successful are shampoos containing cetrimide or selenium sulfide.

deafness

Loss or impairment of hearing. From about the age of 10 to 15 every person begins to lose the hearing acuity of childhood; thus every adult hears slightly less well than children, particularly in the higher frequencies.

The range of frequencies capable of being heard by the human ear are from 16 Hertz (i.e., cycles per second) to 20,000 Hz. Above 20,000 Hz lie the ultrasound frequencies, which are audible to dogs and certain other

animals but not to man. The various types of deafness can best be explained by reference to the normal hearing apparatus of the healthy human.

Sounds come to us by means of vibrations of the air, which enter the ear through the external auditory meatus (earhole). The sound waves travel down the external ear canal and strike the eardrum, a tiny piece of specialized tissue about the size of a piece of confetti. The eardrum vibrates at the same frequency as the sound waves and passes on the vibrations to a tiny bone known as the *malleus* (or hammer) which fits into its rear surface. The malleus is jointed to a second tiny bone known as the *incus* (or anvil), which in turn is jointed to the smallest bone in the human body, the *stapes* (or stirrup; named because of its striking resemblance to a stirrup).

The base of the stapes fits into an oval window in the side of a highly specialized organ, about the size of a pea, known as the *cochlea* (literally, "snail"). The vibrations caused by the original sound waves, much intensified by the three bones—collectively known as the auditory ossicles—are passed by the stapes to the fluid in the cochlea (which forms part of the structures of the inner ear). Finally, within the cochlea is the *organ of Corti*, an elaborate center which transforms the fluid waves into impulses which pass to the brain through the *auditory nerve* (the nerve of hearing).

Specialists generally recognize four types of deafness:

1. *Conductive deafness* is caused by disease of or injury to some part of the hearing apparatus which conducts the sound waves from the eardrum to the fluid of the internal ear (that is, the eardrum or the auditory ossicles).

2. *Sensorineural deafness* (also known as *perceptive* or *nerve deafness*) is caused by damage to the part of the hearing apparatus that perceives the sound, from the cochlea to the brain.

3. *Mixed deafness* is a combination of the two above types.

4. *Functional*, or *psychogenic*, *deafness* is caused by psychological upset or shock in the absence of any organic disease.

Conductive deafness may be caused by a plug of wax in the external auditory meatus or by a direct blow to the ear which injures the eardrum or dislocates the auditory ossicles. A common cause in wartime is explosions that rupture the eardrum, but traffic accidents are now responsible for many cases. *Otic barotrauma* is the cause of a special type of conductive deafness caused by repeated changes in atmospheric pressure in air travel. *Otosclerosis* is a condition in which extra bone grows around the stapes and prevents conduction of sound to the cochlea; a surgical operation can correct this condition (see STAPEDECTOMY).

Sensorineural deafness can result from injury, and

also from constant subjection to loud noises, such as those made by machinery or loud rock music groups. Excessive alcohol consumption interferes with the absorption of vitamin B and this leads to sensorineural deafness. Drugs, in particular streptomycin, have also been involved in many cases of deafness.

About one in a thousand of all children are born deaf, either through heredity, maternal rubella (German measles) or drugs taken during pregnancy. Nearly all cases of congenital deafness are sensorineural.

A large proportion of people over the age of 65 complain of some degree of deafness, due to degenerative changes in the cells of the organs of hearing. This is usually permanent but it can be helped by appropriate hearing aids.

Some of the "miracle cures" of deafness arise from the fourth category, where the condition is caused by autosuggestion or the subconscious. These cases of functional or psychogenic deafness are often cured by psychotherapy.

See also HEARING.

debridement

The removal of foreign material, dead tissue and other debris from a wound. By keeping the wound as clean as possible, infection is discouraged and prompt healing is enhanced.

decompression sickness

A technical name for the BENDS.

defibrillation

The use of electrical energy to stop arrhythmias of the heart, particularly VENTRICULAR FIBRILLATION.

The ventricles are the two chambers which pump blood out of the heart into the arteries. In a normal heart the ventricles are controlled by the *pacemaker*, a bundle of fibers in the right atrium which sends out electrical impulses that control the rate of heartbeat.

In cases of heart disease, particularly where MYOCARDIAL INFARCTION kills part of the heart muscle, this normal rhythm can be disturbed. It is replaced by a form of excitation which causes the muscles of the ventricles to quiver rather than to contract regularly. The ventricles are then unable to perform their task of pumping blood around the body and death quickly follows if the fibrillation is not corrected.

Ventricular fibrillation is a common complication of coronary heart disease. Some 75 to 95% of patients in coronary care units suffer from arrhythmias. The first object of the medical team confronted with this condition is to stop the fibrillation and resume the normal rhythm.

This is done by applying electrodes to the chest (first placing on the skin a paste which increases electrical conductivity) and then passing an electric current through the chest wall to the heart. When open-heart surgery is being performed, the same procedure is carried out, but the electrodes are applied directly to the heart.

The defibrillator is a machine which gathers electrical charge in capacitors and then discharges it in a fraction of a second. The energy level is usually about 400 watts per second, which is sufficient to stop the heart quivering and give it a chance to resume its normal rhythm under the control of the pacemaker. Defibrillation is now a routine procedure in any well-equipped medical center; the overall success rate for termination of arrhythmias should approach 90%.

Complications are seen in about 15% of cases, but this figure does not include minor skin burns and transient arrhythmias. One of the most common complications is a change in concentration of enzymes in the body, which may be seen in one case out of ten.

deficiency diseases

Diseases caused by the shortage of an essential nutrient in the diet.

Humans require protein, carbohydrates, fat, vitamins and trace elements to maintain health; prolonged shortage of any one of these may cause a deficiency disease.

The most spectacular is deficiency of protein in children. This is uncommon in developed nations, but is a threat to life in the so-called Third World, where it is known as KWASHIORKOR.

Absence of vitamins in the diet can cause a variety of deficiency diseases. Vitamin A deficiency causes night blindness. Vitamin B_1 (thiamine) deficiency leads to beriberi. Vitamin B_2 (riboflavin) deficiency causes skin and eye troubles. One of the most serious deficiency diseases is pernicious anemia (see ANEMIA), which arises from a lack of vitamin B_{12}, and can be treated by regular injections of the vitamin. Pellagra is a deficiency disease caused by lack of niacin, another vitamin of the B complex. Rickets is caused by lack of vitamin D, and scurvy by a deficiency of vitamin C.

Among the trace elements, iron is the most commonly deficient; the result is ANEMIA, a lack in the blood of hemoglobin, which depends on iron for its production.

degenerative diseases

A group of disorders caused by aging of the structures of the body, with loss of elasticity, a reduction in the number of active cells and an increase in the proportion of fibrous connective tissue.

A major difficulty in the consideration of degenerative diseases lies in making the distinction between symptoms due to a disease and the universal effects of aging. If the rate of decline is faster in one organ than in the rest of the body, then the diagnosis is likely to be a degenerative disease. Doctors regard OSTEOARTHRITIS and ATHEROSCLEROSIS as diseases, whereas wrinkling of the skin and changes in the sex organs are accepted as normal processes. In part this is a difference of degree: while a family is likely to accept some forgetfulness, irritability and quirky behavior in an elderly grandparent, they will probably seek medical advice if his mental functioning falls below a certain level (and grandpa may well be diagnosed as having *senile dementia*). (See DEMENTIA.)

Although degenerative diseases most commonly afflict the aged, the underlying problem might have been progressing unnoticed for many years. For example, surveys in the United States and Britain have revealed that approximately 10% of people in their early 20s show the characteristic changes of osteoarthritis (noted by x-ray studies) in their joints; by the age of 50, such changes are present in over 80% of the population. However, *symptoms* of osteoarthritis are extremely rare in the 20s and affect only about 20% of people by the age of 50.

In many degenerative diseases there is a hereditary tendency. This factor is difficult to assess in common conditions such as osteoarthritis and atherosclerosis, but is striking in disorders such as CATARACT (which often seems to run in families).

The increasing proportion of old people in the populations of industrialized societies means that degenerative diseases are becoming more important in terms of human suffering and in the burden placed on health services. This has led belatedly to more research into the possible causes and treatment of degenerative disease. As a result, traditional ideas—like osteoarthritis being due to "wear and tear" and senile dementia resulting from atherosclerosis of the cerebral arteries—are now being critically reexamined and found to be inadequate.

The aim of research is to alleviate existing symptoms and possibly to arrest the progress of degenerative diseases. If successful, this would improve the quality of life—although it would probably not significantly increase the life span of man.

dehydration

The state produced by abnormal loss of body water; the deprivation or loss of water from the tissues.

Water at first may not appear to be a very important constituent of our relatively solid-looking bodies, but in fact it forms approximately 65% of the weight of the body. Most of this fluid (about 41% of the body weight) lies within the cells (intracellular fluid), from which it cannot be removed in any quantity without severe disturbance of their metabolic processes. The remaining fluid includes that which lies between the body cells (intercellular fluid), the liquid portion of the blood (blood plasma), the lymph and the fluid in certain cavities of the body (serous cavities). This *extracellular fluid* can be subject to greater variation than the *intracellular fluid*. The plasma component can to some extent use the intercellular water as a reservoir but, to maintain the circulation and other body functions, the total amount of extracellular fluid cannot be greatly reduced.

Dehydration may arise from deprivation of water or an inability to drink either because of difficulty in swallowing (as, for example, in cancer of the esophagus), or because the patient is weak, drowsy or comatose from any cause.

Vomiting may both prevent fluid from being taken and also increase loss of fluid from the body as the secretions of the stomach and intestine are lost. Diarrhea may act in the same way to increase water loss and a combination of vomiting and diarrhea will lead to rapid dehydration.

Dehydration may also be due to excessive secretion of urine despite falling body reserves of water; this occurs in both untreated DIABETES MELLITUS and DIABETES INSIPIDUS and in certain kidney disorders. Finally, excessive sweating in a hot climate will cause rapid dehydration if water is not freely available.

It is unusual for dehydration to occur as an uncomplicated problem. Vomiting, diarrhea, sweating and kidney disease frequently cause simultaneous excessive loss of salt from the body, the gross deficiency of which may be more serious than that of the water itself.

Symptoms of uncontrolled dehydration are thirst, followed by weakness, exhaustion and finally delirium and death.

While a healthy adult may survive weeks without food, complete deprivation of water and food may prove fatal within about three days. If food but not water is available the time will be longer, since most foods contain some water and additional water is produced during their metabolism in the body. Dehydration in small infants is more serious still and death may occur very quickly.

Treatment, if dehydration is the result of water deprivation alone, is by the cautious administration of fluids. If complicated by vomiting, diarrhea or sweating, laboratory tests to determine the extent of any salt deficiency and the administration of intravenous salt solutions may be required.

deja vu

A feeling that some event or experience has happened before; an apparent familiarity with what are in reality new events, strange surroundings or people.

Literally translated from the French, the expression means "already seen." Deja vu is experienced by normal individuals from time to time, especially when fatigued. However, it can be a prominent feature in the phobic anxiety type of neurosis or it may herald an attack of psychomotor EPILEPSY.

Deja vu usually occurs at a time of decreased consciousness and is often described as a dreamlike experience. It may be accompanied by other distorted perceptions, such as a feeling of depersonalization. The underlying mechanism of deja vu is not understood, but in epileptic cases an abnormality can frequently be demonstrated in the brain.

An analogous phenomenon of "jamais vu" (never seen), where objects appear unreal or very distant, can also be a symptom of temporal lobe epilepsy.

delirium

A clouding of consciousness in which attention and perception are disordered and the patient is extremely restless. Hallucinations frequently interrupt mental activity and add to the patient's general anxiety.

Usually the onset of delirium is abrupt and the condition lasts for a few days. There is remarkable variability in the patient's mental state from hour to hour, so that he might experience occasional islands of recognition in the sea of confusion and incomprehension.

Some individuals are thought to be more prone to delirium than others, but virtually anyone will develop delirium if subjected to certain intensive physical insults to the body—such as some infections, drugs, head trauma and destructive brain lesions (including hemorrhage).

In bacterial infections such as MENINGITIS, TYPHOID FEVER and PNEUMONIA, the accompanying delirium is thought to result from the action of toxins on certain parts of the brain. A similar "toxic" effect results from overdoses of amphetamines "speed" or certain antidepressants. By contrast, abrupt withdrawal of alcohol or barbiturates—drugs which have a strong inhibitory effect on the brain—leads to delirium.

The exact site of the brain's malfunction in delirium has not been identified, but there is strong evidence implicating the "reticular system" (which intricately controls the level of consciousness).

Treatment of delirium involves control of the underlying cause and reassurance by quiet, careful nursing; sedatives prevent self-injury or exhaustion.

delirium tremens (DTs)

A form of DELIRIUM due to sudden withdrawal of alcohol following a long period of intoxication. It is the most dramatic complication of ALCOHOLISM.

The condition is preceded by a generalized epileptic fit in about 25% of cases; there is often increasing tremulousness ("the shakes"), wakefulness and hallucination for a day or so beforehand.

In a full-blown attack the patient has many symptoms common to other types of delirium, but the special features of delirium tremens are (1) a fine tremor of the tongue, lips and hands; (2) an increased pulse rate and profuse sweating and (3) terrifying auditory and visual hallucinations (often of little animals).

In most cases, delirium tremens terminates in a deep sleep following three or four days of relentless activity. The patient normally awakes hungry, exhausted and clear minded—but with very little memory of the delirium.

Sedatives and anticonvulsants may be given during an attack, but they are only a prelude to the long-term treatment of chronic alcoholism. About 10% of cases of delirium tremens end fatally.

delusion

A false belief out of keeping with a person's educational, cultural and religious background.

A *primary* delusion occurs when a normal perception is abnormally interpreted so that it takes on an inexplicable personal meaning or significance. For example, a man sitting next to you in a bus lights a cigarette and this immediately conveys to you that he is having an affair with your wife. Such primary delusions appear suddenly and cannot be refuted by rational argument. They are one form of thought disorder typically encountered in schizophrenic patients.

In a *secondary* delusion, the false belief may be based on an abnormal initial perception (hallucination) or it might form part of an elaborate delusional system, the origin of which is not clear even to the patient. Secondary delusions are less specific to the diagnosis of schizophrenia than primary delusions because they are found in most other psychotic diseases, notably manic depressive psychosis.

A schizophrenic patient might construct a tortuous system of delusions on the basis of what voices in his head have told him. Often these delusions persecute the patient; they may have a political, erotic or religious theme. Delusions of grandeur also occur in schizophrenia, although historically they were associated with general paralysis of the insane (the final stage of syphilis).

In *depressive illness*, delusions are commonly hypochondriacal: the patient is convinced that his body is decomposing or that he has cancer. Alternatively delusions of guilt, unworthiness or poverty can haunt him. By contrast, in the *manic* phase of depression the delusions are of grandeur and omnipotence.

dementia

Literally "loss of mind."

Dementia can have many possible causes and mechanisms, but the constant feature is loss of memory, particularly for recent events.

The earliest signs of dementia are often very subtle and can be detected only by an observant relative or employer. There may be a mood change or a minor shortcoming at work, often attributed to depression by the doctor. However, as the underlying brain disease of dementia progresses over months or years, the patient loses all intellectual powers and emotional control, with the result that his personality is completely degraded. This total deterioration can be prevented in a few cases, so that it is important to try and establish the cause of every dementia.

Senile dementia is a degenerative condition of the nerve cells of the brain, particularly those of the cerebral cortex. The brain shrinks, the natural cavities (ventricles) within it enlarge and the surface convolutions begin to waste away (atrophy). Senile dementia is not just an exaggeration of the normal aging processes; its effects are more pronounced than the ordinary blunting of intellectual faculties.

ALZHEIMER'S DISEASE is an identical progressive dementia but it begins long before old age and results in early death.

In old people, disease of the brain's blood vessels causes *arteriosclerotic dementia*, which can be impossible to differentiate from senile dementia: indeed, the two conditions can coexist.

No specific therapy is available for the above dementias. Conditions such as subdural hematoma (a blood clot beneath the outer covering membrane of the brain), tumors of the frontal lobe of the brain, hypothyroidism and neurosyphilis can all give rise to a similar progressive intellectual deterioration, which is treatable by treatment of the underlying disease.

(*Dementia praecox* is an obsolete term for SCHIZOPHRENIA.)

demyelination

Loss of the protective fatty coating (myelin sheath) that surrounds the nerve fibers.

In order for the nervous system to function swiftly and efficiently, the nerves have to be insulated from each other. In many nerves this is achieved by a sheath of

DEMYELINATION

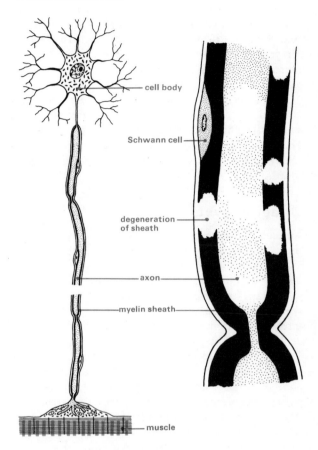

Nerve fibers are wrapped in a fatty myelin sheath which acts as an insulator and allows nerve impulses to travel at very high speeds. In certain diseases, for example, multiple sclerosis, the loss of insulation (demyelination) causes neurological disorders such as paralysis and numbness.

fatty material called myelin around each nerve fiber. (The "white matter" of the brain and spinal cord owes its appearance to this glistening myelin coating.) The loss of myelin is the common feature in "demyelinating diseases" of the central nervous system.

Such diseases may be acute (where the demyelination can occur within a few days) or chronic (where the condition progresses over several years).

Acute disseminated encephalomyelitis (see ENCEPHALOMYELITIS) can occur after various viral diseases (such as measles, chickenpox, smallpox and rubella) or after vaccination against smallpox or rabies. The vaccination-type tends to occur in older children and adults, about ten days after the vaccination. The outlook is grave because there is a high mortality rate and survivors usually have permanent neurological defects. The disease is thought to result from a type of allergic response or hypersensitivity reaction.

MULTIPLE SCLEROSIS—an example of a chronic demyelinating disease—shows a similar pattern of focal demyelination. Many experts believe that it, too, is caused by an allergic response to a viral infection, perhaps after a gap of several years.

Diffuse cerebral sclerosis—another chronic form of myelin loss—comprises a group of rare diseases (the leukodystrophies) which occasionally run in families. There is massive demyelination of the cerebral hemispheres due to defects in the metabolism of the myelin sheath fats.

dengue fever

An acute and often epidemic disease caused by infection with Arbor B group viruses. (The disease is also known as "breakbone fever.") It is transmitted to man by the *Aedes* mosquito and is found throughout the tropics, particularly in the mosquitoes' active season. When symptoms develop, 3 to 15 days after the bite, one of three broad clinical patterns may be seen: classical dengue, a mild atypical form or hemorrhagic fever.

In the *classical* form, a runny nose or conjunctivitis is followed within hours by a severe headache ("breakbone"), pain behind the eyes, backache, leg and joint pains and depression. The fever may be of a characteristic "saddle back" type: a raised temperature for about 3 days followed by several hours when the symptoms and fever disappear before returning for another day. During the second phase of fever, swollen glands and a characteristic berry-like rash are frequently present. Classical dengue fever usually lasts only 5 to 6 days and is never fatal. Treatment involves only the relief of symptoms (strong analgesics may be required). The patient commonly feels depressed and tired for several weeks.

The *atypical* mild form of dengue fever usually lasts less than 72 hours.

Dengue *hemorrhagic* fever occurs mainly in Southeast Asia, particularly in infants. The initial symptoms are similar to those of the classical fever, but damage to blood vessels leads to more severe problems. Again, treatment can only be supportive (relief of symptoms). Mortality rates of up to 20% have been reported in some epidemics.

dentistry

The profession that treats diseases of the teeth in particular and also supervises the general health of the mouth.

Common problems confronting dentists are caries (tooth decay), periodontitis (inflammation of surround-

DENTISTRY

PERMANENT TEETH OF RIGHT SIDE OF JAW

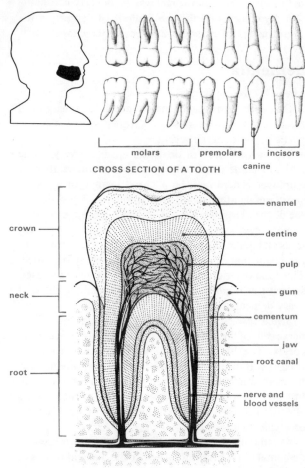

The root of every tooth is securely fixed into a bony socket, and the blood vessels and nerve enter at this site. Enamel, the hardest substance in the body, covers each crown and allows it to endure years of biting, chewing and grinding of foodstuffs.

ing tissue, especially the gums) and malposition of teeth. Dental caries is the most common disease of man. In modern society, caries predominantly affects the tooth enamel, although the roots may be affected in adults when the gums have receded. Caries results from the acid dissolution of calcium salts in enamel and cement. Bacteria which colonize the mouth ferment sugars from food to produce various acids. These acids attack the enamel, especially where there are pits or fissures in the surface of the tooth. Although it is agreed that certain foodstuffs, such as cakes and candy, are more conducive to caries than others, there is no simple relationship between sugar composition and the amount of enamel demineralization. Free sucrose is removed from the mouth faster than sucrose combined with starch and seems to be less damaging to the enamel.

The treatment of dental caries has a long history. Extraction was practiced in ancient Greece, and the first attempts at restoring carious teeth were made in the Middle Ages. The earliest fillings used were resins and waxes; lead and gold fillings were introduced about 1450. Silver amalgam (a mixture of silver and other metals) appeared in 1828 and by 1910 had largely replaced gold because it was cheaper and easier to apply. There are now about 150 varieties of silver amalgam available, but subtle differences in composition are less important than correct manipulation of the amalgam by the dentist and his assistant. Over the years, silver amalgams have become smoother, faster setting and more durable.

Preventive dentistry has only been practiced since 1910, but is now recognized as being of fundamental importance. Fluoride is taken up by enamel and in dilute solutions has been shown to reduce caries significantly. Addition of fluoride in trace amounts to the water supply is the simplest method of giving this protection to the population. However, pressure groups have prevented fluoridation of water supplies in many areas because they fear it constitutes a health risk. To date there has been no convincing scientific evidence to support these fears, and surveys in America, England and Italy have found no relationship between fluoride and the incidence of cancer. Fluoride has also been shown to be effective when applied locally in toothpastes or mouthwashes. Fissures in the occlusal (chewing) surface of teeth have also been sealed as a measure to prevent caries. It has been appreciated for 900 years that removing calculus from the teeth improves the health of gums. We now know that removal of microbial plaque from teeth prevents periodontitis. Despite these facts, few people know how to use a toothbrush and dental floss effectively.

The British Dental Association (BDA) is the national organization which represents the dental profession in all spheres of practice, including general, hospital and community dental services. The profession is regulated by the General Dental Council. Recognized specialities in the U.K. are orthodonics, oral surgery and restorative dentistry.

Dental surgeons carry out extractions of impacted teeth, treat facial trauma, reconstruct jaws, correct congenital abnormalities such as cleft palate and remove benign cysts and malignant tumors of the mouth. Orthodontists are concerned with the rectification of irregular teeth causing malocclusion; although traction by means of a dental brace is the most common treatment, severe cases may require surgical correction. Periodontists were originally concerned with the treatment of soft-tissue disease in the mouth, especially gingivitis (chronic inflammation of

the gums). Recently they have tended to become oral diagnosticians, since the gums can be affected by many systemic diseases and drugs.

Prosthodontics is the art of replacing natural teeth with artificial parts so that the functions of chewing and speech are preserved and the best esthetic result is obtained. Dentures may be fixed or removable, partial or a complete set. Crowns and bridges are fixed partial dentures. More extensive prostheses for the upper jaw can be constructed from acrylic resin and other materials, and are fitted after major surgery for oral cancer.

See also CARIES.

deoxyribonucleic acid

See DNA/RNA.

depilation

The removal of unwanted body hair.

Unwanted hair is a common cosmetic problem, especially affecting women. If hair growth is excessive, a physician should examine the individual before any treatment is undertaken because there may occasionally be an underlying disorder of the ovaries, pituitary or adrenal glands. In most cases, however, no such problem exists and hormonal treatment is both ineffective and potentially dangerous.

A variety of local treatments are available to remove hairs without unnecessary damage to the skin. Depilatory pastes can be applied to the area but must be used in the correct concentration and not left on too long. Alternatively, the skin can be dusted with powder and hot wax applied. When the wax has hardened it is pulled off, bringing the hairs with it. Both depilatory creams and wax treatment are only temporary solutions; the hairs reappear within a month or so.

Permanent removal of superfluous hair may be achieved by electrolysis. This technique, first used by Hardaway of St. Louis in 1877, destroys the papilla which carries nutrients to the hair follicle in the skin. In the hands of a skilled operator, electrolysis should be virtually painless and not leave visible scars.

depression

Depression may be a normal reaction (probably experienced by everyone at some stage in life) or it may be a pathological state. There is no clear cut boundary between the two; a diagnosis of depressive illness is usually made when the degree or duration of symptoms is out of proportion to the apparent cause.

Depressive illness accounts for approximately 12% of all hospital admissions in the United States.

Psychiatrists have traditionally divided depression into three types. The first type, *reactive depression*, is precipitated by physical or emotional factors such as chronic illness or bereavement. These would sadden anyone, but some people become overwhelmed by them or even by an apparently trivial event.

In the second type, *endogenous depression*, there is no obvious precipitating cause but a family history of depression may exist. There may be pure depression or curious mood swings between despair and elation—the condition known as *manic-depressive psychosis*.

The third variety is *involutional melancholia*, an agitated depression which sometimes occurs in middle age or in the elderly.

Often these three conditions cannot be distinguished clinically and the diagnosis of involutional melancholia rather than endogenous depression is often made solely on the patient's age.

The main symptom of all depression is a persistent unhappy mood. According to a set of criteria established by psychiatrists in 1972, the patient should have in addition at least five of the following eight symptoms: poor appetite, sleep difficulty, loss of energy, slowness of thought, poor concentration, feelings of guilt, loss of interest in usual activities (particularly sex) and recurrent thoughts of death or suicide.

Treatment does not depend much on an exact psychiatric classification of the depression; both psychological support and drugs are important. There is some evidence that endogenous depression results from a depletion of substances called biogenic amines (particularly norepinephrine) in the nerve cells of the brain.

Two of the most widely used groups of antidepressant drugs—the tricyclics and the monoamine oxidase inhibitors—both conserve norepinephrine and this is thought to be the basis of their efficacy.

Lithium carbonate, a simple salt, has recently proved extremely useful in the treatment of manic-depressive psychosis. Electroconvulsive therapy (commonly called "shock treatment") is used by some psychiatrists in the treatment of depression that is refractory (unresponsive to any other treatment) and severe, but its use is controversial.

dermabrasion

A technique to scrape away areas of skin.

Dermabrasion is mostly used to remove the pitted scars of acne from the face. Sandpaper was the first abrasive employed, but it has been replaced by special high-speed, rotary steel brushes.

The aim of the treatment is to plane down the epidermis (the outer layer of skin) in the scarred area. As long as the glands in the underlying dermis are not damaged, the epidermis will soon grow again.

Local anesthesia is achieved by spraying the skin with a "freezing" fluid such as Freon. Skin abrasion then takes only a few minutes, although it is followed by superficial bleeding for 15 to 20 minutes. A dry dressing is applied for the first day but subsequently the wound is left open, so that dry crusts form and peel off after about 10 days. For the first month after the procedure, the skin should not be exposed to sunlight or cosmetics.

Dermabrasion has also been used to remove facial tattoos, some types of birthmarks and warts and (in selected cases) wrinkles.

dermatitis

An inflammation of the skin.

It may be the result of an infection or an allergic reaction or contact with a strong chemical or contact with the leaves of certain plants (such as poison ivy, poison oak or poison sumac). Although the term "dermatitis" covers a large number of conditions—which in themselves may arise from a bewildering number of causes—the pathological changes are remarkably constant.

Like any other inflammation, dermatitis can be classified as acute, subacute or chronic. The initial or acute stage is characterized by redness and swelling of the skin with the formation of vesicles (tiny blisters) in the outer layer. As the acute stage subsides, there are fewer vesicles and the skin becomes thickened and scaly. In chronic dermatitis, where the process has persisted for many weeks or months, there are usually no vesicles but the epidermis often becomes much thicker and leathery in appearance.

While the classification of many apparently different skin conditions under the heading of dermatitis is an oversimplification, it does avoid a multiplicity of terms which would otherwise be needed to denote minor variations.

Much confusion exists in the usage of the terms "dermatitis" and "eczema." In the United States, chronic recurrent skin inflammations are called "eczema" and more acute self-limited ones "dermatitis." In Britain, on the other hand, it has been customary to restrict the term "eczema" to those inflammatory skin conditions with no apparent external cause. The trend now is to regard the two terms as synonymous.

All of the individual types of dermatitis described below can be aggravated by the following factors: scratching; application of irritating medications which might have no effect on normal skin; infection due to a change in the bacterial population on an area of inflamed skin and blockage of the sweat ducts, which can cause a secondary heat rash.

Acute contact dermatitis—probably the single most

common type of dermatitis—is a reaction to external agents. The causative agent is often an irritant such as a strong acid or alkali; the skin reaction appears within 24 hours of contact. Alternatively, sensitizing agents such as nickel or rubber penetrate the epidermis and link with a tissue protein to form an antigen. The sensitized individual then experiences a delayed allergic response to this skin antigen over a period of days or years, leading eventually to dermatitis.

Primary irritants in sufficient concentrations will cause dermatitis in everyone, but sensitizing agents present in low concentrations over prolonged periods will cause a reaction only in susceptible individuals.

The sensitizing agent can be very difficult to identify, but the site of the dermatitis often gives a clue. For example, hair dyes and shampoo affect the scalp; airborne sprays or dusts, volatile chemicals and cosmetics involve the face; clothing and deodorants affect the armpits; and glue, industrial chemicals, plants and rubber produce a reaction on the hands. Many ointments, especially antibiotics, can cause contact dermatitis.

If dermatitis is recurrent and has no known cause, patch testing of the patient's skin with potential sensitizers can be carried out.

The first step is the removal of the offending agent. In severe cases a cortisone-like steroid drug, such as hydrocortisone, may be applied to the skin.

Atopic dermatitis runs in families and is closely associated with hay fever and asthma. About 10% of the population are *atopic* (that is allergic) because they are predisposed to form high concentrations of "IgE" type antibodies in their serum, although there is little evidence that these are directly responsible for the dermatitis.

Eczema usually starts in infancy and often disappears before adolescence. No cure is available but the intense itching can be relieved with creams.

Nummular (coin-shaped) eczema is a subacute dermatitis which begins in middle age.

Seborrheic dermatitis, often an inherited condition, is characterized by greasy scaling of the skin—not only of the scalp but around the eyebrows, behind the ears, between the shoulders and other skin folds. In mild cases the dandruff can be controlled by frequent shampooing, but more extensive involvement may require steroid ointment. Since bacterial infection may occur, an antibiotic is sometimes combined with the steroid in treating this condition.

dermatomyositis

Inflammation of the muscles accompanied by a rash over the eyelids, cheeks, chest and knuckles.

It affects females more commonly than males and may occur at any age, although two thirds of patients. are over 30 years old.

A slowly progressive weakness develops during a period of 3 to 12 months, particularly affecting muscles around the shoulders and hips. The patient may notice difficulty in climbing stairs or in raising his arms above his head. The skin rash may appear before, during or after the onset of weakness.

Up to 50% of patients with dermatomyositis also show signs of a COLLAGEN DISEASE (rheumatoid arthritis, systemic lupus erythematosus or scleroderma). There is also some association with cancer, especially among older patients.

The exact cause of dermatomyositis is unknown but it is thought to be an autoimmune disorder (see AUTOIMMUNE DISEASE). Antibodies against their own muscle have been found in the blood of many patients. Most patients improve on high doses of corticosteroids and the chances of a cure are good in young patients.

dermatosis

A nonspecific name for any skin disorder.

Skin diseases are usually diagnosed by their visual appearance and the following terms are common.

A *macule* is a flat area of altered color, common to many rashes.

A round solid elevation of the skin is called a *papule* when it is less than 1 cm (2/5 inch) in diameter, and a *nodule* when over 1 cm.

A *plaque* is a raised flat patch of skin of any color; typical plaques occur in psoriasis.

A *vesicle* is a small fluid-containing blister, many of which are seen in the acute forms of dermatitis.

Bullae are larger fluid-filled spaces found in conditions such as pemphigus.

desensitization

1. A treatment used to suppress some forms of allergy such as hay fever or asthma. For uncontrollable hay fever, for example, after tests to determine which variety of pollen is responsible, repeated injections of minute doses are given for perhaps three to six months before the pollen season. It is unclear whether desensitization works by damping down the formation of antibodies to the allergen or by inducing "blocking antibodies" (which in effect neutralize pollen antigens before they reach the cells that produce the reaction). Desensitization is highly effective in some cases but it needs to be repeated each year and the same result may not be obtained on later occasions. Some individuals find, however, that after several years of treatment their symptoms disappear completely.

2. Desensitization is also the name of a method

used by psychiatrists to reduce "phobic anxiety" by slowly accustoming the patient to the source of his fears while he is relaxed—often with the help of an intravenous injection of a tranquilizer.

In the first stage, the patient is asked to think of a small aspect of his phobia until it no longer provokes fear. For instance, if the phobia concerns air travel he might be asked to imagine himself taking a taxi to the airport. Then he has to imagine progressively more frightening situations until he can tolerate the whole idea of air travel. The next stage is to go through the same steps in real life. Desensitization is a painstaking and lengthy technique, but it can be effective in selected cases.

desquamation

Normal loss of the very outer layer of the skin (epidermis).

The epidermis consists of several layers of squamous (scale-like) cells covered by a layer of keratin. Squamous cells are thin flat cells which fit together to form a continuous membrane.

The cells in the deepest layer of the epidermis divide and move toward the surface. As they approach the surface, these cells are transformed into keratin—a tough waterproof protein, which forms a protective covering for the skin. Keratin is continuously being renewed by this transformation of cells rising to the surface of the skin while the superficial layer sloughs off. This sloughing of keratin is desquamation.

detached retina

In this condition there is not an actual detachment of the retina (the light-sensitive "screen" at the back of the eye) from the underlying tissues, but a collection of fluid between two layers of the retina. This fluid can come either from blood vessels or, more commonly, from the vitreous humor (fluid within the eye) through a hole in the retina.

When the detachment begins, the patient may notice flashes or streaks of light and clouding of vision. There has often been some recent injury; although this is directly responsible in only a small proportion of cases, it does accelerate detachment which has been developing over a long time.

Inflammation and tumors in the eye, high blood pressure, vitreous hemorrhage and myopia all predispose to retinal detachment.

The detached part of the retina can be "sealed" against the underlying tissues by means of an intense beam of light (such as a laser). It is directed into the eye in an extremely narrow column (about the size of a pinpoint), focused for a fraction of a second and

DETACHED RETINA

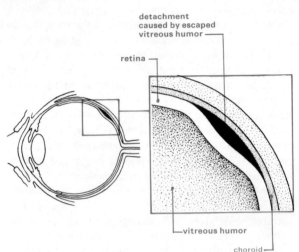

The retina is the film at the back of the eye which contains the light-sensitive receptors of the optic nerve. Detached retina results from a tear in this delicate film; the jellylike vitreous humor squeezes through the hole and separates the retina from the underlying choroid. Prompt treatment is vital.

automatically shut off. The inflammatory reaction this produces causes the detachment to fuse with the underlying tissues.

Unless surgery is undertaken quickly, the detachment extends progressively and sight in the affected eye may be irretrievably lost. Prophylactic surgery can be carried out in the unaffected eye if it is thought to be at risk of future detachment.

dhobie itch

A fungus infection of the crotch. See TINEA.

diabetes insipidus

This is a rare condition in which an individual passes substantial quantities of urine and is constantly thirsty.

Part of the pituitary gland (at the base of the brain) normally secretes a hormone called vasopressin or *antidiuretic hormone* (ADH), which is carried by the blood to the kidneys; there it limits the outflow of water in the urine. Diabetes insipidus is caused by ADH deficiency and leads to the passage of large quantities of pale, dilute urine with consequent dehydration and excessive thirst.

The great majority of cases are due to a tumor or inflammation in the region of the pituitary gland, thereby suppressing ADH production. Trauma, whether a fracture of the base of the skull or surgery in the pituitary area, can also cause diabetes insipidus. In addition, there is a rare inherited form of diabetes insipidus where the production of ADH is normal but the kidneys do not respond to the circulating hormone.

The condition is unrelated to the more familiar form of diabetes (DIABETES MELLITUS).

diabetes mellitus

A syndrome in which the basic defect is absence or shortage of the pancreatic hormone *insulin*. There are two major types of diabetes—which are thought to differ in their cause, onset and response to treatment.

Juvenile-onset diabetes usually comes on very suddenly with excessive thirst and appetite and an unusually high daily output of urine. In addition to raised blood sugar levels, weight loss is often apparent. These children or young adults are totally dependent on regular insulin injections plus a strict diet to control their blood sugar levels. Unlike the grim fate before insulin therapy became available in the 1920s, however, their life expectancy is not drastically shortened.

Maturity-onset diabetes has a slower onset, in middle age or later years, and can usually be controlled by diet alone or with special tablets. In fact the mild symptoms of maturity onset diabetes mean that it often goes unrecognized. In Britain 1.5% of the population suffers from diabetes melitus, and the number worldwide is rising markedly each year; about 25% of known diabetics need treatment with insulin.

Diabetes runs in families, although there is no simple pattern of inheritance. Close relatives of diabetics stand a two and a half times increased chance of developing diabetes. Recent studies on identical twins have tended to reverse the traditional ideas about the cause. Juvenile-onset diabetes was thought to be mainly genetic, but autoimmune processes and viral infections are now being postulated as causes. By contrast, maturity onset diabetes was long held to be the result of obesity and other environmental factors; it is now thought to have a stronger genetic basis than the juvenile type.

In a small number of patients diabetes mellitus is associated with some other predisposing disease—such as ACROMEGALY, CUSHING'S SYNDROME or HEMOCHROMATOSIS—or with the effects of drugs.

Although insulin primarily controls the metabolism of carbohydrates, fat metabolism is also disordered in diabetes. The latter defect leads to the appearance of ATHEROSCLEROSIS at an unusually early age in diabetics and may account for many of the complications (such as diseases of the kidneys and retina, gangrene of the feet, and nerve disorders).

A diabetic patient will lose consciousness if the level of sugar (glucose) in his blood is too high or too low.

Hyperglycemia (too much glucose) can occur in an undiagnosed diabetic or in one who has omitted to take his insulin; this can lead to a very dangerous condition marked by coma. Hypoglycemia (too little glucose) is very common and usually results from overactivity, undereating or insulin overdose. It produces sweating, nervousness, weakness, irrational behavior and then rapid loss of consciousness, and, sometimes, it produces convulsive seizures. Sugar given by mouth during the brief period of warning symptoms will prevent the unconsciousness.

dialysis

A technique to remove waste products from the blood when the kidneys are unable to perform this task (also called *hemodialysis*).

The most important functions of the kidneys are to excrete the waste products of the body's metabolism and maintain the correct electrolyte balance of the blood. When both kidneys are failing, these functions have to be maintained artificially.

Dialysis is based on the simple principle of osmosis: many chemical substances will diffuse through a membrane from a strong to a weak solution.

Blood from a patient in renal failure contains high concentrations of urea and other toxic substances and low concentrations of essential electrolytes such as sodium. During dialysis the patient's blood and the dialyzing fluid (containing the correct concentrations of electrolytes) flow in opposite directions on either side of a membrane. The blood cells are too large to cross the membrane, but the toxic substances diffuse into the dialyzing fluid while electrolytes pass from the fluid into the blood.

In the familiar kidney machine (*hemodialyzer*) the membrane is made of a synthetic substance such as cellophane. In *peritoneal* dialysis the dialyzing fluid is introduced into the patient's peritoneal cavity where the peritoneal membrane serves as the barrier. It is only used in cases where the renal failure is expected to reverse quickly or as a holding operation until a kidney machine becomes available.

Although a kidney machine can maintain life for many years, it is not a perfect replacement for the natural kidney. A patient on long-term hemodialysis tends to develop ancillary medical problems and experience severe psychological stress. Successful kidney transplantation is the best treatment of chronic renal failure; most patients are maintained on dialysis only until a suitable donor kidney becomes available. In the event of transplantation failure, the patient can return to dialysis.

The treatment of chronic renal failure is governed by its enormous cost; unfortunately, the vast majority of patients die without being offered dialysis or transplantation. In an effort to reduce the expense, patients are now encouraged to dialyze at home rather than in the hospital. In addition, being at home means the patient can dialyze at convenient times; most choose to do so three nights a week during their sleep, thereby freeing their waking hours.

diarrhea

The frequent passage of loose stools.

A sudden change in bowel habit to voluminous, watery stools, as in acute diarrhea, is an unmistakable symptom. Intermittent bouts of loose stools extending over a period of months (chronic diarrhea) usually presents a more difficult diagnostic problem.

Acute diarrhea in a previously healthy person is nearly always due to infection; it is occasionally possible to identify a particular meal as the source of infection, especially when other people contract the same illness. If diarrhea occurs within 24 hours of eating the meal, it is probably due to ingestion of a bacterial toxin. "Traveler's diarrhea," the scourge of tourists everywhere, is a self-limiting condition which lasts up to three days. It can be due to a pathogenic strain of the bacterium *Escherichia coli* or might result from the normal bacteria in the bowel being changed to unaccustomed strains.

If the diarrhea is bloodstained, dysentery due to *Shigella* bacteria or the protozoon *Entamoeba histolytica* may be responsible. The *Salmonella* group of bacteria produce either typical food poisoning with diarrhea about 72 hours after ingestion or the much more serious TYPHOID FEVER and PARATYPHOID FEVER, in which diarrhea is a late symptom.

The prevention of acute diarrhea by strict hygiene is more effective than its treatment, which in the self-limiting disease consists of salt and water replacement, perhaps with drugs such as Lomotil. Antibiotics are of value only in prolonged illnesses such as typhoid.

In chronic diarrhea it is the change in bowel habit which is important, rather than the number of visits to the bathroom daily or the consistency of the stools. Associated signs or symptoms might reveal that the diarrhea is one feature of a generalized disease, such as thyrotoxicosis. In the majority of patients, however, chronic diarrhea results from inflammation or irritation of the bowel. Such irritation occurs in ulcerative colitis, Crohn's disease, diverticular disease and tumors of the large bowel. In the absence of any positive physical findings, the diagnosis of IRRITABLE BOWEL SYNDROME is often made.

Some drugs, such as penicillin, ampicillin, tetracycline, and a number of others, can cause diarrhea as a side effect.

diastole

Each of the four chambers of the heart acts as a pump, contracting and expanding alternately. Diastole is the period when a chamber expands and fills with blood.

The period of ventricular diastole corresponds to the period when the atria are contracting (SYSTOLE) and discharging blood into the ventricles.

When the ventricles contract to pump blood around the body, the atria are in diastole, the right filling up with blood from the general circulation and the left with blood from the lungs. Nonreturn valves between the atria and the ventricles prevent backflow.

When the term *diastolic blood pressure* is used, it refers to the pressure in large arteries during ventricular diastole.

See also BLOOD PRESSURE.

diathermy

The generation of heat in body tissues by means of an electric current. Diathermy is one form of CAUTERY.

The heat produced in tissues by the passage of the current may be sufficient to destroy them. This technique is used in surgery to seal blood vessels as they are cut and in the destruction of certain tumors.

Short wave diathermy uses current of a much higher frequency than that used in cauterization. It produces insufficient heat to destroy tissue but enough to dilate blood vessels and relax muscles. It is frequently used to relieve the pain and stiffness of rheumatic conditions of joints or muscles. Commonly the heat treatment is applied for about half an hour, several times a week.

digestion

The process whereby food is broken down into its constituent nutrients ready for absorption into the bloodstream.

Digestion of complex food molecules into smaller, absorbable molecules begins in the mouth and is completed by the time the food reaches the end of the small intestine. Apart from the mechanical processes of chewing and swallowing, the journey of food through the alimentary canal and its digestion take place without any voluntary control, but the activity of the digestive organs is very susceptible to emotion such as excitement, fear and anger.

Digestive juices are produced in the mouth, stomach, intestine and pancreas, under the control of nerves and hormones, and fat-embolizing bile is secreted by the liver and stored in the gallbladder. Enzymes in these juices encourage the breakdown of large molecules into smaller ones. Each digestive enzyme is responsible for the chemical splitting of a particular type of nutrient.

DIGESTIVE TRACT

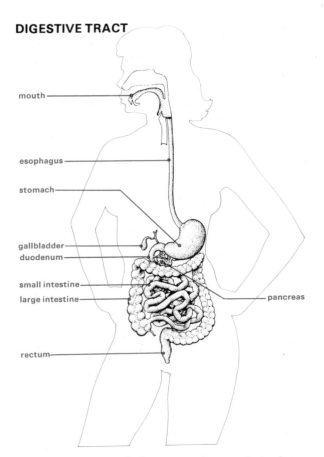

mouth

esophagus

stomach

gallbladder
duodenum

small intestine
large intestine

pancreas

rectum

Digestion starts with chewing in the mouth; in the stomach the food is churned for several hours and mixed with acid and pepsin (a protein-breaking enzyme) so that it becomes liquid. Small amounts of this liquid are released into the duodenum where enzymes from the pancreas complete the digestive process.

Digestion of carbohydrates (starch and sugars) begins in the mouth under the influence of saliva and continues in the stomach and small intestine. The large molecules are split into smaller fragments, eventually yielding simple sugars such as glucose. In the same way, proteins are digested into their constituent amino acids by a series of enzymes secreted by the stomach, small intestine and pancreas.

Dietary fat is digested into smaller units in the small intestine, where these are mixed with bile salts which enable them to be absorbed as an emulsion.

Almost all the nutrients in the food—including minerals and vitamins as well as the end products of enzymatic digestion—are absorbed in the small intestine. The liquid waste is then passed into the large intestine (colon) where most of the water is absorbed and the solid feces stored in the lower part of the bowel (rectum) until it is convenient to discharge them.

Apart from the rare cases of absence of one or more of the digestive enzymes, most of the diseases of the gastrointestinal tract are due to physical damage to the organs concerned. The most common cause of indigestion is unwise eating or drinking—especially the excessive consumption of alcohol. The modern Western diet is mostly made up of highly refined foods—white flour, white sugar—and contains few unrefined cereals or raw vegetables. The lack of vegetable fiber ("roughage") in such a diet is known to slow the transit of food through the intestines and is now thought to be largely responsible for chronic digestive disorders such as constipation and diverticular disease (see DIVERTICULITIS and DIVERTICULOSIS). The lining of the stomach and intestine may also be irritated and inflamed by virus and bacterial infections and by toxins (as in some forms of food poisoning). More serious digestive disorders may be due to ulceration of the stomach or the colon, as well as to chronic inflammation of the intestine (such as in CROHN'S DISEASE) and tumors.

See also BOWEL AND BOWEL MOVEMENTS and METABOLISM.

dilatation

The expansion of a cavity or the widening of an opening, tube or passageway.

Dilatation may occur naturally under hormonal or nervous control. For example, blood vessels dilate in order to supply tissues with more blood when necessary; and the pupil of the eye dilates when it needs to admit more light in dim conditions.

Dilatation may also be part of a disease process or an adaptation to a disease. In heart failure the ventricles dilate as the heart is unable to pump blood out of them; again, when a tube such as the ureter is obstructed the part of the urinary tube before the obstruction is forced to dilate.

In some circumstances dilatation is used as a therapeutic procedure. A narrowed urethra, which makes passage of urine difficult, may be mechanically dilated; or the cervix may be dilated to provide access for a curette in the procedure of DILATATION AND CURETTAGE.

The opposite of dilatation is constriction.

dilatation and curettage (D & C)

A minor gynecological procedure performed to obtain tissue for examination or to treat certain disorders. The cervix (neck of the uterus) is dilated and a spoon-shaped scraping instrument (curette) passed in.

D & C is carried out under general anesthesia. A series of gradually widening dilators, metal rods of increasing

DILATATION AND CURETTAGE (D & C)

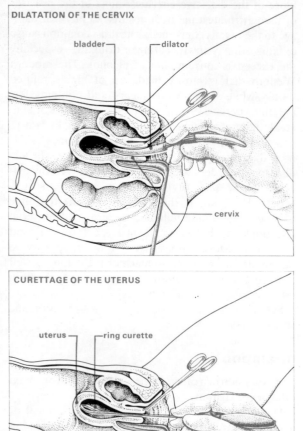

DILATATION OF THE CERVIX

bladder — dilator

cervix

CURETTAGE OF THE UTERUS

uterus — ring curette

A dilatation and curettage (D & C) is the most commonly performed gynecological operation. It is used both for diagnosis (in cases of abnormal bleeding from the uterus) and treatment (for example, after abortions). Progressively larger dilators are used to open the cervix, and then the lining of the uterus is scraped with a ring curette.

diameter, are passed via the vagina to dilate the cervix. When it is sufficiently dilated, a curette is passed into the uterine cavity.

A curette is a rod with a scraping device at one end, to scrape the lining of the womb (endometrium). A sample of endometrium is then sent to the laboratory for examination.

D & C is useful in establishing the diagnosis of menstrual disorders, pelvic tuberculosis and endometrial cancer, as well as for the investigation of infertility.

As a treatment procedure, D & C is sometimes used to procure abortion. When remnants of placenta are left in the uterus following childbirth or spontaneous or induced abortion, a D & C may be used to remove them and halt any associated bleeding.

Dilation and curettage is also used to remove POLYPS and for temporary relief during the occurrence of severe menstrual pain (dysmenorrhea). It may be used as well to insert radioactive radium into the uterus in the treatment of gynecological cancer.

discoid lupus erythematosus

See LUPUS ERYTHEMATOSUS.

disease

A condition in which the normal function of part of the body, or a bodily function, is impaired. It is not an entity, but the description of a pattern of symptoms and physical signs which enables the observer to foretell the probable course of events. Construction and identification of the pattern depends on degrees of probability in correlating the signs and symptoms; in some cases the data lead clearly to a diagnosis, in others there is no single discriminating factor.

The interpretation of signs and symptoms depends on knowledge of anatomy, physiology and pathology—the way the body is constructed, the way it works and the ways in which disease occur. In general, diseases are divided into four basic groups; congenital, traumatic, inflammatory and neoplastic. They may be acute (quickly appearing and soon over) or chronic (slow and long-lasting). They may be determined by genetic influences or by the environment (infections, injuries, reaction to chemicals or radiation, allergic reactions). They may have no known cause, as in the majority of new growths. Disease may be a consequence of genetic or environmental factors, or a combination of both.

Patterns of disease and the incidence of diseases alter in time, both because of advances in treatment and prevention (poliomyelitis and smallpox) and because of changes in the way people live. In the last century the prevalence of infectious disease, which had been by far the most common cause of sickness, began to give way to an increased incidence of chronic respiratory disease, heart disease and new growths (cancers). Infant mortality fell dramatically in the industrialized countries; but the incidence of road accidents as a cause of death and disability rose. It has been said that the occurrence of mental illness is no greater now than in the past; but as physical illnesses become less common, mental disturbances become more obvious.

Only about one third of illnesses occurring in the general population of industrialized countries receives medical attention, but most people see the doctor three or four times a year. The most common diseases are those affecting the respiratory system, which outnumber by far injuries and infections elsewhere which are the second most common acute conditions. The leading causes of death are heart disease, malignant growths and cerebrovascular disease.

dislocation

The displacement of a part of the body—most commonly a joint—from its normal position.

Injury is the usual cause of dislocation of a joint. The severity of the condition depends on whether the displaced joint presses on a neighboring artery or nerve.

The dislocated joint can be put back in position by skilled mechanical handling, a maneuver that is quick and safe in experienced hands but can cause great pain if attempted by the unskilled. The joint may afterwards be

DISLOCATION

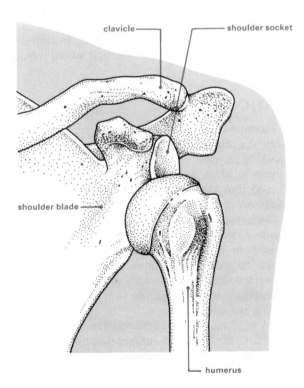

clavicle — shoulder socket

shoulder blade

humerus

Dislocation is due to trauma and results in the complete separation of the two bones which make up a joint. The shoulder joint becomes dislocated relatively frequently, because the socket into which the humerus fits is shallow. Because of the pull of the muscles, the humerus usually dislocates forwards and inwards as shown.

splinted to help it stabilize in the correct position. Joint dislocation sometimes tends to recur; in such cases an operation may be necessary to tighten the ligaments and thus help hold the joint in place.

CONGENITAL DISLOCATION OF THE HIP, as the name implies, is present from birth. It is due to a genetic or acquired structural deformity or to lax ligaments. All babies today are examined for "CDH" so that cases can be corrected immediately. Otherwise they might not be detected until the child attempts to walk, by which time irreversible damage may have occurred. Uncorrected CDH also carries an increased risk of osteoarthritis in later life.

Chronic inflammation may rarely cause joint dislocation.

disseminated lupus erythematosus

Another term for *systemic lupus erythematosus* (see LUPUS ERYTHEMATOSUS).

diuresis

The passing of abnormally large quantities of urine. It may be a symptom of disease, or it may be deliberately induced to treat certain conditions in which the body has too much water.

Urine is a concentrated solution of waste products which the body needs to excrete. Normally the amount of water in the solution is carefully controlled so the body is neither dehydrated nor waterlogged.

Diuresis occurs in certain diseases when the concentration mechanism in the kidney fails. It may also be a symptom of diabetes, since the kidney needs to excrete large quantities of water to carry the excess glucose out of the body.

Normally diuresis occurs if the body contains a lot of fluid—for example, if the person has drunk large quantities of fluid, especially alcoholic drinks.

Sometimes doctors give drugs called diuretics to remove excess fluid and salt from the body in conditions such as high blood pressure, heart failure or cirrhosis. They are also used to treat edema (swelling, usually of the feet or legs) and kidney disease. Diuretics may also be used to flush out poisons or drugs when an overdose has been taken.

diverticulitis

Diverticula (small pouches which can form in the walls of any hollow organ) are commonly found in the large intestines of people after middle age. (This condition is known as DIVERTICULOSIS.) Diverticulitis is the term for an inflammation of these pouches.

The inflammation may affect one diverticulum or

many diverticula along a considerable length of the colon. Attacks tend to be recurrent. Symptoms are usually mild and consist of recurrent attacks of pain in the left side of the lower part of the abdomen, associated with constipation or bouts of diarrhea. This may continue for months or years.

Sometimes an acute attack supervenes, characterized by pain and tenderness in the left side of the lower part of the abdomen, often accompanied by fever. In an acute attack a diverticulum may perforate to produce a generalized PERITONITIS. One complication of recurrent attacks of inflammation is fibrosis and narrowing of the colon, which can result in complete obstruction of the colon.

Another complication is that the inflammation may extend to adjacent structures—most commonly the bladder, sometimes other parts of the small bowel, and rarely the uterus and vagina. The inflamed areas between these structures may break down resulting in abnormal passageways (fistulae) between the colon and the organs affected. Hemorrhage is another complication of diverticulitis and can sometimes be massive.

The diagnosis of diverticulitis is confirmed by a barium enema (see BARIUM MEAL/BARIUM ENEMA). Treatment consists of giving a bulk laxative to produce bulky and soft stools, while pain produced by spasm of the colon may be relieved by the administration of an antispasmodic drug. Acute attacks may require bed rest and broad-spectrum antibiotics. Surgery is indicated when attacks are frequent and crippling, when hemorrhage is severe or when other complications occur.

diverticulosis

Small pouches (diverticula) lined by mucous membrane in the walls of the large intestine, found in about a third of the population of industrialized countries after middle age. It is thought that contractions of the large bowel increase the pressure inside to a degree where the mucous membrane is forced through the muscular walls of the intestine at points of weakness where blood vessels run.

The condition is rare in countries where the normal diet contains much roughage (dietary fiber). The part of the large intestine most commonly affected is the sigmoid flexure of the colon, which lies in the lower left hand side of the abdominal cavity. Normally they give rise to no trouble, but in a minority of cases they become inflamed and give rise to the disease known as DIVERTICULITIS.

dizziness

Strictly, a sense of rotation—either of oneself or of the environment.

Such a symptom is also known as a true VERTIGO, indicating a disorder of parts of the nervous system concerned with maintaining balance: these are located in the eyes and the vestibular system of the ears, as well as in the brain.

Dizziness is often aggravated by movements of the head and in severe cases may be accompanied by nausea and vomiting.

Except for travel sickness, in which the cause is obvious, special tests are commonly required to establish the nervous fault responsible for the symptom.

People commonly use the term dizziness more loosely to mean any one of a range of symptoms including faintness, lightheadedness, a swimming sensation, uncertainty or strange feelings such as a sensation of walking on air. These symptoms are classified as "pseudovertigo" and are often experienced by neurotic or very introspective people. There is usually no underlying physical cause.

Dizziness of this type may, however, be a symptom of temporary lack of oxygen or nutrients to the brain. It is therefore common when a person suddenly gets up from a reclining to a standing position, during hunger, or as an accompaniment of anemia or disease of the heart or lungs. If dizziness is not associated with an obvious cause, and is unrelieved by rest, medical advice should be sought.

DNA/RNA

The chemical chains in all living cells which hold and activate the genetic code.

DNA (deoxyribonucleic acid) holds all the genetic information which ensures that the descendants of a cell—and thus the descendants of a whole plant or animal—are of the correct type for that species. Watson and Crick discovered in 1953 that the DNA molecule consists of two extremely long chains spiraled around each other to form a double helix. The arrangement of the chemicals called "bases" in each chain is the secret of the genetic code; it determines the exact order in which amino acids are joined together to form cell proteins, including enzymes.

RNA (ribonucleic acid) transfers the genetic information from the DNA in the chromosome to the part of the cell where protein is synthesized and also controls its synthesis.

double vision

Normally when an object is viewed with both eyes, a single image is seen because eye movements are coordinated by complex brain reflexes which ensure that light from an object falls on corresponding points on the two retinae. These reflexes involve several nerves and muscles. Any condition which affects these nerves or causes paralysis of one of the eye muscles can result in double vision (also known as *diplopia*).

Diplopia is rarely encountered in children under five, even if they have strabismus (cross-eye), because the brain is still able to ignore one of the images. Beyond this age it is difficult to suppress the second image.

If the cause of the diplopia is not treatable, the condition can be relieved by covering one eye with a patch.

DNA

THE CHEMICAL STRUCTURE OF DNA
—a double helix

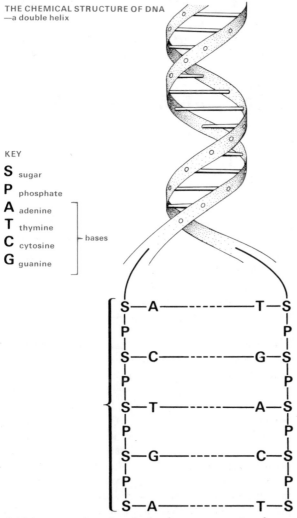

KEY

S sugar

P phosphate

A adenine

T thymine ⎫ bases

C cytosine

G guanine ⎭

DNA, a complex chemical substance, carries the genetic information which determines all the characteristics of an organism—bacteria, plants, insects and humans alike. Each molecule of DNA consists of two long strands, as shown above, which are held together by chemical bonds between pairs of base substances. The exact sequence of these bases along a strand of DNA forms the "genetic code."

Down's syndrome (mongolism)

A congenital disorder consisting of moderate to severe mental retardation accompanied by a variety of physical abnormalities.

It is also known as *trisomy 21*, because of the precise chromosomal abnormality which is responsible. The normal human complement of chromosomes is 23 pairs. A mongol, however, has an extra chromosome of the type known as number 21 (thus the term "trisomy 21") and a total of 47 chromosomes instead of 46.

In most cases this chromosomal abnormality occurs unpredictably rather than by inheritance, although there may sometimes be a familial tendency. The risk of producing a mongol child in a couple with some family history of the condition, or when the mother is relatively old (the risk increases with age), can be assessed by GENETIC COUNSELING. The overall incidence of the syndrome is 1 in 600 births, rising to 1 in 400 in mothers aged over 40, and 1 in 40 over the age of 45.

The mental deficiency in Down's syndrome does not make the sufferer aggressive or antisocial. Patients can mimic well and can be taught socially acceptable behavior. The average mental age attained is about eight years, a point to remember when dealing with adult mongols. Cases have been reported, however, of mongols given excellent parental help and encouragement who have attained almost normal intellectual capacity.

Physically, the best-known abnormality is the characteristic facial appearance with upward-slanting eyes. Other common physical abnormalities include a protruding tongue, small and badly aligned teeth, broad spade-like hands and feet, a short wide neck, short stature, dry skin, abnormal skin creases and cataracts. Congenital heart defects are also common.

The patient with Down's syndrome is especially prone to infection, and leukemia is at least ten times more common than in normal children. The mongol is also more likely to develop serum HEPATITIS, especially if he is raised in an institution in close contact with other mentally retarded children with poor hygiene.

There is no cure for Down's syndrome. Almost half of all sufferers die in infancy or in childhood, mainly from respiratory and gastrointestinal infections; but with proper care there is no reason why a mongol cannot survive into adulthood.

AMNIOCENTESIS can be used to determine whether a fetus is a mongol. The technique involves aspiration of a small quantity of the amniotic fluid surrounding the fetus in the womb. Fetal cells floating in the fluid are examined, and the presence of an extra chromosome detected. The mother may then be offered the opportunity of a clinical abortion.

Obviously this technique cannot be applied to all

DOWN'S SYNDROME (MONGOLISM)

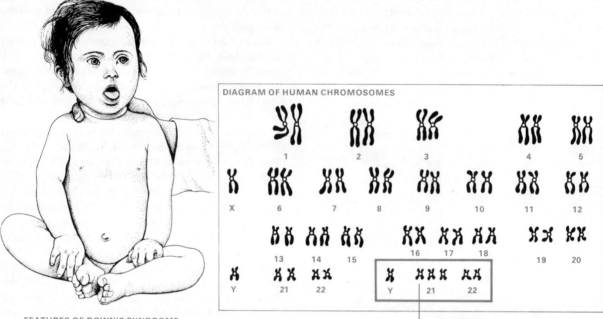

DIAGRAM OF HUMAN CHROMOSOMES

FEATURES OF DOWN'S SYNDROME
IN A ONE-YEAR-OLD BOY

trisomy 21

Down's syndrome, or mongolism, is a congenital condition which produces severe mental retardation as well as many physical abnormalities. The one-year-old boy pictured above shows the more obvious physical signs—slanting eyes, simple ears, large tongue, and squat hands with stubby fingers. All these effects are due to the child having an extra number 21 chromosome (trisomy 21) in his cells, giving him a total of 47 chromosomes.

pregnant mothers, for reasons of both cost and medical risk. It is, however, valuable for women at particular risk.

dreaming

Brain-wave studies have shown that sleep is accompanied by cycles of brain activity. One stage of sleep is called Rapid Eye Movement sleep (*REM sleep*), and it has been established that this is when dreaming occurs.

REM sleep comes on about every 90 minutes in the adult, and lasts for an average of 15 to 20 minutes each time. This represents, in total, up to a third of sleeping time. In infancy, a much greater proportion of sleep is REM sleep; the proportion gradually decreases until it reaches the adult level at about puberty.

REM sleep gets its name because it is characterized by rapid, jerky movements of the eyeballs under closed lids. During REM sleep the brain is active, the heart beats faster, the individual lies quite still with flaccid muscles, and he is more difficult to awaken. A number of other physical signs of REM sleep have been noted; for example, penile erection in the male.

If an individual is awakened during REM sleep he can usually remember his dream in vivid detail. If he is awakened some time after a period of REM sleep he will remember less of it.

Research on REM sleep has revealed several findings that indicate the importance of dreaming, although the exact reason for its importance is still not understood. If, for example, a person is consistently awakened at the start of periods of REM sleep he becomes irritable during the day, even if his total amount of sleep is normal. Moreover, when he is allowed to sleep undisturbed he will devote a greater proportion of the night to REM sleep, as if to make up for lost dreams.

REM sleep is depressed by alcohol, sleeping tablets, tranquilizers and certain other drugs. Again, when a person ceases to take such agents the proportion of his sleep devoted to REM sleep rises above normal for awhile. This is another indication that the body requires its REM sleep, and presumably also its dreams.

But just as the reason for the importance of dreams is not understood, neither is their physiological mechanism. It has been suggested that the characteristic pattern of a dream—a collection of related and unrelated random events strung into a semicoherent story—may reflect the work of the brain in ordering images into memory. There is, however, no real evidence for this or any other explanation, at least at a physiological level.

Psychologists have a special interest in dreams, interpreting them as messages of an individual's subconscious feelings. Freud, Jung and many others have classified dream images in terms of their sexual symbolism. Although modern psychologists are less prepared to accept such strict categorizations, there is little doubt that discussion and interpretation of dreams at least constitute a useful technique in exploring a person's mind through psychoanalysis (whether that is of ultimate value to the patient or not!).

dropsy

An obsolete term for generalized EDEMA.

drug abuse

In the the early years of this century, addiction to opium and hashish was prevalent in the Far East but rare (except in Chinese communities) in the United States and Europe. Sniffing cocaine was briefly fashionable in the 1920s, but drug abuse became a major social problem with the growth of heroin addiction. Heroin—an extract of opium which is usually taken by intravenous injection—is the most powerful and destructive of the drugs of addiction, and its use spread very rapidly in socially deprived areas of inner cities after World War II. Much of the growth of the problem was linked with organized crime.

The 1950s also saw an explosive growth in the prescription of sedatives and stimulants by doctors. As amphetamines, barbiturates and tranquilizers such as meprobamate (Miltown) came into ever wider legitimate use, their abuse also became common. At much the same time, opinion-formers such as Aldous Huxley began to write of the mind-enhancing potential of drugs such as mescaline (peyote), the active ingredient of the mescal cactus, and the current pattern of drug abuse became established.

Experimentation with drugs is now commonplace, especially among high-school children and college students. Many try cannabis (marijuana or "pot") or one of the many minor tranquilizers, especially if these are handed around at a weekend party; experimentation with injected barbiturates or opiates such as heroin or morphine is less common. Whether or not experimentation leads to addiction depends on many variables, including the addictive potential of the drug (high for heroin, amphetamine and tobacco; low or nonexistent for cannabis) and the personality and social environment of the individual. Hardcore addicts come mostly from socially deprived areas; in addition, many have disturbed or unstable family backgrounds.

Psychological dependence on drugs is common. Most people are mildly dependent on coffee or tea; a similar but stronger dependence may develop on sleeping pills or tranquilizers. Dependence on cannabis is of this kind. But serious addiction is much more likely when the drug concerned causes physical dependence, when deprivation of the drug causes physical symptoms (see ADDICTION). In the case of heroin, for example, an addict who is deprived of the drug will within a few hours develop severe abdominal pains, sweating and tremors. Alcoholics have a similar strong physical dependence on their "drug."

Drug addiction causes problems partly from its socially disruptive effects, and in particular from the effects of chronic addiction on an individual's ability to live and work normally. Many addicts turn to crime to find money to pay for their supplies. Addiction to drugs such as heroin also carries a substantial hazard to health, particularly from intravenous injections given without sterile precautions. Addicts have a high mortality rate from hepatitis (inflammation of the liver) and blood poisoning, as well as from drug overdosage.

Treatment of established addiction is unrewarding. When heavy physical dependence exists, the risk of relapse is very high. The complex interactions of psychological and social factors which promote drug abuse are still little understood.

duodenal ulcer

The duodenum—the first and shortest part of the small intestine, connecting with the outlet of the stomach—is the most common site for *peptic ulcers*. Peptic ulcers include those that affect the lower part of the esophagus, the stomach and the first part of the duodenum. They are erosions of the lining of these structures produced by the action of digestive juices (acid and pepsin) secreted by the stomach. Normally the lining is able to withstand the action of these digestive secretions.

Duodenal ulcer affects about 10% of the population. Symptoms may start at any age, but usually begin in young adulthood. Males are affected four times as frequently as females. Symptoms may be vague, absent or atypical, but usually the patient complains of upper abdominal pain—which has variously been described as gnawing, burning, cramplike or boring. Typically the pain starts an hour or two after a meal and is relieved in about half an hour by food or milk. Diagnosis of a duodenal ulcer is confirmed through the use of a barium meal or by gastroscopy. (See also BARIUM MEAL/BARIUM ENEMA.) The aim of drug treatment is to reduce the secretion of the digestive juices, to neutralize the acid after it has been secreted or to increase the resistance of the gastrointestinal lining to the action of acid and pepsin. Stress and anxiety are thought to play a part in producing ulcers in some patients; thus, a sedative may also be prescribed.

It is no longer considered necessary to adhere strictly to a bland diet. Most patients would know what foods aggravate symptoms in their own cases, and these should be avoided. It is advisable to avoid foods which stimulate excessive acid secretion—such as tea, coffee, cola drinks and alcohol. Smoking encourages ulceration and delays healing and should be avoided. Meals, however, should be regular and frequent to neutralize the acid that is produced.

Symptoms tend to be recurrent despite treatment. In about 5–10% of cases, symptoms persist despite drug treatment and surgery may prove necessary. When complications such as hemorrhage, perforation of the duodenum or stenosis (narrowing or obstruction due to fibrosis) occur, the need for surgical treatment becomes urgent.

Dupuytren's contracture

An inherited deformity of the hand, almost exclusively affecting men of European descent.

Tendons of some finger muscles lie within the palm side of the hand. In Dupuytren's contracture, which usually starts after middle age, the covering of such a tendon contracts into a fibrous nodule. In doing so it causes the relevant finger to bend toward the palm. The fibrous nodule also causes a puckering of the skin of the palm.

In the early stages there is pain on grasping. Later the pain disappears but the grip becomes weak and the patient finds it difficult to release objects. In severe cases the fingernails dig into the palm.

Usually both hands are affected, one more severely than the other, and the condition may also afflict the feet.

Treatment is by surgical operation, which can produce reasonable results but does not always effect a complete correction of the deformity. Recurrence may take place (especially in younger patients) within a year or two of the operation.

Dupuytren's contracture is also associated with some cases of epilepsy and alcoholic cirrhosis of the liver.

dwarfism

See ACHONDROPLASIA.

dysentery

Dysentery is an infection of the colon which causes painful diarrhea with mucus and blood in the stools. It may be caused by bacterial or amoebic infection.

Bacillary dysentery is the result of infection of the large intestine by bacteria of the genus *Shigella*—*Shigella sonnei*, *Sh. flexneri*, *Sh. dysenteriae* and *Sh. boydii*, the last three flourishing in tropical and subtropical countries. Infection with *Sh. sonnei* is usually relatively mild, the other infections tending to produce severe loss of fluids and prostration. The incubation period of all is usually two or three days. Infection is spread by food contaminated by feces, being the result of poor standards of personal hygiene and sanitation. Flies may spread the infection. Diagnosis is made by isolation of the infecting organisms from the stools; treatment depends on the severity of the condition, ranging from simple kaolin mixtures in mild cases to suitable antibiotics and intravenous fluid therapy in those patients suffering from serious fluid loss.

Amoebic dysentery, also spread by faulty hygiene, results from infection with protozoa of the species *Entamoeba histolytica*. The disease is found all over the world, particularly in poor communities, and produces symptoms of varying severity ranging from mild abdominal discomfort with loose stools to severe and acute bloody diarrhea with frequent abdominal pain. The condition may become chronic, and may be mistaken for other gastric and intestinal disorders. But in time large numbers of amoebae may multiply in the liver and give rise to a dangerous abscess, which may burst into the abdominal cavity, the chest or through the wall of the abdomen or chest. Diagnosis is made by microscopic examination of the feces for *E. histolytica*, by endoscopy of the large bowel (which when infected shows typical ulceration) or by serological techniques. Treatment includes administration of diloxanide, injections of emetine and the use of tetracycline and chloroquine. Abscess formation in the liver may require surgical treatment.

It is important to note that both bacillary and amoebic infections can be spread by "carriers," infected persons who show no signs of having the disease but carry live organisms in their intestines. Unexplained outbreaks of dysentery in institutions are sometimes traced to such a carrier by examination of the stools of apparently healthy kitchen workers.

dyslexia

Word blindness; extreme difficulty in understanding the spoken or written word.

Dyslexia covers a wide range of language difficulties; in general, sufferers cannot grasp the meaning of sequences of letters, words or symbols or the concept of direction.

The condition can affect people of otherwise normal intelligence and of every socioeconomic group.

Sometimes there is a family history; sometimes the condition arises from brain damage. But often the cause is obscure.

In severe cases the dyslexic individual is unable to read, makes bizarre errors in spelling, cannot name colors or "left" and "right" and has difficulty putting a name to a picture. Milder cases show less extreme forms of the same difficulties and may go unrecognized.

Indeed, even severe dyslexia is often not diagnosed as the root of a person's problem; the sufferer may therefore be considered lazy, stupid, mentally handicapped, inattentive or obstinate. In fact he may be of normal intelligence but frustrated with his inability to comprehend words.

Signs that a child may be dyslexic include late language development, clumsiness, no preference for one hand or the other, a tendency to alter the sequence of syllables in words (like "efelant" for elephant) or of words in a sentence. Any of these signs in an otherwise bright child may raise the suspicion of dyslexia.

Treatment—which is most successful when the condition is diagnosed early—requires painstaking special teaching techniques.

dysmenorrhea

Pain associated with MENSTRUATION.

The most common type is *primary dysmenorrhea*, which is an extreme form of the discomfort most women feel in the first few hours or days of a period. The lower abdominal pain may be continuous or spasmodic and is sometimes accompanied by pain in the lower back or down the legs. In severe cases the woman may vomit or faint.

Dysmenorrhea is common in women who have not had a pregnancy. It is no reason to fear serious gynecological problems or eventual sterility. The pain is thought to be due to a reduction in blood supply to the uterus when its powerful contractions at the start of a period constrict the blood vessels. Childbirth usually cures the condition because extra blood vessels develop during pregnancy. Even in women who remain childless, dysmenorrhea tends to ease after the age of about 25 and disappear by 30.

A healthy active life helps prevent primary dysmenorrhea. Simple analgesics such as aspirin or paracetamol can usually relieve the pain. Rest in bed with a hot-water bottle is a traditional and often successful treatment.

If such measures are ineffective, a doctor may prescribe the oral contraceptive pill for chronic sufferers, since it prevents ovulation (only periods following normal ovulation are painful). Temporary relief may be obtained by dilatation of the cervix, but ordinarily this maneuver would only be undertaken for

more serious gynecological disorders.

Secondary dysmenorrhea is a symptom of disease rather than a problem on its own. Diseases causing painful menstruation include chronic pelvic inflammatory disease, endometriosis, fibroids and many other gynecological conditions.

The pain usually starts about a week before menstruation and increases in intensity until the start of the period. It may then be relieved once bleeding starts or may worsen in some cases. Treatment is directed at the underlying disease.

Although many gynecological disorders produce dysmenorrhea, it should be stressed that dysmenorrhea does not necessarily indicate the presence of a disorder; very commonly it can be primary. Therefore it is not a symptom that should cause undue anxiety.

On the other hand, in persistent cases medical advice should be sought; the doctor may be able to relieve the pain and exclude the possibility of any underlying disorder.

dyspareunia

Difficult and painful sexual intercourse experienced by a woman. There is often incomplete vaginal penetration by the penis because of the pain or discomfort felt by the woman.

In most cases the embarrassment and sensitivity felt by the woman leads to frigidity. There are many causes of this condition, both physical and psychological.

Physical causes include extreme obesity of either partner, injuries of the hip joint leading to difficulty in wide separation of the legs, a thick hymen ("maidenhead"), a scarred vagina (as a result of episiotomies or gynecological surgery) and inelastic vaginal walls in those who marry relatively late in life.

Among psychological causes are clumsiness in the male, previous experience of pain and fear of pregnancy. In these circumstances the vaginal muscles can go into spasm (VAGINISMUS) and prevent entry of the penis.

Infections or inflammation of the pelvic organs (ovary, uterus, or Fallopian tubes), PROLAPSE of the uterus and ovarian cysts make intercourse painful. The complaint of dyspareunia may lead to the diagnosis of such conditions when they were previously asymptomatic.

Approximately 20% of women experience dyspareunia at some time in their lives. The treatment of physical causes is fairly simple: for example, eradicating the infection, correcting the prolapse or removing a cyst.

Psychologically, confidence may be less easily restored but education of both partners in sex techniques, and the use of lubricants and vaginal dilators, is necessary and usually successful.

dyspepsia

Literally, "difficulty in digesting."

Dyspepsia is experienced by most people at some time in their lives, since INDIGESTION is extremely common. It is ordinarily not a serious problem unless it is either constant or prolonged for many weeks. It can be associated with irregular meals, alcoholic excess or eating foods to which you are unaccustomed.

The symptoms include belching, a feeling of distension in the upper part of the abdomen, an acidic taste in the mouth, stomach pains and sometimes nausea. Common causes include eating fatty foods (especially when fried), foods which contain sulfur (such as eggs, cucumbers, onions and salads) or strongly acid foods (fruit and wines). Dyspepsia is sometimes associated with smoking on an empty stomach, skipping meals and chronic anxiety—thus provoking excess secretions of gastric acid.

If dyspepsia is continual, regularly causes disruption of sleep or occurs after every meal it may be a symptom of a developing ulcer (see GASTRIC ULCER and DUODENAL ULCER). Prompt medical attention should be sought to confirm the diagnosis and permit early treatment.

In mild cases the most effective treatment is the use of oral antacids—particularly the effervescent types—which will usually relieve the discomfort and bring up gas. A glass of milk is sometimes equally effective. Salicylate drugs such as aspirin, however, should never be taken because they can irritate the stomach lining; if an ulcer is the cause of the dyspepsia, aspirin can aggravate the condition or even lead to massive bleeding of the stomach lining. If the cause is related to dietary indiscretion, a change in the types of foods regularly eaten may be necessary to bring persistent dyspepsia under control.

dyspnea

Breathlessness or shortness of breath after slight physical effort, along with consciousness of the necessity to breathe.

The symptoms can occur in people who are otherwise healthy, often as a result of obesity, lack of physical fitness or excessive smoking. Respiratory or cardiac disease may be a cause, but as dyspnea is a subjective complaint it cannot be correlated closely with the extent of the disease.

In general the lungs have a diminished capacity to cope with the demands made of them—perhaps because of heart failure causing pulmonary congestion or chronic lung disease causing heart strain—but sufferers show a varying tolerance that depends on the anxiety level produced by the experience of breathlessness.

Rest, appropriate treatment of any underlying disease, dietary control and carefully graded physical training may improve the condition.

When it is not caused by organic disease, dyspnea may be related to anxiety—a common complaint.

dysuria

Painful or difficult urination, which may have a number of causes.

E

earache

Pain in the ear may come from the hearing mechanisms themselves—the eardrum, inner ear, outer canal, or the deeper bone structure—whenever they are subject to trauma or inflammation.

For example, acute earache is felt when flying because of the unequal air pressure within the ear; cabin pressurization outside the ear stretches the eardrum. Similarly, coughs and colds may put pressure on the inner ear. Ear infections cause pain because of the swelling of the inflamed tissue and a consequent rise in pressure within the ear itself.

Because the cranial nerves of the neck, face, jaw and scalp all collect sensory branches from the ear, earache can be caused by disorders such as dental disease, tonsillitis, nasal congestion, jaw inflammation and cervical spine (neck) injury. Eruption of the wisdom teeth is often marked by coincident earache in adolescents and the growth of teeth of infants is frequently accompanied by earache.

Diagnosis of the cause is important to ensure there is no serious ear disease. Treatment, apart from relief of pain, may include the administration of antibiotic drops for the ear, the removal of excess wax, or dental assessment.

In young children otitis (inflammation of the ear) is a common cause of earache and appropriate treatment is necessary to prevent the complications of chronic infection that may damage hearing.

earwax

Accumulated secretions of the minute glands in the skin which lines the external auditory canal of the ear. These secretions protect the eardrum and maintain elasticity. Excessive secretions, however, form a brownish-yellow mass which can block the canal and cause sudden or progressive impairment of hearing or even deafness. The wax then requires removal.

It is usually softened first with drops that dissolve fat (or with warm olive oil); later it can be gently and painlessly syringed out with warm water by a nurse or physician.

Working in a dusty, humid atmosphere or the frequent wearing of earphones increases wax secretion and some individuals require ear syringing regularly.

ecchymosis

A purplish-brown patch of flat bruising due to bleeding under the skin.

It may be due to fragility of the blood vessels, blood clotting defects, or minor trauma. Ecchymoses are very common in the elderly and are a normal part of aging— even where there is no evidence of other circulatory disorders, nutritional deficiency or blood disease.

In young people ecchymoses are rare unless they are associated with a serious blood defect, scurvy, hemophilia, or the effects of various drugs or chemicals.

Ecchymoses resolve themselves without treatment (by absorption of the "leaked" blood) usually within a week of their appearance. Frequent recurrence indicates the need for special blood tests.

ECG (or EKG; electrocardiogram)

A tracing that represents the contraction and relaxation of the heart muscle as it beats. The tracing is an electrocardio*gram;* the instrument used is an electro-cardio*graph.*

All muscular contraction emits very small electrical discharges. Over a hundred years ago it was discovered that heart muscle activity could be detected by electrodes placed on the chest wall and the limbs. Electronic sensitivity has improved dramatically since then, and nearly every physician now has access to an ECG machine. As a routine test to assess a patient's cardiac efficiency, the ECG is now a standard part of any comprehensive physical examination.

The ECG can alert physicians to a wide range of abnormalities: changes in heart size due to congenital defects or to hypertension; coronary thrombosis; arrhythmias; pericarditis; and many other conditions that alter the wave patterns of the electrical activity of the heart. However, the graph must always be interpreted in conjunction with a physical examination. An ECG may show various changes that are perfectly normal in some individuals but not in others.

The ECG can be traced either on paper or shown on an oscilloscope. The latter technique is an essential part of intensive care and major surgery, where doctors must constantly assess the state of the patient's heart. Some oscilloscopes sound an automatic early warning bell if there is any variation in the wave pattern, in order to alert the medical and nursing staff.

Fetal electrocardiography can be used before and during the induction of labor to assess the state of the baby's heart and give warning of FETAL DISTRESS (lack of oxygen in the fetus during the process of labor). It is achieved by attaching electrodes across the mother's abdomen.

ECHO viruses

A group of viruses responsible for several mild diseases such as summer flu, diarrhea of the newborn and certain skin rashes. (The name is derived from viruses which belong to the so-called *E*nteric *C*ytopathogenic *H*uman *O*rphan group.)

They attack young children mainly, although not exclusively, and are more active during the warm months of the year. Often they cause minor epidemics in which several children in a neighborhood become infected with the virus. The symptoms include a higher fever, headache, pains in the limbs and a sore throat.

One group of the ECHO viruses can produce blisters of the mouth or soft palate, while another causes chest pains similar to those seen in pleurisy; this is called *Bornholm disease*, after the island in the Baltic where the first epidemic was reported. Some other ECHO viruses produce ORCHITIS (inflammation of the testicles); a further group are responsible for a serious form of MENINGITIS (inflammation of the membranes that surround the brain).

This last type of ECHO virus infection is one of only two which require hospitalization, the other being the highly infectious diarrhea sometimes seen in newborn babies.

Many cases of ECHO virus infection go unrecognized. The patient tends to assume that it is a cold, chill, or sore throat. As a result of these mild infections, most people develop immunity to the ECHO viruses by the time they reach adulthood.

The treatment of mild infection is simple home nursing care. The illness seldom lasts more than a few days.

ECT (electroconvulsive therapy)

A form of psychiatric treatment to alleviate serious depressive illness.

A current of 85 to 110 volts A.C. is passed between electrodes placed on either side of the head for up to half a second. There are many technical variations, but usually a muscle-relaxant drug and a general anesthetic are given to spare the patient the distress produced by involuntary muscular convulsion.

ECT is usually given in courses of up to three a week, restricted to 10 to 12 treatments in all. It produces some damage to brain tissue and can impair memory and concentration (often for several weeks after the end of treatment). It can also dull both imagination and perception, but these effects may be beneficial if the patient has been disabled by fear, nightmares, delusions or desperate suicidal wishes.

ECT can be safely used on the old or the young, the physically fit or those with physical diseases. In all cases, however, it is now used only as a last resort since drug treatment of psychiatric disease has dramatically improved in recent years. Where drug treatment fails, however, the benefits of electroconvulsive therapy can be helpful to the desperately disturbed psychiatric patient.

ectopic pregnancy

Pregnancy in which the fertilized egg is implanted somewhere other than the womb.

Normally the fertilized egg passes down the Fallopian tube and grows into a fetus in the wall of the uterine cavity. An ectopic pregnancy occurs when it fails to do so and starts to develop in another area, such as the abdominal cavity, Fallopian tube, ovary, ligaments of the uterus, or in a rudimentary "extra" cavity of a deformed uterus. By far the most common site for an ectopic pregnancy, however, is the Fallopian tube; this is alternatively called a "tubal" pregnancy. About one in every thousand pregnancies is ectopic.

The space for the embryo to grow is limited and the result is an acute surgical emergency at any time from the sixth week onwards. An ectopic pregnancy rarely proceeds beyond the 16th week without provoking a crisis.

The usual cause is blockage of the uterine tube as a result of a previous infection (SALPINGITIS), surgery, the use of an intrauterine contraceptive device, or ENDOMETRIOSIS.

The symptoms of early pregnancy are normal; then acute abdominal pain occurs, with shock (often because the tube has ruptured), collapse and vaginal bleeding. Surgery is then necessary to remove the damaged tissues and the fetus. Unfortunately, the tube usually has to be removed; only about 30% of women who suffer an ectopic pregnancy are subsequently able to conceive satisfactorily.

eczema

A noninfectious inflammatory disease of the skin that takes the form of redness, blistering, crusting and scaling.

The well-known type of eczema seen in infancy and childhood, medically called *atopic eczema*, tends to run in families where there is asthma, migraine or hay fever.

ECTOPIC PREGNANCY

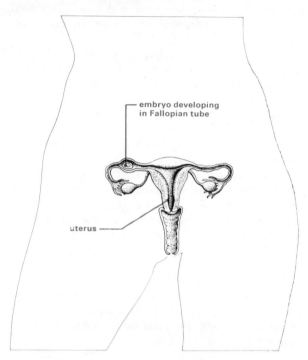

embryo developing in Fallopian tube

uterus

An ectopic pregnancy occurs when a fertilized egg becomes implanted somewhere outside the uterus. A Fallopian tube pregnancy is the most common variety, and usually occurs following infection of the tube.

The skin typically breaks out in eczematous patches—particularly on the forearms, the backs of the knees and the face.

There are other types of eczema: *allergic eczema* is usually due to food allergy. Identification and avoidance of the cause, which may be anything from cow's milk to seafood, cures the problem. *Varicose eczema* occurs around varicose ulcers on the legs in people with circulatory deficiency. *Occupational eczema* may be caused by skin irritants such as mineral oils, detergents and degreasing agents. Liquid detergents and soap powders are a common cause of this type of eczema in housewives. In other cases the eczema may be caused by the application of ointments that produce a sensitivity reaction.

"Eczema" and "dermatitis" are often interchangeable words, especially in the sensitivity type of inflammation.

Eczema is fundamentally a reaction to irritants. Even atopic eczema may be due to an inherited metabolic disorder causing biochemical disturbance of the skin. Eczema is common, affecting 20% of the population at some time in their lives and is more frequent in whites than in blacks.

In treatment, the patient is advised to avoid any external skin irritants. At the same time, medications are used to suppress the inflammatory response in the skin. This is best achieved with creams, lotions and dressings which contain cortisone-like steroids.

Sedatives or antihistamines may be used to relieve the symptoms of itching and burning, and antibiotics prevent infection of the damaged skin.

Many young children with atopic eczema grow out of the worst manifestations of the disease by the time they reach puberty, but not everyone is completely cleared.

For successful treatment of the child with atopic eczema, the frequent attention of a dermatologist may be required.

edema

Swelling of a part of the body due to congestion with an excess of retained tissue fluid.

If you press a finger into tissues that are excessively edematous, a "pit" mark remains afterwards. It is a sign of a disorder or disease rather than a disease itself.

Edema is most obviously seen in the legs of people with varicose veins or mild heart disease. Edematous swelling of the ankles can occur even in healthy people during hot weather or during pregnancy. Local edema is also seen around wounds or insect bites, or in eczema where the skin cells are injured and there is local "puffiness."

Excess body water is normally removed by the

ECZEMA

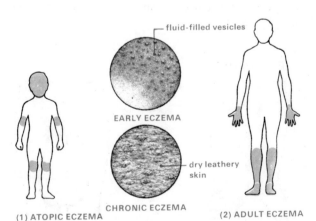

fluid-filled vesicles

EARLY ECZEMA

dry leathery skin

CHRONIC ECZEMA

(1) ATOPIC ECZEMA   (2) ADULT ECZEMA

Eczema may run in families ("atopic eczema") or result from an external irritant. Atopic eczema may start in infancy, when the face is particularly affected, and later tends to be confined to the hollows of the elbows and behind the knees (1). In adults, hands are often affected in certain occupations, and eczema over the legs develops with bad varicose veins (2).

EDEMA

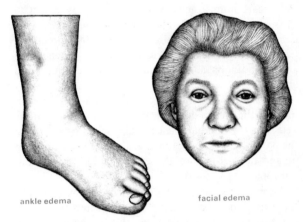

ankle edema   facial edema

Edema is the distension of the soft tissues by excess fluid which has seeped out of the circulation. Ankle edema usually results from poor drainage by the veins and is seen in congestive heart failure and pregnancy. Facial edema is a characteristic of kidney disease and is especially noticeable after a night's sleep.

circulation of the blood and excreted via the kidneys, so disease of either the heart or the kidneys characteristically results in edema. The patient may retain 10 to 20 pounds of excess water before edema is detectable. Ankle swelling is usually the first sign, although in bedbound patients the first swelling commonly appears in the lower back. The congestion impairs pulmonary efficiency since the lung tissue also becomes waterlogged; the patient then has difficulty in breathing.

Edema is often an early sign of toxemia of pregnancy, reflecting impaired kidney function and salt retention. It is also seen in severe malnutrition due to deficiencies of B vitamins or protein.

Edema does not cause pain, but it must be treated because it is a manifestation of some disorder and it can cause problems of its own. Drugs which stimulate kidney excretion (diuretics) are used to correct edema, in combination with cardiac muscle stimulants and a low-sodium diet. Potassium supplements have to be taken with some diuretics because they cause the kidneys to excrete this mineral along with the excess water.

The control of edema is an essential part of the treatment of chronic heart failure.

EEG (electroencephalogram)

A tracing of the brain's electrical activity obtained by the application of very sensitive electrodes to the skull. The instrument used is an electroencephalo*graph*; the tracing is an electroencephalo*gram*.

All the brain function involves electrical activity

which is detectable through the skull, in the same way that heart muscle activity is detectable by an ECG through the chest wall. The tracing of an EEG is very complicated and requires skilled interpretation. Changes from the normal can aid in the diagnosis of such conditions as brain tumors, brain injury and epilepsy.

Brain wave patterns of patients with seizures can indicate the type of disorder (petit mal or grand mal) by detecting the buildup of electrical discharge even when the patient has no symptoms, so the EEG is a common diagnostic method for those with a history of convulsions.

Attempts to interpret thought patterns by means of the EEG, so it could serve as a lie-detector or as a measurement of intellectual ability, have proved unsuccessful.

The EEG has also been used to define BRAIN DEATH.

Electra complex

See OEDIPUS COMPLEX.

electric shock

The effect of the passage of an electric current through the body.

An electric shock with a voltage of 85 to 110 and a current of about half an ampere is commonly used to treat mental patients suffering from depression and other disorders. But in general electric shocks to the body, especially those caused by a higher current and voltage, can be dangerous and even fatal (electrocution); 110 volts is particularly dangerous in triggering cardiac arrhythmias. Every effort should be made at all times to avoid contact with live electrical wires, for the domestic supply can give a fatal shock, but even so a great deal can be done by way of first aid to bring help to victims.

The first measure to take is to switch off the supply as near to the main power line as possible, even if circuit breakers or fuses have blown. If this is not possible, stand on a rubber mat or other insulating material and maneuver the victim away from the source of the current with the aid of a nonconducting article such as a broomstick. Loosen the clothing to facilitate breathing. The victim may be unconscious and the heart may have stopped, so it will be necessary to give mouth to mouth resuscitation or (if you have received special training) external cardiac massage. Where the current entered and left the body there may be burns which will almost certainly be worse than they look. So even if an electric shock victim recovers quickly, medical aid should always be called.

Where an overhead cable or industrial supply is involved, no move to rescue the victim should be made until it is absolutely certain that the supply has been completely cut off.

electrocardiogram

See ECG.

electrocution

Death by electric shock. See ELECTRIC SHOCK.

electroencephalogram

See EEG.

elephantiasis

Dramatic swelling of the tissues caused by severe blockage of the lymphatic vessels by tiny threadlike worms (filariae).

These microscopic worms are transmitted to humans in tropical and subtropical zones of the world largely by a particular species of mosquito (*Culex fatigans*). Obstructive filariasis, to use its proper name, is commonly known as elephantiasis because it causes such marked and chronic swelling of the legs, scrotum, arms, breasts and vulva that the huge deformities look elephantine in their disproportion.

This severe form of filariasis develops slowly only after years of chronic reinfection and is seen in less than 0.2% of those infected with the worms. Treatment of the early infection is successful with drugs; once chronic obstruction has developed, however, surgical treatment may be necessary.

ELEPHANTIASIS

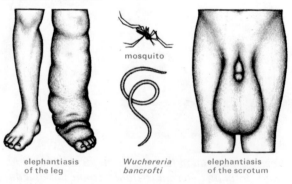

elephantiasis of the leg

Wuchereria bancrofti

mosquito

elephantiasis of the scrotum

Elephantiasis is a state of severe swelling caused by the human filarial worm Wuchereria bancrofti, *which blocks the lymphatic channels draining the legs, arms, breast or scrotum. The worms enter the body as eggs which emerge from a mosquito's mouthparts when it bites.*

embolism/embolus

Blockage of a blood vessel by material transported in the blood circulation. The condition is called *embolism;* the blocking material is an *embolus.*

An embolus is often a piece of solid matter that forces its way through the circulatory system until it becomes wedged in and blocks a small blood vessel. It may be a clot of blood, a globule of fat, or a piece of tumor tissue that has eroded a blood vessel. Or it may be a bubble of air admitted during an intravenous injection.

The most common cause of embolism is the breaking away of a thrombus (the formation of a blood clot within the heart or blood vessels). It may occur in an artery, a vein, or the chambers of the heart. When a fragment of the thrombus breaks off it becomes the embolus, which eventually may lodge in a smaller blood vessel.

Pulmonary (lung) *embolism*—obstruction of the pulmonary artery or one of its branches—is so serious as to cause death in approximately 5% of cases. Most emboli arise from the veins of the legs and pelvis, and are a well-recognized complication of pregnancy, post-operative recovery, or extended bed rest.

Fat embolisms may occur after injury to the long bones and the consequent release of bone marrow fat into the bloodstream. *Air embolism,* as a consequence of unskilled intravenous injection, is commonly seen in drug addicts.

The effect of an embolism is to deprive the involved tissues of their blood supply (ISCHEMIA), which can cause irreparable damage or even death of those tissues. *Cerebral embolism*—where an embolus has lodged in an artery of the brain—may produce signs of a STROKE. In an arterial embolism (most often seen in the legs), the area beyond the blockage becomes white, cold and painful. If an air embolus lodges in the heart, cardiac arrest and death can occur instantly.

Vascular surgeons can often successfully remove an arterial thrombus (see THROMBOSIS/THROMBUS), especially if they operate soon after the diagnosis. Small venous embolisms may be bypassed in time with the development of new channels for the flow of blood. Their recurrence can be prevented by anticoagulant drugs.

emesis

The technical word for VOMITING.

emphysema

The abnormal presence of air in certain parts of the body, particularly in the lungs *(pulmonary emphysema).* Air may enter tissues by a variety of means, such as trauma or surgery; but in clinical practice the term emphysema is virtually confined to a lung condition characterized by distension of the air sacs (alveoli). This may occur as a consequence of other diseases, such as bronchitis or whooping cough, in which alveoli are damaged and merge into larger spaces. This results in a decrease in the efficiency of respiration, with a consequent strain on the heart, breathlessness and edema. The chest may become barrel-shaped and wheezy breathing is particularly common.

Treatment of this basically irreversible condition consists of protecting the patient from infection and preserving his or her general health for as long as possible.

empyema

A fluid-filled abscess in the chest.

It is a fairly rare complication of a primary infection of the lungs (e.g., pneumonia, tuberculosis, pulmonary abscess, or pleurisy). The inflamed tissue is "walled off" by the body's defense mechanisms and pus begins to accumulate within the chest.

The natural course of empyema is for the contained pus and fluid to burst and discharge itself outward through the chest wall or inward into the bronchus. Before this happens, however, the condition may be manifested by fever, sweating, and either lung collapse or visible fluid levels in the chest x ray.

Empyema has been virtually eradicated by antibiotic therapy. Formerly it occurred in at least 5% of cases of severe pneumonia; the only treatment then available was surgical drainage.

EMBOLUS

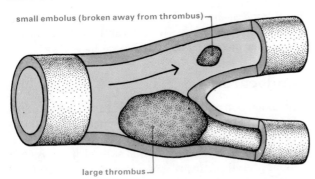

small embolus (broken away from thrombus)

large thrombus

An embolus is any abnormal particle circulating in the blood. The most common type is a fragment of blood clot which has broken off from a larger thrombus as pictured here. The embolus travels along until it blocks a small blood vessel, thus cutting off the supply to an area of tissue. Embolisms can be fatal, especially when they lodge in the circulation of the lung or brain.

encephalitis

Inflammation of the brain, usually caused by a viral infection (some cases are known to be bacterial in origin).

Certain viruses that attack man—a few of them transmitted by insects—show a tendency to localize their effects in the brain and the membranes surrounding the brain (meninges). All these tissues may become inflamed, swollen and edematous; the resulting vascular congestion sometimes leads to small hemorrhages. The patient is then suffering from encephalitis (sometimes called "brain fever").

Encephalitis can be a part of other virus diseases that have a developing stage of widespread viremia (viruses in the general blood circulation) before settling into their more obvious clinical manifestations. Examples are the early stages of measles, mumps, chickenpox and poliomyelitis. The symptoms are fever, headache, a stiff neck, photophobia (abnormal sensitivity of the eyes to light), irritability, and sometimes convulsions.

Epidemics of encephalitis have occurred in certain areas of the world, such as St. Louis, Japan, Russia and Australia's Murray Valley. These are spread by mosquitoes in the early spring and summer and mainly attack children. Adults are thought to develop immunity. The death rate is high, perhaps 20% in the undernourished and the very young. Attempts to produce a vaccine have been only partly successful. Thus the prevention of epidemics depends on public health measures to control insects and to stop them from breeding.

The treatment of encephalitis is mainly careful nursing: control of fever, analgesics for the relief of headache, rest and prolonged convalescence.

encephalitis lethargica

A disease which first occurred in the wake of the pandemic of influenza during and for about 10 years after World War I. Nothing like this disease is recorded from before 1914 and few if any cases have been recorded in America and Western Europe since 1930. Also known as *von Economo's disease*.

Although the organism was never identified, the disease was typical of a viral infection. Patients usually suffered from pronounced somnolence together with ophthalmoplegia (paralysis of the eye muscles), although a minority were hyperactive. Disorders of movement, headache, insomnia, dizziness, tiredness and confusion were common. More than 20% of the victims died within a few weeks and a high proportion of the survivors developed PARKINSON'S DISEASE. Some children developed psychopathic personality with compulsive behavior.

encephalomyelitis

Diffuse inflammation of both the brain (ENCEPHALITIS) and spinal cord (MYELITIS). It can be caused by a number of agents, including viral infections and syphilis; bacterial encephalomyelitis rarely occurs.

endarterectomy

The surgical removal of part of the inner layers of an artery together with anything that is impairing the blood flow—such as a clot or fatty deposits (atheromas) on the arterial walls. Also called *thromboendarterectomy*.

The surgeon uses a "coring out" process which leaves behind the smooth inner lining of the arterial wall to act as the new channel for the blood circulation.

It was first performed in 1957 by American cardiac surgeons on the coronary arteries of the heart, in an attempt to increase blood flow to the heart muscle. But the entire length of the coronary artery is usually affected in patients with ATHEROSCLEROSIS and it is technically impossible to remove all of the lining of long, convoluted and tiny blood vessels. So endarterectomy did not prove successful for every patient with coronary artery disease. The technique is more successful with the larger arteries, such as those of the limbs.

It was not until the venous bypass operations on the coronary arteries became possible in the late 1960s, using grafts of leg vein tissue, that surgery for coronary atherosclerosis came into general favor. Since then a number of techniques have been combined: joining together blood vessels from inside the chest wall, bypass, and endarterectomy. Some 20,000 such operations for coronary disease are now undertaken annually in the U.S.A.

Carotid endarterectomy, to improve the blood flow to the brain by "coring out" the carotid arteries in the neck, has proved moderately successful.

endocarditis

Inflammation of the surface of the heart valves or of the lining of the heart chambers. Most often endocarditis is caused by bacterial infection; it may also be a complication of COLLAGEN DISEASES such as systemic lupus erythematosus or rheumatoid arthritis. *Thrombotic endocarditis* is a possible complication of the terminal stages of any fatal illness.

Infective endocarditis is usually an illness of slow onset, and weeks of unexplained ill health may pass before an accurate diagnosis is made. The initial symptoms include fever, sweating and loss of weight; later, small painful nodules may develop in the hands and feet and there may be bleeding beneath the fingernails. Untreated, the damage to the heart valves from multiplication of bacteria on their surface causes distortion of their shape, leading to heart failure. Treatment depends on recognition of the condition and laboratory culture of the microorganisms responsible from the bloodstream (which can include certain species of fungi in addition to bacteria). Prolonged therapy with an appropriate antibiotic should eradicate the infection, especially if begun at a relatively early stage in the disease.

Bacterial endocarditis is unusual in persons with normal hearts. The infection starts most often in persons with a heart defect associated with a congenital heart disease or in those with a heart valve which has been scarred by RHEUMATIC HEART DISEASE (a possible complication of RHEUMATIC FEVER during childhood).

Patients known to have a heart disease are usually given antibiotics to protect them from bacterial endocarditis on occasions (such as before a tooth extraction or other forms of dental surgery) when bacteria may be released into the bloodstream.

endocrine glands

The ductless glands of the body, which secrete HORMONES directly into the bloodstream. Included among these glands are the pituitary, the adrenal and thyroid glands.

endometriosis

The internal lining of the uterus, the *endometrium*, is normally confined to the cavity of the organ, but in some women "islands," or fragments, of endometrial tissue are to be found on the ovary or in various places within the abdominal cavity. These patches of endometrium respond in the same way as the normal lining of the uterus to the hormonal changes of each menstrual cycle. The internal bleeding that occurs with each cycle leads to the formation of blood-filled ("chocolate") cysts in the affected organs.

Endometriosis may be silent or it may produce symptoms, usually between the ages of 30 and 40. Lower abdominal discomfort or pain (worse at the time of the menstrual period), pain during sexual intercourse (dyspareunia), and disordered menstruation all suggest the possibility of endometriosis.

The condition may be one cause of infertility; but as it is often found in women who marry and conceive later in life, and less often in those who have early pregnancies (so that the pregnancy may be said to protect against endometriosis), the relationship is obscure. Symptoms certainly improve during pregnancy and disappear at the menopause.

Treatment includes surgical removal of the abnormally sited endometrial tissue or the administration of ovarian sex steroids.

endometritis

Inflammation of the endometrium (the lining of the uterus), usually caused by a bacterial infection.

The disease may occur spontaneously or follow a septic abortion or injury involving the pelvic organs. It may be acute or chronic; the chronic form of the disease is usually the result of repeated acute attacks.

Acute endometritis is characterized by pain in the lower part of the back, low abdominal pain and disorders of menstruation (such as DYSMENORRHEA and MENORRHAGIA).

Diagnosis may require DILATATION AND CURETTAGE (D & C), followed by microscopic examination of a sample of the affected tissues and culture and identification of the causative microorganisms. Once the cause of the inflammation of the endometrium is established, the appropriate antibiotic therapy can be initiated.

ENDOMETRITIS

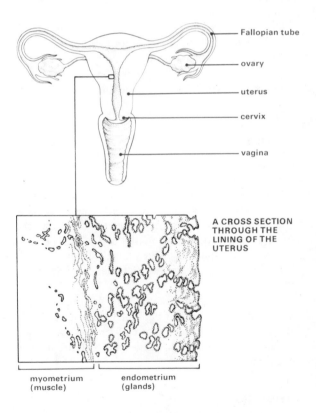

- Fallopian tube
- ovary
- uterus
- cervix
- vagina

A CROSS SECTION THROUGH THE LINING OF THE UTERUS

myometrium (muscle)

endometrium (glands)

The endometrium—the glandular lining of the uterus—grows rapidly in thickness under the influence of estrogens during every menstrual cycle, in preparation for a possible pregnancy. Endometritis, inflammation of the endometrium, is rare but can occur after childbirth or in old age.

endoscopy

The examination of the interior of the body through optical instruments inserted into the interior of hollow organs by way of natural passages or, in some cases, through special incisions. It is possible through endoscopes to inspect the esophagus ("gullet"), stomach, large intestine, bladder, the air passages of the lungs (bronchi), the peritoneal cavity, the interior of joints and even the ventricles of the brain (cavities containing cerebrospinal fluid).

The basic technique was invented in the 19th century, but instruments were relatively clumsy because they depended on straight optical pathways demanding rigid shafts bearing an inspection lens and a light at the end. With the invention of fibers capable of conducting light (fiberoptics), the shaft of the endoscope no longer had to be rigid. Because of this flexibility, modern instruments make it possible to inspect structures formerly inaccessible. Photographs can be taken through the endoscope, and in many cases a fragment of suspected abnormal tissue can be removed through the endoscope for microscopic examination (BIOPSY).

Although the procedure is somewhat uncomfortable for the patient, endoscopy is not painful nor is it dangerous when performed by specially trained physicians. It does not require a general anesthetic and, in many cases, it is not necessary to admit the patient to the hospital.

enema

A fluid introduced into the rectum through the anus. Water or oil may be used.

An enema may be necessary to: (1) clear the bowels of feces in severe constipation, or where the feces have become impacted, or before labor; (2) clean out the bowels before an operation on that part of the body; (3) replace body fluid in mild dehydration; and (4) administer drugs, as in the treatment of ulcerative colitis.

The enema nozzle is inserted up to three or four inches. As much as eight pints of fluid can be slowly introduced into the lower bowel. For a simple bowel evacuation the usual amount is two to four pints of soapy water.

enteritis

Inflammation of the intestines, particularly the small intestine.

There may be a number of causes. The most usual one is bacterial or viral infection after consuming contaminated food or water, as when on vacation in a strange country.

Outbreaks of food poisoning occasionally produce serious attacks of GASTROENTERITIS lasting a few days, with headaches, fever and severe diarrhea. Public health measures may be required to track down the offending organism, which often originates in a specific restaurant or institution. Gastroenteritis in babies is serious as it may cause rapid dehydration.

Acute gastroenteritis may also result from food allergies and excess alcohol.

Regional enteritis, or CROHN'S DISEASE, is an inflammatory disease of an isolated segment of the intestine, characterized by recurrent cramplike pains, weight loss and chronic diarrhea. Special diets and the elimination of stress may be required as well as steroid drugs, sulfonamides, or surgery.

enuresis

The technical name for BEDWETTING.

epidemic parotitis

The technical name for MUMPS.

epidemic pleurodynia

An infectious disease characterized by the sudden onset of severe abdominal pain or chest pain (or both), fever and headache. Also known as *epidemic myalgia, devil's grip* and *Bornholm disease* (after the Danish island of Bornholm where a study of an epidemic was made in 1930).

Epidemic pleurodynia usually occurs in outbreaks in the summer and fall, but it may also occur in single cases. It is most common in children and young adults and is caused by a virus of the Coxsackie B group. The first symptom is usually severe abdominal pain, made worse by movement, or pleuritic chest pain (see PLEURISY). A few patients have a preceding illness of a few days of a "head cold," with headaches and muscle pains—all eventually have headaches and a fever. The pattern of symptoms varies from one outbreak to another.

The diagnosis is easily made in an outbreak, but single cases are more difficult to diagnose and the condition may be initially confused with serious illnesses such as acute appendicitis or myocardial infarction ("heart attack").

There is no specific treatment. Bed rest, and the relief of pain and fever by drugs such as aspirin are all that can be offered. Death has never been reported and serious complications are very rare. The disease usually lasts for only a few days, but some patients may have lingering after effects of tiredness and weakness, with only a gradual return to full health.

epidural anesthesia

A form of regional anesthesia achieved by injecting the anesthetic agent between the spines of the vertebrae into the space (extradural space) just outside the outermost covering membrane (dura mater) of the spinal cord. Also called *peridural anesthesia.*

Compare CAUDAL ANESTHESIA.

epilepsy

Disorganized electrical activity in the brain leading to transient attacks of disturbed sensory or motor functions. Some forms of epilepsy are characterized by convulsions (epileptic seizures or "fits").

In what is known as *symptomatic* epilepsy, the convulsions may be traced to one of several definite causes. These include structural disorders of the brain, such as a tumor or abscess which causes pressure on sensitive brain tissue; disease of the blood vessels of the brain; poisoning by drugs, or injury to the brain. Children very often experience fits during infections in which there is a high fever.

More common, however, is *idiopathic* epilepsy where abnormal brain cell activity arises for no apparent reason. It is this condition which most people think of as epilepsy. Many physicians believe that this type may also be symptomatic but that the cause (a tiny scar in the brain tissue for instance) has gone unrecognized.

It is also possible that some people are more susceptible than others to minor irritation of brain cells. In support of this "lower threshold" theory is the fact that some children have childhood seizures which they grow out of, just as others grow out of having convulsions with high fevers.

Warning symptoms may be noticed: headaches, drowsiness, giddiness, yawning. These are followed by the "aura" which is really the beginning of the seizure. There may be tingling sensations in the limbs with disturbances of taste and smell.

The attack itself falls into one of three main types.

Petit mal attacks are quite difficult to recognize clinically, particularly in children, in whom they mainly occur. The child may simply appear to be vacantly daydreaming for a few seconds. If he is standing, he may sway slightly and fall to the ground. Observers are often unaware that anything has happened.

Grand mal attacks are usually preceded by warning symptoms and the aura. As consciousness is lost, the patient may fall and sometimes emits a characteristic "epileptic cry" as the larynx goes into spasm. The muscles contract rigidly and the jaws clamp shut with tremendous pressure. Sometimes the patient bites his tongue. Then the muscles start to jerk violently and the patient may look blue until the convulsion passes and normal breathing is resumed.

As the fit passes off the patient may fall into a deep sleep (from which he should not be disturbed) or may go into a trancelike state. It is important that epileptics are not left face downward or in a position where they could swallow their own vomit.

Focal seizures (or "Jacksonian seizures") usually result from organic disease or brain injury. The attack starts in a localized group of muscles and does not usually lead to loss of consciousness.

Many people are able to lead fully normal lives with their epilepsy controlled by special drugs. Epilepsy is not thought to be inherited, although there is sometimes a tendency for it to run in families. It is quite reasonable for epileptics to marry and have children.

Many jobs are open to epileptics. They cannot drive cars or operate dangerous machinery, unless the epilepsy is well controlled. Intellectual capacity is unimpaired in most epileptics. In only a small proportion, repeated attacks lead to mental deterioration.

Children tend to grow out of their epileptic seizures, although in some the condition may later recur. Many adults, especially those with a mild form of epilepsy, keep the seizures totally under control with drugs. Phenobarbital was formerly used in epilepsy, but has now been very largely replaced by superior modern drugs which exert better control, without causing drowsiness. After a period of trial and error the correct dose is worked out for each individual.

If the patient has not had a seizure after two years or so, the dose is slowly reduced. Some patients appear to be completely cured.

Because of general ignorance of the condition, epilepsy still has not lost its stigma. In earlier times it was thought to be associated with possession by evil or even divine spirits. Even in this century it has been erroneously linked with insanity. In fact it is a disease like any other; epileptics are otherwise as normal as people with high blood pressure or diabetes.

epinephrine

A hormone secreted by the ADRENAL GLANDS.

episiotomy

A small surgical incision in the perineal area (which lies between the back of the vagina and the anus) made to assist childbirth.

During delivery the perineal skin becomes very stretched, particularly if the baby's head is large; as a result, jagged tears of skin and muscles may occur. Many gynecologists believe it is better to prevent this by making a small incision to enlarge the entrance to the vagina just before delivery.

EPISIOTOMY

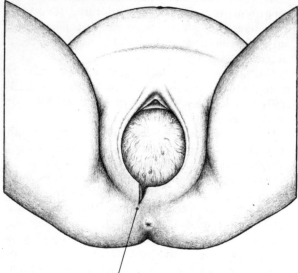

episiotomy

An episiotomy—a small cut made at the bottom of the vagina at the moment of delivery of the baby's head—is performed where there is a risk that the baby's head will tear the mother's perineal tissues. The cut is placed to avoid vital structures such as the anus and the supports of the uterus.

Little or no pain is felt because of the previously administered local anesthetic or general anesthesia. The surgical wound is stitched up following delivery. It heals rapidly, often with very little discomfort.

Episiotomies are essential to aid forceps or breech deliveries, although many experts do not think they should be a matter of routine for all births. Those in favor of the procedure point out that the stretching and damage (without the incision) may be severe enough to affect the future sex life of the mother and possibly predispose the woman to other gynecological complications.

epistaxis

The technical name for NOSEBLEED.

epithelioma

A type of tumor of the skin: there are various types with different degrees of severity.

Malignant ulcers may be caused by overexposure to sunlight; their incidence in such people as farmers, sportsmen and sun worshippers is directly linked with exposure to the sun. Fair-skinned people are more susceptible.

RODENT ULCERS are common and often occur on the face. There may be a small ulcer which heals centrally but continues its cancerous growth at the edges. Growth may be rapid or it may take several years for a spread of no more than one centimeter. But gradually deeper tissue will be invaded. The success of treatment of this condition by simple surgery is excellent.

Tumors known as *squamous cell epitheliomas* may suddenly start to grow after a long latent period. They look like papules or plaques which develop into crusted ulcers or fungal growths. The mucous membranes of the mouth, nose and vulva may be affected as well as the skin.

Unusual nodules, bumps and ulcers on the skin should always be reported to the doctor. After early diagnosis, treatment by surgery or irradiation is very successful.

Epstein-Barr virus

A virus, named after its discoverers, that is responsible for causing INFECTIOUS MONONUCLEOSIS and is strongly implicated as a cause of BURKITT'S LYMPHOMA. Also known as the *Ebb virus*.

ergotism

A serious but fortunately rare disease caused by eating bread made from rye that is contaminated with a certain parasitic fungus.

The symptoms are severe muscle pains, cold skin, vomiting, diarrhea, weakness and severe mental confusion.

The fungus contains a number of powerful chemicals called alkaloids, some of which are now used as therapeutic drugs. One, known as *ergometrine*, is used for the treatment of bleeding following childbirth. Another, *ergotamine*, is used for the relief of migraine. These ergot alkaloids are related chemically to the hallucinogenic drug lysergic acid diethylamide (LSD).

erysipelas

A dangerous skin disease, caused by infection with the bacterium *Streptococcus pyogenes*. Erysipelas (also known as "St. Anthony's fire") produces a bright red inflammation and swelling of the skin, together with fever, chills and sometimes nausea and vomiting.

The condition may originate from infection following a minor scratch or from contamination of a surgical wound. Infection with the streptococci causes a red, glistening swelling of the skin with a clearly demarcated edge. The inflammation may spread rapidly and in untreated cases may progress to collapse and death. Sulfa drugs or antibiotics are highly effective, however, and the disease is now rarely seen in its florid form.

erythema

Redness of the skin, caused by congestion of the tiny blood vessels (capillaries) near the surface. The capillaries may become dilated and congested with blood as the result of many factors, including some nervous mechanism or as the result of exposure to an external stimulus—such as heat, cold, ultraviolet rays (as in SUNBURN) or ionizing (high-energy) radiation—such as x rays or gamma rays. Among other causes of erythema are reactions to certain drugs, insect bites or stings, and certain viral infections that produce an erythematous rash (such as MEASLES). Patchy erythema may also occur in chronic diseases such as systemic LUPUS ERYTHEMATOSUS.

Specific types of erythema are often indicated in medical practice by a modifying term: for example, *erythema nodosum* is an acute inflammatory skin disease, thought to be caused by various types of allergic reactions, characterized by the formation of red nodules.

erythrocyte sedimentation rate: ESR

If a sample of blood (treated with an anticoagulant to prevent clotting) is placed in a tall narrow tube which is set up in a vertical position, the red cells slowly settle toward the bottom of the tube. In a normal person, in good health, the process of sedimentation is slow; by the end of an hour the top of the red cell column will have dropped by only 5 to 10 millimeters.

In many diseases in which the blood proteins are abnormal the rate is increased—with figures as high as 100 to 150 millimeters per hour. This constitutes a simple but useful test for the presence of various organic diseases. However, since it provides little information about the *type* of disease present, it is quite nonspecific.

eschar

An area of dead tissue produced by the action of corrosive substances or by burning.

Escharotics are substances employed to treat warts, the most commonly used being trichloroacetic acid and nitric acid. Their action is unpredictable and the area burned may exceed that desired.

esophageal varices

Enlarged and tortuous veins in the lower part of the esophagus, found in association with raised blood pressure in the abdominal veins (*portal hypertension*)—a complication of CIRRHOSIS of the liver.

In the United States, portal hypertension is most commonly caused by alcoholic cirrhosis, but it may occur in cirrhosis secondary to HEPATITIS or to other causes. The branches of the veins in the esophagus near the stomach form links with the portal vein. The varices are potentially dangerous because they are often the site of bleeding. This may be massive and sudden or there may be minor bleeding for days before the condition is discovered.

It is often difficult to diagnose the source of this hemorrhage, since bleeding in the stomach may be due to an acute or chronic peptic ulcer. Treatment is also difficult. Injection of vasopressin, which causes the blood vessels to contract, is sometimes effective. If this fails it may be necessary to use "balloon tamponade," in which an inflatable device is inserted into the esophagus and pressed against the site of the bleeding. Finally, a surgical operation may be needed to seal the veins and so stop the bleeding directly. In cases of recurrent bleeding the portal hypertension may be treated by diverting the blood from the portal vein into the vena cava.

See also LIVER DISEASE.

esophagitis

Inflammation of the esophagus ("gullet"), often caused by the flow of small amounts of gastric juice up from the stomach. This reflux is sometimes known as "heartburn" and may appear after large meals or in the presence of a hiatus hernia—an abnormal protrusion into the chest cavity of the top part of the stomach through a gap, or "hiatus," in the diaphragm (see HERNIA). Because of the abnormal displacement and relaxation of the normally closed muscular ring at the base of the esophagus (known as the "cardiac sphincter"), some of the acid contents of the stomach may flow up to irritate and inflame the esophageal lining.

estrogens

One of the two types of female sex hormone, secreted by the ovary. There have been more than 20 different estrogens identified biochemically but estrone, estradiol and estriol are the three main ones of clinical interest.

Estrogens are responsible for the regeneration of the uterine lining immediately after menstruation, and their withdrawal (as the ovarian follicle degenerates) provokes menstrual bleeding and the onset of a period. After the menopause the production of estrogens is considerably diminished; many of the unwanted symptoms of this time in a woman's life are related to the reduced amounts of estrogens circulating in the blood following the ovary's cessation of activity.

In pregnancy, estrogens are secreted by the placenta to stimulate breast growth and to maintain uterine growth and receptivity to the fetal demands. Measurements of plasma and urinary levels offer a useful assessment of placental efficiency where the baby is "small for dates," or where there is doubt about the prognosis for the pregnancy (i.e., after threatened labor or hemorrhage).

Estrogens, synthetically produced, are a constituent of the combination type of oral contraceptive used to suppress ovulation. Therapeutically they are used in hormonal creams or pessaries for the treatment of postmenopausal vaginitis, and as "depot" (i.e., long-acting) injections or as tablets in hormone replacement therapy ("HRT") for the menopausal woman. Used cosmetically to rejuvenate aging skin they have no value. Excessive doses are associated with an increase in blood-clotting and in recent years the dosage used in oral contraception has been reduced.

For a number of years replacement therapy with estrogens has been widely recommended in cases where the menopause is accompanied by troublesome symptoms, but recent work demonstrates that there is a slightly increased tendency for women who have taken estrogens for a long time to develop cancer of the endometrium (lining of the womb). It is also possible that the incidence of cancer of the breast could be similarly increased, but the evidence is not clear. The likely incidence of cancer of the womb has been given as 1 per thousand; the incidence with estrogen replacement 4 per thousand.

The conclusion must be that it is unwise to use estrogens as a routine in women who are undergoing the menopause, and that if they are used it must only be under medical supervision.

exophthalmic goiter

HYPERTHYROIDISM that is accompanied by abnormal protrusion of the eyeballs (exophthalmos) and GOITER.

extrasystole

The heart normally beats in a regular rhythm which is controlled by specialized tissue in the heart known as the conducting system. The beat is generated by a small mass of tissue belonging to this system, which is known as the *sinoatrial node*. From there, an impulse spreads and travels along the rest of the conducting system and through heart muscle to cause other parts of the heart muscle to contract in a well-defined order.

However, impulses are sometimes generated outside the sinoatrial node so that extra beats (or extrasystoles) occur. This may occur in normal health as a result of excessive stress or excitement, or it may be due to heart disease, or to drugs.

The patient may notice a "skipped beat," or a flutter, or extra beats. The significance of extrasystoles depends on the underlying cause of the extra beats and on their frequency; too many extra beats prevent the heart from pumping blood around the body efficiently. Treatment depends on the cause and on the type of extrasystole.

F

faecalith

see FECALITH.

faeces

see FECES.

fainting

Complete or partial loss of consciousness due to a temporary lack of blood supply to the brain.

Fainting can be brought about by a physiological reaction to overwhelming pain, an emotional shock, or extreme fear. These cause stimulation and overactivity of the *vagus nerve*, resulting in a slow pulse and reduction of the output of the heart, accompanied by dilation of the blood vessels in the muscles and pooling of the blood (which thus fails to reach the brain in sufficient amounts).

The person about to faint feels weak and nauseated; the skin breaks out in a sweat and feels cold, and there is yawning or deep sighing. In a little while the complexion becomes deathly pale and consciousness slips away.

Some individuals may show small involuntary movements during a simple faint which can be mistaken for an epileptic attack. Fainting can also be induced by a close hot atmosphere, prolonged lack of food, or by standing still in one position too long so that the blood pools in the vessels of the legs.

Recovery quickly ensues once the patient's head is lowered in relation to the rest of the body. Lowering of the head permits a prompt return of the blood to the brain followed by a return to consciousness.

Fallopian tube

The tube through which the female egg cell travels from the ovary to the uterus. There is one on each side of the uterus.

In each monthly cycle a *Graafian follicle* forms in an ovary and eventually ruptures, releasing an ovum into one of the tubes. It is during the passage of the ovum through the Fallopian tube (which takes several days) that fertilization by a sperm cell can occur. After fertilization the fertilized egg continues its journey through the tube to the uterus and is eventually implanted in the wall of the womb.

Sometimes the embryo remains in the tube and develops there—a condition known as ECTOPIC PREGNANCY.

Sterilization in women is most often performed by ligation of the tubes, which prevents ova from descending from the ovaries. The Fallopian tubes may be blocked by disease with the same effect, making the woman infertile.

farmer's lung

A disease associated with heavy exposure to organic dusts, particularly those given off by moldy hay, grain and other vegetable matter. It is also known as *acute interstitial pneumonitis* or "thresher's lung."

Characteristically it begins suddenly with night sweats, cough, fever, difficulty in breathing, headache and chest pains. Most sufferers recover soon after being removed from the environment in which they are exposed to hay and grain. With repeated attacks, however, more serious lung conditions such as emphysema may develop with potentially fatal consequences.

Farmer's lung is thought to be due to sensitivity to antigens in the molds.

fecalith

A concretion in the large intestine formed from hardened feces and calcium salts.

The condition is a relatively rare but potentially serious complication of chronic constipation. If the concretion blocks the intestine, surgical removal of the hardened mass may be necessary.

feces

The solid waste matter eliminated from the body after the digestion of food. Feces, like urine, are often a useful aid in the diagnosis of various diseases.

The process of digestion takes place in the stomach and small intestine. The indigestible residue passes through the large intestine, where its water content is largely reabsorbed, and collects in the rectum—together with large quantities of bacteria which have assisted in the process of digestion and coloring matter such as bile. The normal dark brown color of the feces is derived from a bile pigment known as stercobilin.

For most people, one daily bowel movement is normal; but the "normal"can range from several times a day to once every several days. A sudden change in bowel habits may be a warning sign of disease.

The shape of feces ("stools") should be cylindrical and the consistency should be firm without being hard. Many physicians believe that modern Western diets lack essential fiber ("roughage") and that added fiber is needed to ensure a healthy digestive system.

The two most common departures from the norm are diarrhea and constipation. Each can be a sign of a number of different diseases; if either is prolonged medical attention should be sought. Blood in the feces can be a sign of conditions as diverse as hemorrhoids and tumors, and is an even more important reason to seek medical attention.

Fecal fat is often measured during hospital laboratory investigations since it provides an indication of the efficiency of digestion and absorption.

felon

Any acute inflammation of the deep-seated tissues of the fingers, usually one that exudes pus. The term may also be applied to an inflammation of the toes. Also called *whitlow*.

The structure which is affected may be the root of the nail, the pulp of the finger or toe tip, the bone, or the sheaths of the tendons that run along the back and front of the fingers or toes. Usually, the felon begins either as a small abscess at the root of the nail or as an abscess in the tissues (both fatty and fibrous) that make up the pulp of the digit.

Inflammation of bones in the fingers or toes is rare, but a felon may originate in the sheath of the tendon.

Treatment involves incision and drainage of the lesion (usually by a surgeon who specializes in treating disorders of the hand) and the administration of antibiotics or other appropriate drugs.

fertility

Fertility—as measured by the number of children a couple have during the woman's reproductive lifetime—depends on a combination of biological and social factors. In societies such as the Hutterite communities, in which there are no social constraints on childbearing within marriage, couples commonly have 11 or 12 children. A woman's potential for childbearing is determined by her age at the MENARCHE (the onset of menstrual cycles) and at the MENOPAUSE, on the time spent recovering between pregnancies and on the frequency of sexual intercourse. A woman in good health in her 20s is estimated to have a 25% chance of conceiving from intercourse at the fertile midpoint of a single menstrual cycle.

Male fertility is less easily measured, but most men retain their fertility as long as they remain sexually potent, often well into the 70s or later. About one in every ten couples is infertile due to sterility in one or the other partner (see INFERTILITY). The infertile partner is just as likely to be the man as the woman.

In practice most societies have limited the number of children either by social means—late marriage and abstention from sexual intercourse within marriage—or by infanticide, abortion, or contraception. Even so, most countries in the world today have growing populations as the numbers of births exceed deaths. This is due to a dramatic fall in infant and childhood mortality worldwide with the control of diseases such as smallpox, malaria and tuberculosis, and better nutrition.

Most couples in the developing world, however, still want a large family—especially of sons—to help work the land. Despite campaigns by the International Planned Parenthood Federation many communities are slow to accept contraception.

fertilization

The process by which the egg cell (ovum) is fertilized by a sperm cell. It is believed to take place in a Fallopian tube, down which the egg cell descends after ovulation. Sperm cells swim up through the uterus into the Fallopian tube to meet the egg. When they do so they release an enzyme to soften the outer layer of the ovum, thus making it possible for one sperm to penetrate it.

Of the millions of sperms produced during coitus, only one is required to fertilize the ovum: the first one to reach the goal immediately forms a barrier membrane around itself to prevent further penetrations. At this point, in a small minority of cases, the fertilized ovum may split in two and so bring about the conception of identical (homozygous) twins. Nonidentical (heterozygous) twins are conceived as a result of the simultaneous fertilization of two separate ova. (The release of more than one ovum, ordinarily a rare event, became more common with advent of the so-called *fertility drugs*.)

Upon fertilization, the nucleus of the sperm fuses with the nucleus of the ovum, forming a single cell which contains the 46 chromosomes necessary for human development. Division of the cell proceeds while the ovum is descending the tube into the uterus, where it arrives as a *blastocyst* containing many new cells. The process of fertilization may be said to be complete when the blastocyst implants itself into the lining of the uterus, where it will develop for the rest of the pregnancy.

fetal distress

The term used to describe the signs of lack of oxygen in the fetus during the process of labor. When the obstetrician detects evidence of fetal distress he will take steps to deliver the baby very quickly—by forceps or vacuum extraction, or by Cesarean section.

During the early stages of labor the obstetrician monitors the state of the fetus by recording its heartbeat, either by listening through a stethoscope or by an electronic instrument that records the fetal heartbeat continuously. The pattern of the change in the heart rate with each contraction can give an early warning of fetal distress.

Blood samples from the fetus may also be taken for direct measurement of its oxygen content and the acidity. When these techniques of fetal monitoring are used any lack of oxygen can be detected before any serious fetal distress occurs. Their introduction has led to a substantial fall in the numbers of stillbirths and of babies who have difficulty in breathing immediately after birth.

fever

A body temperature above the normal average of 98.6°F (about 37°C). The term is also used to describe a disease in which there is an elevation of body temperature above

FERTILIZATION

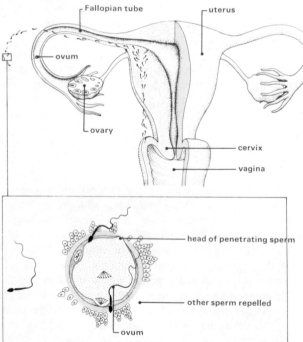

When a sperm meets the ovum, it releases enzymes which digest the membranes surrounding the egg allowing the head of the sperm to penetrate it. After successful union, no other sperm can penetrate this barrier; the fertilized egg implants in the uterine lining about one week after ovulation.

normal. Fever is one of the body's defense mechanisms against bacterial and viral infection: indeed as recently as 40 years ago patients with syphilis were treated by "fever therapy" in which they were deliberately given malaria to cause a high fever.

The autonomic nervous system, controlled by centers in the brainstem, regulates temperature in the body; the part of the brain called the *hypothalamus* is the biological "thermostat." On a hot day the hypothalamus senses the greater heat production and directs an increased flow of blood to the skin so that the capillaries dilate, sweat glands become active and heat is lost. On a cold day the hypothalamus directs the muscles to contract rapidly, or shiver, and heat production increases.

During an infection the thermostat sets itself at a higher level than normal, and thus may be enough to eliminate the microorganisms responsible for the illness. Fever may also be due to a noninfective cause—some brain diseases, neoplasms such as Hodgkin's disease, and metabolic disorders such as thyrotoxicosis may all cause a rise in body temperature, as may excessive exposure to heat.

The early symptoms of a fever may include a feeling of heat and discomfort, flushed skin or rash, increased pulse and respiration rates, nervous restlessness and insomnia. The simplest and most effective drug to control fever is aspirin, but if the fever rises above 104°F additional cooling may be provided by ice packs, fans, and sponging with tepid water.

fibrillation

The action of the heart muscle is normally coordinated so that the heart can pump blood efficiently. When the muscle relaxes, the chambers of the heart are filled by blood flowing into them—in the case of the right side, from the great veins, and on the left from the lungs.

Contraction normally occurs in an ordered sequence: the atria contract just before the ventricles to complete ventricular filling just before the ventricles themselves contract and expel the blood under pressure. Backward flow of blood is prevented by the heart valves.

There is a natural pacemaker in the wall of the right atrium, the *sinoatrial node*, from which a wave of excitation spreads through the muscle of the atria. A specialized bundle of fibers (Purkinje fibers) originates at another node, the *atrioventricular node* (also in the right atrium, but lower down and nearer the ventricle than the sinoatrial node). Through this bundle the wave of excitation is conducted at 400 to 500 centimeters per second to the right and left ventricular muscle. If contraction becomes disorganized the muscle contracts and relaxes irregularly throughout its mass and is effectively paralyzed. This condition is called *fibril-*

lation: the fibers going up to make the muscle mass contract and relax independently and circulation ceases in the part of the heart affected.

Fibrillation may affect the atria or the ventricles. In the latter case, death follows quickly unless treatment is immediate (see VENTRICULAR FIBRILLATION).

fibroadenoma

A benign tumor containing a mixture of fibrous and glandular tissue. Fibroadenomas may be found in many organs, but they are especially common in the breast.

The condition is probably much more common than is revealed by cases coming to the attention of surgeons: one study showed that even in "normal" breasts unsuspected fibroadenomas (often just visible to the naked eye) were present on biopsy in 25% of all patients.

Four out of every five women who have a lump removed from the breast are found *not* to have cancer, and fibroadenomas account for many of these benign tumors. Unfortunately they are sometimes recurrent, and some women have several removed over a period of years. Even so, any swelling or lump detected in the breast should be examined medically to exclude the possibility of cancer.

See also BREAST CANCER.

fibrocystic disease

Another term for CYSTIC FIBROSIS.

fibroids

Tumors of the womb consisting of muscle and some fibrous tissue.

Fibroids are benign and are the most common of all uterine tumors. Their cause is unknown.

They are more correctly known as *myomas*, since they rarely contain much fibrous material and consist almost entirely of smooth muscle. Fibroids are three times more common among black American women than among whites and are also more common in childless women. About one woman in five over the age of 35 has them, but the vast majority are benign and cause no symptoms. The fibroids range in size from microscopic lesions to multiple tumors weighing several pounds. Abnormal bleeding is the most common symptom.

In most cases the tumors require no treatment—particularly when there are no symptoms and when the patient is past the menopause. Once fibroids have been diagnosed the doctor will normally perform an examination every 6 or 12 months to make sure there is no increase in size. Some gynecologists have a rule that fibroids should be removed only when they are bigger than a pregnant uterus of 12 to 14 weeks. However, cervical myomas larger than $1\frac{1}{2}$ in. (3-4 cm) in diameter should usually be removed surgically.

Total hysterectomy is rarely necessary; it is performed only when the fibroids are large and multiple. Smaller fibroids may be removed by "shelling" them out (*myomectomy*).

Surgical removal is not normally attempted when a woman with fibroids is pregnant, unless there is a definite risk that the size of the fibroids may cause spontaneous abortion.

fibroma

A benign tumor composed principally of white fibrous connective tissue; almost any part of the body may be affected, but fibromas are especially common in the ovaries, nerves and skin. On the skin they can be seen as firm slowly growing nodules. They are reddish, yellow or bluish-black and found most often on the limbs.

Neurofibromas affect the nerve sheaths and contain nerve elements as well as fibrous tissue. When neurofibromas are present in large numbers the condition is known as *neurofibromatosis* (VON RECKLINGHAUSEN'S DISEASE). The tumors may cause symptoms from pressure on the nerves, especially in and around the spinal canal.

Odontogenic fibroma can lead to the development of benign tumors in the gums.

fibrosarcoma

A type of cancer in which the tumor contains collagen fibers.

Various kinds of fibrosarcoma affect different tissues, including the nerves, teeth and breast.

fibrosis

Damaged tissues are normally repaired by fibrosis, the formation of fibrous, or scar, tissue.

Fibrous repair restores the continuity of the damaged part, but fibrous tissue cannot function as part of the repaired organ; moreover, it contracts as the scar is formed and can interfere with normal function. Such contractures are often seen after the skin has been extensively damaged by burning, and may be severe enough to require plastic surgery.

Continued irritation of tissue may promote fibrosis. Examples include the fibrosis of lung substance produced by the inhalation of particles of silica in PNEUMOCONIOSIS, and the extensive fibrosis found in cases of ASBESTOSIS, when respiratory function is grossly impaired.

CYSTIC FIBROSIS is a condition found in about 1 in 2,500 live births. It is a disease affecting the exocrine glands, especially those which secrete mucus. (Exocrine glands, as opposed to endocrine glands, release their secretions onto the surface of epithelial tissue—either directly or by means of ducts; the endocrine glands are ductless.) The secretions from the glands are abnormally viscid, and there is a high concentration of chloride, potassium and sodium in the sweat. About 10% of babies affected die in the first few days from obstruction of the intestine. Later, the duct of the pancreas may become blocked with thick mucus; the substance of the gland becomes "cystic" because the secreting tubules dilate and a fibrous reaction follows. The children are very prone to develop infection of the lungs, and may suffer from repeated attacks of bronchitis and bronchopneumonia. Lack of normal intestinal secretions leads to constipation, and progressive destruction of pancreatic tissue may eventually produce diabetes. Diagnosis is made on analysis of the sweat and of pancreatic juice. Treatment may include a surgical operation to relieve obstruction, administration by mouth of pancreatic enzymes and fat-soluble vitamins, salt supplements, and the management of lung infections with wide-spectrum antibiotics and physical therapy. The disease is hereditary.

fibrositis

A general term for an aching condition of the muscles. (Also called *muscular rheumatism*.)

The condition was given the name because it was wrongly believed to result from inflammation ("–itis") of the fibrous tissue that binds the muscles together.

The pain described as fibrositis is sharp—particularly in the muscles of the back, shoulder and neck.

The connection between tension or stress and fibrositis is well known. It probably occurs because nervous tension can lead to tensed muscles. Cold is occasionally mentioned as a cause of fibrositis; this may also be due to the tensing of muscles, a natural reflex to cold conditions. Professional sportsmen, such as golfers and baseball players, seem to be particularly vulnerable but this may be an illusion—an attack is more costly and more widely noticed when a sportsman is involved.

Treatment consists of rest (with occasional moderate exercise if the pain is not too severe) and some form of heat treatment, which may be as simple as warming the affected area with hot towels.

fistula

An abnormal opening or passage between two hollow organs or structures, or between an organ or part and the exterior. The condition may be present from birth (congenital fistula) or may be a complication of an acquired disorder or disease process.

FISTULA

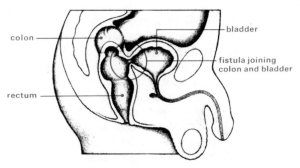

A fistula is an abnormal connection between any two hollow organs or between a hollow organ and the skin. Fistulas occur in Crohn's disease, cancers, as a result of inflammation (for example a rectal abscess) and as postoperative complications. A fistula between the colon and bladder, as pictured above, would let air and infecting bacteria into the bladder, and the patient might have the bizarre symptom of a whistling noise whenever he passes urine.

fits

See SEIZURES.

flatulence

The presence of gas in the stomach or intestines.

Swallowing air is a common cause. Flatulence may also be caused by bacterial fermentation of food. Cellulose in vegetables is broken down to produce methane and hydrogen, while eggs, peas and beans are responsible for sulfurated hydrogen and carbon disulfide.

Individuals who are particularly prone to flatulence should avoid foods that cause it.

Excessive swallowing of air (*aerophagia*) can occur when gulping down food or be associated with emotional stress. When the gas is in the stomach it is belched out through the mouth; in the bowels it causes rumbling, discomfort, and "breaking of wind."

Close control of the diet and attention to any air-swallowing habit are essential for the successful control of flatulence.

fleas

Wingless blood-sucking insects of the order Siphonaptera.

Several fleas are of medical importance because they can act as both host and transmitters of disease organisms.

The human flea, *Pulex irritans*, is parasitic on the skin of man. It is a host of the larval stage of *Dipylidium caninum*, the common tapeworm of dogs which can be passed on to man. It also transmits *Hymenolepsis diminuta*, the dwarf tapeworm. The bites of *Pulex* can cause dermatitis and it may on occasions pass plague from one victim to another. Like all fleas, it is susceptible to DDT and to more recent insecticides such as malathion.

More important as a disease vector is the rat flea, *Xenopsylla cheopsis*. In addition to the dwarf tapeworm, it passes on to rats and man the microorganism that causes bubonic plague, *Pasteurella pestis*, and the cause of murine typhus, *Rickettsia mooseri*.

Two species of flea commonly infest pet animals: *Ctenocephalides canis* in dogs and *Ctenocephalides felis* in cats. Many pet owners find that these fleas, while normally confined to the coats of animals, make the transition to human hosts quite freely. Frequent use of flea-killing preparations on pets may be necessary to avoid the irritation and threat to health that infestation can bring.

Apart from the general undesirability of harboring a parasite that feeds on human blood, fleas should be eradicated because they are a common cause of papular urticaria in children. This condition—a rash of red blotches and white weals—is caused by animal fleas rather than *Pulex irritans* and is an allergic reaction to the protein of the fleas' bodies, whether dead or alive.

Any unduly sensitive child should not be allowed

FLEA

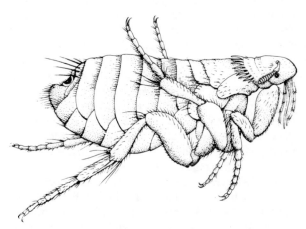

The flea is a wingless parasite which feeds solely on the blood of mammals and birds. There are over 1,500 different species of flea known, including the common rat flea (illustrated above). This little insect (length 2–3mm) was responsible for millions of deaths in the Middle Ages, as it transmitted the bacteria which caused the Black Death from rat to man.

close contact with pets that may be infested. Several proprietary preparations containing the latest effective pesticides against fleas are on sale at any drugstore.

Cat or dog fleas are rarely bothersome to humans where cats or dogs are around (since they really *prefer* cats or dogs); but when a cat or dog dies or is suddenly removed from the house, the house may suddenly appear massively infested and even become uninhabitable without the aid of professional pest control measures on two or three successive weeks. Also, fleas can stay active in an empty house for months without any host present.

flukes

Minute flatworms of the Trematoda family, which may infest man and other animals as parasites.

Flukes can invade many organs of the body and cause a number of diseases, the most important of which is SCHISTOSOMIASIS (or bilharziasis), which affects about 200 million of the world's population, most of them in Africa. Three types of fluke can cause the disease: *Schistosoma hematobium* and *S. mansoni* in Africa, Arabia and neighboring countries, and *S. japonicum* in China, Japan, the Phillipines, Taiwan and Indo-China. *S. hematobium* infestations mainly affect the bladder, *S. mansoni* and *S. japonicum* the intestinal tract.

Flukes have at least two hosts in their life cycle: as adults they live in vertebrates, while they develop in invertebrates, usually some sort of snail, often leaving the snail as free-swimming *cercariae* which lie in wait in the water until they are attracted to their next host by the agitation he produces by swimming or walking nearby. They penetrate his skin, leaving an irritating papule which blisters and then dries up in about two days. This is known as *swimmer's itch*. Fortunately, flukes do not multiply in the vertebrate host and the severity of the disease depends on the number of cercariae able to gain entry. Schistosomes become mature and mate in the veins of the liver; the eggs, which carry spines, are laid in the veins of the intestines or bladder where by ulceration they make their way into the cavity of the organ and pass to the exterior via the excreta. In water, the eggs develop into larval stage, known as a *miracidium*, which must gain entry into a suitable snail within 30 hours or die.

Flukes other than Schistosoma which cause human disease are *Clonorchis sinensis*, which may be eaten in raw or pickled freshwater fish in the Far East; *Opisthorchis felineus*, which also infects freshwater fish but is found in Southeastern Europe and parts of Asia; and the lung fluke *Paragonimus westermani*, which develops in crabs and crayfish. *Fasciola hepatica* is a liver fluke commonly found in cattle and sheep which may affect man, while a similar organism, *Fasciolopsis buski*, occurs in the Far East, usually in pigs.

fluoridation

Addition of fluoride (a compound of the chemical element fluorine) to the public water supply in order to prevent dental decay, especially in children. It is one of the simplest and most effective health measures available today, and it costs only a few cents per person a year. Yet it has been strongly resisted by some critics who maintain that it represents compulsory medical treatment and that fluoride is poisonous.

The incidence of dental caries is lower in districts where fluoride is a natural component of the water supply than in areas where it is not. Reputable scientific studies have established that adjustment of the fluoride level in water to one part per million can reduce caries by half: the reason is that the fluoride becomes incorporated in the mineral structure of the teeth and strengthens their resistance to caries.

Medical and dental authorities in favor of fluoridation agree that excessive levels of fluoride can cause mottling of teeth, but the proposed levels are not high enough to do so. Other alleged side effects, including even cancer, are easily dismissed.

An alternative way to obtain fluoride is in the form of toothpastes, mouthwashes, or tablets. For the maximum protection fluoride should be ingested with drinking water throughout tooth development.

folliculitis

Inflammation of the hair follicles of the skin or the scalp. It is usually caused by bacterial infection, the commonest organism being staphylococcus.

It may take a variety of forms. Acute infection originating in a hair follicle may develop into a boil or carbuncle. When the infection affects the hair follicles in the beard area, the patient has *sycosis barbae* or "barber's rash."

Pseudofolliculitis gives a similar appearance but is not directly due to infection. It is caused by damage to the surrounding tissues by the sharp tips of shaved hairs entering the skin around the follicle. Milder cases of folliculitis may occur on the legs or arms as a reddish rash corresponding to the distribution of hair follicles. This condition may be caused by infection, but irritants such as oil or chemicals coming into contact with the skin may also produce it.

Treatment is by attention to skin hygiene and, if severe, by the administration of antibiotics.

food poisoning

Food contaminated by bacteria or bacterial toxins can produce dramatic and swift intestinal disorders, characterized by vomiting and diarrhea.

Staphylococci growing on food—commonly dairy products, or cooked meat and fish—release a toxin which reduces the victim to a state of miserable shock in a few hours, but the attack passes off relatively quickly. Bacteria of the Salmonella group can contaminate various sorts of food; they produce symptoms which take longer to appear but which last longer. The patient may suffer from headache, shivering and prostration as well as diarrhea and vomiting. The illness may be extremely severe.

A rare but very dangerous disease—BOTULISM—is produced by the organism *Clostridium botulinis*, which grows without oxygen at low temperatures and can survive as spores resistant to boiling. The processes of home canning are often insufficiently stringent to kill this organism, which multiplies in preserved food and releases a toxin which can be absorbed by the intestine and taken up by the central nervous system. Botulism is characterized by double vision, dilated pupils, paralysis of the face, difficulty in swallowing and eventually paralysis of the muscles of respiration and arrest of the heart. Hospital treatment is essential, but even when this is provided the disease may prove fatal. A small but continuing number of cases have been recorded in recent years in the United States.

The treatment of staphylococcal food poisoning is directed toward relief of the symptoms, for the disease is not caused by the living organism itself. Salmonella food poisoning is a true infection, and severe cases may require the use of antibiotics.

Prevention is more important than cure. In tropical and subtropical climates it is important to remember that all food, particularly vegetables, may be contaminated and should only be eaten fresh after washing. Food must be stored in cool, well-ventilated places free from flies and dirt. All persons who handle food must be very careful in their personal hygiene. Home canned and preserved food must not be eaten if there is any suspicion that it has deteriorated, and processed food must not be kept too long.

foreign bodies

"Foreign body" is the term given to any extraneous object lodged in a part of the human body. This is generally accidental; occasionally it happens deliberately from ignorance or from abnormal action. Foreign bodies can range from bullets to badly swallowed food.

In the eyes dust, grit, hairs or filings flung from a lathe may move under the lids or become embedded in the eyeball. The condition is painful and may be a threat to sight unless expertly and promptly dealt with. Simple first-aid measures can be used for removal of those particles that are loose under the lids. In any case, the eyes should never be rubbed.

Ears and nostrils are sites where small children experimentally poke up beads or small toys, which they then cannot remove. They may forget about them or be too scared to tell their parents. If the objects remain, the subsequent inflammation and infection will eventually require medical attention, at which time the doctor will remove them. Sometimes insects can get inside these cavities and be unable to escape, especially if the region is hairy. The irritation they cause is out of proportion to their size. First-aid methods can help to extract insects from the ear, but all other cases need a doctor's help. Probing is likely to drive objects further in and should be avoided.

Objects swallowed generally give little trouble, moving smoothly from the stomach through the bowel to be passed with the stools. This often can be helped by the doctor's prescription of smooth mucilaginous preparations. Surgery is very rarely needed, although it may be indicated if repeated x-ray checks show that the object appears stationary within the digestive tract.

In the throat and airways foreign bodies can cause great irritation and may constitute a serious medical emergency. The fishbone caught in the throat is painful, especially on swallowing movements; amateur attempts to dislodge it are likely to drive it back further. Larger objects—including hard candy, toys or small dentures—can cause severe choking and need rapid first aid. The most serious ASPHYXIA arises from a big bolus of food caught in the windpipe, blocking it entirely. This is a life-threatening emergency to be dealt with immediately by a technique of pressure on the abdomen just below the diaphragm to eject the object. The technique is known as the *Heimlich maneuver* and should be learned by everyone.

The urethra, bladder, rectum and vagina are occasionally the sites of foreign bodies lodged after having been inserted. They are unlikely to free themselves and may cause great trouble. There must be no hesitation in seeking medical help.

fracture

A break in a bone.

The signs and symptoms may include pain, swelling, deformity, shortening of the limb, loss of power, abnormal movement and a grating noise between the fractured ends. In severe cases there may be shock increased by loss of blood.

The obvious cause is direct violence, such as a blow from a heavy object. But there are indirect causes: for example, falling on the hand may cause a fracture of the collarbone; or a sudden violent contraction of muscles may fracture the kneecap. X rays are used to confirm the diagnosis.

FOUR TYPES OF FRACTURE

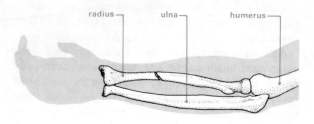

radius — ulna — humerus —

1 simple—skin intact over fracture

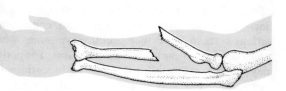

2 open—bone exposed to infection

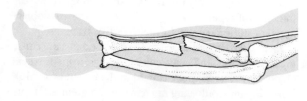

3 complicated—artery torn causing hemorrhage

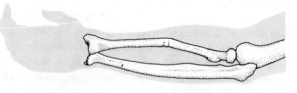

4 greenstick—incomplete break common in children

Bones may break in many different ways depending on the type of injury and on the age and general health of the person. Children have relatively soft, elastic bones which often break on one side only—a greenstick fracture (4). Elderly people have brittle bones which tend to be fractured by trivial forces. The most important complications of fractures are infection (2) and damage to structures adjacent to the fractured bone such as nerves, blood vessels (3), or internal organs.

In young children the break may be incomplete and is referred to as a *greenstick* fracture.

A *closed* fracture is one where the skin is not broken, while an *open,* or *compound,* fracture is one in which the broken bones pierce the skin. If the fractured end protrudes through the skin, bacteria may gain access.

The fracture is said to be *complicated* when it is associated with injury to an important structure such as the brain, major blood vessels, nerves, lungs, or liver; or when the fracture is associated with a dislocation of a joint.

Pathological fractures may be the result of bone disease; for example, a cyst or tumor may cause preliminary softening, which leads to a break.

An *impacted* fracture occurs when one fragment is driven into the other and locked into position.

In first aid, do not move the patient unless he is in immediate danger. After an accident the priorities are to make sure the patient is breathing and not bleeding heavily. Any wound should be dressed, using improvized bandages if necessary. The injured parts can be supported to prevent further damage.

The fracture and the joint (if any) on either side of it should be immobilized. This can be done by securing the broken part firmly to the nearest firm and convenient part of the patient's body. A broken leg is tied to the sound one, an arm to the chest wall. Whenever possible the uninjured part should be moved to the injured part and not the other way around.

If the fractured limb or other part has to be moved it should be given steady support so as to disturb it as little as possible. Padding is put between a limb and the part to which it is secured. Towels, belts and scarves make good emergency bandages.

In cases of a suspected fracture of the spine the patient must be kept absolutely still until experienced help is at hand. Suspect a fractured vertebra after any forceful fall or blow followed by pain in the neck and back.

frigidity

Lack of sexual desire in women or failure to respond to sexual intercourse. This inability to experience sexual satisfaction may be a permanent feature or may persist for a time and then under favorable conditions be replaced by a more normal sexual response.

The cause is often psychological. Poor general health may also diminish sexual interest.

Ignorance of the basic techniques of sexual intercourse—especially, lack of knowledge by one or both partners of the essential role of the clitoris in governing the female sexual response—or poor communication about sexual needs may contribute to frigidity. Many women are aroused sexually more slowly than men and may be left unsatisfied and disappointed.

Concepts of feminity and masculinity, attitudes toward marriage, fear of pregnancy or genital injury can all affect sexual fulfillment.

If a teenage girl receives faulty sexual instruction she can come to believe that sexual matters are shameful or distasteful and this attitude of mind may be difficult to counter.

The time and energy a couple are able to devote to the sexual side of their relationship may also be significant. The pressures of life can seriously dampen a woman's response to intercourse.

Reassurance and education are essential in the treatment of frigidity. A sympathetic interview by a physician can frequently bring to light problems and mistaken attitudes. An alcoholic drink taken by the woman before intercourse can be relaxing and helpful, but despite popular belief there are no such things as aphrodisiacs.

In particularly severe cases of frigidity some form of psychiatric counseling or psychotherapy may be useful. In addition, many excellent books exist (which the family physician can recommend) that help dispel ignorance concerning sexual techniques and which have proved profitable to many more than the authors and publishers. However, one of the best treatment modes is patience, understanding and tenderness on the part of the male partner.

frostbite

Injury or death of a part of the body due to extreme cold.

Frostbite is caused by the direct effect of freezing on the tissues, made worse by the lack of blood to the area (ischemia). The ischemia itself is made worse by the effect of freezing, since blood clots form in the blood vessels and impede blood flow. *Wet* cold is more of a danger than *dry* cold in the induction of frostbite—which most commonly affects the ears, nose, chin, fingers and toes. The sufferer may not notice it, especially on the face, and companions in cold environments need to watch each other for frostbite.

The skin first takes on a pallid color, progressing later to reddish violet, and ultimately to black' as the tissue dies. The black color is also derived from decomposition of hemoglobin from blood cells that have escaped from the circulation.

Skin and nails that slough off may regrow later, although there is often a permanent loss of movement.

Frostbite can be avoided by full protection of the face, hands and feet. Clothes should not be so tight as to restrict circulation. In any cold climate it is best to wear several layers of clothes to maintain body heat. The outer clothing should be waterproof to prevent the most damaging coldness induced by wet clothes.

Prevention of frostbite is better than treatment. As soon as it is noticed the area should be rewarmed by placing a fur glove over it. Cold hands and feet should be placed against a warm part of the body—either the victim's own body or a companion's.

The affected part must not be rubbed (especially not with snow!) and should be rewarmed gently and slowly, not rapidly.

furuncle

The technical name for a BOIL.

G

gallstones

Stones in the gallbladder or the bile ducts. They are present in 10–20% of all autopsies, and are more common in females than males below the age of 50. Women who have had children are more commonly affected than those who have not. The incidence increases with age; gallstones are very rare in infancy and childhood.

The mechanisms underlying the formation of gallstones are poorly understood, but they are often associated with infection of the gallbladder. There are three main types of stone; mixed stones, made of bile pigments, calcium and cholesterol; pure cholesterol stones; and those made up of bile pigments alone, which are rare. Cholesterol stones are usually solitary and large—up to $1\frac{1}{2}$ in. (4 cm) or more in diameter—while mixed stones and those composed of bile pigments are small and multiple.

The stones may be silent, producing no symptoms, or they may be associated with recurrent infection of the gallbladder following obstruction of the cystic duct. Obstruction of the common bile duct by a stone may lead to obstructive JAUNDICE. In obstruction of either duct the gallbladder first shows a noninfective inflammation of its wall secondary to the retention under pressure of bile, and then secondary infection by

GALLSTONES

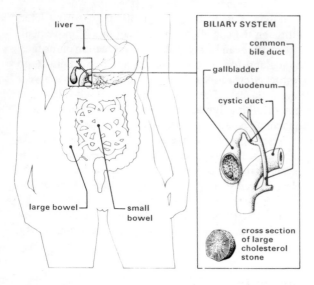

liver

BILIARY SYSTEM

common
bile duct

gallbladder

duodenum

cystic duct

large bowel

small
bowel

cross section
of large
cholesterol
stone

*The gallbladder stores and concentrates bile,
which is a mixture of substances manufactured in
the liver. Most gallstones form because the
concentration of cholesterol in the bile is too high,
although the pure "cholesterol solitaire" shown
above is unusual. If gallstones produce symptoms
of jaundice, pain or fever, the gallbladder
should be removed.*

organisms from the intestines. The patient develops an
acute pain in the upper part of the abdomen, usually
traveling from the midline to become concentrated
under the right ribs. Pain may be felt in the back and in
the right shoulder, and may be accompanied by fever,
nausea and vomiting.

Most cases settle with bed rest, a light fat-free diet and
antibiotics. Subsequent plain x rays may demonstrate
radiopaque stones; but only about 10% of stones
contain enough calcium to produce a strong shadow on
the x ray, and in most cases it is necessary to carry out
"contrast radiography." If the gallbladder is shown to
contain stones, and especially if its function is deficient,
it may be necessary to remove the gallbladder and the
stones by surgical operation. Some acute cases require
urgent operation, but often surgery is best left until the
acute attack has subsided and the inflammation died
down.

ganglion

1. A swelling on a nerve at the site of the junction of
nerve fibers. There are ganglions on the roots of each
pair of sensory nerves as they emerge from the spinal
cord; they also occur at major branching points of some
of the cranial nerves.

2. A soft, painless swelling on the hand or foot due to
a cyst developing from a tendon. The condition is
harmless, but if the swelling causes inconvenience it may
be removed surgically.

gangrene

Death of an area of tissue.

Gangrene may affect a small area, such as a fingertip
or toe, or may spread to involve a whole limb.

Dry gangrene occurs without infection. It is caused by
failure of the arterial blood supply to the affected part,
as the result of injury to the artery, blockage due to
disease, or frostbite. At first the area is painful and pale;
later it becomes discolored and eventually black. There
is a red line between the dead and living areas which
moves as the gangrene spreads. Spread of dry gangrene
is slow.

In *moist gangrene* infection plays a part and the
changes are caused by tissue putrefaction. Poor blood
supply is also a factor, perhaps due to infective
thrombosis or pressure on blood vessels from a hernia.
In addition to the unpleasant gangrenous area the
patient may suffer all the signs of a generalized blood
infection. Surgical removal of the gangrenous part may
be necessary to save life.

Gangrene quite commonly develops in the legs of
elderly people and of diabetics, because of an impaired
blood supply. It should always be considered in people
who have varicose ulcers or bedsores. If gangrene does
occur the area must be kept free from infection.

Gas gangrene is due to infection with the bacterium
Clostridium. It occurs as the result of entry of the
bacteria into a wound, without any predisposing
shortage of blood supply.

The bacteria are anaerobic—that is, they thrive in
conditions where oxygen is absent. They are therefore
found in dirty conditions as well as in cultivated soil.
(Gas gangrene is a common complication of war
wounds.) When they enter the body through a dirty
wound they produce gas and toxins. The wound
becomes green or black and has a very offensive
discharge. The tissues crackle because of the presence of
gas.

The infected tissue must be removed and the wound
opened to admit oxygen. It may be irrigated with
hydrogen peroxide to ensure oxygenation. In addition,
anti-gas gangrene serum may be given by injection,
together with local and systemic antibiotics.

gastrectomy

Surgical removal of all or part of the stomach. The
extent of the operation depends on the condition for
which it is being performed.

Gastrectomy may be indicated in cases of ulceration of the stomach and duodenum which have not responded to adequate medical treatment (see DUODENAL ULCER), in cases of uncontrollable bleeding from ulcers, in the treatment of cancer of the stomach, and for the relief of obstruction to the emptying of the stomach caused by old ulceration near the outlet of the stomach (pylorus)—scarring may narrow the passage from the stomach to the duodenum (the first part of the small intestine).

If the operation has been carried out in a suitable case the results are usually good, but there may be unwanted after effects such as loss of weight, anemia, recurrent ulcers, or the *dumping syndrome*. In the last-named, the patient either becomes faint and pale about five minutes after a meal and suffers from abdominal rumbling and distention with vomiting and diarrhea, or finds these symptoms coming on about half an hour after his meal. In the first case, symptoms are due to the rapid passage of food into the small intestine; in the latter case, which is far less common, the quick passage of food produces a sharp rise of blood sugar followed by an outpouring of insulin which leads to an abnormally low blood sugar (hypoglycemia). Relief may be obtained by taking small meals, lying down after meals and learning to take appropriate doses of glucose at the right time.

gastric ulcer

Ulceration of the lining of the stomach. Gastric ulcer most commonly occurs in the 60 to 70 age group, slightly more often in men than women. Gastric ulcers are slightly less common today than they were several years ago, but no one knows why. Whereas the "ulcer" was once the businessman's likely complaint through overwork, it has now been largely replaced by the "coronary."

Indigestion is present episodically with acute attacks lasting from two weeks to two months, with free intervals from two to twelve months. Pain usually occurs within two hours of eating. Weight loss is not uncommon and vomiting is a frequent feature.

X-ray examination following a BARIUM MEAL may assist the diagnosis. The ulcer may actually be seen directly on the stomach lining, however, through a *fiberoptic endoscope* (a special illuminated instrument passed into the stomach through the mouth and esophagus).

Bed rest in the hospital and refraining from smoking help gastric ulcers to heal. Milky diets and antacids do not speed healing but they may help to relieve the symptoms. There has been considerable controversy over the use of special diets. Many clinicians now feel that the patient himself is the best judge of what he should eat. But regular frequent meals which avoid highly seasoned and greasy foods may be of some benefit. Surgery (for example, GASTRECTOMY) may have to be considered in cases that do not respond to drugs.

Possible complications of gastric ulceration are hemorrhage, anemia, obstruction and perforation of the stomach wall.

gastroenteritis

Inflammation of the lining of the stomach and intestine.

It is usually due to infection and begins suddenly with a feeling of general discomfort, loss of appetite, vomiting, abdominal cramps and diarrhea. Persistent vomiting and diarrhea may result in severe dehydration and shock, requiring immediate medical attention. Acute alcoholism is also a frequent cause, as is overindulgence in highly spiced or other unsuitable foods. Other causes include food poisoning, arsenic or mercury poisoning and the excessive use of harsh laxatives or other drugs—such as aspirin or broad-spectrum antibiotics.

In adults the symptoms usually subside. All that may be necessary is bed rest with plenty of fluids to drink until diarrhea and vomiting have stopped; thereafter, a bland diet can be given. If symptoms do not disappear within 48 hours, stool examination and culture are needed to discover a possible causative organism.

Organisms called *rotaviruses* have recently been shown to account for about half the cases of gastroenteritis in children. Bacteria have been isolated from the stools in about 15% of infants with the acute form, which may be highly infective. Gastroenteritis often damages the villi (the absorptive cells of the intestine), preventing the absorption of milk sugar which then attracts water into the intestines and causes frequent and fluid stools.

The most serious danger in infants is that dehydration may lead to death, which can occur rapidly in a small baby. Signs of dehydration are failure to pass urine, sunken eyes, inelastic skin and a dry tongue.

Admission to the hospital is usually essential. Milk and solids are withheld from the diet initially; instead, clear fluids (such as 5% glucose solution) are given.

Gaucher's disease

An inherited disease seen most commonly in Ashkenazi Jews and due to an enzyme deficiency which results in the accumulation of a fatty compound in the liver, spleen and bone marrow. In a severe variant of the disease the brain is also affected, and the child dies in infancy. More commonly, however, the disease has a slow onset with the first symptoms coming on in adult life due to swelling of the spleen. Yellowish-brown discoloration of the skin is another frequent feature.

The effects on the spleen and bone marrow may lead to reduction in the number of blood cells: red cells, white cells and platelets. Nose bleeds and other hemorrhages tend to occur.

There is no specific treatment, although surgical removal of the spleen and blood transfusions may help correct the blood pattern.

General Medical Council

This is the body, elected from within the medical profession, responsible for the licensing of, and maintenance of discipline amongst, members of the profession. It also produces an annual register of doctors.

It is often confused by laymen with the British Medical Association which is an association to which doctors may or may not belong as they choose.

genes

Geneticists use the word gene to signify a factor which controls the inheritance of a specific physical characteristic.

Genes are carried by structures in the cell nucleus called chromosomes, which are made up of deoxyribonucleic acid (DNA), and a gene may be regarded as a region of the very long spiral DNA molecule.

Each mammalian species has a characteristic number of chromosomes: in man the number is 46, arranged as 23 pairs. When cells divide the chromosomes split, so that each of the daughter cells still has 46. In the formation of the sex cells, or gametes, however, the chromosomes do not split, but go half to one cell and half to another; the ovum and the sperm thus have 23 chromosomes each, and the fertilized ovum the full 46. In this way characteristics are inherited from each parent in a very subtle and complicated way—studied by the science of genetics, initiated by the Austrian monk Gregor Mendel (1822-1884).

See also CHROMOSOMES, DNA/RNA.

genetic counseling

Advice to parents about inheritable diseases, especially concerning the likelihood of passing them on to their children. Genetic counselors also give information on alternatives to natural conception, such as artificial insemination and adoption.

They will also advise on AMNIOCENTESIS (a test on the uterine fluid to detect fetal abnormality) and ABORTION.

Counseling is commonly offered to a couple when either the man or woman is known to have a genetic disorder, or to a woman who becomes pregnant at a relatively old age (when the fetus is more at risk).

Part of the process of counseling consists of building up a family pedigree. Sometimes it is necessary to go back over the obstetric history and family history of several previous generations. Often the best results are obtained when patients acquire the family information they need, at the doctor's request, from the family "matriarch."

Medical records may also be consulted for details of earlier illnesses, and causes of death and stillbirths.

Conducted carefully, the procedure usually produces a realistic assessment of the risk of the genetic disorder recurring. This will be expressed as "odds." For example, the couple may have a one in ten risk of producing an abnormal child, which would obviously cause them to think carefully; on the other hand, a risk of one in several hundred would be worth taking, even though there is no guarantee of a normal child.

In simple dominant conditions such as Huntington's CHOREA, the risk of inheritance from one affected parent is as high as fifty-fifty. In recessive conditions such as CYSTIC FIBROSIS the risk may reach one in four if both parents are carriers.

With many common genetic diseases the mechanisms of inheritance are not simple to calculate; estimates must be made on the basis of past medical experience and observation.

genetic disorders

Any disease or malformation that may be passed from one generation to the next by inheritance.

In relatively straightforward diseases such as HEMOPHILIA, the risk of inheritance can be understood because the disease is known to be associated with a particular chromosome.

In many other diseases, however, only observation has established a tendency for families to suffer; in such cases the mechanisms of inheritance are not understood. They are certainly complicated and therefore difficult to quantify. Examples of this type include CLEFT LIP/CLEFT PALATE, SPINA BIFIDA, congenital heart defects, and CLUBFOOT.

Not all genetic disorders take the form of obvious physical malformation. Many are metabolic disorders, from the relatively common DIABETES MELLITUS to extremely rare enzyme defects.

Genetic disorder may not be the same as *congenital disorder,* which means any abnormality present from birth, whether inherited or not.

The risk of genetic disorders is assessed and the parents advised in the process of GENETIC COUNSELING.

German measles

An acute viral disease, common in childhood, which is

contagious but in most cases fairly mild. Also known as *rubella*. The importance of rubella as a public health problem is not in its effects on the sufferers but in the fact that if it is contracted by a pregnant woman during her pregnancy there may be congenital defects in the baby.

Defects can be multiple and include congenital CATARACT in both eyes, heart disease, deaf mutism, mental retardation and microcephaly (an abnormally small head).

No woman should embark on a pregnancy without natural immunity to the disease as a result of a previous infection, or vaccination. However, if infection occurs in pregnancy, an intramuscular injection of *gamma globulin* (a special protein formed in the blood, which is associated with the ability to resist infection) may be effective in diminishing the risk of abnormalities. The rubella virus appears to cause a major epidemic of the disease every seven years or so; formerly, in epidemic years before strong preventive measures were taken, it was responsible for thousands of fetal deaths and abnormalities.

In children, rubella is a mild disease with an incubation period of 14 to 21 days. Symptoms include slight fever, a moderate rash (which first appears on the face and neck and then spreads to the body and limbs), and some enlargement of the glands behind the ears. The child can infect others who have not had rubella until the fever and rash have subsided. The child should get plenty of rest and be given light meals and drinks. One attack of rubella usually provides immunity for life.

giardia

A common intestinal parasite, found especially in warm climates, which can cause acute attacks of diarrhea and abdominal pain.

The microorganism responsible, *Giardia lamblia*, is a pear-shaped protozoan parasite. The disease (known as *giardiasis*) is most prevalent in areas of poor sanitation and in institutions, but outbreaks have been reported due to contaminated water supplies. About 3,000 cases a year occur in England and Wales.

Infection leads to multiplication of the protozoa within the bowel. There may be no symptoms, but heavy infections produce diarrhea, abdominal cramps, bloating, anemia, fatigue and weight loss. Undigested fat may be present in the stools. Drugs such as metronidazole are highly effective in clearing up the condition.

gigantism

Overgrowth caused by excessive secretion of growth hormone before puberty (that is, before the long bones of the body have grown together naturally; their ends

and shafts are originally separated by an area of cartilage).

Both the skeleton and the soft tissues hypertrophy with the result that there is an increase both in height and in overall size above the normal. The underlying cause is generally an ADENOMA of the anterior lobe of the PITUITARY GLAND, sometimes detectable in x rays of the skull. At the beginning of the illness the patient is typically strong and alert, but later is likely to develop pituitary insufficiency with weakness and a tendency to tire easily. Later there may be the added complication of hypogonadism (underdevelopment of the genitalia) due to reduction in the amount of gonadotropin secreted.

Treatment is by surgery to remove the tumor (see ACROMEGALY) and the administration of adrenal hormones, thyroid hormones, and gonadal hormones to combat hypopituitarism (underactivity of the pituitary gland).

Gilles de la Tourette disease

A bizarre psychiatric disorder of unknown cause, beginning in childhood and characterized by the tendency to swear obscenely, and progessively violent jerking movements of the face, shoulder and limbs. The patient grunts and makes explosive noises. The disease can be controlled with tranquilizing drugs.

gingivitis

Inflammation of the gums, causing pain and often minor bleeding when cleaning the teeth or eating hard food such as apples.

Gingivitis is the most common oral disease in adult life; children are more likely to have symptoms from caries ("cavities"). It is most often due to a combination of a soft, sugary diet and poor dental hygiene, but it may also occur as a complication of debilitating diseases and of vitamin deficiencies. Rarely a severe form of gingivitis (trench mouth) may result from infection with the organisms of VINCENT'S ANGINA.

Gingivitis is best treated by a dental surgeon, who may cut away damaged, overgrown portions of the gum (gingivectomy) in addition to giving advice on better dental hygiene and the use of a mouthwash.

glandular fever

Another name for INFECTIOUS MONONUCLEOSIS.

glaucoma

Impairment of vision due to a rise in the fluid pressure within the eye. One of the most important causes of blindness in middle age, it affects an estimated 1–2%

GINGIVITIS

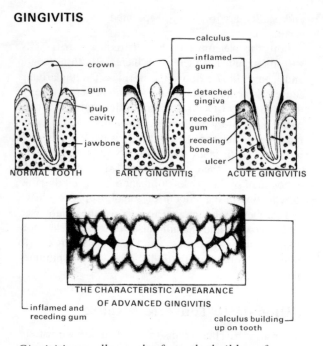

NORMAL TOOTH — crown, gum, pulp cavity, jawbone

EARLY GINGIVITIS — calculus, inflamed gum, detached gingiva, receding gum, receding bone, ulcer

ACUTE GINGIVITIS

THE CHARACTERISTIC APPEARANCE OF ADVANCED GINGIVITIS

inflamed and receding gum

calculus building up on tooth

Gingivitis usually results from the buildup of calculus (tartar) near the junction of teeth and gums. It causes varying degrees of redness, swelling, and bleeding of the gums, as well as halitosis (bad breath). If left untreated, teeth may eventually become loose and fall out.

of persons over the age of 40.

There are several distinct types of glaucoma. The most common and most insidious is *chronic simple glaucoma*, in which the rise in pressure within the eye occurs over a period of months or years without causing any symptoms. The gradual narrowing of the field of vision (so that only objects directly in front of the eyes are visualized) may pass unnoticed unless the eyes are examined by an ophthalmologist. Without treatment chronic simple glaucoma will eventually cause total blindness.

Acute glaucoma, in contrast, usually develops very suddenly, with severe pain in the eye, which becomes extremely hard, red and tender. Urgent treatment is needed to lower the pressure within the eye if vision is to be saved.

Glaucoma may also be *symptomatic*, in which the rise in pressure is secondary to some other disease in the eye.

Whatever the type of glaucoma, the underlying cause is a defect in the mechanism which removes fluid continuously formed in the front chamber of the eyeball. In acute glaucoma there is a physical block due to narrowing of the angle at the edge of the iris; in chronic glaucoma the blockage is thought to be in the meshwork of vessels that should absorb the fluid.

Treatment depends on the cause: *narrow angle*

glaucoma is usually relieved by a minor surgical operation, whereas *chronic glaucoma* is treated with drugs that reduce the rate of the formation of fluid.

Anyone with a family background of glaucoma should have the eyes examined regularly.

glioma

A type of tumor of the brain or spinal cord.

Most gliomas are malignant (cancerous), but they seldom spread to other parts of the body. As with other brain tumors the symptoms include headache, vomiting and pressure upon the optic nerve (papilledema). There may be progressive mental or physical deterioration, such as deafness, partial blindness, or personality change. Other symptoms suggestive of tumor are giddiness and convulsions.

The diagnosis can be confirmed by skull x rays, electroencephalography (see EEG) or brain scanning.

The intracranial pressure may be relieved by cutting into the skull (craniotomy). A glioma cannot usually be removed completely; the usual treatment is partial removal followed by radiotherapy.

globulin

The second major type of protein in the blood plasma. (The first is ALBUMIN.) Globulins are of several kinds. The types can be separated by modern methods of physicochemical analysis.

Alpha and *beta globulins* combine loosely with other important body chemicals to carry them around in the blood. *Alpha—1* globulin contains a fraction that binds bilirubin, and another responsible for the carriages of steroids and lipids. *Alpha—2* globulin combines with free hemoglobin in the plasma.

Beta globulins include some responsible for transporting lipids, and others that bind copper and iron for transport. Prothrombin, one of the blood-clotting factors, is a beta globulin.

The *gamma globulins* are extremely important in the body's IMMUNE SYSTEM: they are alternatively known as *immunoglobulins* and are subdivided into classes (IgA, IgE, IgM, etc.) according to their function.

The overall pattern of alpha, beta and gamma globulins may be measured to assess the progress of many different types of disease and treatment, since they are quite commonly affected. The specific immunoglobulins are also a useful diagnostic indicator.

glomerulonephritis

Inflammation of the glomeruli—the tiny clumps of blood vessels which act as filters to form the urine within the substance of the kidney. The condition may be acute or chronic and is an important cause of kidney failure: glomerular disease accounts for approximately two thirds of all patients dying of kidney disease.

Acute glomerulonephritis is most often a complication of infection of the throat or elsewhere in the body with one form of bacterium, a streptococcus. The immune defenses against the infection produce antibodies which also damage the glomeruli. This reaction usually occurs two to three weeks after the bacterial infection. The damage to the kidneys reduces the output of urine, which may become dark from the presence of blood. Typically, the ankles swell and the face becomes pale and puffy. Most often (in approximately 90% of cases in children) the symptoms of acute glomerulonephritis resolve within a few weeks. But in a minority of patients, the kidney failure may become total; without specific treatment by DIALYSIS or a kidney transplant the outcome is fatal. In another small proportion of cases, although the recovery appears complete, the inflammation within the kidneys grumbles on and the condition then becomes chronic. Over a period of years the kidneys become scarred and contracted, and again

GLOMERULONEPHRITIS

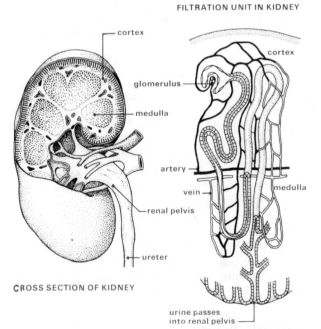

FILTRATION UNIT IN KIDNEY

cortex

cortex

glomerulus

medulla

artery

vein

medulla

renal pelvis

ureter

CROSS SECTION OF KIDNEY

urine passes
into renal pelvis

Glomerulonephritis is a complex disease resulting from the production of antibodies which damage the glomeruli in the kidney. Blood plasma passes through the glomeruli in the first stage of urine formation. In glomerulonephritis, proteins and red blood cells leak through as well so that the urine is said to resemble cola.

the end result may be kidney failure.

The glomeruli may also be damaged by chronic diseases such as diabetes mellitus, by high blood pressure, and by connective tissue disorders such as systemic lupus erythematosus. Whatever the underlying cause, loss of a substantial proportion of the two million glomeruli (one million in each kidney) leads to kidney failure.

See also KIDNEY DISEASES for further information on glomerulonephritis.

glossitis

Inflammation of the tongue.

Glossitis may be caused by an infection such as SCARLET FEVER, in which the red taste buds (papillae) protrude through a white coat or fur. Later the "fur" disappears, leaving the swollen papillae projecting from a bright red "strawberry tongue."

A smooth, bald tongue type of glossitis occurs in deficiency of some vitamins—for example, PELLAGRA (deficiency of niacin) and pernicious anemia (deficiency of vitamin B_{12}—see ANEMIA). A similar appearance is seen in CELIAC DISEASE and in the severe anemia of STARVATION.

Syphilis causes a chronic superficial glossitis. There are areas of opaque, white, thickened skin and in between a scarred surface without papillae.

Patchy tongue furring with smooth, well-defined red patches is known to doctors as "geographical tongue" because of its maplike appearance, and is not of any medical importance.

glycogen storage disease

The general name for a group of rare inherited diseases (about a dozen varieties are now known) in which the body is unable to store carbohydrate in the normal way.

Glucose, the body's principal carbohydrate, can only be stored in the liver and the muscle cells in the form of glycogen. A series of biochemical reactions is needed to control the formation and release of glycogen. Enzyme defects at various stages of this process account for the various subtypes of glycogen storage disease.

The symptoms of the disease vary widely, but the muscles are often weak—especially after exercise. Symptoms may begin immediately after birth or be delayed until the teens. Newborn infants may suffer convulsions because of a low blood sugar; in other cases the first sign may be an enlarged liver in a symptomless child several months old.

No treatment is possible for most varieties of the disease; when symptoms occur in infancy they may be reduced in severity by adjustment of the diet with frequent small feeds.

glycosuria

The presence of sugar (glucose) in the urine.

Glycosuria is the major sign of DIABETES MELLITUS, although not everyone with glycosuria necessarily has diabetes.

Doctors can detect glucose in a specimen of urine by means of a simple "dip" test. Similar tests are used by diabetics to detect and measure glucose in their own urine, thus permitting them to determine if their disease is under control.

Normal urine contains no glucose. It appears when the amount in the blood exceeds the "renal threshold"— that is, the quantity above which the kidneys cannot prevent it escaping in the urine. The threshold may be low, in which case glycosuria occurs in a nondiabetic. In diabetes the threshold is exceeded because of the high level of glucose in the blood.

Once glycosuria is detected, a *glucose tolerance test* is used to determine whether the patient is diabetic or merely has a low renal threshold requiring no treatment. In this test the patient drinks a standard amount of the sugar and the quantity remaining in the blood is measured hourly for a few hours.

goiter

A swelling of the thyroid gland on the neck.

It may be caused by too little iodine in the diet, or by an excess of certain foods (such as soya or cabbage) which prevent the gland from making the thyroid hormones, or it can arise without any known cause.

Iodine-deficiency goiter occurs in areas where the soil and water are virtually free of iodine. It is then called *endemic goiter*. In England the so-called "Derbyshire Neck" was due to a simple goiter caused by lack of iodine in the Derbyshire area. The introduction of iodized salt caused this disease to die out. It is still seen, however, in the Austrian Tyrol and in many mountainous districts, including the Andes and the Himalayas. An estimated 200 million people in the world suffer from simple iron-deficiency goiter.

The only sign of endemic goiter is a gradual enlargement of the neck. Where iodine deficiency is slight the disease is usually confined to young women. Men and preadolescent children are only affected when the deficiency is severe. In such areas CRETINISM is common.

Once formed, goiters do not respond to iodine treatment—indeed, iodine may make the condition worse by encouraging thyroid overactivity. Endemic goiter does not appear to lead to cancer of the gland.

Simple nonendemic goiter usually occurs in adolescent girls as a smooth swelling in the neck, which may disappear in a few years. but it may proceed slowly to

GOITER

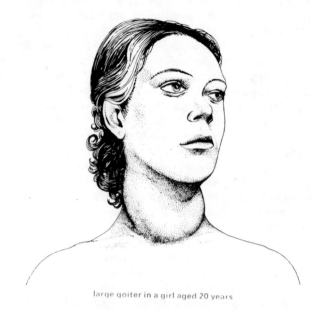

large goiter in a girl aged 20 years

A goiter is a swelling in the neck due to an enlarged thyroid gland. Surgical removal of goiters is only performed when drug treatment has failed, unless there is an acute emergency such as a respiratory obstruction due to a large goiter (above) or if it seems a cancer might develop.

become "nodular" (with small lumps) in middle age and finally "toxic" in old age, when signs of increased thyroid activity arise. Thyroid overactivity in the elderly with goiter often results in heart failure. In less than 2% of patients nonendemic goiter may become cancerous.

The treatment of early cases is by thyroid hormone preparations. Most cases of nonendemic simple goiter need no treatment, but follow-up is necessary. The thyroid enlargement may cause pressure on the windpipe or other structures in the neck, causing difficulty in breathing, swallowing or talking. Growth of a nodule may indicate a malignant (cancerous) change. Surgical removal is usually successful, although recurrent goiter is common after surgery. Surgeons, however, are able to give thyroid preparations postoperatively to prevent it.

gonadotropins

Any hormone capable of stimulating the gonads (sex glands); especially, certain female sex hormones.

The female reproductive system depends on these hormones, which are secreted from the pituitary gland at the base of the brain. Immediately after menstruation the first of the gonadotropins—*follicle-stimulating hormone* (FSH)—passes into the bloodstream. The ovary responds by ripening a small area on its surface, called a Graafian follicle, which contains an ovum.

The second gonadotropin—*luteinizing hormone* (LH)—starts flowing some days after FSH. The follicle then begins to produce the hormone *estrogen*.

After two weeks a sudden surge of LH induces the follicle to rupture, expelling the ovum from the ovary into the Fallopian tube. The follicle, now termed the "corpus luteum," produces the hormone *progesterone* which encourages correct implantation of the ovum into the uterine wall after fertilization.

The production of progesterone from the corpus luteum depends on continuous pituitary secretion of LH. If conception does not occur, the pituitary secretion of gonadotropins falls and the ovarian production of both estrogen and progesterone drops correspondingly. This results in the menstrual shedding of the uterine lining, which has responded to the hormones by thickening.

If fertilized, the ovum produces a third gonadotropin—called *chorionic gonadotropin*—which maintains the corpus luteum for the first three months of pregnancy and ensures the safe continuance of the pregnancy. It is this hormone which is detected in the urine in pregnancy tests.

In men, FSH promotes the growth of the sperm-forming tubes within the testicles and of the sperms themselves; LH ensures that the testicles produce androgens, the male sex hormones.

See also MENSTRUATION.

gonorrhea

A common venereal disease.

Gonorrhea is an infection of the genital organs and urinary outlet by the bacterium *Neisseria gonorrhoeae*. It can spread to other organs if the infection is left untreated—for example the joints, tendons, muscles, heart and brain—but this is relatively rare since the advent of antibiotics.

No one really knows the incidence of gonorrhea since the disease tends to be under-reported. Many patients treat themselves and many infected women have no symptoms. But one study showed that 6% of pregnant women in the United States were carriers of the disease. About 70–80 million new cases occur worldwide each year.

Who gets the disease? Most patients are between 15 and 25 years of age. Among men, gonorrhea tends to be seen in the armed forces, in men whose occupation requires a great deal of travel (such as migrant workers and seamen), and in homosexuals. In women, similar lifestyles may predispose to the disease; prostitutes are also commonly infected—it is estimated that between

10 and 35% are carriers of the disease.

Although sexual intercourse is by far the most common means of transmission, gonorrhea does spread in other ways. Babies can be infected at birth if the mother is infected. In such cases the disease causes a severe conjunctivitis which can lead to blindness. Until recently this was a principal cause of blindness, but it was largely eradicated when doctors began the routine procedure of instilling protective ointments into the eyes of the newborn.

In very rare cases infants and young children may contract the disease from their parents by close contact. In some institutions, outbreaks have occasionally been blamed on infected towels.

The incubation period of gonorrhea is between two and ten days. The illness starts suddenly in men, with a repeated urgent desire to pass urine and severe pain during urination. Considerable quantities of pus are discharged from the penis. At this stage infection is so obvious that the patient cannot fail to recognize the need for treatment. If the disease is not treated it can spread to the prostate gland and testicles, giving rise to fever and perhaps involuntary retention of urine. Eventually it will subside, even without treatment, but may leave strictures of the urinary outlet and cause sterility.

In women the disease is milder and may produce no symptoms at all—which is dangerous, since the woman may not realize she is infected. In other cases there may be urgency and pain on urination, discharge of pus and the formation of abscesses. Even when these resolve, the infecting bacteria remain to infect the woman's sexual partners unless she is properly treated with antibiotics.

Penicillin is the mainstay of treatment for patients with gonorrhea, although higher doses and longer courses have become necessary over the years as the gonococcus has developed resistance. Some strains now fail to respond to penicillin at all, in any dosage, and must be treated by other less effective antibiotics. In every case all sexual partners should be contacted and treated.

A condom provides some barrier to the spread of gonococcal infection, but is not completely protective.

gout

Almost everyone knows of gout as a cause of attacks of extremely painful arthritis (inflammation of a joint), but in fact the disease is essentially a chemical defect which causes the accumulation in the bloodstream of a waste product of metabolism known as *uric acid*. It is the deposition of crystals of uric acid (urate or sodium urate) in the skin, joints and kidneys which is responsible for the symptoms.

The disease has four major aspects: (1) gouty arthritis; (2) the formation of tophi (lumps of urate under the

GOUT

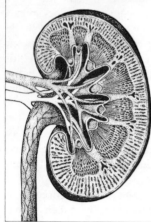

CRYSTALS CAN
DAMAGE KIDNEYS

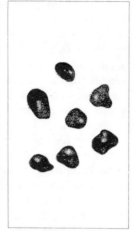

URIC ACID CRYSTALS

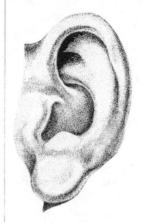

CRYSTALS DEPOSITED
IN EARS AS "TOPHI"

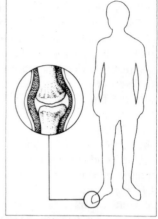

GOUT CAUSES HOT,
SWOLLEN, PAINFUL JOINTS

Gout is an extremely painful condition which predominantly affects men. It is caused by an excess of uric acid which forms needle-sharp crystals in the joints, ears and kidneys. Gout is in part a hereditary disease, but is also exacerbated by high-protein food.

skin, especially in the fleshy rim of the ear); (3) the formation of kidney stones composed of crystals of uric acid; and (4) kidney failure (caused by blockage of the kidneys with stones).

Symptoms usually appear in men in middle age. The disease is much less common in women and rarely appears before the menopause. In Europe and the United States the incidence of gout is about 0.3%, and accounts for 5 in every 100 cases of arthritis. Gout is usually first manifest with a sudden and extremely painful attack affecting a single joint—most often the first joint of the big toe. The initial attack commonly occurs during sleep and may occur without warning or be precipitated by some stress such as the excessive consumption of alcohol a few hours earlier, or by unaccustomed exercise or an injury sustained earlier the same day.

An attack of gout can cause such severe pain that many sufferers are unable even to bear the weight of light sheets over the affected joint. The tissues around the joint are also inflamed in most cases—producing heat, swelling, redness and excruciating pain and tenderness. After the first attack, more can be expected—usually before a year has passed—in the absence of treatment.

Tophi, the second main feature of gout, develop in chronic untreated cases. They consist of creamy white lumps of insoluble sodium urate under the skin, seen (in addition to the rims of the outer ears) in the hands, feet

and elbows. Tophi can become massive and disabling, sometimes ulcerating and discharging.

About 15-20% of patients with chronic gout have kidney stones, the symptoms of which are occasionally the first evidence of the disease. Urate crystals in the kidneys may lead to death as the result of kidney failure in untreated cases.

The treatment of gout used to be based on relief of symptoms by administration of the traditional herbal drug *colchicine*. Now that the underlying chemical cause of gout is clear, however, the treatment has changed. Although colchicine may still be used in acute attacks, the symptoms of an acute attack are now usually relieved by the administration of anti-inflammatory drugs such as phenylbutazone or indomethacin. (Both of these drugs can exert potentially serious side effects, especially if administered over prolonged periods; thus, their use must be under close medical supervision.) More important, once the acute attack has been controlled, is the prevention of future attacks. The drug allopurinol (Zyloprim) can prevent the formation of excess amounts of uric acid and thus prevent acute attacks. Other classes of drugs, known as *uricosurics*, can act to control the symptoms of gout by hastening the excretion of uric acid by the kidneys (however, they must not be used in the presence of known kidney damage). Allopurinol, which interferes with the production of uric acid, must usually be taken for years to control the blood levels of uric acid—the excessive production of which is known as *hyperuricemia*.

granuloma

A slowly growing inflammatory swelling, usually due to infection but sometimes arising from noninfectious foreign bodies.

Granulomas can cause various problems depending on their site and cause. They can vary from lumps in the skin following immunization (such as the triple vaccines given to infants) to masses within the brain.

Granulomas differ from abscesses in that they are solid—filled with inflammatory cells and tissue, but without pus. Diseases in which granulomas are common include tuberculosis, syphilis, fungal infections, sarcoidosis and parasitic disorders. They may be solitary or widespread.

Symptoms occur if the granuloma is in a vital area, such as the brain, or can be seen in the skin. Treatment of infective granuloma is directed toward eliminating the infecting organism, often by antibiotics. Surgery is sometimes necessary.

Lethal middle granuloma is a rare but terrible disease in which the tissues of the middle of the face are slowly eaten away by inflammation. The nose, eyelids, skin and finally the bones are destroyed and the patient (usually a man in early or middle adult life) succumbs eventually from infection. Radiation or anticancer drugs may help.

Wegener's granuloma, also rare, is another slowly progressive disease. It first affects the nose and sinuses, later spreading to the lungs and kidneys. Drugs to suppress immunity may be of help.

granuloma inguinale

A chronic bacterial disease, widespread in tropical and subtropical areas, in which an ulcerating infection spreads slowly over the skin of the genital organs and groin. The highest incidence is between the ages of 20 and 40.

It is thought to be transmitted during sexual intercourse or other close contact and is caused by microorganisms commonly known as *Donovan bodies* (technical name: *Calymmatobacterium granulomatis*). In rare cases the disease has been known to spread from the genitals to joints or bones in other parts of the body, due to invasion of the lymphatics and blood circulation.

Granuloma inguinale is usually not painful, but it is very destructive as it spreads over the genitals and the surrounding skin. Secondary infection with other bacteria is almost inevitable. Doctors can distinguish the disease from syphilis by microscopic identification of the Donovan bodies.

Two weeks of antibiotic treatment usually cures granuloma inguinale, although severe cases may take longer to heal. The disease can probably be prevented by washing the genital organs thoroughly after sexual intercourse.

Graves' disease

Another name for HYPERTHYROIDISM.

green monkey disease

Another name for MARBURG VIRUS DISEASE (also known as *green monkey fever*).

growth hormone

See SOMATOTROPIN.

Guillain-Barré syndrome

An inflammation of the nerves and (less commonly) the spinal cord, of unknown cause. It usually follows 10 to 21 days after an infection of the upper respiratory tract (such as the common cold) or a gastrointestinal infection.

Guillain-Barré syndrome starts slowly with weakness of both legs. Later the weakness becomes a paralysis affecting muscles of the trunk, arms and occasionally the face. The condition was formerly thought to be caused by a viral infection of the nerves, but specific evidence is lacking.

Eventually the paralysis and accompanying loss of sensation reaches a plateau which may last for several weeks. Then a gradual return to normal health occurs, though this also may take weeks or even months.

About 10% of patients are left with some weakness.

Intensive care is given in the early stages of the condition because there is a risk of paralysis of the muscles that control breathing.

There was considerable interest in an outbreak of Guillain-Barré syndrome which appeared to follow the mass influenza vaccination program in the United States in the winter of 1976/77. About one in every 125,000 Americans vaccinated developed the syndrome—an incidence ten times the normal.

Other countries—for example, Britain and Holland—found no increase in Guillain-Barré cases after their vaccination campaigns in the same winter. The link between influenza, influenza vaccination and Guillain-Barré syndrome is therefore not established.

Guthrie test

A test for the disease PHENYLKETONURIA in newborn babies.

A few drops of blood taken from the baby's heel can ensure that the disorder of phenylketonuria is recognized early enough to prevent brain damage.

About one British child in 20,000 has phenylketonuria, an inherited disease in which an amino acid, phenylalanine, accumulates in the blood. Untreated, it causes irreversible mental retardation by the fourth month of life. Early treatment with a special diet may allow the child to develop normally.

The test is performed when the baby is three to six days old. If the results are positive, other blood tests are performed to confirm the diagnosis. If the initial results are negative they should be confirmed by a follow-up urine test three to six weeks later.

In Scotland the Guthrie Test is also used to rule out the presence of at least five other diseases.

gynecomastia

Excessive enlargement of the breasts in a boy or man.

Some enlargement of the breasts is a normal, transient occurence in newborn boys, whose breasts are engorged and swollen in response to their mothers' hormone levels. It may also be seen temporarily during adolescence, when it is of no significance except as a minor embarrassment. Fat boys may appear to have enlarged breasts—but this is not *true* gynecomastia, which is related to hormonal imbalance.

Boys with persisting gynecomastia may have the rare chromosomal abnormality known as KLINEFELTER'S SYNDROME—characterized by small testicles, disproportionately long limbs and a feminine body shape. Similar enlargement of the male breast occurs in some generalized skin disorders, malnutrition, overactivity of the pituitary or thyroid glands, lung and testicular tumors and failure of the liver or kidneys.

Gynecomastia also occurs occasionally as a side effect of certain drugs, including the heart drug digitalis, or estrogens given to control acne or breast cancer.

GYNECOMASTIA

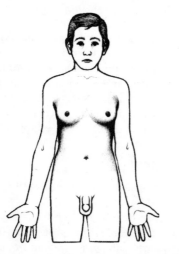

Gynecomastia results from an excess of the hormone estrogen. It is common in newborn boys, and the high estrogen levels in breast milk can prolong it for months. Gynecomastia is also normal around puberty, but at other ages it can be due to one of a number of diseases or drugs.

H

haem-

For words beginning HAEM- see HEM-.

hair (diseases of)

The basic facts are that the growth of hair is cyclical, and that all the hair follicles are present at birth.

There are three types of hair: (1) *lanugo*, the hair which covers the fetus and is shed at about eight months; (2) *vellus*, fine hair up to 3 cm long which covers the body surface before puberty, except for the scalp, eyelashes and eyebrows; and (3) *terminal* hair, which appears on the scalp during childhood and in the pubic region at puberty; later it grows in the armpits and over the thighs, legs, forearms, chest, arms, shoulders and buttocks.

Loss of hair from the scalp (*alopecia*—see BALDNESS) may occur after general illness dampens down the activity of the hair follicles, in various specific illnesses such as hypothyroidism, in protein deficiency and in anemia. But the most common cause of patchy loss of hair is *alopecia areata*, where localized bald patches spread on the scalp for about three to six months, being followed by spontaneous recovery. The condition may recur, and the advice of a dermatologist is helpful.

Baldness in men is very common, and is due to a combination of factors—heredity, stimulation by the male hormone, and aging. The hair recedes, possibly starting soon after puberty, and the gradual loss proceeds until nearly all the scalp may be bald. No really effective treatment is known.

halitosis

Bad-smelling breath arising either from the mouth or from the lungs.

Many people have a faint sweetish halitosis in the morning, accompanied by a bad taste in the mouth; both can be relieved by proper brushing of the teeth.

Halitosis can arise from poor oral hygiene (e.g., failure to brush away particles of food lodged between the teeth), decayed teeth, or pockets of diseased and overgrown gums. The breath is often foul after dental surgery, particularly when there is bleeding. Less often halitosis can be associated with an oral infection such as trench mouth.

Causes of halitosis outside the mouth include chronic infections of the sinuses or lungs (see BRONCHIECTASIS) or a lung abscess. More commonly halitosis results from foods such as garlic, whose chemical odors are excreted in the breath. Poor diabetic control leads to a characteristically sweet smell of acetone on the breath; kidney failure may cause a smell of ammonia. On corrective treatment the smell usually disappears.

hallucination

The perception of false sensations in the absence of any physical cause.

Hallucinations can affect any or all of the senses: they may be seen, heard, tasted, smelled or felt. They vary greatly, from simple flashes of light to sensations of highly specific and identifiable objects or sounds. Normal people under severe stress may share a hallucination, as when victims of a shipwreck together see a nonexistent shore.

Hallucinations may be a sign of a mental disorder, such as schizophrenia or severe depression, or may occur as a result of physical illness. Epileptics often experience hallucinations just before a seizure. In states of clouded consciousness—caused, for example, by high fever, chronic alcoholism, a head injury, liver failure, or senile brain degeneration—repeated and often terrifying hallucinations are common. Tumors of the brain can also cause hallucinations of taste, vision, or hearing, depending on the site of the brain tumor.

Some drugs, especially narcotics, can be powerful hallucinogens. The cocaine user may feel insects crawling under the skin. Drugs such as mescaline and LSD are classed as hallucinogenic because of the vivid and unpredictable nature of the visual hallucinations that they induce.

Hallucinations can best be suppressed by treating the underlying disease. The hallucinations seen in delirium associated with typhoid fever, for example, disappear as the body temperature returns to normal; the alcoholic with delirium tremens stops seeing terrifying animals following sedative treatment.

hare lip

See CLEFT PALATE/HARE LIP.

Hashimoto's disease

A chronic form of THYROIDITIS. Also known as *struma lymphomatosa* and *Hashimoto's struma*.

hay fever

An allergic disease of the membranes of the nose, throat and eyes, (also known as pollinosis). It is caused by increased sensitivity to airborne pollens and is therefore usually seasonal—occurring only when the air contains pollen of a specific type, not necessarily from hay.

Hay fever is an allergy similar to infantile eczema, asthma and some food allergies, all of which may be inherited.

Pollens that produce hay fever are usually light and scattered by the wind from grasses, weeds or trees. The pollen of plants pollinated by insects (which is heavy and sticky) rarely causes the disease.

In Britain the Meteorological Office releases daily information about the pollen count during the spring and summer months. The condition is likely to become clinically distressing whenever the count rises above 30.

Although hay fever affects many, most of the sufferers are relatively mildly affected and need no special treatment. The nose, eyes and throat itch and are congested and reddened, and the eyes water. Even the ears may itch. Most distressing are the bouts of uncontrollable sneezing. Coughing, breathlessness and wheezing often indicate that allergic ASTHMA is manifest.

The diagnosis is usually obvious: the seasonal timing, the worsening of symptoms on dry windy days and their relief during rain, and their onset in many fellow sufferers at the same time leave little doubt. The diagnosis can be confirmed by applying extremely weak extracts of pollens to the skin under strictly controlled conditions.

Patients with hay fever should try to avoid the provoking pollen. Certain drugs can prevent the reaction, or "desensitizing" injections of pollen extracts may be given three to four months before the season starts.

Hay fever, once contracted, is typically a lifelong problem but not a life-threatening one. Asthma may occur in up to one in three patients.

headache

Most headaches arise in tissues outside the skull. Probably the most common type is the "tension" or "nervous" headache caused by contractions of the muscles of the scalp and the back of the neck. Pain spreads from the back of the head to the top of the eyes and is associated with feelings of pressure and tension. The headache is relieved when the muscle contractions cease.

MIGRAINE arises from dilation and constriction of blood vessels in the scalp, temple and face. Migrainous headaches are usually one-sided, sudden, very intense and associated with visual disturbances. People who are migraine sufferers often know beforehand when an attack is imminent.

But not all migraines follow this pattern. Sometimes the headache is accompanied by temporary paralysis of one arm and leg, or of the eyes. *Cluster headache,* another migraine variant, combines one-sided headache with sweating, flushing, watering of the eyes and a runny nose. It lasts only a short time, but is nevertheless very unpleasant. Some "tension" and migraine headaches may occur together.

Congestion and inflammation of the nasal sinuses may give rise to headache in the forehead and face, usually with tightness and irritation in the nose. People often blame eye strain as a cause of headache, but it seldom is. Increase in pressure within the eye may cause headache—as in sudden-onset GLAUCOMA—and so may infection and inflammation of the eye. Poor light or prolonged reading are seldom responsible, in themselves, for headaches.

Headache may arise from disease of the teeth, ears, or nerves, and from the bones, muscles and joints of the neck and jaw.

Chronic severe headache may follow head injury—either because of tenderness at the point of injury or because of the contraction of muscles around it. Vascular (migraine-type) headaches are common after injury. Less common are "delusional" headaches, complained of when there is no damage. (They may miraculously disappear when financial compensation for the accident is paid!)

Trigeminal neuralgia is a stabbing, exceptionally severe pain in one side of the face, along the distribution of the fifth cranial nerve. It occurs sporadically, perhaps many times over a few hours, then disappears for a few months. Specific drugs are available to relieve trigeminal neuralgia; surgical interruption of the nerve is a last resort.

One form of headache in the elderly is particularly important, since failure to recognize and treat it early may lead to total and permanent blindness. In this condition, *cranial arteritis,* there is a structural change as well as inflammation in the major arteries of the temples. The patient has sudden severe pain in the temple and the scalp is particularly tender to the slightest touch. The tongue may be pale and tender. The artery itself is usually thickened and tortuous, but may be pulseless and difficult to locate. If the disease is allowed to continue, the artery to the retina may become blocked and blindness will inevitably follow. The condition can usually be arrested and blindness prevented by high doses of steroid drugs.

One condition popularly associated with headache is high blood pressure. Surprisingly, only one in ten patients with high blood pressure complains of headache (usually of the tension or migrainous type).

Headaches arising from within the skull are uncommon, but are often more important than those arising outside it. Headache in fevers and infectious diseases is caused by distension of the arteries in the brain. Tumors of the brain may press upon pain-sensitive nerve fibers.

Treatment of headache, if possible, should be directed at the cause. Where quick relief is required, most cases of simple headache respond quickly to aspirin or other analgesics.

head injury

Head injury is the most common cause of unconsciousness in patients seen in hospital emergency departments. The usual causes are violence and automobile accidents—often when under the influence of alcohol—and the outlook may be serious.

Anyone who witnesses a head injury should act quickly to obtain medical help, especially if the patient is unconscious. It may not be clear whether or not the patient is unconscious; if in doubt, assume that he is.

CONCUSSION is the state of mild confusion after a head injury, and can occur without loss of consciousness. A concussed person may answer questions quite reasonably or even volunteer information, but in other cases may be slow in his responses. The severely concussed patient repeats himself. On recovery, he usually cannot remember the incident or the events before and after it. Following a severe head injury consciousness may be dulled, but the patient can often answer questions in monosyllables and appreciate sound, touch and pain.

An annoying or aggressive "drunk" with a head injury may be merely drunk, or he may be suffering the effects of a concussion. Only overnight observation can distinguish between the two; thus the need for prompt medical attention.

The more deeply unconscious patient may still respond to painful stimuli—by attempting to push away the attendant's hand—and may blink when his eyelid is touched.

When even these responses are absent the outlook is grave, though not hopeless. Deep unconsciousness may be produced by hemorrhage within the brain, requiring surgical treatment.

A person found unconscious should be laid on his side and his tongue should be pulled forward: these maneuvers are to prevent the inhalation of vomit, which can be fatal. False teeth should be removed.

As well as performing these first aid measures and calling for medical help, the bystander who witnesses a head injury can be of considerable help if he has an accurate picture of the incident. The duration of loss of consciousness, the amount of blood lost, and the time of the incident can all be crucially important.

Since some head injuries follow fits or faints due to brain disease, particularly in the elderly, a description of the fall may be very important to the exact diagnosis of a particular case.

HEARING

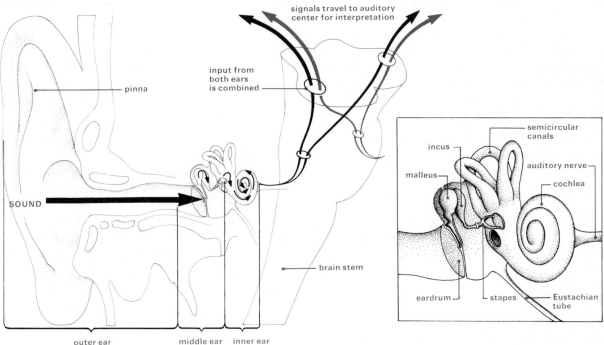

signals travel to auditory center for interpretation

input from both ears is combined

pinna

SOUND

brain stem

outer ear — middle ear — inner ear

semicircular canals

incus

malleus

auditory nerve

cochlea

eardrum — stapes — Eustachian tube

Hearing, the perception of sounds, involves mechanical and nervous mechanisms. Sound waves cause vibrations in the tense eardrum, which are transmitted and magnified by the chain of bones in the middle ear. The spiral cochlea contains delicate hair cells arranged along a membrane and they are stimulated by movements of the stapes to send signals up the auditory nerve to the brain.

hearing

Sound waves in the air are converted by the ear into impulses which travel in the auditory nerve to the brain, where they are perceived as sound. The outer ear canal *(external auditory meatus)* conducts the sound waves to the eardrum, on the inner side of which three small bones *(ossicles)* amplify the vibrations and conduct them to the organ of hearing *(cochlea)* in the inner ear. Nerve endings in the cochlea transmit the vibrations as impulses through the auditory nerve to the brain.

Hearing may be impaired by obstructions in the external ear canal such as wax, by disturbances in the middle ear (when the defect is called conductive deafness), or by disease of the inner ear (perceptive or sensorineural deafness).

Hearing is examined by a number of tests which vary from the simple one of whispering in the patient's ear while the other ear is covered up, through the use of the tuning fork, to the use of the audiometer (an instrument which produces sounds of selected frequency and pitch).

By the use of an audiometer the threshold of hearing can be measured at each desired frequency by reducing the intensity until it is inaudible. A recently introduced audiometric device can be used to measure brain waves to determine hearing deficit. This instrument, used while the patient is asleep, is particularly useful for very young children or mentally retarded patients.

Conduction through the air and through the bones of the skull can be measured. The degree of deafness is measured for both means of conduction in *decibels;* it represents the increased intensity of sound required for hearing in the deaf ear compared to a normal ear. Speech audiometry is very useful, as it measures the intensity of sound necessary for the understanding of recorded speech. It can be used to help in the diagnosis between conductive and perceptive deafness.

The range of sound technically capable of being heard by the normal ear is from about 16 to 20,000 Hertz (cycles per second). The discrimination of speech sounds primarily involves frequencies between about 500 and 5,000 Hertz; therefore the loss of the ability to hear higher frequencies does not present any problems in communication.

See also DEAFNESS.

heartburn

A burning sensation felt behind the breastbone, sometimes radiating into the neck or the back. Technical name: *pyrosis.*

It is a common complaint, produced by the presence of gastric secretions in the lower part of the esophagus. It is usually made worse by bending down or lying down.

Normally the contents of the stomach do not regurgitate into the esophagus, both because of the shape of the upper part of the stomach and because the muscles of the diaphragm act as a sphincter. But in some cases, particularly where the patient is obese or pregnant, the upper part of the stomach may herniate upward through the opening of the diaphragm and form a hiatus HERNIA. In such cases heartburn is liable to follow a heavy meal, especially if the patient goes to bed; it may be relieved by sitting up.

The use of antacids (and the avoidance of heavy meals) is usually enough to relieve the symptoms, but in some cases surgical treatment may prove necessary. Hiatus hernia is present in about 50% of people over the age of 60, but in many it is "silent" (produces no discomfort).

heart disease

Heart disease affects persons of all ages: the baby born with congenital structural abnormalities, the teenager and young adult with rheumatic heart disease, the older patient with ischemic heart disease due to coronary artery blockage or high blood pressure. Ischemic heart disease is now the most common cause of death in adult Britons.

Disorders of the heart affect its ability to pump blood around the body. Infants with mild congenital heart disease may show this by failing to grow as quickly as other children, or by becoming easily breathless or tired on exertion. More severe congenital heart disorders in which arterial and venous blood are mixed in "shunts" between the chambers of the heart, produce a blue coloration (CYANOSIS), of the lips and extremities. Infants with congenital heart disease may even be born with heart failure; they are pale, fretful infants unable to feed and constantly breathless. Their care is a surgical specialty in itself.

Congenital heart disease is not necessarily inherited. Maternal German measles infection during pregnancy may cause multiple heart abnormalities, and most children born with abnormal hearts have a normal genetic makeup. Their mothers can be reassured that future babies will be healthy.

Rheumatic heart disease in the older teenager and adult stems from throat infections with bacterium *Group A hemolytic streptococcus;* the body's reaction to this leads to rheumatic fever. Half the patients with rheumatic fever develop an acute heart illness which on subsiding leaves a slowly progressing disorder of the heart valves and the muscular walls of the heart. Heart failure from narrowing or incompetence of the valves may follow between 5 and 20 years after the attack of rheumatic fever.

Penicillin by mouth soon destroys the streptococcus, so that early and effective treatment of streptococcal sore throats prevents both rheumatic fever and the subsequent heart disease. Antibiotics have no effect on rheumatic fever itself. Its incidence has fallen steeply since the 1940s, so that rheumatic heart disease is becoming rare.

Even those with established rheumatic heart disease can take comfort from the great strides in heart surgery since the 1950s. Narrowed valves can often be reopened or replaced with artificial valves at minimal risk to the patient, and sophisticated drug therapy helps control possible complications.

The symptoms of ischemic heart disease arise from failure of the coronary arteries (which supply blood to the heart muscle itself) to deliver oxygen to the heart muscle. The result is ANGINA PECTORIS—a deep aching, crushing or vicelike pain in the chest, radiating perhaps to the arm, or the neck and jaw. It is fairly common in men in their 40s and older whose arteries have been seriously narrowed by ATHEROSCLEROSIS. The condition may progress to complete blockage of the arteries, and so to a myocardial infarction ("heart attack") with death or *infarction* of the muscle area supplied by the blocked vessel.

Factors leading to the present high death rate from ischemic heart disease have been investigated all over the world. The highest incidence is in Eastern Finland, where both blood fat levels and blood pressures are unusually high. Smoking, stress, lack of exercise and obesity are also considered to predispose to heart disease, but the evidence is less clear-cut. The Japanese male smokes as much and is subjected to as much stress as his American counterpart, but he has much lower blood cholesterol levels, and rarely has ischemic heart disease.

Recognition that heart disease results from over-indulgence, at least in the Western World, and can only be prevented by people themselves, has led already to fewer "heart" deaths. People are exercising more, smoking less, aware of their blood pressures and seeking treatment sooner. Once severe ischemic heart disease is present, drugs or surgery can help, but prevention is far more effective than cure.

Heart disease may be secondary to other disorders, notably high blood pressure (hypertension). Because the left ventricle has an additional load placed on it by the high pressure in the arterial system, it may in time fail. At first it becomes enlarged, but then incapable of supporting the increased strain; the symptoms of left heart failure supervene, with breathlessness from edema of the lungs as the pressure in the venous circulation of the lungs, and eventual extravasation (escape) of fluid.

Moreover, the heart of a patient with an important degree of hypertension is liable to show the changes of ischemic disease which render it less able to withstand the increased arterial pressure.

Chronic bronchitis and emphysema may lead to such impairment of gaseous interchange in the lungs that there is a lack of oxygen in the blood (hypoxia) and an excess of carbon dioxide. Under these conditions, the function of the kidneys is impaired with retention of salt and water and an increase of blood volume. The hypoxia also produces constriction of the small arteries of the lungs; this, together with the circulatory changes, produces an increase of pressure in the vessels of the lungs. The right ventricle then is subject to increased strain, and may also be affected by the general low level of circulating oxygen; if it fails, there is increasing edema of the dependent parts as well as congestion of the veins.

Cardiovascular disease that is secondary to disorder of the substance of the lung is referred to as COR PULMONALE.

heart failure

The function of the heart is to pump the blood around the body, and to pump blood through the lungs. The left side of the heart is concerned with the systemic circulation, the right side with the pulmonary circulation.

Failure may be predominantly right- or left-sided, and may be caused by congenital or acquired disease. The most common kind of failure is left-sided heart failure following coronary artery disease, high blood pressure, or disease and incompetency of the mitral or aortic valves of the heart. Chronic disease of the lungs and congenital heart disease lead more often to right-sided failure.

The first symptom of left-sided failure is usually shortness of breath on exertion, which may progress so that the patient finds it difficult to make any exertion. He may find it easier to breathe sitting up rather than lying down. He feels tired and may complain of a feeling of tightness in the chest. There may be attacks of severe breathlessness at night. When the right side of the heart fails, the return of venous blood is impaired and the tissues tend to become waterlogged—the site of the swelling (edema) being determined by gravity. If the patient is up, the ankles swell; if he is in bed the swelling is most obvious over the sacrum (base of the spine). The liver may be swollen and the stomach and intestines congested so that there is discomfort in the abdomen and a sense of nausea.

The most important single factor in the treatment of heart failure is rest, which must be absolute in very severe cases but in milder cases proportionate to the

A CROSS SECTION THROUGH THE HEART

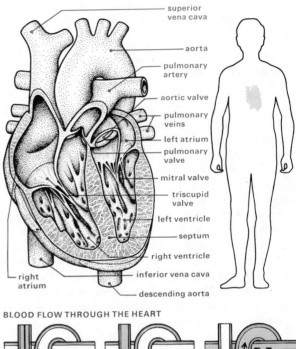

- superior vena cava
- aorta
- pulmonary artery
- aortic valve
- pulmonary veins
- left atrium
- pulmonary valve
- mitral valve
- triscupid valve
- left ventricle
- septum
- right ventricle
- inferior vena cava
- descending aorta
- right atrium

BLOOD FLOW THROUGH THE HEART

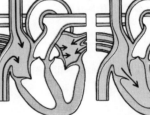
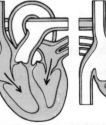
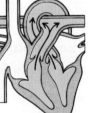

1 Relaxation: venous blood fills atria.

2 Contraction: phase 1– atria contract forcing blood into ventricles, which are still relaxed.

3 Contraction: phase 2– ventricles contract forcing blood into arteries.

The heart pumps out approximately 1⅓ gallons of blood every minute, and it can double this amount when necessary during exercise. As the ventricles relax the valves open (1), allowing blood to flow down from the atria. When the ventricles contract (3), the valves are slammed shut, and blood from the right ventricle enters the pulmonary artery to go to the lungs, while the left ventricle pumps blood into the aorta; from there it is transported around the body in the arterial system.

degree of failure. It is dangerous to let old people become completely bedridden, as they may develop bedsores or infection of the lungs. The administration of digitalis is a major component of therapy in treating patients with chronic heart failure. Its primary effect is to increase the force of contraction of the heart muscle and slow the pulse rate. The excessive use of salt in the diet must be avoided, and in most cases the use of a diuretic helps in the excretion of excess water from the body tissues. The administration of morphine is specific in treating acute congestive heart failure. Some other drugs (such as aminophylline and propranolol) are also useful.

heart murmur

Two basic sounds can be heard through a stethoscope with each beat of the healthy heart. The first is the sound of the closure of the valves between the atria and the ventricles (the mitral and tricuspid valves), which is duller and longer than the second sound, produced by the shutting of the pulmonary and aortic valves.

Heart murmurs are extra sounds between, or even replacing, the usual sounds. They do not necessarily denote heart disease. *Functional murmurs,* arising from the flow of the blood through the heart, are not related to structural defects. *Organic murmurs* arise from obstruction to the flow of blood through a narrowed valve, or from regurgitation through an incompletely closed valve. Murmurs in childhood may arise from defects in the walls between the chambers of the heart (see HOLE IN THE HEART).

See also AUSCULTATION, STETHOSCOPE.

heart rhythms

See ARRHYTHMIA, FIBRILLATION and VENTRICULAR FIBRILLATION.

heart surgery

The first operation on the heart to relieve symptoms caused by a diseased heart valve was attempted on an aortic valve in 1894. An attempt was made to correct the action of a diseased mitral valve in 1924, but it was not until the 1950s that surgeons began to operate successfully for stenosis (abnormal constriction or narrowing) of the mitral valve.

At first, operations were carried out on the beating heart. But the development of heart-lung machines, capable of sustaining the circulation, made it possible to operate on the heart while the blood was bypassed. Techniques of "open-heart" surgery then advanced rapidly.

It is now possible to replace heart valves with artificial valves, to carry out grafting operations on impaired coronary arteries, and to transplant complete hearts—although the problems associated with rejection of grafted heart muscle are far from solved. The correction of congenital heart malformations is in many cases possible, and there has been a remarkable improvement in mortality and morbidity figures.

Surgery involving opening the heart or the grafting of new vessels to its arterial tree requires use of heart-lung bypass technology. In babies with congenital heart malformations who would not survive their first year without surgery, techniques of surface cooling and total circulatory arrest (introduced in 1967, but not adopted generally until the 1970s), have enabled surgeons to operate on still hearts. This has allowed complete correction of complex abnormalities in a single operation, and led to dramatic improvements in results.

The less severely affected child, not requiring surgery in the first year, can wait until just before entering school before undergoing his or her one-stage surgical correction. The diagnosis and ongoing assessment of heart disorders not only have improved technically but are much more humane for the child, so that regular follow-up investigations are no longer a source of fear.

Surgery for valvular heart disease has shown a steady fall in operative deaths and very worthwhile improvement in deaths and illness from heart disease after operation. Surgeons are still searching for the perfect valve, but even the valves inserted in the early 1960s and now considered obsolete are associated with very good survival figures. The original artificial valves carried a higher risk of infection and clot formation on their surface than the newer ones. Nevertheless, patients undergoing replacement (particularly of a rheumatic mitral valve) are still given drugs to minimize the danger of blood clotting after the operation.

In the first decade of rheumatic valve replacement surgery, some deaths occurred from sudden heart attacks due to ischemic coronary artery disease. The recognition that both ischemic and rheumatic disease may occur together has led to routine x-ray examination of the coronary arteries before valve surgery. This has enabled surgeons to operate upon both valve and artery and has considerably reduced risk.

Replacement of diseased coronary arteries by vein grafts has become the most frequent heart operation in the United States. One 1976 report from Kansas City showed that 67.5% of heart operations performed in a community hospital unit were vein BYPASS procedures for coronary artery disease.

Coronary bypass surgery involves replacing a blocked artery with a length of vein taken from another part of the body. The precise area to be bypassed is measured by angiogram (x ray of the artery) before surgery. Even in the most severe cases success (particularly in relieving pain) can be startling, and the opportunity it gives to remove areas of the heart wall that has become thinned by previous infarction may prolong life by years.

heat exhaustion

A serious disorder of the circulation following exposure to dry hot climatic conditions, caused by severe water and salt loss.

Symptoms start with headache, confusion, fatigue and drowsiness. The patient is pale, sweating profusely, with a low blood pressure, but usually no significant rise in body temperature. Loss of appetite, disturbance of vision and vomiting follow. If no treatment is given, the patient collapses into coma.

As the symptoms of the first stage are usually quickly obvious, a fatal outcome is almost always avoided by prompt, early treatment. The patient should be put to bed in cool surroundings and given copious amounts of salt and water. The patient who is either vomiting or comatose has to be given saline solution by intravenous infusion.

heat rash

A common name for MILIARIA.

Heberden's nodes

These common swellings of the last joints of the fingers affect ten times as many women as men, and involve both bone and cartilage. They are inherited, with sisters of affected women having twice the incidence of such nodes than the general population. Similar swellings can occur in baseball players and bowlers. They are commonly associated with generalized osteoarthritis.

Heberden's nodes develop without symptoms, over several years, but can arise suddenly and be painful and tender. They form on the top of the knuckles on each side of the midline. Only when the nodes are very large is the movement of the joint affected. Treatment is rarely needed, except to relieve pain. Aspirin reduces pain and inflammation, as does the application of heat.

hemangioma

A malformation made up of small blood vessels, which are distended and thin walled. They are seen in the skin of newborn infants as "port wine" stains, which tend to be permanent, or "strawberry" birthmarks or nevi, which commonly disappear as the child grows older.

Hemangiomas also occur in the brain, bone, liver, lungs, spleen and other organs. Patients may have multiple hemangiomas of the lips and intestines, which can cause bleeding, but most hemangiomas cause cosmetic rather than medical anxiety.

See also NEVUS.

hematemesis

The vomiting of blood. Hematemesis may be simply caused by irritation of the stomach (for example, by aspirin or alcohol) or be a sign of more serious illness, such as ulcers, cancer, or varicose veins at the lower end

of the esophagus often associated with liver disease (see ESOPHAGEAL VARICES).

About one third of hematemeses originates from chronic duodenal ulcers; another quarter is from acute ulcers of the stomach or duodenum. Bleeding from the junction of the stomach with the esophagus, or from the esophagus itself, is usually bright red; that from the stomach or duodenum is similar to coffee grounds in appearance. Endoscopy and x-ray studies are used to determine the site of bleeding.

Treatment depends on the diagnosis and may include blood transfusion, medical treatment or surgery

hematoma

A swelling composed of blood which has escaped from an injured, diseased or abnormally fragile vessel into the tissues—in other words, a bruise. The vast majority of hematomas subside in their own time, usually about a week, without need for treatment, changing color from

HEMATOMA

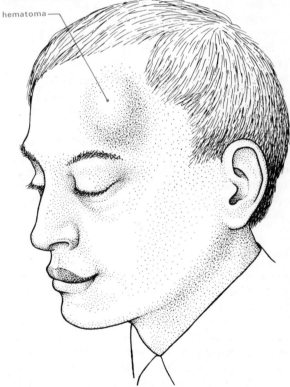

hematoma

Hematomas can become infected and this is particularly dangerous around the nose and eyes, because it can spread through the skull to cause meningitis. If somebody started to behave strangely or complain of severe headaches some days after an injury, he should be taken to the hospital for immediate medical evaluation.

purple to brown, to green-yellow, as the spilled hemoglobin is altered and taken back into the circulation.

Internal hematomas may follow severe injury, the effects depending on the site of the blow. After head injuries, hematomas may rarely occur over the surface of the brain or within its substance. A typical case involves a patient who recovers quickly from a knockout blow on the head, then some hours later develops headache, drowsiness, perhaps one-sided paralysis, then coma. This can occur in the absence of skull fracture, and even when the patient considers the blow to have been light and the resulting unconsciousness brief. Unless treated surgically, death can follow from pressure on the brain by the expanding hematoma. Injury-induced hematoma of the lung or kidney is much less serious, ·usually resolving without treatment in about three weeks.

hematuria

The passing of blood in the urine. Its cause, especially when painless, must always be fully investigated. It may vary from simple infection of the urethra, bladder, or kidneys, to more serious disease of any part of the urinary system. Rarely, it is a sign of inherited cysts of the kidneys or of disorders of bleeding or blood vessels. The presence of a stone in any part of the urinary system may cause hematuria—usually, but not always, in association with pain.

Investigation includes microscopic and bacteriological study of the urine, endoscopy and x rays. In children nephritis and pyelonephritis are common findings; in adult life cystitis, pyelonephritis and stones are common; and in the elderly, tumor and prostatic disease are frequent.

hemianopia

Blindness for half the visual field. It may be *bitemporal,* in which both eyes are blind for the outer half of their field of vision; *nasal,* in which the eye cannot see the inner half of the visual field; or *homonymous,* in which each eye is blind for the same half visual field. The type of hemianopia depends on the site of interruption of the optic nerve pathway from the eye to the brain.

Light, received in the retina of each eye, is translated by receptor cells into electrical impulses which pass along the optic nerves—there is one for each eye—to the surface of the brain. Behind the eyes, on the floor of the skull just above the pituitary gland, the optic nerves meet, then part again in a cross-shaped structure, the optic *chiasma.* Here the fibers from the inner half of each retina, carrying perception of the outer half of the field of vision, cross over to the opposite sides of the brain.

Those from the outer half of the retina remain on the same side.

Interruption of either nerve between the eyeball and the optic chiasma will make that eye blind. A pituitary tumor, exerting pressure on the optic chiasma, produces bitemporal hemianopia. Interruption behind the chiasma leads to homonymous hemianopia. Hemianopias may arise from strokes, injuries, congenital abnormalities or tumor, and all require neurological investigation. Recovery of sight is rare.

hemiparesis

Weakness of the muscles on one side of the body, usually the sign of damage or disease affecting that part of the brain which controls the nerves which direct movement (motor nerves). The site of the damage is often the *internal capsule,* where the motor fibers run closely packed together on their way from the cerebral cortex to the spinal cord. The underlying cause of hemiparesis is usually cerebrovascular disease.

hemiplegia

Paralysis of one side of the body, as the result of damage or disease of the part of the brain that controls the motor nervous system; the left side of the brain controls the right side of the body, and the right side the left.

Damage can arise from injury, either at birth or as the consequence of accidents or wounds, and in such cases recovery is at best partial. The most common cause of hemiplegia is cerebrovascular disease leading to clotting of the cerebral arteries or bleeding from the diseased arterial wall. The most common site affected is the *internal capsule,* the part of the brain where nerve fibers descending from the cortex to the spinal cord are packed together. There are cases where the internal carotid arteries or the basilar artery are partially blocked, and here the paralysis may be transitory.

After a STROKE the limbs are at first limp, but they soon become stiff and may suffer cramps. The reflexes are exaggerated. Improvement may follow the most complete paralysis, and it is important to keep the limbs as flexible as possible and to avoid contractures. Some improvement is possible up to two years after the initial paralysis.

Slowly increasing paralysis of one side of the body is seen in cases where the brain is the seat of a tumor. Proper treatment depends on the exact nature of the growth.

hemochromatosis

A chronic illness in which iron is deposited in body tissues, causing FIBROSIS and malformation of the organs concerned. The liver and pancreas are mainly involved, their iron concentrations being between 50 and 100 times the normal level, but the heart muscle, endocrine glands and skin are also affected. The patient gets bronzed as the iron deposits become more dense.

Hemochromatosis is caused by the body's inability to prevent the absorption of large amounts of iron in the diet, a process usually controlled by the cells of the intestinal wall. Treatment aims at removing the iron by repeated blood letting or by injections of a chelating agent. Supplementary B vitamins may help.

hemodialysis

See DIALYSIS.

hemoglobin

Hemoglobin, the pigment carried in the red blood cells, is a complex protein containing iron; its specific function is to transport oxygen in the blood. Hemoglobin has a high affinity for oxygen and will absorb a large amount of the gas when the blood passes through the lungs. On reaching the tissues, where the oxygen level is much lower, hemoglobin is able to release its absorbed oxygen equally freely. Normal blood contains around 14 to 15 grams of hemoglobin in each 100 milliliters, although slightly lower levels are normal in women and children. A fall in hemoglobin below the normal lower limit for the individual constitutes ANEMIA.

In most persons, the hemoglobin is of a fixed and unvarying chemical composition and is referred to as *adult hemoglobin* (or *Hemoglobin A*). In newborn infants, a different chemical type of hemoglobin is present—better adapted to the needs of the baby while still in the womb—and is known as *fetal hemoglobin* (or *Hemoglobin F*). All normal blood also contains a trace of a third type of naturally occurring hemoglobin *(Hemoglobin A2)*.

In certain individuals, however, a small but important chemical and structural abnormality is present in their hemoglobin molecule *(mutant* or *variant hemoglobin)*.

In sickle cell disease, for example, most of the hemoglobin is in the form of *Hemoglobin S*. This causes the red cells to become distorted (sickle shaped when seen under the microscope) when they give up their oxygen, and they are easily destroyed. The symptoms of sickle cell disease include anemia and episodes of severe pain and fever due to the sickled cells blocking the small blood vessels in the bones and other organs. (See SICKLE CELL ANEMIA.)

Other hemoglobinopathies include thalassemia (affecting mainly peoples of Greek, Italian, or North African origin) and diseases associated with rarer abnormal hemoglobin such as Hemoglobins C, D and E.

hemophilia

Hemophilia is perhaps the best known of the inherited bleeding disorders. Although comparatively rare, it is still much more common than other similar disorders. In addition, its historical association with the royal families of Europe in the 19th and 20th centuries has made it familiar to many.

Hemophilia affects two to three people per 100,000 of the population. It is caused by an inherited deficiency of a specific clotting factor in the blood *(antihemophilic globulin,* also referred to as *Factor VIII)*. The mode of inheritance of this clotting factor deficiency is unusual as it is a "sex-linked recessive" and carried on one of the chromosomes that determine sex (the X chromosome). Affected male hemophiliacs (XY) have only one X chromosome, the defective one; thus they have very low levels of Factor VIII and are susceptible to the fully developed disease. Female carriers of the disorder (XX) have one normal and one abnormal X chromosome and do not usually show any clinical abnormality, although they may have somewhat reduced levels of Factor VIII.

A male hemophiliac cannot pass the abnormality to his sons (to whom he passes only a Y chromosome). His daughters, however, must all receive his only X chromosome—a defective one—and must, therefore, become carriers of the disorder. A female carrier may transmit *either* one of her two X chromosomes (one of which is normal and one abnormal) to a son or a daughter. There is thus a 50/50 chance of a son being affected or a daughter being a carrier.

Clinically, the disorder may occur in either a mild or severe form; there may also be some variation within a family or a single generation. Patients bruise easily and large bruises characteristically occur in the deeper tissues rather than in the skin. Hemorrhage into joints may occur. Small injuries may result in excessive bleeding for long periods; the abnormality may first be revealed during surgery or the extraction of a tooth, although in many cases the problem will be discovered by means of preoperative tests to determine the clotting time. Severe cases may be identified for the first time in infancy when the baby starts to crawl (and is more prone to injuries). Diagnosis depends on the patient's medical history and on the results of specific blood tests which will reveal the absence of the clotting factor.

Treatment is now greatly improved but remains a complex problem which requires the supervision of a unit specializing in the management of bleeding disorders. Replacement of the missing factor with concentrated Factor VIII (obtained from human donor blood) is the mainstay of therapy. An effort is made to arrange home treatment so that the patient may lead a more normal life, especially with regard to education and job opportunities.

hemoptysis

The coughing or spitting up of blood. The amount of blood involved may vary from a small streak seen in a piece of phlegm coughed into a handkerchief, to a quantity that over even a limited period may be large enough to endanger life, to massive hemorrhage associated with tuberculosis or lung cancer.

Hemoptysis is a characteristic symptom in certain serious diseases, such as pulmonary tuberculosis or cancer of the lung; its occurrence should always be an indication to seek medical advice. It must be remembered, however, that hemoptysis can occur in much less serious conditions affecting the lungs, windpipe and larynx. It may also come from sites such as the nose and throat; the blood may trickle down the back of the throat and then appear to have been coughed up from within the chest (particularly in children).

hemorrhage

The technical term for bleeding.

In accidents and injuries the blood loss may occur from any tissue or part, but hemorrhage may also be caused by disease such as internal ulceration. Bleeding from the nose *(epistaxis)*, bleeding from the stomach and intestines with passage of blood in the stools *(melena)*, and bleeding from the kidney or urinary tract with passage of blood in the urine *(hematuria)* are all common examples of hemorrhage. In certain disorders—such as leukemia, hemophilia, or when there is a shortage of platelets in the blood *(thrombocytopenia)*—the blood-clotting mechanism is disturbed; in such cases bleeding may occur in any site, including bleeding into an internal organ (often with serious consequences).

*The effects of hemorrhage depend on the site involved and the amount of blood loss. The loss of two or three pints of blood over a short period will produce a rapid pulse, palpitations, dizziness, faintness and often collapse and shock. The patient becomes pale, cold and sweaty; the blood pressure drops, the pulse rate rises, and, if the blood loss continues, death may occur.

The first-aid treatment of hemorrhage is pressure: a cloth pad pressed firmly over the bleeding point will usually halt the flow of blood. Anyone who is bleeding or has bled heavily should be admitted to the hospital, where (if necessary) the lost blood can be replaced by transfusion; if the bleeding continues it can be treated surgically either by ligation of the bleeding vessels or by electrocoagulation.

The chronic loss of small amounts of blood every day, possibly into the bowel or stomach (in which case it may pass unnoticed by the patient), can only be replaced by the body itself if the patient's reserve stores of iron are not exhausted. Men may have reserves of iron which will allow the natural replacement of several pints of blood, but many women of childbearing age may have little or no iron reserves because of their regular blood loss in menstruation. When reserves are exhausted, an *iron-deficiency anemia* appears; this will worsen unless iron is supplied, the bleeding is stopped, or transfusion blood is supplied.

hemorrhoids

Hemorrhoids (or "piles") is a condition in which the veins around the anus or in the anal canal are abnormally dilated. There is much argument about the cause. In certain cases, as in pregnancy, obstruction to the flow of blood in the veins of the rectum is the cause. In others, factors such as constipation, straining at stool, lack of dietary fiber, obesity, heavy lifting, athletic exertions and a hereditary predisposition have all been implicated.

Whatever the cause, the first symptom of hemorrhoids is usually bleeding from the anus, particularly during a bowel movement. Bleeding may be severe or only a slight trace of blood may be seen on the toilet

HEMORRHOIDS

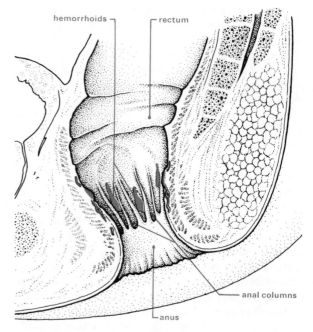

Hemorrhoids are abnormally swollen veins in the lining of the anal canal. They are extremely common but opinions vary as to their cause. Small hemorrhoids may go unnoticed while large ones protrude through the anus and require surgical removal.

paper. Irritation and itching commonly occur. The hemorrhoids, if large, may come to project through the anus *(prolapsed piles),* where they are constricted by its contraction and become very painful.

Hemmorrhoids is a very common condition. The treatment is as controversial as the cause. In severe cases the dilated veins may be removed surgically and the remaining parts of the veins tied off *(hemorrhoidectomy);* or, in less severe cases, the dilated veins may be injected with chemical solutions which will cause obliteration of the affected vessels by clot formation. The condition may also be treated by local freezing *(cryosurgery)* or the anus may be dilated and stretched under an anesthetic to relieve the pressure on the veins and allow them to return to normal.

All these methods of treatment are moderately successful, even though they are often uncomfortable for the patient. Surgical removal of the veins and cryosurgery usually require admission to the hospital, but injection and dilatation may be performed on an outpatient basis. Various suppositories and creams may provide temporary local relief but will not cure the condition, which may, however, regress by itself. Constipation and diarrhea both aggravate piles.

hepatitis

Inflammation of the liver; unless further qualified, the term is usually taken to refer to the virus infection of the liver referred to as "infectious hepatitis."

Virus hepatitis occurs in two basic forms, one of which is called *infectious hepatitis* (or *hepatitis A*) and the other *serum hepatitis* (or *hepatitis B*), which is also "infectious." It is fairly certain that these two conditions, although clinically similar, are caused by different viruses. There are other differences as well, including the length of the incubation period and the means by which the virus is spread. In hepatitis B, this appears to be mainly by the injection or transfusion of contaminated blood or blood products, or by accidental skin pricks or other injuries caused by contaminated needles or other sharp objects. Transmission also occurs from inadequately sterilized hypodermic needles, syringes, surgical and dental instruments, tattooing instruments and razors. It is common among narcotic addicts and others who use unsterile syringes for drug injections.

The virus which causes hepatitis A, by contrast, is present in the feces; although it can be spread by blood transfusion, the main route is from infective feces to the mouth via the hands or objects contaminated with feces.

The patient with hepatitis may notice little or nothing wrong, as many cases are very mild and occur without JAUNDICE (a yellowing of the skin). In more severe cases the patient will have fever, headache, nausea and vomiting, a severe loss of appetite and aching in the muscles. The jaundice, caused by an accumulation of yellow bile pigment in the blood, appears after a few days or, in some cases, a week or two from the onset of the symptoms. The liver may become enlarged and tender. With the appearance of jaundice, the symptoms may be temporarily increased but soon diminish. Convalescence may be prolonged and complicated by mental depression.

More acute or "fulminant" cases occasionally occur and may eventually lead to death from liver failure. A few patients will remain jaundiced, with an enlarged liver, for some months but in most cases they recover. Some patients may recover but ultimately develop CIRRHOSIS of the liver. This appears to be more common with hepatitis B, as is the condition of *chronic active hepatitis* in which liver damage continues over a long period and requires specific treatment.

An uncomplicated case requires only bed rest at home and care in the handling of infected excreta. Alcoholic beverages should be rigorously avoided. Injections of *gamma globulin* may temporarily protect against hepatitis A infections in those contemplating travel to high-risk areas.

Toxic hepatitis is caused by poisoning of the liver with various chemicals (such as industrial solvents), drugs, or (rarely) general anesthetics. Hepatitis is also occasionally caused as a result of a bacterial, protozoal, or other microbial infection. In such cases the treatment is directed toward the underlying cause.

hepatoma

A primary tumor of the liver, often malignant. It must be distinguished from the much more common secondary tumors of the liver which arise from the spread (metastasis) of cancer cells from other parts of the body, especially from organs within the abdominal cavity.

Primary tumors of the liver usually occur as a terminal complication of CIRRHOSIS of the liver. They are difficult to treat since the organ is already diseased and surgery rendered difficult. Tumors confined to one lobe of the liver, however, have been successfully removed and some anticancer ("cytotoxic") drugs may be useful. Liver transplantation has had a limited success.

Benign (nonmalignant) hepatomas that occur occasionally in women may be related to long-term use of oral contraceptives.

heredity

The transmission of physical and mental characteristics from parent to offspring. The study of heredity is known as genetics.

Each characteristic is carried by a gene—the basic unit of heredity. GENES, which are found in every cell, are fragments of a complex protein molecule known as DNA (see DNA/RNA). Genes are carried on chromosomes, rodlike structures found in the nuclei of cells. Each human cell (except ova and spermatozoa) normally has 46 chromosomes, arranged in 23 pairs. One pair consists of the sex chromosomes, which determine the sex of the individual; they may also carry genes for other characteristics. For example, the gene for hemophilia is carried on the female chromosome, and hemophilia is known as a sex-linked disease. The other 22 pairs are known as autosomes, which can be differentiated from each other under the microscope.

Genes are arranged along the chromosomes in linear order, each gene having its own position. Genes which occupy corresponding positions on a pair of chromosomes carry the trait for the same feature (for example, color of the eyes) and are known as *alleles* for that feature. If the alleles are identical—for example, both determine that the eyes should be brown—then the individual is *homozygous* for the color of the eyes, and will have brown eyes. If the alleles are not identical—for example, one gene dictates blue eyes and the other brown—the individual is *heterozygous* for that characteristic, and the color of his eyes will be that of the dominant gene (brown). Blue eyes are a recessive trait, and will only manifest themselves if the person is homozygous for blue eyes.

An individual gets half his genes from one parent and half from the other, because during the maturation of the sperm and the ovum the two halves of a pair of chromosomes separate from each other so that only one of a pair is transmitted to the offspring.

Not all features are determined in a clearcut manner by a single gene. Some have a familiar basis—for example, the tendency to develop diabetes mellitus or hypertension—but there is no clearly defined pattern of inheritance.

Genes may change spontaneously, a process known as *mutation*. If a mutation affects the gene in a sperm or ovum, the offspring that is produced may have characteristics carried by neither parent.

See GENETIC DISORDERS. GENETIC COUNSELING.

hernia

The protrusion of part of the abdominal contents through a defect in the wall of the abdominal cavity. The hernia, or rupture, may escape so that it lies under the skin or it may in the case of a diaphragmatic or *hiatus hernia* pass out of the abdominal cavity into the thorax.

The most common site for a hernia is the groin, at the point where the spermatic cord in a man or the round ligament of the uterus in a female passes out of the

abdomen to enter the scrotum or the labium majus. This hernia is much commoner in men than women, and it may pass down into the scrotum itself to form a considerable swelling.

The hernias that follow the path of the spermatic cord are called *indirect inguinal hernias;* those which make their way through a weakened abdominal wall behind the cord to form a bulge are called *direct inguinal hernias.*

Commoner in women than men is a type of hernia which appears in the upper part of the thigh just below the groin; it makes its way out of the abdomen on the inner side of the canal through which the major blood vessels pass into the leg. This is called a *femoral hernia.*

Less common than inguinal or femoral hernias, a third type emerges at the navel—an *umbilical hernia.* It may be found at birth, caused by failure of part of the bowel to return within the abdominal cavity from its developmental position within the umbilical cord; or, more rarely, it may be the result of infection of the umbilicus soon after birth. Hernias are found in adults near the umbilicus, but they pass through a weak area of the abdominal wall just above or below the umbilicus itself and are called *para-umbilical hernias.*

Incisional hernias are the result of weakening or incomplete healing of a surgical wound in the abdominal wall, usually in the midline below the umbilicus. They may follow sepsis of the wound, and are more

HERNIA

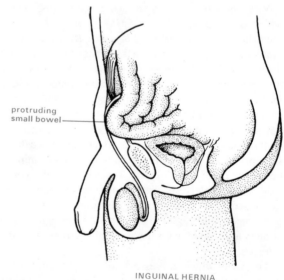

protruding
small bowel

INGUINAL HERNIA

A hernia is any protrusion of an internal organ through the wall of the cavity which normally contains it. Most hernias involve the gut, the most common form being the inguinal hernia which causes a lump in the groin. Inguinal hernias should always be repaired by surgery.

likely to develop in obese persons with weakened abdominal muscles.

The only common hernia in which the abdominal organs escape into another body cavity is the *diaphragmatic hernia*. Occasionally such a hernia forms in the newborn as a result of a developmental defect in the diaphragm, but in adults the protrusion of a part of the stomach through the esophageal opening of the diaphragm is often found, especially in those who are overweight. Usually, this *hiatus hernia* produces no symptoms, but it may mimic peptic ulcer and result in pain in the upper part of the abdomen or behind the lower part of the breastbone (sternum). It may also lead to an uncomfortable "heartburn," caused by the reflux of food or gastric juices into the esophagus, especially when the patient is lying down after a heavy meal.

Signs and symptoms of hernias in the abdominal wall include uncomfortable swelling and often pain on straining. It is often possible to return them with steady pressure into the abdominal cavity; if this cannot be achieved, it may mean that the hernia has become trapped. This is potentially dangerous, for once trapped the contents of the hernia tend to swell and if left unreduced may become gangrenous.

It follows that the best treatment for a hernia is a surgical operation designed to replace the herniated contents into the abdominal cavity and repair the defect in the abdominal wall. The attempt to hold a hernia in place with an old-fashioned truss is both insufficient and potentially dangerous.

Treatment for a hiatus hernia is much the same as that for peptic ulcer, except that it is reasonable to sleep with the head of the bed raised, and often possible to gain relief by sitting up when troubled at night. Only in severe cases is an operation justifiable.

herniated disk

Another name for SLIPPED DISK.

herpes simplex

A virus which causes crusted sores, commonly around the lips and mouth ("cold sores") and the genitalia. The infectious condition itself is also known as herpes simplex.

Many people suffer repeated attacks of cold sores whenever they have a fever, a rise in skin temperature, or are exposed to sunlight. Antibody studies have shown, however, that 90% of adults have immunity which prevents the spread of the virus in the body beyond the local site of attack. Herpes simplex is intermittently present in the mouths of healthy carriers and is spread by personal contact; genital herpes is spread by sexual contact with an infected person and is a venereal disease.

An attack begins with itching of the skin in the affected area, quickly followed by redness and swelling. Within a few hours fragile blisters (vesicles) appear and rupture to exude a sticky serum-like fluid which rapidly crusts. Unless secondary infection with bacteria occurs, the lesions heal without scarring within about a week.

The diagnosis can be confirmed by virus culture from the exudate, but this is both complicated and expensive. The appearance of the rash is so characteristic as to make the diagnosis obvious in most cases of herpes affecting the face. There are no serious complications of oral herpes simplex except for the unsightly appearance. When the conjunctiva is involved, however, there is a danger of corneal ulceration.

Antibiotics may be administered to prevent bacterial infection. Some success in reducing the spread of the virus has been achieved with the antiviral drug iododeoxyuridine (IDU), particularly in reducing the complications of conjunctivitis.

Genital herpes infections may cause a painful cervicitis (inflammation of the cervix) in women, with ulceration and a vaginal discharge. In men the genital infection is usually less severe. The results of recent research studies have suggested that women who develop herpes cervicitis may have an increased risk of developing cancer of the cervix in later years. The condition is now seen as a reason for regular screening by Pap smears, which can detect early cancerous changes at a stage when treatment is simple and curative.

herpes zoster (shingles)

A viral infection with the same virus (varicella-zoster virus) which causes chickenpox. It is characterized by a rash preceded by pain and skin irritation.

"Zoster" develops from reddened raised areas into blisters which join together and rapidly rupture and crust. The affected areas are always along the course of one or more of the spinal nerves beneath the skin. The rash typically progresses in a band around one side of the chest, trunk or abdomen. The virus may also attack the ophthalmic cranial nerve, causing a rash that stretches from the eyelid across the forehead into the hairline.

Once the rash appears, the diagnosis is obvious and needs no laboratory investigations. Zoster most commonly attacks adults between the ages of 40 and 70, often after contact with a child suffering from chickenpox. It can also arise in times of stress. One theory is that the virus may lie dormant in the body for many years before the infection erupts.

The main patient complaint following an attack of herpes zoster is pain (due to irritation of the affected nerve below the skin), which can be severe and particularly distressing in the elderly. The rash usually disappears within two weeks or so, although the pain can persist for many weeks thereafter. The patient may require frequent doses of analgesics (pain-killing drugs). As with most viral infections, there is no specific treatment for herpes zoster. Soothing dressings of calamine lotion help to dry up the crusts and antihistamines can relieve the itching. More commonly it is the pain that requires relief with strong analgesics. Recurrent attacks of shingles are very uncommon but do occur.

hiccup

Hiccup (or *hiccough*) is caused by an involuntary spasm of the muscle of the diaphragm, which separates the chest cavity from the abdomen.

This spasm sucks air down the windpipe, but the inhalation is checked by sudden closure of the glottis at the back of the throat. The result is the characteristic jerk and sound. As everyone has experienced, hiccups usually occur in repeated spasms and soon subside.

The reason for the spasm of the diaphragm is irritation of the nerve which supplies it (phrenic nerve), the irritation usually being provoked by eating or drinking too rapidly. Hiccup is of no medical significance unless it persists, in which case some disorder of the stomach, diaphragm, or chest may be responsible.

In a normal attack of hiccups the most effective cure is to hold the breath for as long as possible in order to suppress the response of the diaphragm. A number of treatments have been attempted for rare cases of very persistent hiccups, from dry sugar to numerous powerful drugs. A guaranteed treatment, which is undertaken if the hiccup is severe and persistent enough to merit it, is crushing of the phrenic nerve in a surgical operation.

high blood pressure

See BLOOD PRESSURE.

hip replacement

Osteoarthritis of the hip is a very common cause of severe disability, particularly in the elderly. It is caused by wear and tear, but any injury or disease that damages the joint surfaces tends to accelerate the development of osteoarthritis. Where the cartilage wears away there is considerable pain, made worse by walking, and increasing stiffness develops in the joint. For mild cases, medication and physical therapy may make life tolerable, but a worn-out joint cannot be regrown. However, there are two main types of operation for the surgical replacement of an artificial joint.

Cup arthroplasty is where the joint socket (acetabulum) on the pelvis is smoothed out and a highly polished metal cup (often of titanium) is placed over the head of the thighbone (femur) to serve as a replacement lining for the joint.

In *total replacement* the head of the femur is removed and replaced by a metal prosthesis permanently embedded in the shaft of the bone. The socket is deepened and a rigid plastic cup is cemented to the bone with an acrylic compound. This operation has fewer complications and is increasingly used. There is rapid convalescence, immediate pain relief and a dramatic improvement in movement range. Many thousands of hip replacements are now being performed each year in the United States and the duration of the new joint's activity is known to be at least a decade.

Hirschprung's disease (congenital megacolon)

A rare congenital disorder of the colon causing severe constipation in babies.

The baby, more commonly male than female, is born with a defect in the nerves that normally control the muscles of a specific area of the colon. That part of the colon therefore cannot relax to permit the passage of feces, so the intestine just above it becomes grossly distended.

The child may vomit and appear to have difficulty in passing feces soon after birth. For a while further trouble may be avoided since the baby is on a liquid diet, but as soon as he starts to eat solid food the bulkiness of the stools leads to more and more obstruction of the intestine; weeks may elapse without a bowel movement.

The disorder can be distinguished from a normal bout of persistent constipation because the latter responds to alterations in diet or to laxatives. Also, the abdomen of the baby with Hirschprung's disease becomes extremely distended and growth is retarded.

Once the diagnosis is confirmed by x ray and biopsy (examination of a sample of colon tissue), the affected area of the colon is removed surgically and the remaining ends rejoined. The outcome of the operation is usually excellent.

hirsutism

The growth of unwanted hair on the body. The term is nearly always used to describe excessive hair growth in women, which creates upsetting cosmetic problems.

Typical of hirsutism are growth of the pubic hair up towards the navel, growth of hair around the nipples and hair in the "shaving" areas of the face. There may be some demonstrable hormone change that can be related to the woman's change of life (menopause), but such hormone problems are found only in about one case in a hundred.

Some rare genetic, hormonal and metabolic diseases cause hirsutism.

In the majority of cases, however, there is no explanation and little point in detailed hormonal investigations. What is required is skilled treatment for the cosmetic problem of the unwanted hair.

Hormone therapy cannot be used, as a rule, because it would cause too many other undesirable effects. The basis of treatment, therefore, is disguise or removal of the excessive growth of hair.

Unwanted hair can be disguised by bleaching or dyeing it a light color; shaving of the hair seems to encourage renewed growth. Removal can be effected by depilatory creams, abrasives, shaving waxes, or electrolysis. The advice of a skilled beautician is recommended.

Electrolysis—removing the individual hairs by cautery of their roots—is expensive and may leave scars, but for small patches of strong growth it is ideal.

histocompatibility antigens

The antigens responsible for an individual's "tissue type," which is important in matching for transplantation.

An antigen is a protein substance that provokes an antibody response from the host through the mechanisms of the IMMUNE SYSTEM. All human cells have antigens on their surface, which can be recognized by the body as "self" but which, if transferred to another individual, would be recognized as "nonself." If too many of the antigens (termed "HL-A antigens" or "transplantation antigens") are dissimilar in the recipient of a donated organ his body is likely to reject it.

Unlike blood group matching—where A, B, AB and O groups can be accurately matched—histocompatibility antigens are far more complex.

When testing the suitability of a donor organ for transplantation, an attempt is usually made to match at least two of the four HL-A antigens. The chances of success are known to correspond to the closeness of the match. However, a minor degree of mismatching is not of crucial importance, since treatment with immunosuppressive drugs can damp down the rejection mechanisms.

histoplasmosis

A fungal disease of the lungs caused by the inhalation of contaminated dust.

The parasitic fungus responsible *(Histoplasma capsulatum)* is found particularly in the dust from chicken houses and other areas contaminated by bird dung.

Once inhaled it spreads through the lungs to cause a severe and persistent cough, shortness of breath, chest pain, fever and a feeling of being unwell.

Fortunately histoplasmosis is usually a mild and self-limiting disease. However, some severe and untreated cases can be extremely serious. The treatment of choice is the antibiotic agent *amphotericin B,* usually administered intravenously.

There is a world-wide distribution of histoplasmosis, but it is endemic in certain areas, e.g. the Mississippi Valley, while x-ray and immunological-tests have shown that as many as 80% of the population of the Eastern and Midwestern U.S. have been in contact with the disease at some time in their lives.

hives

A popular name for URTICARIA, a skin eruption in which raised red-and-white patches on the skin are seen on the trunk and face.

HLA (human leukocyte antigens)

See HISTOCOMPATIBILITY ANTIGENS.

Hodgkin's disease

A malignant disease of the LYMPHATIC SYSTEM.

The lymph glands affected by this cancer, situated in many parts of the body and with an important role in immunity, enlarge and can eventually cause pressure on adjacent structures; cancer cells may also invade the spleen and liver and cause them to enlarge. The disease is not painful in the early stages, although there is fever, weight loss, malaise (a general feeling of being unwell), anemia and sometimes itching of the skin.

Hodgkin's disease affects twice as many males as females and is seen most often between the ages of 15 and 35 and after the age of 50. Modern treatment is prolonging the lives of many patients with this potentially fatal condition.

The reason why the whole lymphatic system is affected by malignant growth is unknown. A viral cause for Hodgkin's disease has been suspected but not proved.

The glands in the neck, groin and armpit first draw attention to the condition, usually because they do not settle after an infection in the normal way. Chest x rays show lymph gland enlargement in the chest; superficial lymph glands feel tense and rubbery as they grow over a period of weeks and become entangled in neighboring glands.

The disease is treated by a combination of radiation and chemotherapy; newer combinations of anticancer drugs are being tried constantly with increasing success.

Survival is now often measured in years rather than months and there are many long-term survivors.

The prognosis is best if the disease is detected early, as with all types of malignant disease.

hole in the heart

A common name for a congenital heart defect in which two of the chambers of the heart are not properly separated.

The term "hole in the heart" is in fact an accurate description of the condition, which may occur on its own or with other congenital deformities in the cardiovascular system. The hole may be between the two upper chambers (an *atrial septal defect*) or the two lower chambers (*ventricular septal defect*). In either case the hole allows blood to pass directly from one side of the heart to the other, so that unoxygenated blood may pass around the circulation without going via the lungs. In consequence the sufferer may have a blue appearance due to the high proportion of unoxygenated blood in the circulation.

Congenital heart defects of this kind affect about one child in every 1000. The diagnosis is usually made by the pediatrician's detection of a heart murmur—although it must be stressed that not all heart murmurs are ominous. Occasionally a minor deformity may not be detected until much later in life, if at all.

If surgical treatment is planned, the diagnosis will be confirmed and the severity of the defect measured by cardiac catheterization: a thin flexible tube is passed via blood vessels into the chambers of the heart; the movement of blood within the heart is charted by the pressure in the chambers and by x-ray films. Many septal defects are isolated lesions, but in a minority of cases there are other anomalies in the heart, making surgical repair more difficult.

With advances in heart surgery such as the use of the heart-lung bypass to allow the surgeon time to work, most cases of hole in the heart can now be satisfactorily corrected. If the hole is large it is covered either by tissue taken from elsewhere in the patient's body or by an artificial fiber patch. Usually correction of the defect allows the child to return to normal or near normal life.

homeopathy

A system of medical treatment based on the principle that "like (in small doses) cures like."

Homeopathy was introduced in Europe at the beginning of the 19th century by a German physician, Samuel Hahnemann (1755–1843). Its basic tenet, quoted as "similia similibus curentur," was that the cure of a disease could be effected by very small amounts of a drug capable in larger doses of producing, in a healthy

HOLE IN THE HEART

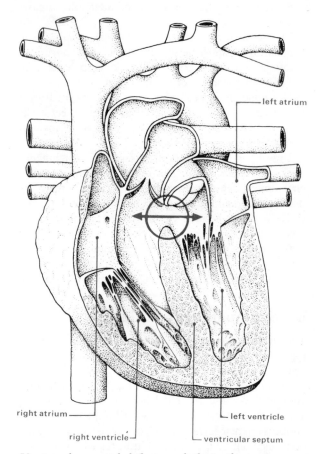

left atrium

right atrium

right ventricle

left ventricle

ventricular septum

Ventricular septal defect—a hole in the septum between the two ventricles of the heart—is the most common type of congenital heart disease. Fortunately, most of these holes are small and close of their own accord, but larger defects and holes associated with other heart malformations require cardiac surgery to correct them.

subject, symptoms similar to those of the disease to be treated.

Dr. Hahnemann's original treatise, "Organon" (1796), provoked considerable controversy. It claimed that this type of therapy had been recommended by Hippocrates; its principles were contrary to those of its day. Minute doses were recommended, the agent being distilled and diluted until its final concentration might be less than a millionth part of the solution. Only a single drug was to be given at a time and many current practices were forbidden.

"Homeopathy," wrote Hahnemann, "sheds not a drop of blood, administers no emetics, purgatives or laxatives ... and applies no mustard plasters."

At the time, leeches were being applied by orthodox

doctors in cases of pneumonia, massive doses of opium were given to children, mercury was used as a teething powder and many other bizarre remedies—now known to be highly toxic—were prescribed by the most respected physicians.

In that context, it can be seen how the revolutionary philosophy of homeopathy as a purification of attitudes managed to attract its devotees. Hospitals for homeopathic treatment were established in Leipzig, Vienna and London.

The remedies have not, however, stood the test of modern scientific pharmacology. Some, like iodine for goiter, are established orthodox treatments today. But many others are regarded by a majority of the medical profession as pointless.

homocystinuria

A rare inherited disorder of metabolism.

Like other inborn errors of metabolism it is due to the deficiency of an enzyme, and is characterized by the appearance of an unusual substance—in this case homocystine—in the urine.

Patients are often mentally retarded and die young from THROMBOEMBOLISM. A diet low in the amino acid methionine may help if it is instituted virtually from birth.

hookworm

A human parasite which is endemic in certain parts of the world.

The adult hookworm lives attached to the inside of the human intestine, from where it releases as many as 10,000 eggs daily which pass out with the feces. Eggs deposited on warm moist soil develop into larvae. Many weeks later the larvae may penetrate the skin of another person, enter a blood vessel and subsequently be carried to the lungs.

The larvae break out of the lung tissue and migrate up the bronchi to the throat, where they are swallowed and eventually reach the intestine to develop into adults. About six weeks elapse between skin penetration and the first appearance of eggs in the feces, but the adult can remain in the intestine for many years once it is established there.

Hookworm infection is endemic in many parts of the world where the climate is suitable; it is usually confined to rural areas where sanitation is relatively poor and many people go barefoot, but even though it is relatively rare in the U.K., there were still 1,687 cases identified in England and Wales in 1979.

Since the hookworm feeds on blood it causes a severe ANEMIA. At the site of entry there is severe itching, with local redness and swelling. A heavy larval infestation will frequently cause symptoms of bronchitis.

Any inexplicable case of anemia, especially in someone who has returned from abroad or who lives in an endemic area, should be investigated for hookworms. The diagnosis is made by examination of the stools for egg cells.

A single dose of specific antihookworm drugs will kill all the adults in the intestine; it is usual to check the feces two weeks later to be sure. Thereafter, iron therapy progressively corrects anemia.

Prevention of hookworm infestation requires the proper disposal of human excreta, at least by deep burial, and the avoidance of any possibility of skin penetration by the wearing of shoes in all contaminated areas.

hormones

Hormones are very complex chemical substances, secreted by the ductless (endocrine) glands to serve as blood-borne "messengers" which regulate cell function elsewhere in the body. They form a communications system in the body and can bring about extraordinary changes in cell activity.

The transformation of a tadpole into a frog due to the influence of growth hormone is no more remarkable than the cure brought about in a person suffering from myxedema when treated with thyroid hormone. Similarly, the immature child of prepubertal years is changed by the influence of growth and sex hormones to become a sexually mature adult.

In therapy hormones are used as replacement where the patient is deficient (e.g., insulin for the diabetic), as treatment to overcome disease (e.g., cortisone for arthritis or asthma) and as controlling agents to divert natural functions (e.g., sex hormones as contraceptives). Synthetic compounds resembling the natural products, but achieving enhanced or differing affects, have gradually become available since the 1930s and in recent years an explosive increase in the knowledge of their benefits—and their disadvantages—in medicine has been achieved.

The nervous and endocrine systems of the body actually function as a single interrelated system. The central nervous system, particularly the hypothalamus, plays a crucial role in controlling hormone secretion; conversely, hormones markedly alter neural function. No hormone is secreted at a constant rate, and most hormones are either degraded by the liver or excreted by the kidneys. The investigation of endocrine disease therefore depends on assays of excretion rates (e.g., 24-hour urine samples) and circulating serum levels; but since many of these chemical messengers are bound to protein in the blood plasma, the diagnostic tests are particularly complicated and expensive.

Hormones exert their effects by altering the rates at which specific cellular processes proceed. For example, insulin promotes glucose (sugar) uptake by cells that require energy, follicle-stimulating hormone provokes the ovary into producing an ovum, and testosterone enhances the production of spermatozoa in the testes. They do this by combining with enzymes, or by enhancing enzyme production in the cell through a chemical effect on the RNA (ribonucleic acid) of the cell. The result in the body depends on the target organ cell of the hormone and its function: the table below illustrates some of the major hormones and their effects.

Disease in the endocrine system is revealed by a physiological defect in the expected effects of the target organ cells. For example, growth fails to occur, ovulation is inadequate, or myxedema occurs because of inadequate function of the thyroid gland. Less frequently the disorder may be that of excessive hormonal secretion, for example, virilization in a female patient from a pituitary tumor, or thyrotoxicosis from a thyroid tumor.

The treatment of hormonal disorder is undertaken by an endocrinologist for it involves the achievement of balance in the supplements administered; diabetic control by the appropriate daily dosage of insulin is the clearest example of this.

Considerable improvements in the effectiveness of hormone treatment and replacement therapy have been achieved in recent years; but the accurate elucidation of each hormone's multiple influences on human physiology is a continued challenge.

Horner's syndrome

Dilatation of the pupil and drooping of the upper eyelid as a result of facial nerve damage.

Other features of the syndrome are a red face (due to vasodilatation) and often the absence of normal sweating. The eyeball seems more prominent than usual, probably because the patient is trying to overcome the effect of the droopy eyelid by contracting the forehead muscles.

Horner's syndrome almost always occurs only on one side of the face. The nerve damage causing it may arise for many reasons—including trauma, brain tumor, thrombosis, or neurological disease. Treatment is directed at the underlying disorder.

housemaid's knee

Inflammation and swelling of the bursa in front of the kneecap (a form of BURSITIS), caused by prolonged kneeling on a hard surface.

Hurler's syndrome (gargoylism)

A rare disease due to an error of metabolism which can be inherited.

The physical manifestations include a grotesque appearance due to a disproportionately large head and coarse facial expression, with a flat nose and thick lips. Bone changes lead to shortness of stature, chest deformities, marked limitation in the extensibility of

Gland	Hormone	Effect
anterior pituitary	growth hormone	increase in body size
	thyroid-stimulating hormone	enhanced metabolism
	adrenocorticotropic hormone (ACTH)	response to physical stress
	gonadotropic hormones	growth of gonads (sex glands)
	prolactin	breast development
posterior pituitary	oxytocin	uterine contraction
	antidiuretic hormone	excretion control
thyroid	thyroxine	metabolic rate increase
adrenal cortex	cortisone	defense against disease
	aldosterone	excretion rate control
ovary	estrogen	maintenance of
	progesterone	sexually reproductive
testes	testosterone	function
parathyroids	parathormone	calcium uptake by bone
pancreas	insulin	glucose uptake by cell

limbs and "spade-like" hands.

Other features include an enlarged tongue, liver and spleen, skin changes, mental deficiency, blindness, deafness, disease of the heart valves, congestive heart failure and angina pectoris.

No active treatment exists at present for Hurler's syndrome.

hyaline membrane disease

A disease of the newborn, also known as the *respiratory distress syndrome,* which usually develops within the first four hours after birth. It is characterized by difficulty in breathing, a bluish appearance of the skin caused by imperfect oxygenation of the blood (cyanosis), and easy collapsibility of the air sacs (alveoli) of the lungs. It is due to a lack of *pulmonary surfactant,* a substance which normally serves to reduce "stickiness" within the air sacs.

When the disease persists for more than a few hours a thick *hyaline* (glassy or translucent) membrane is formed lining the air sacs and their ducts. Approximately 25,000 babies die each year in the United States from this disease, which has a mortality rate of from 30 to 50%.

Essentially, hyaline membrane disease is the result of premature birth. The lungs of a fetus do not contain enough surfactant for normal respiration until the last quarter of pregnancy. Prevention of the disease therefore depends on the prevention of premature births. When there are medical reasons (such as diabetes) for inducing labor prematurely, it is vital that this should be delayed until the fetal lungs contain surfactant. It is now possible to test the amniotic fluid (which surrounds the developing fetus) to determine whether or not the fetus is mature enough to avoid hyaline membrane disease; use of this test is reducing the incidence of the condition. When cases do occur, the infant may be treated by a special form of artificial respiration (intermittent positive pressure respiration) which helps support the lungs for the critical period until surfactant is formed normally. Even so, the condition remains the most important threat to the life of very small babies.

HORMONES

ENDOCRINE GLANDS WHICH PRODUCE THE BODY'S HORMONES

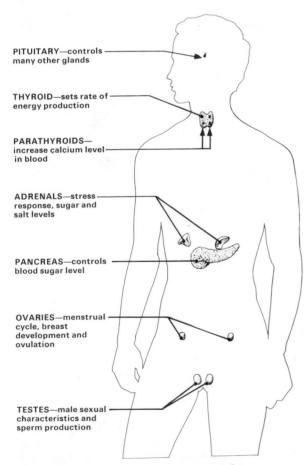

PITUITARY—controls many other glands

THYROID—sets rate of energy production

PARATHYROIDS—increase calcium level in blood

ADRENALS—stress response, sugar and salt levels

PANCREAS—controls blood sugar level

OVARIES—menstrual cycle, breast development and ovulation

TESTES—male sexual characteristics and sperm production

Hormones are chemical messenger substances secreted directly into the bloodstream by the endocrine glands shown above. They travel in the blood to different "target organs" where they control the rate of cell activity.

hydatidiform mole

An abnormality occurring about once in every 2,000 pregnancies, in which the ovum dies but does not miscarry. The placenta continues to grow, forming a swelling—or "mole"—which mimics a normal pregnancy. The condition is more common in Asian than in European women and the risk increases with age.

The first sign of hydatidiform mole is a rapid increase in the size of the womb shortly after conception—often much larger than it would normally grow at that stage of gestation. Other suspicious signs include vaginal bleeding and lack of fetal movement.

On investigation, the doctor will be unable to detect a fetal heartbeat; x-ray examination will fail to show bone formation after the 12th week, when it would normally be seen. Further tests, such as ultrasonic scanning, will confirm the diagnosis.

The mole will then be removed and the gynecologist will conduct further examinations at regular intervals to make sure that all fragments have been removed. The serious risk with a "molar pregnancy" is that the growth may be or become malignant: this variant, the CHORIONEPITHELIOMA, occurs about one in every 40 cases of hydatidiform mole.

If evacuation of the cyst reveals abnormal cells, or

if there is any suggestion of recurrence of the growth, then anticancer drugs such as methotrexate and dactinomycin may be administered. With early treatment the chances of cure of chorionepithelioma are close to 100%.

In view of the high risk of complications, many gynecologists advise more radical treatment of molar pregnancies, and in women over the age of 30 an immediate hysterectomy (surgical removal of the uterus) may be performed. However, in a younger woman such treatment may be unacceptable, since once recovery is complete—and followup for at least a year will be necessary—there is no reason why another, normal pregnancy should not follow.

hydatidosis

Formation of cysts *(hydatids)* in the internal organs due to infestation with the larval stages of the dog tapeworm *(Echinococcus granulosus)*. The condition occurs most often in agricultural communities where dogs mix closely with human families and where the dogs eat raw entrails.

The parasite is transmitted to man by the ingestion of food and water contaminated with the feces of infected animals, by hand-to-mouth transfer of dog feces and through objects soiled with feces. Eggs may survive for several years in farmland, gardens and households.

Ingested eggs hatch in the intestine and the larvae migrate to various organs to produce cysts, most often in the liver and lungs. Less commonly they occur in the kidney, heart, bone, central nervous system and thyroid gland. Humans do not harbor the adult tapeworm, which is about a quarter of an inch long and lives in the intestines of infected dogs.

The symptoms of hydatidosis are variable and depend on the location of the slowly growing cysts. Cysts in the liver may reach a considerable size without causing symptoms. Sometimes there is a "dragging pain" in the abdomen, and pressure on the bile duct may cause jaundice.

When the cyst is in the lungs there may again be no evidence of the disease, except perhaps for a cough and sometimes bloodstained sputum. Long-standing cysts may become calcified. In vital organs the cysts can cause severe symptoms, and may need to be removed surgically.

Effective preventive measures are education of schoolchildren and the public about the hazard and rigid control of the slaughter of herbivorous animals, so that dogs have no access to uncooked entrails.

hydrocele

This is an accumulation of clear fluid within the tunica vaginalis (covering) of the testis. The cause is most often unknown, though occasionally it can be secondary to some disease of the testis, or to trauma.

Generally, a hydrocele is dealt with by a simple operation to remove the sac, though sometimes in patients who would be a poor risk under anaesthesia, or in the elderly, the hydrocele is simply 'tapped' with a wide-bore needle and the fluid aspirated. Since the fluid has a strong tendency to recur, this procedure generally has to be repeated every few months.

hydrocephalus

An abnormal collection of cerebrospinal fluid around the brain or in the brain cavities, leading to enlargement of the skull. The condition is known colloquially as "water on the brain." The clear, watery cerebrospinal fluid is normally formed within a cavity (ventricle) in the brain. It passes along a channel (the aqueduct) through the brain substance to reach its surface, where the fluid is

HYDROCEPHALUS

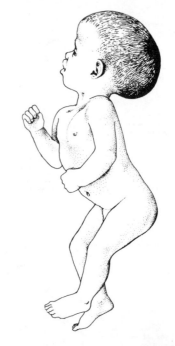

hydrocephalus in a nine-month-old baby

Hydrocephalus, or "water on the brain," is caused by obstruction to the circulation of cerebrospinal fluid in the brain. In babies, the resulting increase in pressure leads to expansion of the head. Hydrocephalus is often present at birth (usually combined with spina bifida), but may occur in an older infant due to a brain tumor (above).

absorbed into the bloodstream.

Hydrocephalus may be congenital due to a defect such as blocking of the aqueduct or acquired from inflammation of the membranes covering the brain. It is often associated with SPINA BIFIDA.

When hydrocephalus afflicts an infant the skull is still distensible and rapid enlargement of the head will take place in the first few weeks of life. The forehead bulges outward and the eyes turn down. If the circulation of cerebrospinal fluid is impaired in an adult the skull does not distend: instead the fluid pressure rises, causing damage to the brain and especially the eyes.

The condition can sometimes be relieved by a drainage operation. For instance, one end of a tube may be placed into a brain space and the other end into the jugular vein (in the neck). A device known as a Spitz-Holter valve (invented by an engineer whose child suffered from hydrocephalus) is included to permit the flow of cerebrospinal fluid out of the brain but prevent the flow of blood into it.

Without drainage, hydrocephalus causes progressive brain damage and may be fatal.

hydrops

The abnormal accumulation of clear fluid in body tissues or cavities.

See EDEMA.

hyperemesis gravidarum

A potentially serious form of MORNING SICKNESS in which excessive vomiting during pregnancy may lead to weight loss and complications such as ACIDOSIS.

Affected patients are typically (but not necessarily) of a highly sensitive or nervous disposition.

In most cases treatment involves only the administration of antiemetic drugs (to control vomiting), rest in bed, mild sedation and special dietary management.

hyperglycemia

The level of sugar in the blood, mainly in the form of glucose, is carefully controlled by a variety of mechanisms, including the action of insulin and other hormones. In DIABETES MELLITUS this control is defective and the blood sugar level rises beyond normal limits, a condition described as *hyperglycemia*.

Above a certain level of blood sugar, the sugar overflows into the urine, producing the condition of GLYCOSURIA; this can be detected with a common urine test. Measurement of the blood sugar level provides a confirmatory test for diabetes and is also valuable in adjusting treatment.

Compare HYPOGLYCEMIA.

hyperparathyroidism

Overactivity of the parathyroid glands, in which parathyroid hormone is produced in amounts greater than normal.

The hormone controls the level of calcium in the blood, and overactivity leads to a rise in blood calcium. If this is marked, the patient complains of lassitude, depression, loss of appetite, weakness, nausea, vomiting, constipation and occasionally excessive thirst. Calcium is removed from the bones; pain and tenderness may follow, and the bones (being fragile) are more prone to fracture. This may lead to diagnosis of the condition, for the x-ray appearances of the bones alter.

Increased excretion of calcium in the urine often leads to the formation of kidney stones; about 5% of patients with kidney stones are likely to show features of hyperparathyroidism.

There are four parathyroid glands, one pair situated on each side of the thyroid gland (see the illustration at THYROID) and are normally about the size of a pea. Overactivity may be due to the development of a tumor of one of the glands (primary hyperparathyroidism) or may be the result of a chronically low level of calcium in the blood—such as occurs in kidney disease or deficient absorption of calcium from the intestine. Treatment of primary hyperparathyroidism is surgical removal of the tumor; treatment of secondary hyperparathyroidism requires correction of the underlying condition. It is possible to raise the blood calcium level by reducing the phosphate level, so that in chronic kidney failure a diet that is low in protein and phosphorus, with additional aluminum hydroxide and vitamin D, may be recommended.

hypertension

The technical name for high blood pressure.

See BLOOD PRESSURE.

hyperthyroidism

Excessive activity of the thyroid gland leading to oversecretion of the thyroid hormone. This produces a characteristic clinical picture first described by Dr. Parry in 1786, and later described independently by Graves and Basedow (who gave their names to the disease). It is also known as *thyrotoxicosis, exophthalmic goiter* or *toxic goiter*.

About five times as many women as men are affected; it can occur at any age, with a marked peak between the ages of 20 and 40. The onset of the disease is insidious. It may first be recognized when the condition is made worse by emotional stress, hot weather or an infection. The patient is hot, sweats excessively, and dislikes hot weather and heavy clothes. Sometimes he or she becomes very thirsty, loses weight, suffers from palpitations and breathlessness, becomes anxious and shows a fine tremor of the hands. Emotional instability is common, as is muscular weakness, and the patient may be subject to diarrhea or vomiting. The menstrual periods in female patients may be scanty or absent, and in many cases there is an obvious GOITER. The upper eyelids become drawn up to reveal more of the eye than normal, sometimes being so far retracted that the white of the eye is seen above the cornea. The eyeball itself may move forward in the orbit (its bony casing) and become unduly protuberant; this condition is called *exophthalmos*. Infiltration of the tissues behind the eyeball by white blood cells, as well as edema of the connective tissue, may produce partial paralysis of the muscles that move the eye. It may prove necessary to relieve the condition by a surgical operation to decompress the orbit.

Hyperthyroidism may be treated in three basic ways, all of which are designed to reduce the amount of thyroid hormone circulating in the bloodstream. Part of the thyroid gland may be removed surgically *(partial thyroidectomy)*; a proportion of the cells making up the thyroid gland may be destroyed by radioactive iodine (I^{131}) introduced into the body; or specific drugs can be administered which interfere with the synthesis of thyroid hormone. Antithyroid drugs are commonly tried first; but if they fail and the patient's condition relapses (as it does in about 50% of cases), it may be necessary to remove part of the thyroid surgically, particularly in people under the age of 40. In older patients, the physician may administer carefully calculated doses of radioactive iodine, which are taken up by the thyroid cells and produce partial destruction of the gland over a period of approximately one to three months.

See also HYPOTHYROIDISM.

hypnosis

A passive state of mind induced artificially without the use of drugs during which the subject shows increased obedience to suggestions or even commands.

The hypnotic state is brought about in susceptible subjects by placing them in a quiet environment at rest; they are asked to concentrate on a monotonous stimulus while listening to the voice of the hypnotist, who delivers his "patter" quietly and insistently. It is possible to hypnotize a subject by making him stare at a pin stuck into the wall while a tape recording of the hypnotist's voice is played through a loudspeaker.

About 15% of people cannot be hypnotized, and about 1 in 20 is exceptionally prone to hypnotic suggestion. It is not possible to make a person under hypnosis carry out any order or suggestion that conflicts with his or her conscious or unconscious wishes (although it may be possible to trick him or her into thinking that some harmful act is harmless).

Orthodox medicine makes relatively little use of hypnosis because the depth of hypnosis induced is variable and it takes a fairly long time to hypnotize the patient. Although hypnotic suggestion has produced suppression of pain sufficient to allow the extraction of teeth or the performance of certain surgical operations, it is not a reliable method of anesthesia.

Hypnosis is sometimes used to explore repressed memories in mentally disturbed patients, and it has been used for centuries in the treatment of warts. A carefully controlled series of cases concerned with the treatment of warts was recently published, in which it was suggested to patients that the warts on one side of the body would disappear while those on the other side would remain. Out of 14 patients, 9 showed disappearance of warts on one side of the body. It was thought that the phenomenon was related to the depth of hypnosis induced. In another recent scientific paper, a number of warts on a patient's hands were induced to disappear after treatment by hypnosis for about ten months. The reason for these results is not known.

hypocalcemia

An abnormal decrease in the concentration of free calcium ions in the blood circulation.

Although 98% of the calcium in the body is in the skeleton, the small proportion in the blood is essential to health. Results of hypocalcemia include increased neuromuscular irritability, which may lead to TETANY—cramplike involuntary muscle spasms which often spread to all but the eye muscles. Hypocalcemia may be a sign of HYPOPARATHYROIDISM (a deficiency of the parathyroid hormone), or may arise from kidney failure, OSTEOMALACIA, acute nutritional deficiency, MALABSORPTION and PANCREATITIS—although tetany does not appear in all these diseases. The aim of the treatment is twofold: first, an attempt is made to restore calcium to normal levels by supplementary dietary calcium and vitamin D, which relieves the symptoms of the neuromuscular irritability; second, correction of the underlying cause of the hypocalcemia is sought.

hypochondria

A neurotic preoccupation by a person with his or her general state of health or the condition and function of a particular organ.

Hypochondria is often linked with obsession and depression, and may be a symptom of a specific mental illness. Complaints usually involve the abdominal organs; the patient insists that there is a malady, against all reassurance by the physician. Often he exaggerates the intensity of normal physical sensations, or describes bizarre discomforts. He cannot admit that his troubles are not due to physical lesions, and rarely agrees to seek psychiatric help. He is always liable to damage himself by excessive medication, and in some severe cases there is a risk of suicide.

Hypochondria is a personality disorder that may become manifest from adolescence onward. However, its origins may lie in childhood experiences, particularly where illness has been used successfully as "emotional blackmail" or to ensure attention.

hypoglycemia

The level of sugar in the blood, mainly in the form of glucose, is carefully controlled by a number of mechanisms including the action of insulin. In DIABETES MELLITUS lack of insulin causes a rise in the blood sugar level and a number of other disturbances of metabolism appear; treatment by the injection of daily doses of insulin is necessary in many cases.

A potential danger of this treatment, however, lies in the fact that too large a dose of insulin will produce an excessive fall in the blood sugar level, giving rise to a condition known as hypoglycemia. The patient becomes weak, shaky and confused and may, without warning, lapse into coma. Hypoglycemia is very common after excessive physical activity in an insulin-dependent diabetic, when too much sugar has been burnt up.

Reversal of these symptoms may be obtained very rapidly by giving sugar by mouth in the early stages, but hypoglycemic *coma* constitutes a serious emergency requiring immediate admission to the hospital in most cases.

Compare HYPERGLYCEMIA.

hypophysectomy

Surgical removal of the pituitary gland. An alternative name for the pituitary gland is the *hypophysis* (or *hypophysis cerebri*); thus the basis for the term *hypophysectomy* (surgical removal of the hypophysis).

The pituitary gland, the size of a pea, is situated beneath the brain behind the eyes. It acts as an intermediary between the brain and the major endocrine glands, controlling the secretion of sex hormones, thyroid hormone, and the adrenal corticosteroids. The pituitary also secretes growth hormone and hormones controlling lactation.

The pituitary may be removed surgically (hypophysectomy) if a tumor forms in the gland—though treat-ment by radiation therapy is often preferred. It is also removed in some cases of advanced breast cancer when the tumor has been shown to be hormone-dependent. Whatever the cause, after removal of the pituitary the normal hormone balance of the body needs to be maintained with synthetic hormones.

hypospadias

A congenital malformation in which the urinary opening is on the underside of the penis.

The urethra fails to extend the full length of the penis and therefore opens somewhere on the under-surface. The farther back the opening, the more serious the condition. Hypospadias occurs with an incidence of about one in every 200 male births.

In mild cases the urethral opening is just under the tip of the penis. No surgical treatment is necessary unless the presence of a fibrous band causes a severe downward curvature of the penis.

The main complication in such cases is the patient's difficulty in directing the urinary stream. He will be capable of normal sexual intercourse, although conception may be difficult since the semen is directed downwards instead of upwards.

When the urethral opening is further back, surgery is only indicated at birth if there is any obstruction to the passage of urine. Otherwise operation is delayed until about two years of age or later. The first procedure is to

HYPOSPADIAS

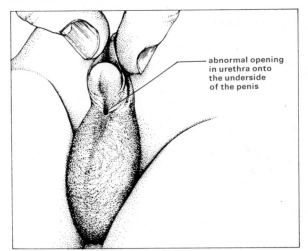

abnormal opening in urethra onto the underside of the penis

During embryonic life the underside of the penis normally closes up like a zipper; hypospadias occurs where this closure is incomplete. Minor degrees of hypospadias do not require treatment, but an opening well down the shaft of the penis interferes with urinary and sexual functions and needs surgical correction.

straighten the shaft of the penis; later, plastic reconstruction of the urethra may be necessary.

Surgical complications include narrowing of the urethra and the development of abnormal routes for the passage of urine, which require further operation.

hypotension

The technical name for low blood pressure.

See BLOOD PRESSURE.

hypothalamus

A very important part of the brain which lies just above the pituitary gland. It is concerned with the vital functions and its integrity is essential for life, for it plays a major part in temperature regulation, sexual function, body weight, fluid balance and blood pressure.

Through the pituitary gland, which produces a wide range of hormones, it influences the activity of the thyroid gland, pancreas, parathyroids, adrenals and the sex glands. The pituitary also produces the growth hormone by which growth in childhood and adolescence is regulated.

It is thought that levels of hormones circulating in the blood are "sensed" by the hypothalamus, which keeps the balance as required through its controlling action on the pituitary. The hypothalamus has complex central connections in the nervous system, and is part of the *limbic system* that controls the physiologic expressions of emotion.

HYPOTHALAMUS

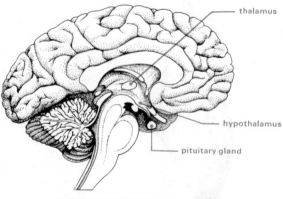

thalamus

hypothalamus

pituitary gland

MIDLINE SECTION THROUGH THE BRAIN

The hypothalamus is a structure deep in the brain which regulates many bodily functions. It is linked to the higher centers via the thalamus and exerts its influence mainly by controlling the output of hormones from the pituitary gland. Tumors in the hypothalamus can disturb appetite, emotion, sexual behavior, blood pressure and sleep.

Disease rarely affects the hypothalamus, but it may be involved in tumors growing nearby or in injuries (sometimes surgical). In such cases there may be excessive thirst or water loss (DIABETES INSIPIDUS), excessive food intake, disorders of growth, loss of temperature control and somnolence.

hypothermia

Hypothermia means abnormally low body temperature. The normal body temperature is maintained at 98.6°F (37°C) and fluctuations around this figure are usually small. Falls in body temperature result from deficient heat production by the body or (more commonly) from excessive loss of body heat.

Patients who are in coma or suffering from extreme exhaustion, and in whom physical movement ceases, are in danger of hypothermia if the condition is prolonged and they are not kept warm. Hypothermia from heat loss occurs classically on immersion in cold water. Without protective clothing, a man in water at around 0°C (32°F) may lose consciousness in as little as five minutes and may be dead in 30 minutes; the actual time will vary with body build, movement and other factors. This has been well recognized in shipwreck victims in cold seas but is less well recognized among amateur sailors. Without protective clothing (a "wet suit," for example), the rescue of a crewman from even normal temperate seas is a matter of urgency. Hypothermia is also a threat to hikers, climbers and others who spend long periods outdoors during cold, damp weather.

Still another situation in which dangerous hypothermia occurs is *accidental hypothermia* in the elderly. This affects elderly persons in cold weather who live alone in underheated houses. Symptoms begin when body temperature falls to 95°F (35°C). The patient is listless and confused and makes little or no effort to keep warm. At 86°F (30°C), serious problems appear, with lowered respiration, pulse and blood pressure.

Treatment of hypothermia is by removing the patient to a warmer environment. If this is not possible, body heat must be conserved by wrapping the patient in insulating materials (such as a "survival bag" for climbers).

In serious cases restoration of body heat must be gradual, under medical supervision; sudden reheating, as in a hot bath, may be fatal.

hypothyroidism

Underactivity of the thyroid gland leading to partial or complete deficiency of thyroid hormone in the circulating blood.

The condition may be the result of some congenital defect of the thyroid gland or be associated with a metabolic disorder. It may be divided into *juvenile* and *adult* types. Adult cases commonly occur in people between the ages of 40 and 60, and in the approximate proportion of six women to one man. Hypothyroidism may be accompanied by a GOITER, and it is common in those parts of the world where simple goiter is endemic because of lack of iodine in the diet. If the condition is not accompanied by a goiter, it is now thought to be due to an AUTOIMMUNE DISEASE. It may also occur as a result of radioactive iodine therapy or surgical removal of part of the thyroid gland in cases of overactivity of the thyroid gland (HYPERTHYROIDISM).

Symptoms of hypothyroidism, which are most likely to be felt when the weather is cold, consist of undue tiredness, a feeling of weakness, a hoarse voice and general slowing down of activity. The patient may experience an unusual weight gain, constipation, impaired memory and shortness of breath. Signs include a gradual change in appearance. The skin becomes thickened, particularly in the hands, feet and face (which typically becomes swollen and pale) and there is very little secretion of sweat. The hair becomes dry and coarse and tends to fall out. Occasionally, mental processes are affected and the patient becomes demented. The condition, when fully developed, is called MYXEDEMA; if medical treatment is not provided, the patient becomes cold and may eventually even fall into a coma. Fortunately, if the condition is not too far advanced, myxedema responds to adequate doses of *thyroxine,* the thyroid hormone.

Hypothyroidism in children is more difficult to recognize because the onset is insidious. Symptoms are similar to those found in adults, except that growth is retarded; at first the child may be thought lazy and careless.

Hypothyroid babies, if untreated, become *cretins:* the face is puffy, the nose snub and obstructed, the tongue too large for the mouth and the skin yellowish, cold and thick; the intelligence is diminished (see CRETINISM). Umbilical hernias are common in such babies and may aid in the diagnosis. The sooner treatment is begun with thyroid hormone, the more likely the infant is to recover; but in many cases lack of thyroid secretion in early development leads to permanent intellectual deficiency.

hypoxia

The condition produced by lack of oxygen. It may be due to lack of sufficient oxygen in the air breathed, and is often associated with mountain climbing, flying at high altitudes, and in other conditions where the oxygen supply is restricted.

Even if oxygen is present in normal amounts in the air, hypoxia may still occur if there is disease of the lungs preventing the oxygen from reaching the blood, or if the circulation to the lungs is reduced by heart failure or obstruction of the blood vessels in the lung. All produce lack of oxygen.

The severely hypoxic patient will be short of breath and may show a bluish tinge to the skin (CYANOSIS) due to an increased proportion of unoxygenated hemoglobin in the blood.

Treatment involves the administration of oxygen by mask or oxygen tent, but it is also necessary for the underlying condition to be treated if lasting relief is to be obtained.

hysterectomy

Surgical removal of the uterus (womb), an operation which while classed as a major operative procedure is not considered dangerous. The uterus may be removed through an incision in the lower part of the abdomen or through the vagina. The most radical operations are carried out for cancer of the womb, and involve removal of not only the uterus but also the Fallopian tubes, the ovaries and the lymphatic glands which drain the area of malignancy. Such complete removals are best carried out through an abdominal incision, but in cases where a less radical clearance is indicated the vaginal approach is used.

The indications for such an operation include fibroid tumors, pelvic infections, endometriosis and excessive uterine hemorrhage. The operation may be advised for a number of other conditions, especially in women past childbearing age, for it is possible to argue that an organ which has no further function is useless and in many cases best removed. Opinion varies, and each case must be assessed on its own merits. Removal of the uterus clearly means that the patient will thereafter be sterile, but adverse physiological effects are kept to a minimum by the preservation of the ovaries where it is possible, and by the vaginal approach which leaves no scar. This approach is doubly indicated in some cases, for it is possible as part of the operation to carry out a repair to the pelvic floor where there is a degree of muscular weakness leading to a rectocele or cystocele. Contrary to popular opinion, sexual desire is not generally lost after the operation.

hysteria

In its widest definition, hysteria means any excessive emotional response. But psychiatrists prefer to define it as a disorder in which the patient develops symptoms of illness (mental, physical, or both) for subconscious reasons. Typically, the development of hysteria allows the patient to escape from an anxious or threatening life situation.

Hysterical illness may take the form of loss of memory, hysterical fits, or sleepwalking. *Conversion hysteria* takes the form of loss of function of some part of the body. There may be sudden and complete paralysis or loss of sensation in the legs or other parts of the body, blindness, deafness, or vomiting. Such symptoms are dramatic, but they are totally reversible—recovery is just as sudden as the onset of the disability.

The treatment of hysterical symptoms is often delayed while x rays and laboratory investigations are performed to exclude the possibility that there is an underlying physical disease. Once the psychological basis is clear, treatment may be given with psychotherapy tranquilizers, and more specific measures to remove the emotional stresses that precipitated the illness.

I

iatrogenic disorder

Any adverse mental or physical state or condition induced in a patient by his physician's or surgeon's attitudes, words, oversights, actions or treatments.

ichthyosis

A hereditary condition characterized by thick, scaly and very dry skin.

Keratin, the horny substance on the surface of the skin, is normally shed and replaced continuously throughout life. In ichthyosis, there seems to be an imbalance in the rates of replacement and shedding; that is, there is either an overproduction of keratin or it is shed relatively slowly.

The condition usually becomes apparent in the first few weeks or months of life. Mild cases may pass off as merely dry skin, but in severe cases the skin looks like fish skin or alligator hide. The scalp may also be affected, but usually not the palms and soles. Warm weather seems to have a beneficial effect.

Treatment consists of measures like protecting the skin against the cold, avoiding the handling of detergents, and lubricating the skin daily with lanolin or ointments based on petroleum jelly.

In winter it is advisable to have daily or twice daily baths in weak salt water to hydrate the skin, followed immediately by the application of ointments which impede the evaporation of water. Some people claim that vitamin A taken in the winter months is helpful.

All these measures may improve the condition and appearance of the skin temporarily, but a permanent cure is unlikely.

icterus

Another word for JAUNDICE.

idiopathic disease

Any disease in which the cause is unknown or not clear.

ileitis

Inflammation of the ileum, the third and last part of the small intestine.

By far the most common cause of ileitis is a condition variously called *regional enteritis, regional ileitis* or *Crohn's disease.* Although the ileum is the site most frequently affected by Crohn's disease, any other part of the intestine may be affected, especially the colon.

In Crohn's disease, the inflammation characteristically affects one or more clearly demarcated segments of the intestine, producing rigidity and thickening of the affected length of bowel and a narrowing of the lumen.

The cause of the disease is unknown. It usually starts between the ages of 10 to 40 with intermittent bouts of right-sided lower abdominal pain, accompanied by a low-grade fever and diarrhea alternating with constipation. Sometimes the disease starts with a sudden flareup and may be mistaken for appendicitis, in which case the diagnosis is made at the time of surgical investigation (laparotomy).

In most cases the disease progresses, continuously or intermittently, producing mild to severe disability and complications such as perianal fistulas or fistulas into other organs. Rarely, perforation of the intestine or hemorrhage may occur. In severe and long-standing cases, malnutrition results.

Diagnosis rests on barium studies of the intestine. Treatment consists of rest in bed during the acute phase, with a high-calorie, high-protein and vitamin-rich diet, excluding raw fruit and vegetables. In severe cases, drugs may be given to suppress the inflammation; but if symptoms persist or worsen and complications occur, an operation may be required to remove the affected portions of the intestine.

ileostomy

The surgical formation of an opening through the abdominal wall into the ileum (the lower part of the small intestine). The operation is performed whenever the colon has to be removed; the opening then acts as an artificial anus through which the contents of the small intestine are discharged instead of passing along the colon to the natural anus.

The opening does not have muscles like the opening of

ILEOSTOMY

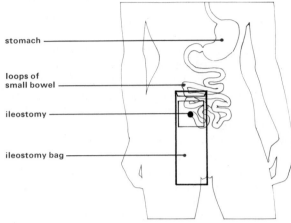

stomach

loops of
small bowel

ileostomy

ileostomy bag

*An ileostomy is an opening made in the ileum
(the last part of the small bowel) in order to
divert fecal material to the exterior, where it is
collected in a bag. Ileostomies are necessary
where the colon and rectum have been removed.*

the natural anus, so patients with ileostomies have to
wear a bag continually to collect the excreta. This
sounds unpleasant, but in fact an ileostomy is perfectly
compatible with a normal life.

The colon (large intestine) absorbs water from the
intestinal contents. But the waste products discharged
through an ileostomy have not passed along the colon;
thus they are watery, especially when the colon is first
removed. Later the body adapts and the excreta
gradually become more formed, although never
completely solid.

Minor dietary modifications, which vary from patient
to patient, may be required to alter the consistency of the
stools or to reduce odor.

Patients learn how to look after their ileostomies at
the hospital where the operation is performed.
Additional help may be obtained from the United
Ostomy Association or its chapters which exist in all
states of the United States. With such assistance
patients can adapt more easily to their condition.

ileus

Paralysis of the intestine. Peristalsis, the wavelike
rhythmic movement which propels food, along the
gastrointestinal tract, ceases and the effect is a non-
mechanical obstruction of the intestine.

The most common cause of ileus is PERITONITIS.
Cessation of peristalsis in such a situation helps to
localize infection, which could spread very rapidly if
peristalsis continued. Another fairly common cause of
ileus is an abdominal operation, which usually results in
a temporary ileus lasting about 48 hours.

Ileus may also occur when the blood supply to the
intestine is cut off, or following severe injuries to the
abdomen or spine. Generally, when there is a mechanical obstruction the part of the intestine above the site of
obstruction contracts vigorously in an attempt to overcome the obstruction; but if this persists an ileus may
result.

The symptoms of ileus are abdominal distension and
vomiting. Pain is not a prominent feature.

No food should be taken by mouth when there is an
ileus. During this time, the patient is fed intravenously
and a tube is passed into the stomach to remove the
digestive juices which continue to be secreted. Salts lost
in this way have to be replaced in the intravenous feeds.
If there is peritonitis, antibiotics are essential. Otherwise
treatment is that of the underlying cause of the ileus.

immune system

The body's defense mechanism against "foreign invaders."

The most common are infectious microorganisms,
which are obviously a different species from humans.
But human tissue may also be treated as foreign when it
is introduced for medical reasons, such as occurs with
blood transfusions (blood is technically one of the
"tissues" of the body), skin grafting, or organ transplantation. This is because every individual is born with a set
of "identification marks" or "immune markers" which
makes his body regard any tissue that contains different
markers as foreign or "non-self."

There are numerous possible combinations of the
markers which make up an individual's set; that is why it
is so difficult to find a suitable donor who is immu-
nologically compatible with a patient who requires a
transplant.

Since the markers are inherited, the chances of finding
a compatible donor (or the least incompatible donor)
are better among the patient's relatives. (The ideal
donor would be the patient's identical twin.)
Compatibility or a good match between two individuals
is determined by tests known as tissue typing.

These markers, which are found on the surface of
cells, are called *antigens*. An individual's immune system
is quick to recognize any foreign marker and responds
by the production of *antibodies*.

Antibodies are substances which counteract antigens;
they are produced by lymphocytes (a type of white blood
cell). Each type of antibody is formed in response to
invasion by a particular antigen and is able to act only
against that type of antigen.

In *circulating* or *humoral* immunity, antibodies are
released into the circulation and travel around the body.
Their primary role is defense against infection by
bacteria, which they attack so that they can be more

easily engulfed and digested by special cells known as phagocytes.

Some bacteria, such as the tubercle and leprosy bacilli, are able to live and grow within the cell which has engulfed them. In such cases the body has another immune mechanism, called *cellular* immunity, for dealing with them. In the newborn and during early childhood special lymphocytes are processed in the thymus gland (in the neck) to enable them to carry antibodies on their surface. They migrate to the area where they are needed, to surround and help to overcome the "invader."

This cellular (or "cell-mediated" or "delayed") immunity is responsible for rejecting transplants.

Several conditions arise from disorders of the immune system. Allergies, for example, are the result of an unusually sensitive immune system; people with allergies are more likely to react badly to immunization or to develop drug reactions.

On the other hand, those with abnormalities of the thymus or of the lymphocytes have a very poor immune response, the most important effect of which is a high susceptibility to infection.

The immune system may be depressed by a number of chronic debilitating diseases, including cancer and chronic kidney failure. It may also be suppressed by a number of drugs known collectively as *immuno-suppressive* agents. These drugs are useful in the treatment of a variety of conditions, but patients receiving them become very prone to infections.

An abnormality of the immune system is believed to be responsible for a group of diseases known as the *autoimmune* disorders, which include the COLLAGEN DISEASES. They are currently thought to be due to an allergy to one's own tissues, but are not yet well understood.

IMMUNIZATION is the deliberate stimulation of antibody production. The infecting organism (in a modified form) is introduced into the body, which begins almost immediately to form antibodies against it. These antibodies, in common with those produced in response to natural invasion, remain in the circulation for some time (often for the lifetime of the individual) and are therefore always ready in case the actual disease should attack.

It is a feature of the immune system that a second attack by an antigen is always repulsed more vigorously than the first attack—because the antibodies are ready and the body has "learned" to make more of that particular antibody quickly. Subsequent attacks are repulsed even more efficiently. This can be an advantage in that it prevents second attacks of certain diseases, but it can be a disadvantage for allergic people because allergies can produce increasingly severe attacks with every exposure.

immunization

The process by which resistance to infection is artificially induced.

Normally the body resists infection by producing substances called antibodies, which act against infectious organisms. Each infectious organism has on its body surface a substance called an antigen which the body recognizes as "foreign." Whenever an infectious agent invades the body, the body starts to produce antibodies against this type of organism. The antibodies produced are released into the blood circulation so that they can reach the site of infection.

Each type of organism has its own particular type of antigen, and antibodies produced in response to infection by one type are specific only against that type of antigen. (See ANTIBODY/ANTIGEN.)

Often after recovery from an infection sufficient antibody remains in the circulation to protect against further infection by the same organism. This type of resistance is known as *naturally acquired immunity*.

Artificial immunization can be produced in two ways, active and passive. In active immunization the antibodies are produced in response to antigens deliberately introduced into the body, usually by injection but sometimes by swallowing. These antigens may come in the form of dead organisms, or organisms so weakened (by laboratory methods) that they cannot cause disease but can stimulate antibody production.

If the disease is caused by toxins (poisons) produced by infectious organisms, *antitoxin* production may be artificially stimulated by injecting chemically modified toxins, known as *toxoids*.

In *passive immunization*, ready-made antibodies against a particular organism are injected. These antibodies may have come from the blood of someone who has previously been infected or immunized, or from animals which have been deliberately immunized so that their antibodies can be harvested for use in passive immunization. Passive immunization provides quicker but only temporary immunity. Active immunization may require a few weeks before antibodies are produced, but the effect is longer-lasting, the degree and duration of immunity varying with different diseases. Sometimes the antigen has to be given in two or three doses to ensure the production of a reasonable quantity of antibody.

Immunization may sometimes produce unpleasant reactions, but this varies with the type of immunization. People who have allergies are more likely to suffer from adverse reactions.

Immunization against several specific diseases of childhood is advisable; not only does this protect the individual child, but it protects the whole community, because if a large proportion of the susceptible population is immune to a disease an epidemic cannot get under way—so that even those who are not, or cannot be, immunized are to some extent protected.

The age at which a child gives the best response to a vaccine varies with the type of immunization, and the following schedule is the one adopted in the United Kingdom:

Age	Immunization	
3 months	1st diphtheria injection	by
	1st whooping cough injection	single
	1st tetanus injection	injection
5 months	2nd – as above	
11 months	3rd – as above	
15 months	measles—if required	
4–5 years	booster of diphtheria and tetanus	

NB. Whooping cough (pertussis) injection should *not* be given in the following circumstances:
1. Where there are any signs or symptoms in the first few days after birth which suggest that the child may be brain damaged.
2. Where there is a history of fits.
3. Where the first injection has produced an allergic reaction in the child.

Smallpox vaccination is no longer given to children in Britain, though it may still be required for entry into certain countries in spite of the fact that the World Health Organization claims that endemic smallpox has been eliminated from the world. Other infections for which immunization is required when traveling include cholera, yellow fever, plague and typhoid. The requirements vary from time to time and from country to country, so they should be checked whenever a trip outside the country is planned.

Prospective travelers may obtain information from shipping and airline offices, local health authorities, or from branches of the Public Health Department. Inquiries should be made and vaccination obtained several weeks in advance of leaving the country partly because vaccination certificates become valid only 6–10 days after the vaccination (depending on the type of vaccination) and because, if more than one vaccination is required, it is probably a sensible precaution to allow a two-week interval between vaccinations.

It is also wise to inquire about what type of immunization is required for specific reentry into the United Kingdom.

impetigo

A highly contagious bacterial infection of the superficial layers of the skin. The organism most commonly re-

sponsible for the infection is the *Staphylococcus aureus;* less frequently, the infection is caused by streptococci. Impetigo may occur at any age, but is most common in the newborn and in children.

The lesions start as a reddening of the skin, but soon become clusters of blisters and pustules which break to leave sores with straw-colored or honey-colored crusts. The only symptom is itching. The lesions may be found anywhere on the body, but are most common over the face and limbs.

Treatment should be started promptly or the infection may spread rapidly to other areas of the skin. In babies, especially those who are ill or are premature, the infection may spread to other structures such as the bones or lungs. Occasionally, nephritis (inflammation of the kidneys) occurs a few weeks after the skin infection has settled.

Treatment consists of rupturing the blisters and pustules, and of removing the crusts by washing gently with water and an antiseptic agent. If necessary, the crusts may have to be soaked with wet dressings to make them easier to remove. Antibiotics are applied locally to the lesions, but if there is no improvement in three or four days, or if the infection is severe, antibiotics may have to be given by mouth or by injection.

To prevent the spread of infection to other areas of the skin or to other people, the patient should wash his hands frequently and take care not to touch or scratch the lesions.

impotence

The inability to attain or sustain erection of the penis in the presence of sexual desire.

Transient impotence is fairly common and does not imply a physical or psychological disorder. It is often related to mild degrees of anxiety, depression, preoccupation, or fatigue associated with ordinary problems of daily living.

Chronic impotence, on the other hand, is due to either physical or psychological reasons; emotional problems account for an estimated 90% of cases.

Physical factors should be ruled out first. These include aging (it has been estimated that 50% of men over the age of 65 are impotent), chronic debilitating disease, alcoholism, drug addiction, diabetic neuropathy, disease of the nervous system (such as spinal cord damage and multiple sclerosis), endocrine disorders (such as those of the pituitary gland, the thyroid or the gonads), damage to the urethra, and large hydroceles or hernias. Various drugs, including certain antihypertensive drugs, antidepressants and tranquilizers, may produce impotence in some men; the problem is solved when the drug is discontinued.

Whether or not impotence due to physical factors can

be treated depends on the underlying cause. If it is due to hormonal imbalance, improvement is usually possible; but if the nerves are affected, little can be done.

Psychological reasons for chronic impotence often include guilt and anxiety about the sexual act itself, hostility toward the partner, unwillingness to assume responsibility for all that goes with marriage and children, a mother fixation, or various neurotic tendencies. For people with such problems, psychosexual counseling may be of help.

incontinence

Lack of voluntary control over urination and bowel movements.

Incontinence is normal in young children, since voluntary control must be learned. It is usually achieved by the age of three, although some physically normal children do not become fully continent until five or six—or occasionally, in the case of urinary incontinence, not until the late teens. After this age urinary or fecal incontinence is often due to disease, such as cystitis, or to psychological reasons.

In adult life loss of control over urination may occur as a result of injuries to the mother during childbirth which weaken the muscles of the pelvic floor; this may also occur during pregnancy, or may be the result of surgical operations on the urethra or prostate gland. It may also occur when obstruction to the passage of urine leads to retention of urine in the bladder, with eventual overflow.

Neurological conditions and damage to the spinal cord may lead to loss of control over the passage of both urine and feces by interruption of the nervous pathways which control these functions. The elderly may become incontinent because of lack of sensation or confusion. In some cases severe constipation leads to the retention of hard masses of feces which cause irritation and obstruction, with the development of a paradoxical uncontrollable diarrhea. Such causes of apparent incontinence of feces are liable to be overlooked.

Treatment depends on the cause and may involve the administration of certain drugs, or surgery. When cure is not possible, incontinence bags may be used; however, no satisfactory bag has yet been devised for females. Sometimes mechanical or electronic devices are used to increase the pressure around the urethra to prevent the escape of urine, but all of these are still subject to various disadvantages.

See also BEDWETTING.

indigestion

A popular term used to describe a multitude of vague symptoms thought to be associated with food intake or otherwise arising in the digestive system. Also called *dyspepsia*.

Indigestion is a nonspecific term that has a different meaning for different people. It may be used to mean abdominal discomfort, fullness, pressure, pain, heartburn, belching, distension, flatulence or nausea. Some even use it to mean constipation or diarrhea.

All these symptoms may be produced by disease in the gastrointestinal tract. Thus, if symptoms are severe or persist, a doctor should be consulted. Often, however, they are the result of consistently poor eating habits. They may also sometimes be psychogenic in origin, especially in those who always complain of "nervousness," or who are very bowel-conscious and frequently resort to laxatives. Eating habits which give rise to indigestion include overeating, gulping down food, or eating when the appetite is depressed by anger or worry.

A person may notice that certain foods bring on symptoms. There may be a reason for this. It could be that the person lacks the enzyme which deals with the digestion of that particular foodstuff; for example, people who lack lactase may get "indigestion" with milk which contains lactose. In such cases, which can be confirmed by special tests, the offending food should be avoided. But in most cases all that is necessary to avoid indigestion is to take regular, unhurried meals.

Often indigestion is due to increased quantities of gas in the gastrointestinal tract. Most of this gas is swallowed, the rest being produced by bacterial fermentation of carbohydrate and proteins—often from raw fruit and vegetables. Swallowing of air (aerophagia) is normal, but with chronic anxiety or poor eating habits more air tends to be swallowed. Fatty meals may aggravate symptoms due to gas because they slow down emptying of the stomach, so delaying the passage of gas down the gastrointestinal tract.

If there is no recognized disease causing the symptoms, and regulating the eating habits does not help, a number of drugs may relieve symptoms—usually those which neutralize gastric acid (antacids) or those which calm the gut. Rarely, psychotherapy may help.

induction of childbirth

The use of artificial means to start off the process of childbirth, or labor. This is sometimes carried out when it appears safer for the fetus or mother that pregnancy be terminated as soon as possible. The timing should be such that the fetus is mature enough to have at least as good a chance of survival outside the uterus (even if in an incubator) as inside it.

Sometimes labor is induced not for obstetric problems, but so that it can take place at a convenient time for both mother and doctor. The desirability of such induced abortions is highly debatable.

Labor can be induced in two basic ways. One is the use of drugs, given intravenously, to stimulate the uterus to contract. The other is artificial rupture of the membranes surrounding the fetus. The release of fluid produced by rupture of the membranes sets off uterine contractions. Sometimes artificial rupture of membranes is used in conjunction with induction by drugs.

Induction of labor carries some risk. The uterus may respond to induction by contracting too violently (in which case the uterus may even rupture), or it may not respond sufficiently. The fetus may turn out to be too premature, or it may not withstand the process of childbirth and show signs of FETAL DISTRESS. If the membranes have been ruptured, there is also a risk of infection.

Thus, very careful observation of mother and fetus has to take place throughout an induced labor and, if necessary, a Cesarean section may have to be carried out if things do not go well.

See also CHILDBIRTH.

infarct/infarction

An *infarct* is an area of dead tissue (see NECROSIS) surrounded by healthy tissue, caused by a blockage of blood flow to the affected area. In addition to meaning the same as infarct, *infarction* also refers to the formation of an infarct or the process which leads to it.

When the heart muscle is the site of the infarct, the condition is known as a *myocardial infarction* ("heart attack"). Most infarcts are caused by interruption of the blood flow by a thrombus or embolus (see EMBOLUS/EMBOLISM, THROMBOSIS/THROMBUS).

infectious mononucleosis

An acute viral infection, also known as *glandular fever*. It is caused by the *Epstein-Barr virus,* which is present worldwide. Some cases are associated with cytomegalovirus infection. Most infections with the Epstein-Barr virus occur in childhood and usually go unrecognized; the virus may be found in the throats of healthy people.

Infectious mononucleosis can affect any age group, but most commonly those between 10 and 35. The incubation period is uncertain but probably lies between four to seven weeks. The mode of spread is also uncertain, but there is evidence that it is transmitted in the saliva either by kissing or by sharing drinking vessels. The virus remains in the patient's throat for several months after recovery.

The disease affects many parts of the body and manifests itself in a number of ways. The typical patient has fever, a general feeling of being unwell (malaise), loss of appetite, aches and pains all over the body, enlarged lymph nodes felt as slightly painful lumps (particularly around the neck) and a sore throat. Approximately half the patients have a rash; half may also have an enlarged spleen, which does not produce symptoms but which can be felt (palpated) by the doctor. About 5–25% have jaundice, and in a smaller proportion the heart, kidney or lungs may be affected without producing symptoms, although the involvement can be detected by laboratory tests. In a smaller proportion still, the nervous system is affected and patients may develop meningitis, encephalitis or neuritis.

Because of the wide variety of ways in which the disease presents itself, blood tests may be required before the diagnosis can be confirmed. As the name suggests, the blood contains atypical *mononuclear cells.*

There is no specific treatment for the disease. Bed rest is advisable until the fever disappears, and mild antipyretics and analgesics (such as aspirin) may be given to bring down the fever and to relieve aches and pains. Gargles are often helpful in relieving the discomfort of a sore throat.

In uncomplicated cases, the fever settles in about ten days and the enlarged lymph nodes and enlarged spleen return to normal in about four weeks. In some cases the disease may linger on for months. Those who have had jaundice should avoid alcohol for about six months. Recovery is usually complete.

infertility

The inability to conceive. In general, infertility can be suspected if pregnancy has not occurred after a year of regular sexual intercourse (without the use of any form of contraception).

The cause of infertility may lie in the male or the female. There are numerous causes of infertility in each sex; sometimes no cause is ever found.

Investigations for causes in the male are safer and simpler; consequently, they are normally performed first to save the woman a series of tests if a cause can be found in the male. Doctors do not ordinarily rush through all the investigations but space them out over six months or so, because sometimes a pregnancy occurs for no apparent reason during the course of investigations.

The cause of infertility may be either structural or due to functions of the reproductive system. There may be no production of sperm or ova, or for some reason the two may not meet to bring about fertilization. Some causes are treatable, with varying degrees of success, by either surgery or drugs. Individual cases should be discussed with a medical expert, who will explain the possibility of any complications associated with the investigations and treatment and the chances of success.

General ill-health, especially chronic diseases or

endocrine abnormalities, can cause infertility. Where no cause can be found, simple measures like reducing obesity or improving physical fitness may help to increase fertility.

Sometimes the oral contraceptive pill produces a period of infertility in women when they stop taking it; this is nearly always temporary and should not be a cause for immediate concern.

inflammation

The way in which living tissue responds to injury—usually to injury by an infectious agent, although the same response is seen with physical, chemical or radiation injuries. It is essentially a protective mechanism by which the tissues attempt to localize infection.

The blood vessels around the site of injury dilate and their walls become permeable, so that white blood cells can leave the vessel and migrate to the site of injury—where they either ingest the infecting organism or release chemical substances to digest damaged tissue.

Local inflammation produces swelling, heat, redness, pain and loss of function of the affected part. Sometimes the effects of inflammation are seen beyond the site of damage, as fever or as changes in the numbers and types of circulating white blood cells.

An acute inflammation usually heals completely, but sometimes a scar results.

influenza

An acute viral infection of the respiratory tract, with symptoms present elsewhere in the body. It can affect people at any age. The consequences in the very young, the elderly, the debilitated, and those with heart or lung disease are particularly dangerous. The infection is spread when infected droplets discharged by an infected person during speaking, coughing or sneezing are inhaled by an uninfected person. There is an incubation period of one to four days before the symptoms appear.

Symptoms appear abruptly and include fever, chills, a dry cough, nasal stuffiness, a running nose, aches and pains all over the body, a sore throat, headache, loss of appetite, nausea, weakness and depression. Mild cases may resemble a common cold, although the weakness and depression are usually greater than would be experienced with a cold.

As with viral infections in general, there is no specific drug treatment for influenza. General measures include rest in bed during the acute phase, followed by a gradual resumption of normal activity. If required, a mild antipyretic and analgesic may be taken to relieve symptoms. In uncomplicated cases, symptoms usually subside within a week.

Influenza reduces the patient's resistance to bacterial infection; superimposed bacterial bronchitis is a common complication, which if left untreated may lead to pneumonia. Other bacterial complications include sinusitis and infections of the middle ear (otitis media).

If the fever persists more than four days and purulent (pus-containing) sputum is brought up on coughing, it is advisable to see a doctor—who may prescribe antibiotics if he feels that a bacterial infection is imminent or is already established. Occasionally, the circulatory system is involved and the heart muscle (myocardium) or its outer covering (pericardium) may be inflamed—producing *myocarditis* or *pericarditis,* respectively.

The simplest way of minimizing the possibility of an attack is to avoid crowds during an epidemic. Some people claim that taking large doses of vitamin C at regular intervals helps both to prevent an attack and to reduce the severity of the symptoms experienced, but the consensus of medical opinion discredits this.

An attack of influenza confers immunity to the particular strain to which the infecting virus belongs. A temporary immunity to one or more strains can be acquired by injection of a vaccine prepared against those strains. Such vaccines take about two weeks after the injection to become effective; it is useless to have the injection once symptoms have appeared. Thus, immunization against influenza is usually given in the autumn to protect against attacks during the winter when influenza is most common.

Some doctors advise immunization only for those who are particularly susceptible. Unfortunately, immunization of the public against known strains of influenza virus does not protect against new strains that crop up periodically and are responsible for the epidemics that appear every few years to threaten individuals and communities.

ingrowing nails

A condition in which the sides of the nail are more curved than usual and grow into the flesh of the nail groove. Although any nail may be affected, usually it is the nail of the big toe which becomes painful. The nail fold is unusually prominent and appears to ride up around the nail as pressure is placed on the toe.

Ingrowth is caused by badly fitting shoes or by cutting the nails too short. It can be prevented by cutting the nail carefully—so that the sides are a little longer than the middle, but without leaving a sharp spicule at the corner. The nail should be left just long enough to project from the nail groove.

If there is pain, the nail should be gently lifted out of the groove by elevating it with a sharp pair of scissors or

INGROWING TOENAIL

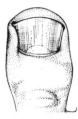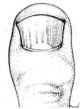

nail growing into skin fold

incorrect cutting—too short and curved

correct cutting—straight across, not too short

An ingrowing nail of the big toe results from a combination of sweaty feet, tight shoes and incorrect cutting. In most cases, correct cutting as shown above will relieve the condition. If unchecked, the top corner of the toenail grows into the skin fold which runs along the side of the nail; this can become infected.

the tip of a nail file placed just under the nail at the outer corner. This should be done for a few minutes each day to encourage the nail to grow out of the groove. Shoes should be roomy.

Toes with ingrown nails are very prone to chronic infection. The nail fold becomes intermittently swollen, red and painful and may discharge pus, while the nail lacks luster and becomes brownish and crumbly. This condition should be treated by a doctor. If antibiotics do not help, the nail may have to be removed. A complete nail will grow again in nine months to a year and should be carefully observed to see that it does not become ingrown again.

insulin

A hormone produced in the PANCREAS and responsible for the control of several body functions, especially carbohydrate metabolism.

Insulin helps the muscles and other tissues to obtain the sugar needed for their activity. A gross deficiency leads to DIABETES MELLITUS, in which the blood sugar is not used by the body and builds up to undesirable levels.

The existence of insulin as an essential component of metabolism was suspected as early as 1909. It was finally isolated in relatively pure form by the two Canadians, Banting and Best, in 1921.

Medical insulin is prepared from the pancreas of sheep or cattle and is injected daily in severe cases of diabetes. Many types of insulin are now available; they differ mainly in the duration of their action. It is estimated that insulin has saved over 30 million lives since it was introduced as a therapy for people who suffer from diabetes.

intelligence quotient (IQ)

A presumed measure of the intelligence of an individual as compared with the total population. The IQ of a person is obtained by means of a suitable series of tests to calculate his mental age, which is then divided by his chronological age and multiplied by 100 to give the IQ. Thus, a person whose mental age is 12 at a chronological age of 10 will be deemed to have an IQ of 120. This means that the IQ of a person of "normal" intelligence will naturally be taken as 100; about half the population score below 100 and the other half above.

Intelligence tests attempt to establish the mental ability of the subject in a number of different fields. Such matters as vocabulary, arithmetic, ability to reason, general knowledge and (somewhat less successfully) creativity are tested by the application of a battery of tests worked out by psychologists. Many intelligence tests now used in the United States and other Western countries have evolved from the pioneering work of the French psychologists Alfred Binet (1857–1911) and Théodore Simon (1873–1961).

In general, the IQ allocated to a child as a result of undergoing intelligence tests correlates well with later achievement in academic work. There is a less close correlation with achievement in later life, presumably because other qualities such as drive and acumen may be as important as sheer intelligence in one's working life.

IQ allocations are also under fire because some critics

INSULIN

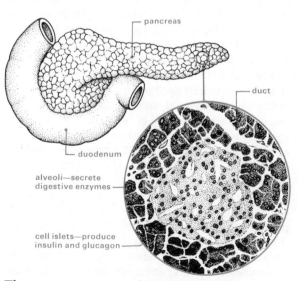

pancreas

duct

duodenum

alveoli—secrete digestive enzymes

cell islets—produce insulin and glucagon

The pancreas is a mixed-function gland. It secretes digestive enzymes through ducts into the duodenum where they break down fats and proteins. It also secretes hormones, most importantly insulin, directly into the bloodstream.

claim that the tests, having been designed by literate, numerate, middle-class white psychologists, do not adequately test the intelligence of children from other sectors of the community. In the most modern tests attempts are made to correct imbalances due to language barriers, reading disabilities or cultural differences. Nevertheless, the use of intelligence tests remains a somewhat controversial subject.

intensive care unit (ICU)

A unit in which especially intense surgical and medical care can be given to patients—widely used in caring for patients in the first few days after suffering from acute myocardial infarction ("heart attack").

Although the use of ICUs has been greatly increased by the application of the principle to the care of coronary patients, and in many people's minds ICUs are identified solely with heart attacks, their use is much more widespread.

ICUs are used to support surgical patients postoperatively, to keep accident victims alive until surgery can be performed on them, and to enable premature babies to survive the first few days of life. They also play a large part in the treatment of burns when the victims are critically ill and cannot undergo surgery until the crisis is over.

In general, it can be said that the objectives of an ICU are the initiation of resuscitation, the administration of electrolytes and fluids, and the prevention of contamination and cross-infection. ICUs designed to deal with coronary patients are usually equipped with a respirator and defibrillator as the basic equipment, and it has been observed that they have been helpful in decreasing the mortality rate from acute myocardial infarction due to the arrhythmias.

As an aid to the main task of keeping the patient alive, ICUs are commonly equipped with a number of monitoring devices; these are designed to keep the medical and nursing staff informed of the state of the patient's heart by displaying his ECG in various ways. An ICU will commonly have facilities for inserting pacemakers in cases where arrhythmias occur, and catheterization of the heart for diagnostic purposes is also common.

The proper use of ICUs has been an important factor in improving survival from heart attacks. The major problem which has arisen is a psychological one, called the "ICU syndrome." It is said to be a confused and agitated state of consciousness possibly related to sensory deprivation. A patient may become emotionally disturbed by the extensive electronic equipment around him, by being in a windowless room, or by hearing cardiac catastrophes occurring to nearby patients. Family and friends are advised to avoid business or other worrying discussions with patients, who should be given daily newspapers, possibly a radio, a clock and a calendar to prevent a feeling of isolation.

intermittent claudication

An intermittent cramp in the muscles of the leg brought on by exercise such as walking. It is caused by reduction in the blood supply of the muscles of the leg brought about by narrowing or obstruction of the arteries supplying the leg. The pain disappears swiftly with rest.

The disease affects nine times more men than women and is most common after the age of 50 to 55. Diabetics are particularly at risk, as are people with high levels of cholesterol in the blood.

The calf muscle is affected most often, but pain may also appear in the buttock and thigh. Other symptoms include tightness, numbness and severe fatigue in the muscles being exercised. The pain of claudication is due to the leg muscles not receiving sufficient oxygen via the blood to work properly. In severe cases the leg may become swollen with dry, shiny, tightly drawn skin. Ulceration may then become a problem.

Diagnosis is helped by the absence or lessening of pulses below the point of obstruction. X rays usually enable the doctor to pinpoint the exact site of arterial damage. In mild cases the patient is advised to lose weight, walk more slowly (but more often), and give up smoking. If the intermittent claudication worsens, or the condition of the affected limb deteriorates, the diseased section of artery may be replaced surgically by a graft of the patient's own blood vessel or synthetic material. Considering the age of these patients, the outlook for prolonged survival is reasonably good.

intersexuality

The state of being intermediate between the sexes; having both male and female characteristics. (The term is descriptive rather than diagnostic.)

Sexual differentiation is determined in the fetus. In the sixth week of gestation the simple gonads begin to develop into testicles if the fetus has male chromosomes. Alternatively, they develop into ovaries in the twelfth week when the fetus has female chromosomes.

Various events may affect this process of differentiation and lead to intersexuality. In the ADRENOGENITAL SYNDROME, the male hormone testosterone is produced by abnormally functioning adrenocortical glands; a girl is born with either an enlarged clitoris or a normal penis with an empty scrotum. A female fetus may also be "virilized" when her mother has a tumor that produces male hormones, or is given progestin treatment (now obsolete). Lack of a specific substance in the fetus may result in a boy being born with a redundant uterus and Fallopian tubes.

Any condition in which the sexual anatomy is improperly or incompletely differentiated is an example of intersexuality. Treatment demands consideration of both psychological and physical factors. Experience over the past few decades has shown that it is not always correct to assign an individual to the sex indicated by the chromosomes. Surgery to correct the anomalies of the sexual organs may be performed at any time; a boy with abnormally small or underdeveloped genital organs (hypogonadism) may have been brought up as a girl and after surgical removal of the genitals may grow to maturity as a woman.

Every case of intersexuality is different and should receive the combined diagnostic and therapeutic expertise of a physician, an endocrinologist and a psychiatrist—as well as a surgeon, in selected patients.

intertrigo

Chafing of the skin where two surfaces, usually moist, rub together.

As a result of the chafing, erythema (redness) or dermatitis (skin inflammation) of the surfaces may occur. Intertrigo may be a particular problem in young infants, since the child does not detect the chafing. The most common sites are the natural folds of skin in the groin, armpits and elbows. Elderly obese people with a greater than normal overlap of tissues may also be especially susceptible.

In general, the condition may be encountered wherever clothes cause pressure or friction, or when individuals walk for long distances.

Retroauricular intertrigo is an inflammatory condition of the skin that develops in the fold where the ear joins the scalp. A painful crack may appear and is sometimes extremely persistent.

Seborrheic intertrigo, a condition similar to retroauricular intertrigo, arises from chafing under heavy breasts or in the folds of the buttocks. Between the scrotum and the thigh is another common site where intertrigo may appear.

Prevention of chafing is best accomplished by keeping the skin clean and dry. Warm water with "superfatted" soap should be used, after which the skin should be carefully dried and sprinkled with dusting powder, such as talcum powder or a mixture of starch, zinc and subnitrate of bismuth. Intertrigo may be aggravated by a fungus infection, which can later become complicated with a secondary bacterial infection.

intoxication

The condition produced by the presence of poison in the body. In everyday speech, intoxication usually refers to the effects of alcohol. In this condition the subject exhibits some or all of the classic symptoms of slurred speech, unsteadiness, nausea, vomiting, unconsciousness and amnesia, according to the stage reached.

Intoxication in severe cases may long outlast a night's sleep, so giving rise to the well-known hangover. It may be said to begin when the alcohol level reaches about 50 milligrams per 100 milliliters of blood, but some people tolerate alcohol more than others, so no universal rule can be applied.

In general terms, intoxication can be used to describe any case of poisoning in which either physical or mental symptoms appear. It may arise from the introduction of any poison externally administered, or in cases of *autointoxication* from toxins secreted by bacteria in the body.

Treatment for intoxication will obviously vary with the circumstances. For all but the most severe cases of alcohol intoxication an undisturbed night's sleep is probably the best treatment. However, alcohol can be fatal if taken in very large quantities. If it is suspected, for instance, that more than a bottle of whisky has been consumed, it may be necessary to apply a stomach pump under medical supervision. In the case of a chronic alcoholic, even such large amounts might be easily tolerated, although not without deleterious long-term effects on the body and mind.

In other cases medical help should be sought and the doctor given all relevant information as to the poison ingested. Bottles, cans or other containers should be handed over to him for identification of their contents.

intrauterine device

A contraceptive device placed in the uterus, several types of which are available.

Also known as an *intrauterine contraceptive device,* an *IUD,* or an *IUCD.* See also CONTRACEPTION.

intrinsic factor

A substance produced by the lining of the stomach which is essential for the absorption of vitamin B_{12}. Intrinsic factor combines with the vitamin to produce an antianemic substance. Because the daily requirement of vitamin B_{12} is so small (1 or 2 micrograms or millionths of a gram), deficiency of this vitamin is almost invariably due to a breakdown of the absorption mechanism. This may be caused by a failure of the stomach to secrete intrinsic factor; or the cells that normally secrete the factor may be replaced by a tumor; or they may be cut out when part of the stomach is removed surgically.

Lack of intrinsic factor for any of these reasons is thought to lead to the type of ANEMIA known as *pernicious anemia*—which can be fatal if the patient is not treated with vitamin B_{12}, iron and a balanced diet.

intubation

The introduction of a tube into a body orifice. The term is usually used to mean the introduction of a tube through the mouth or nose into the windpipe in order to maintain an adequate air passage into the lungs. It is carried out in general anesthesia, in cases of unconsciousness due to other causes, and in cases where the breathing is obstructed.

Gastric intubation, the passage of a tube into the stomach through the esophagus, is necessary in some cases of obstruction to the esophagus or of paralysis of the mechanism of swallowing. It is used in cases of intestinal obstruction so that the contents of the stomach can be aspirated. It is also used to wash the stomach out in cases of poisoning, such as a drug overdose. A gastric tube is passed before operation in many cases of abdominal surgery to guard against regurgitation of gastric contents into the lungs in an unconscious patient.

intussusception

A condition in which one part of the intestine becomes pushed or telescoped into another portion.

It occurs mainly in infants under one year and usually starts at the lower end of the ileum. Overactive wave contractions (peristalsis) of the intestine may be the cause of the condition, driving a loop of the bowel into the one below. The same peristaltic movements may aggravate the condition so that more intestine becomes involved.

Intussusception results in sudden intestinal obstruction, causing severe abdominal pain. The infant has attacks of screaming and draws up its legs. The face becomes very pale when the pain is most intense and brightens in the intervals between spasms. Vomiting starts early and is severe and repeated. After the first bowel movement the infant passes only red jelly-like clots of pure blood and mucus from the bowel.

Examination of the abdomen by the doctor usually reveals a sausage-like mass.

Prompt surgical treatment is necessary to pull the telescoped portion of the intestine back to its normal position. If, as happens in some cases, the intestine is gangrenous, surgical removal of the affected part is necessary.

In adults, intussusception occasionally occurs due to ADENOMA or other abnormality.

iridectomy

Surgical removal of a portion of the iris of the eye. Several types of iridectomy are performed depending on the nature and state of the complaint.

The function of the iris is to act like the adjustable stop of a camera which controls the amount of light allowed to penetrate to the light-sensitive film; it lets in a controlled amount of light to the retina.

A portion of iris is removed to improve sight when for some reason the pupil becomes obscured, or when there is another disease which the procedure may improve.

There are a number of types of iridectomy operation: *basal* or *peripheral,* when a small portion of iris is removed from the base or periphery; *buttonhole,* when only a small portion is removed; *broad,* excision of a large area of the iris including the edge of the pupil, leaving a keyhole type of appearance; *complete,* when the section removed includes the entire width of the iris; *glaucoma* iridectomy, when a wide iridectomy is performed for the relief of congestive glaucoma; *optical* iridectomy, to shape a new pupil and improve vision in cases of central opacities of the cornea or lens; and finally *therapeutic* iridectomy, performed to prevent recurrence of IRITIS (inflammation of the iris).

iritis

Inflammation of the colored part of the eye, the iris. It is characterized by pain, contraction of the pupil and discoloration of the iris itself. Some temporary or permanent decrease in vision may also be involved.

The causes are varied and sometimes unclear. Possible causes include local infection or injury to the eye, tuberculosis, syphilis, collagen disease, REITER'S DISEASE and TOXOPLASMOSIS in infants.

Swelling of the upper eyelid and pain radiating to the temple are common symptoms. There may also be excessive production of tears, intolerance to bright light, blurring of vision and transient near-sightedness.

The eye becomes bloodshot and pus may appear in the anterior chamber of the eye or cover the surface of the lens. Adhesions may form between the iris and the lens, which may be permanent.

The acute form of the condition usually lasts several weeks and tends to recur. Chronic iritis may last considerably longer, with the outcome depending on the severity of the complications.

Early treatment is important. A drug called atropine is used to dilate the pupil so that adhesions are less likely to form between the iris and the lens. Cortisone-like steroid drugs frequently help to deal with the formation of exudates. Underlying causes of iritis are eliminated if possible.

iron

An essential constituent of the body necessary for blood formation and for certain chemical processes in living cells.

IRITIS

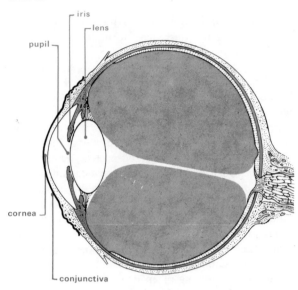

A CROSS SECTION THROUGH THE EYE

The iris is the colored part of the eye which surrounds the pupil. Iritis, inflammation of the iris, causes a painful red eye with a constricted pupil and blurred vision. Although iritis can occur in isolation, it can be a feature of many systemic diseases, for example rheumatoid arthritis, sarcoidosis and syphilis.

About two thirds of the body iron is to be found in hemoglobin—the oxygen-carrying component of red blood cells. The body of an adult contains some 3 to 4 grams of iron. It is lost in small quantities in the urine, feces and sweat, and in larger quantities during menstruation. Hemorrhage can obviously result in more serious loss.

Children require more dietary iron than adults, because of increased growth. Foods rich in iron include meat, eggs and green vegetables. Absorption in the intestine is aided by the presence of vitamin C which is found in many fruits and vegetables.

Extra iron may be given to pregnant women as a precaution against ANEMIA and to ensure healthy supplies for the fetus.

irritable bowel syndrome

The name given to a common syndrome of abdominal pain, alternating bouts of constipation and diarrhea, flatulence and distension of the abdomen. Typically, the stools are small and hard and there may be four to six bowel movements daily. Often the symptoms are made worse by tension, anxiety or emotional disturbances.

The syndrome sometimes appears after an episode of inflammation of the digestive tract (gastroenteritis), but more usually its onset is gradual. Symptoms usually start before the age of 30 and teenagers may be affected.

Although the cause of the irritable bowel syndrome is still disputed, its symptoms often respond dramatically to a change in the diet to one containing more vegetable fiber ("roughage"). The addition of two spoonfuls of bran to the daily food intake—or a switch to a diet containing wholemeal flour and a high proportion of cereals—will double the volume of feces passing through the colon (large intestine). The effect is a reduction in the episodes of spasm and abdominal pain and a return toward normal in the consistency of the stools. A substantial body of medical opinion now believes that the lack of fiber in the modern American diet is one of the main causes underlying the frequency of the syndrome.

ischemia

A reduction in blood supply to a part of the body or an organ, due either to an obstruction in the supplying artery or to a constriction in the diameter of the blood vessels serving the area.

An inadequate blood supply deprives the tissue of oxygen and leads to improper functioning.

Ischemia may give rise to transient symptoms including pain; in more severe cases it may lead to paralysis and death of the affected tissues. For example, the arteries carrying blood to the heart muscle often become narrowed with increasing age and are responsible for the symptoms of ANGINA PECTORIS. Similarly, DIABETES MELLITUS may lead to the narrowing of blood vessels in the legs so that changes occur in the toes which can become cold and ulcerated.

Cerebral ischemia, involving the blood vessels of the brain, can develop into a STROKE.

Control of the symptoms of angina pectoris with drugs can be rapid and effective, but the use of vasodilator drugs for other forms of ischemia is less certain. Sometimes it is possible for surgeons to remove an obstruction in an important blood vessel or bypass the blockage.

Ishihara color test

A test devised by a Japanese ophthalmologist, S. Ishihara (b. 1879), to detect COLOR BLINDNESS.

The subject is asked to examine a set of cards upon which are printed round dots of various sizes, colors and combinations. On each card the dots of one color (or several shades of one color) form a number or letter, while other colors form the background. The numbers or letters can be easily read by those with normal sight. Those who are color blind cannot see them and may in fact detect other patterns which are built into the design.

The tests may be particularly useful in deciding whether a slightly color-blind person can safely be employed in a job where distinguishing between different colors is essential—such as driving a locomotive or connecting color-coded wires in electronic components.

islet cell tumor

A tumor of the insulin-secreting cells in the "islets of Langerhans" of the PANCREAS. These tumors are usually benign but may rarely be malignant. They may produce excess insulin for the body to cope with, or be nonfunctioning.

Associated with excess insulin production is the condition known as *hypoglycemia* (lowered blood sugar), which can have serious consequences for the patient unless treated promptly. Hypoglycemia brought about by the insulin from tumor cells occurs particularly when the patient is fasting, or after exercise.

If excess insulin production is a problem the tumor can be removed surgically. Drug treatment is an alternative if the tumor cannot be located or when surgery is inappropriate or inadvisable because of other factors.

isotopes

Radioactive isotopes are used widely in medicine in both diagnosis and treatment. The isotope of an element differs in its atomic weight but not in its chemical properties, so that a radioactive preparation of iodine, for example, behaves identically to the normal substance except for its emission of radiation.

When a dose of a chemical or drug containing a tiny proportion of the radioactive substance is given (by mouth or injection) it is possible for its pathway through the body to be followed by means of an apparatus similar to a Geiger counter. The extent of the uptake of radioactive iodine by the thyroid gland, for example, gives valuable information on the activity of the gland. Blood cells may be "tagged" with radioactive chromium to measure their survival in the bloodstream after injection. The amounts of radioactivity involved in tests of this kind are tiny—far too small to present any hazard to health.

Larger doses of radioactive isotopes are used in the treatment of some diseases: again, for example, overactivity of the thyroid gland may be treated in this way, as may excessive production of red blood cells by the bone marrow (polycythemia). Radioactive isotopes are also used to treat some tumors: needles of radioactive yttrium, for example, are used to treat some tumors of the pituitary gland.

itching

A sensation of tickling and irritation in the skin, producing a desire to scratch. Itching is known medically as *pruritus*.

The degree of itching can vary widely and may be experienced in only one place or as a general sensation. A mild itch can be almost pleasurable for some people; but, at the opposite extreme, severe and unrelenting pruritus may cause the sufferer to want to attempt suicide. The sensation arises in nerve endings in the skin which are stimulated by released proteolytic enzymes. Substances such as histamine and prostaglandins are thought to be involved. Itching can be caused by chemical, mechanical, thermal or electrical stimuli. For example, the rubbing of an insect bite may prolong itching for a considerable time after the original stimulus has been removed, as the skin remains in a state of increased excitability.

Vigorous scratching of an itch leads to an enlargement of the area involved so that the threshold is further lowered. The damage to the skin may lead to a secondary infection and the formation of fissures or crusts. Long-standing pruritus may be associated with hardening and pigmentation of the skin. Severe itching, often associated with redness and wealing, can be relieved by the administration of antihistamines.

Apart from outside stimuli, the root of the problem may be parasites or skin diseases such as ECZEMA, LICHEN PLANUS and PSORIASIS. Or there may be an underlying disease such as MYXEDEMA, JAUNDICE, KIDNEY DISEASE, LYMPHOMA or internal malignancy.

Pregnancy, the menopause, and drug and food allergies are other possible causes. In addition, psychological or emotional elements are commonly associated with itching.

Treatment sometimes involves only the removal of a specific cause. In other cases more general measures may have to be used, such as the avoidance of very hot baths and a change in the brand of soap or cosmetics. Noninfected itching areas of skin can be treated with external steroid preparations. Drugs such as aspirin, antihistamines, tranquilizers or sedatives may also be valuable.

J

jaundice

A yellow discoloration of the skin and other tissues as the result of deposition of the pigment bilirubin, which is derived from the breakdown of hemoglobin. Bilirubin is normally excreted by the liver in the bile.

There are three causes of jaundice: hepatic, obstructive and hemolytic.

In *hepatic jaundice,* damage to liver cells—as for example in yellow fever or poisoning by phosphorus—prevents normal formation of bile salts from bilirubin so that the level rises in the blood.

In *obstructive jaundice,* blockage of the bile ducts by stones, or tumors of the ducts or pancreas, prevents the normal excretion of bile into the intestine, so that it is reabsorbed into the bloodstream.

In *hemolytic jaundice,* increased breakdown of red blood cells and the release of hemoglobin in excessive amounts may swamp the liver so that the level of blood bilirubin rises.

In hepatic jaundice the urine becomes dark and the color of the stools slowly becomes lighter; in obstructive jaundice the urine is very dark and the stools are as light as clay; and in hemolytic jaundice the stools are dark but the urine is of normal color.

In all cases, it is not the jaundice itself that is treated but the underlying condition.

See also HEPATITIS, LIVER DISEASE.

jet lag

The symptoms which many people experience when they cross several time zones during international air travel.

During a long flight—such as one across the Atlantic—the physiological functions of the body become "desynchronized" from man's artificial time system.

When traveling from East to West, for instance, an airplane may leave one time zone at noon, fly for seven hours, and land in another time zone at 2 pm. The passenger will then usually resume his activities on the false assumption that only two hours have passed. He may carry out normal activities for the remainder of the day until he goes to bed; but in the evening his rhythms are those which would have been appropriate to the period between 7 pm and 3 am, rather than the 2 to 10 pm period of his new time zone. Symptoms include a dry mouth, racing pulse, disorientation, insomnia and often a loss of appetite.

There are certain types of rhythm in the biological system which operate on a period of approximately 24 hours. They include slight fluctuations of body temperature, minor changes in blood levels of salts such as potassium and sodium and changes in hormone secretion. The question of how long it takes to return to normal "circadian" rhythms is one that is still being debated by scientists; it is certainly true that some people are more adaptable than others. However, there is a rough rule of thumb that a passenger should rest for one

day after a flight lasting seven hours. East to West flights are more taxing than West to East because they result in a longer day; passengers often lose sleep in addition to disturbing their circadian rhythm.

There is some evidence that performance is degraded after long flights. Some companies insist that executives should not make important decisions until the lapse of a few days after crossing a few time zones.

Passengers in pressurized airplanes tend to be dehydrated. This is associated both with the extremely dry atmosphere of the cabin and the consumption of alcoholic drinks. This aggravates the symptoms of jet lag. To minimize problems a passenger should have a high fluid intake without alcohol, sleep as much as possible (preferably without sedatives or sleeping pills) and retire to bed at the end of any long journey rather than undertake strenuous activity immediately.

K

keloid

A vascular, hypertrophied scar above the surface of the skin. Keloid is due to an excessive proliferation of the cells known as *fibroblasts* in a wound and it may invade the subcutaneous tissue as well as the skin. Keloid—from the Greek for "crab claw"—is an ugly pinkish elevated scar with clawlike processes.

Patients with burns often become victims of keloid when raw granulating surfaces in deep burns are not resurfaced with a skin graft. It also appears in accidental or operative wounds, or even in such slight traumas as the scar of a boil or abscess, a smallpox vaccination or an ear prick. It is more common in people with dark complexions, in tuberculosis patients and in pregnant women.

Keloid frequently itches and may ulcerate in places. Unlike more common forms of hypertrophied scars, it may grow for months or even years and it is notorious for recurring after surgical excision, but it rarely develops into a malignancy. In its early stages it may be relieved by the application of hydrocortisone ointment and solution. The conventional treatment is to subject the scar to deep x rays in order to diminish the vascularity and to stop the proliferation of the fibroblasts. If surgical excision is undertaken it is usual to cover the area with skin grafts.

keratitis

Inflammation of the cornea (the transparent front layer of the eye). Worldwide, the most common cause is deficiency of vitamin A, but keratitis may also be due to chemical injury or to infection with viruses or bacteria. Exposure to sunlight or ultraviolet light may cause a transient keratitis.

Treatment clearly depends on the cause; correction of the vitamin deficiency will produce a dramatic cure if the condition is not too far advanced. Bacterial infections usually respond to the appropriate antibiotic, but viral infections do not respond to antibiotics or any other drugs. (In such cases a spontaneous remission can only be hoped for.) If the condition is allowed to progress untreated, however, it may eventually lead to blindness.

keratosis

Thickening of the outer horny layer of the skin. It may be caused by constant friction on the soles or the palms, or by pathological processes (particularly in the elderly).

In *senile keratosis,* multiple warty lesions covered by a hard scale form on the forehead, cheeks, lips and on the backs of the hands and forearms following prolonged exposure to sunlight. The condition is also called *actinic* or *solar* keratosis, and those who spend their lives working outdoors in prolonged sunshine may develop the lesions relatively early in life. Its main importance is that it may be precancerous; about 20% of these keratoses are liable to become malignant.

keratosis follicularis

A rare condition in which the outer layer of the skin is marked by overgrowths of the horny layer. Also known as *Darier's disease, White's disease,* or *keratosis vegetans.*

Keratosis follicularis is a form of ICHTHYOSIS, a skin disease in which the surface is very rough and presents a dry, cracked appearance like fish scales. The limbs, neck and face are particularly affected.

The condition appears to be hereditary, typically develops during childhood and is not contagious. No specific treatment or cure exists.

kernicterus

A condition in which the brain of infants suffering from severe jaundice becomes yellow, the nerve centers at the base of the brain (basal ganglia) in particular being susceptible.

If areas in the medulla oblongata are affected the baby may have difficulty in breathing and show twitching of the face and limbs; damage to the basal ganglia is manifest as abnormal writhing movement of the limbs and retarded psychomotor development, while mental defects may become apparent in consequence of damage to the higher cortical centers.

As there is no known treatment for the condition once it has occurred, excess of bile in the blood of an infant must be dealt with by exchange transfusion in the immediate neonatal period. About 75% of cases are due to hemolytic disease (see RH FACTOR), the others often being associated with birth before full term. Preventive treatment requires the early diagnosis and treatment of conditions in the newborn which can cause hemolysis.

Before the introduction of exchange transfusion about one in a thousand babies born alive was liable to develop kernicterus.

ketosis

The presence of excess ketones—a kind of chemical compound—in the body.

Ketones (of which acetone is an example) are normally produced in the liver through the partial oxidation of protein and fat foodstuffs. As a rule they are further oxidized in other tissues.

If, however, ketone production exceeds a certain level (known as the *ketone threshold*) the tissues are unable to cope with them and ketosis results.

The most common condition giving rise to ketosis is DIABETES MELLITUS. Unable to make use of its blood sugar in the normal way, the diabetic body metabolizes fat and produces ketones. It is sometimes possible to smell acetone on the breath of an uncontrolled diabetic; doctors can also test for ketones in the urine.

The patient has fast, panting breathing and may go into a coma. Injection of insulin resolves the diabetic emergency and, with it, the ketosis.

Ketosis is also a feature of starvation, because the body is metabolizing fat from its own stores.

kidney disease

Patients with kidney disease may either develop problems related to urine formation or present a more confusing picture in which the symptoms at first do not seem to involve the kidney.

The main signs and symptoms of disease of the urinary tract are the presence of abnormal constituents in the urine (such as blood and protein), a large increase or decrease in the volume of urine, frequency of urination and pain. The pain may either be a burning sensation on passing urine or low back pain (which has many causes other than kidney disease). Manifestations of kidney disease unrelated to the urinary system include anemia, hypertension, edema, loss of appetite, nausea, weakness, stunted growth in childhood, itching, convulsions, coma and bone disorders.

Apart from URINARY TRACT INFECTION (UTI), most of the kidney diseases mentioned in this article are uncommon. UTI is predominantly a disease of women and is caused by bacteria from the anus spreading up the urinary passages. If the infection is not effectively treated with antibiotics, the kidney is eventually involved in a PYELONEPHRITIS, marked by fever and lumbar pain. In low-grade pyelonephritis there may be no symptoms, yet the disease can progress insidiously to produce small scarred kidneys and chronic renal (kidney) failure.

Chronic renal failure. Chronic renal failure has many possible causes, pyelonephritis being the second most common. The chief cause in children and adults is GLOMERULONEPHRITIS—an inflammatory disease of the kidney which results from disorders in the body's immune defense mechanisms. Damage to the blood vessels of the kidneys, whether from atherosclerosis, hypertension or diabetes, can also result in chronic renal failure. Various congenital abnormalities such as POLYCYSTIC KIDNEY can produce chronic renal failure in adult life. Among the other causes, ingestion of large doses of analgesics such as aspirin over many years could often have been avoided.

Most patients developing chronic renal failure from whatever cause do not notice any symptoms until they have the equivalent of half a single kidney left functioning. The complications which then follow depend on a number of pathological mechanisms: (1) the failing kidney can no longer concentrate urine, leading to frequent voiding and imbalance in the blood levels of sodium, potassium and hydrogen; (2) at a later stage, urine formation falls dramatically so that toxins normally cleared from the blood by the kidney are retained; this state is called UREMIA and is marked by cardiac and neurological disorders; (3) the kidney normally activates vitamin D, which is important for calcium absorption, and when this process fails, bone disorders can occur; (4) hypertension is a common feature of chronic renal failure and the blood pressure may increase rapidly to cause fatal cerebral hemorrhage; (5) the healthy kidney secretes erythropoietin—a hormone which stimulates the bone marrow to produce red blood cells; this mechanism is depressed in chronic renal failure, causing anemia, which is further exacerbated by the state of uremia.

Until recent years the above complications of chronic renal failure were invariably fatal within a short time. Now with techniques of DIALYSIS and surgical TRANSPLANTATION it is possible to prolong life, often for many years, although the problems are formidable.

Acute renal failure. In contrast to the long, insidious buildup in chronic renal failure, acute renal failure is a state where the production of urine falls suddenly to less than a pint every 24 hours. An abrupt reduction in renal blood flow following hemorrhage, crushing muscle injuries (see CRUSH SYNDROME), burns or overwhelming infection can cause such a drop in urine output. If prompt action is taken to restore the blood pressure, the volume of urine produced soon returns to normal. Otherwise, prolonged lack of oxygen kills cells in the kidney tubules and acute renal failure is established. The same picture can result from a variety of drugs and toxins and from the transfusion of incompatible blood. A patient who suddenly stops producing urine completely probably has an obstruction in the urinary tract due to a CALCULUS (stone), blood clot or tumor.

If a patient with acute renal failure survives, he or she passes little urine for the first few weeks and then has a

THE KIDNEYS

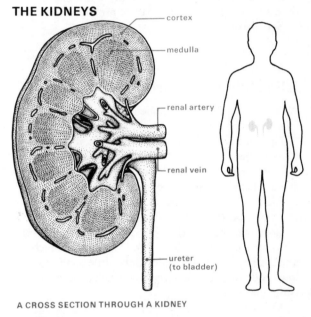

cortex
medulla
renal artery
renal vein
ureter (to bladder)

A CROSS SECTION THROUGH A KIDNEY

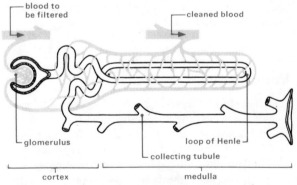

blood to be filtered
cleaned blood
glomerulus
loop of Henle
collecting tubule
cortex
medulla

MAGNIFIED DIAGRAM OF A NEPHRON

The kidneys are paired organs, each about 4 in. long, lying alongside the backbone. Each kidney contains about 1 million functional units or nephrons. *Blood is filtered through glomeruli in the cortex to produce urine, which then flows through the rest of the nephron to the collecting tubules, with great changes in its concentration and chemical composition being made on the way.*

"diuretic phase" when the urine output increases to 6–8 pints per day. With good medical care, renal function usually returns to normal.

Cancer of the kidneys. There are two main types of kidney cancer. *Wilms' tumor* affects young children and in many cases is thought to originate in the fetus. Combination treatment with surgery, irradiation and drugs has recently improved the prognosis for these children. NEPHROMA accounts for less than 2% of all adult cancers and usually affects people over 45 years of age.

NEPHROTIC SYNDROME is mainly a disease of children and is caused by heavy loss of protein in the urine.

See also NEPHRITIS.

Klinefelter's syndrome

A chromosome disorder of men in which partly female characteristics occur.

The normal male has 46 chromosomes, including the two sex chromosomes XY. Females have 46 including XX. Men with Klinefelter's syndrome have 47 chromosomes, including three sex chromosomes XXY.

Patients often have female-type breasts (GYNECOMASTIA) and small testicles with a high output of hormones but which are unable to produce sperm (thus, such patients are infertile). They have a eunuchoid appearance, with long slender limbs, little body hair and low sex drive. Social and psychological disturbances are common.

About 75% of patients exhibit a positive chromatin pattern—that is, their cells contain chromatin, a genetic material normally found only in women.

knock-knee

A deformity of the lower limbs (also known as *genu valgum*) in which the knees turn inward and tend to knock together or touch when walking. When the inner surfaces of the knees are touching, as the child stands in a natural position, the condition leads to the appearance of a gap between the bony protuberances (medial malleoli) of the ankles. The size of this gap is commonly used as a measure of the degree of knock-knee.

After a child begins to walk and before it reaches the age of six years, slight knock-knee is so common that it may be ignored as part of normal development. If, however, it is particularly marked or if it persists to a later age, it may be due to faulty muscular tone. Obesity can aggravate the condition.

Rickets, caused by a deficiency of vitamin D, was formerly responsible for many cases of knock-knee, but the occurrences of rickets are now relatively rare.

Up to the age of seven years, it is not considered necessary to treat knock-knee where the gap between the ankles is less than three inches. Most cases will have become corrected by that age. Splints are used to correct knock-knee in cases where the gap exceeds three inches; in exceptional cases, where it is as much as four inches, or the child is aged nine, an operation may be necessary.

See the illustration at BOWLEG.

kraurosis vulvae

A condition in which the vulva becomes dry, shriveled, red and sore.

Some atrophy of the vulva is normal after the menopause, and kraurosis vulvae probably represents an extreme degree of these normal changes. It is caused by a decrease in the level of circulating estrogens following the menopause; younger women are rarely affected.

Kraurosis vulvae needs treatment for two reasons: it may cause discomfort and it increases the risk of both vulval infections (with CANDIDA or bacteria) and vulval cancer. The treatment is with estrogen, best given in the form of a cream to reduce the risk of side effects.

kwashiorkor

Malnutrition due to a deficiency in the quality and quantity of dietary protein. The condition is common in children in all poor areas of the world.

Kwashiorkor usually develops in children after weaning; as the newborn child is put onto the breast the older baby runs short of food. The principal features are EDEMA of the legs (or even of the whole body), patches of peeling skin, dry and brittle hair, apathy, loss of appetite and failure to grow.

The liver becomes greatly enlarged due to its infiltration with fat and edema fluid collects in the peritoneal cavity, causing the child's abdomen to protrude. Diarrhea is common and usually leads to dehydration and salt imbalance in the body.

Kwashiorkor is treated by gradually restoring regular and well-balanced meals (including all the necessary vitamins), correction of fluid and salt balance, and by administration of antibiotics to control any accompanying infection.

Prevention of kwashiorkor depends upon provision of adequate protein in the diet and the education of parents to make proper use of such a diet for their children. Both of these requirements are lacking in most poor environments; kwashiorkor will continue to be a common disease until these problems are solved and adequate nutrition is provided.

See also DEFICIENCY DISEASES, MALNUTRITION.

kyphosis

An abnormal curvature of the spine, in which its normal curves are exaggerated (compare SCOLIOSIS). It results in the condition commonly referred to as *hunchback* or *humpback*.

See SPINAL CURVATURE.

L

labor

The process by which a baby is expelled from the uterus during childbirth; delivery.

See CHILDBIRTH.

labyrinthitis

A common name for OTITIS INTERNA.

lacrimation

The normal production and discharge of tears. The term is also sometimes used to imply excessive tear production.

Tears wash the eyeball constantly—removing dust, microorganisms and other particles. The composition of tears resembles blood plasma, but also contains an enzyme capable of killing many types of bacteria.

Tears are produced by the lacrimal glands, situated in the outer part of each upper eyelid. They flow over the eyeball to the inner part of each lower eyelid. From here they drain through tiny openings (the lacrimal canaliculi) into the lacrimal sac, which in turn drains through the "nasolacrimal" duct to the nose.

Excessive production of tears may be caused by emotional factors as well as by any condition which irritates the surface of the eyeball—such as conjunctivitis, foreign bodies, or irritant chemicals.

Tear production may appear to be excessive when the drainage apparatus is blocked—the tears spill over to run down the cheek (a condition known as "epiphora"). Blockage is commonly due to infection, but it may also occur from birth due to a failure of development of the drainage apparatus or may be due to a stone in the duct. Epiphora may be caused by paralysis or an outward turning of the lower lid, which prevents normal drainage.

Blocked ducts may be treated by syringing, antibiotics and eyedrops. Surgery is sometimes required; as a last resort, the production of tears may be reduced by injecting alcohol into the lacrimal gland.

Lacrimation is decreased in certain rare conditions. Damage to the surface of the eye may be avoided in such cases by the use of "artificial tear" eyedrops.

lactation

The production and secretion of milk by the female breasts.

See BREAST FEEDING.

laparoscopy

Examination of the contents of the abdominal cavity with an instrument known as a laparoscope (or peritoneoscope).

The patient is commonly given general anesthesia for the examination. Gas (usually carbon dioxide) is introduced into the abdomen through a needle to distend the abdominal cavity and provide room for maneuver of the instrument. A small incision is then made through the abdominal wall below the navel and the laparoscope is inserted through it.

Laparoscopy was first widely used by gynecologists to examine the ovaries, Fallopian tubes and uterus. A good view of these organs can be obtained, often avoiding the need for exploratory surgery. Minor operations can be performed through the laparoscope with special instruments. Female sterilization by cautery of the Fallopian tubes is often achieved in this way.

The laparoscope can be used to examine other abdominal organs—such as the liver, gallbladder and appendix—but the views obtained are often less complete than those of the reproductive organs.

Laparoscopy is relatively safe and has few complications. The minor wound heals rapidly, although the necessary introduction of gas may lead to mild abdominal distension and discomfort for a day or two.

See also LAPAROTOMY.

laparotomy

Any surgical operation in which an incision is made into the abdominal cavity.

Laparotomy may be performed in order to expose for operation any of the organs within the abdomen (stomach, gallbladder, colon, etc.) or for inspection of the abdominal contents (an "exploratory laparotomy"). Exploratory laparotomy is sometimes required to determine the nature of lumps felt in the abdomen, to inspect a suspected tumor and assess whether or not it is operable, and occasionally to seek the cause of an unexplained fever. Modern diagnostic techniques have made exploratory laparotomy a less common procedure than in the past.

See also LAPAROSCOPY.

laryngectomy

Surgical removal of the larynx, performed especially in cases of advanced cancer.

The larynx ("voice-box") is situated in the throat between the pharynx and the trachea. Laryngectomy destroys the power of normal speech, although following this procedure many patients can be taught "esophageal speech." The patient swallows air and then belches it up from the esophagus, moving his lips and tongue at the same time to form words. Artificial "voice-boxes," implanted in place of the removed larynx, have also been fairly successful in restoring speech.

LARYNX

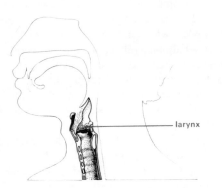

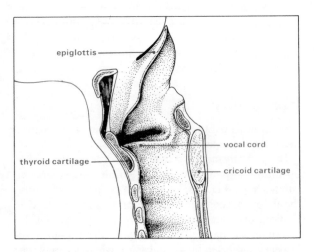

The larynx is the voice-box in the throat: it is an arrangement of cartilages which are connected by ligaments and muscles. Movements of the cartilages sets the tension in the vocal cords and this determines the pitch of the voice.

laryngitis

Inflammation of the larynx, especially the vocal cords, producing huskiness and weakness of the voice.

Acute laryngitis is caused by an infection (usually influenza or another virus) and often occurs in association with inflammation of the throat (pharyngitis) or tonsillitis. It usually causes a harsh dry cough; in young children, it may cause obstructed noisy breathing and CROUP, generally, a complication of a virus or bacterial infection of the upper respiratory tract. As in most infections, the patient has a fever and feels unwell.

Humidified oxygen treatment may be necessary in very young children; steam inhalation may also help to relieve symptoms. A cough suppressant such as codeine may control the dry cough. Antibiotics are often prescribed, but are usually indicated only in the minority of cases where the infection is bacterial. Acute laryngitis commonly resolves spontaneously within a few days.

Chronic laryngitis most often results from overuse or abuse of the voice and is common in preachers, actors, politicians and singers; it is aggravated by smoking. Treatment is absolute rest of the voice for a few days. Rarely, chronic laryngitis may be due to infection with tuberculosis, and the symptoms may also be due to a tumor on the vocal cords. Anyone with persistent change or weakness of the voice should be seen by a laryngologist.

Lassa fever

A serious viral disease, first reported from Lassa, Nigeria in 1969.

The virus is highly contagious and virulent. It can be transmitted to man from domestic rats (the natural host of the virus) and close personal contact with an infected patient. Airborne spread also occurs and infected patients must be treated in isolation.

The symptoms are quite variable. The fever sometimes takes several days to develop and early symptoms may include headache, backache, nausea and vomiting, cough, sore throat, abdominal pain and diarrhea. Examination usually shows inflammation of the throat and a variable range of other abnormalities. Laboratory tests often show a bleeding tendency and the virus can be isolated and identified from blood and other tissue fluids.

Most patients with Lassa fever die without treatment. A specific antiserum offers the best chance of cure and is available in limited supply from centers around the world. Intensive supportive treatment is also essential. Strict "barrier nursing" is necessary to protect doctors and nurses dealing with patients because no prophylactic vaccines or drugs are available.

As of early 1978, no cases of Lassa fever were contracted in the U.S., but rapid air travel makes its transmission by travelers from West Africa a real risk. All such travelers who develop a fever within 17 days (the longest known incubation period for the disease) after leaving the region should seek urgent medical attention.

lead poisoning

Lead may cause acute poisoning when someone swallows a relatively large amount of the metal or one of its compounds; but more commonly symptoms are due to chronic poisoning, since lead acts as a cumulative poison. Lead is not readily excreted in the urine or feces, so that anyone who regularly absorbs even traces of the metal slowly builds up the lead content of the body.

Lead poisoning occurs when water supplies are contaminated—and soft water will dissolve enough of the metal out of lead water pipes to cause problems. It is also common in ghetto areas, where buildings are still covered in lead-containing paints, and the dust from flaking paint work is swallowed, especially by children. Poisoning sometimes occurs from the use of lead-glazed pottery when used to store acidic fluids such as wine or hard cider. Pollution from industrial plants such as smelters may cause lead poisoning in communities around them. The extent of lead pollution from motor vehicle exhausts is disputed, but persons working in close contact with vehicles—traffic policemen, for example—have been shown to have raised blood levels of lead.

In adults mild lead poisoning causes anemia. More severe poisoning may cause cramping pains, especially in the intestines (*lead colic*), discoloration of the gums, and damage to the nerves causing weakness of the muscles, especially in the forearm. This weakness typically affects the muscles controlling the wrist, in which case it is known as "wrist-drop."

In children lead poisoning may cause mental irritability and (in severe cases) mental retardation, convulsions, and eventually death. There is medical disagreement about the effects on children's mental development of *minimal* degrees of lead poisoning: some authorities claim that the lead pollution from paint, vehicle exhausts and industry in inner city areas contributes to the poor intellectual performance of ghetto children (see also PICA).

Once suspected, lead poisoning is diagnosed by laboratory tests on the blood. Treatment—apart from prevention of further exposure—depends on removal of the lead from the body by *chelating agents*—drugs, such as calcium sodium edetate, which become chemically bound to the lead to form compounds which are readily excreted in the urine.

left ventricular failure

Failure of the left ventricle (left lower chamber) of the heart to pump blood adequately for the needs of the body.

Left ventricular failure (LVF) is most commonly caused by coronary artery disease, hypertension (high blood pressure), or disease of the heart valves.

The major symptom is breathlessness, caused by the pooling of blood and fluid in the lungs. At first the patient is short of breath only on exertion, but the condition gradually becomes worse. Shortness of breath is often worse when the patient is lying down and frightening attacks may occur during sleep. Ultimately, the untreated patient's lungs become so "waterlogged" that he can no longer breathe adequately and may lapse into a coma from lack of oxygen.

Acute or *severe LVF* requires urgent treatment with digoxin to aid heart function and diuretics to get rid of excess body fluid. The patient should sit up and receive oxygen. Other drugs are sometimes needed.

Chronic LVF requires treatment with the same drugs and an adjustment of the patient's life-style to suit his condition. Hypertension is controlled and diseased heart valves and blocked coronary arteries may require surgical treatment.

Effective treatment of hypertension has reduced the frequency of LVF and heart-valve disease associated with previous rheumatic fever is becoming far less common. Coronary artery disease, however, is frighteningly common, and statistics show that this disease is presently the major cause of LVF in the Western world.

legionnaire's disease

An acute infectious disease usually producing a form of pneumonia. It received its name from a large outbreak of the disease at an American Legion convention in Philadelphia in 1976, where 29 legionnaires died and scores of others were hospitalized. There had been reports of sporadic cases before that time, however; confirmation was made by the discovery of specific antibodies in blood samples that were stored for just such later tests.

The cause of the disease was at first a mystery, but it has now been identified as a previously unknown rod-shaped bacterium, initially referred to as *legionnaire's agent,* which can grow in the laboratory only under special conditions. The disease is more likely to affect those whose resistance to infection is already reduced. In the United States, one reservoir for the bacteria was found to be the stagnant water in cooling towers and commercial air-conditioning systems.

Symptoms, which are nonspecific but which first

resemble those of influenza, appear after an incubation period of two to ten days, usually with a high fever, malaise, muscle pains, headache and diarrhea. A severe and extensive pneumonia usually develops within a week and may produce symptoms like cough with blood-stained sputum or pain in the chest on coughing because of inflammation of the pleura. The diagnosis is made by finding the organism in specimens of the lung or from the pleural fluid or by detecting antibodies to legionnaire's agent in the blood. The disease has a high mortality rate. Most antibiotics are ineffective. So far, erythromycin seems to be the antibiotic of choice.

Leishmaniasis

A group of diseases caused by infection with protozoa (single-celled animals) of the genus *Leishmania*.

The organisms live within human body cells; they multiply until the cells ultimately burst, releasing a great number of new parasites to infect other cells. They are transmitted from one person to another by the bite of sandflies, in whose bodies further development and multiplication occurs. Animals such as dogs and rats act as "reservoirs" from which the sandflies can transmit the infection to man.

Visceral leishmaniasis ("kala-azar") occurs principally in India, the Near and Far East, around the Mediterranean, and in parts of South America. It has an incubation period of two to six months. The symptoms are often vague. There is usually an irregular fever of long duration and the patient gradually becomes emaciated. The spleen and often the liver enlarge greatly, and blood tests show anemia and high levels of globulins in the blood. Victims are very susceptible to other infections, which may cause additional symptoms and dangers.

The majority of patients with kala-azar die for lack of treatment (usually within two years of onset), although treatment with special drugs can slowly cure up to 98% of patients.

Cutaneous leishmaniasis ("oriental sore") is less serious than visceral leishmaniasis. It occurs in many tropical and subtropical regions and in every country in Central and South America except Chile. The main symptom is dry or moist ulcers of the skin, which may last for many months before healing spontaneously. Secondary infection of the ulcers may require treatment.

American mucocutaneous leishmaniasis is confined to Central and South America. It is similar to cutaneous leishmaniasis, but also causes ulcers of the nose, mouth and pharynx. Severe disfigurement may result from widespread destruction of the tissues of the nose and mouth, so early treatment is required. American mucocutaneous leishmaniasis is more resistant to treatment than the other varieties are, and prolonged treatment with several drugs is very often required.

All types of leishmaniasis are common in the areas in which they occur. The diseases can best be prevented by control of the sandfly vectors and by the individual use of insect repellants to prevent their bites. Elimination of "reservoir animals" has also succeeded in some areas. There are no specific preventive measures.

lens

Any device which causes a beam of light to converge or diverge as it passes through.

The lens of the eye (*crystalline lens*) consists of elongated fibers enclosed in a transparent elastic capsule, suspended by a ligament behind the iris. The ligament is attached to the circular ciliary muscle. Contraction and relaxation of the muscles change the shape of the lens, so altering its focusing power; this is the mechanism that allows us to make a sharp image of objects at variable distances from the eye.

The lens becomes stiffer with age and the range of focusing decreases. Most people over the age of 45 need glasses with weak convex lenses for reading to compensate for this. The lens normally becomes slightly opaque from the age of 60 onward, but impaired vision due to opacity of the lens (CATARACT) may occur at any age.

A penetrating injury of the lens can cause opacity. The lens may also be dislocated from its ligament by external injury to the eye.

Manmade lenses of glass or plastic are used in the manufacture of glasses and contact lenses. They compensate for inadequacies in the focusing ability of the lens of the eye (*presbyopia*), an uneven curvature of the cornea or lens (*astigmatism*), or for long or short sight that is caused by abnormalities in the shape of the eyeball.

leprosy

A chronic but only mildly contagious disease caused by infection with bacteria of the species *Mycobacterium leprae*. Also known as Hansen's disease.

Leprosy occurs mainly in countries between the thirtieth parallels of latitude, but also in Japan, Korea, South China and South Africa. In the United States the disease occurs mainly in those states bordering the Gulf of Mexico and in Hawaii.

Leprosy damages the cooler tissues of the body: skin, superficial nerves, nose, pharynx, larynx and occasionally the eyes and testicles.

There are two main types of leprosy: lepromatous and tuberculoid.

In *lepromatous leprosy* the patient's resistance to infection is low. Many red painful swellings appear on the skin of the face and elsewhere. These harden and coalesce, causing the great disfigurement which has been feared and loathed since Biblical times. The patient has chronic ill-health; he rarely dies from leprosy itself, but death from a secondary infection is common.

In *tuberculoid leprosy* the patient's resistance is high. Unfortunately, his main reaction to the disease occurs in nerves. The "battle" itself causes numbness, tingling and loss of sensation in the areas these nerves supply. Deformities such as wrist-drop, foot-drop or claw-toes may result; the anesthetic areas may be painlessly damaged with ulceration and even the gradual disappearance of the ends of fingers and toes.

Tuberculoid leprosy is not contagious; even lepromatous sufferers are infectious only to those with whom they are in prolonged intimate contact. Contrary to popular belief, isolation of patients is unnecessary. The medical emphasis is now on early detection and treatment.

Leprosy is usually treated with dapsone, a relatively safe drug which may have to be taken for many years. Tuberculoid leprosy responds well, but lepromatous leprosy is not so predictable. Surgery may sometimes be required for some patients with leprosy to correct deformities.

leukemia

A progressive malignant disease (or cancer) of the white cells in the circulating blood and bone marrow. Proliferation of the cancerous cells crowds out the normal healthy white and red blood cells and blood platelets, causing anemia and bleeding disorders and lowering the natural defenses against infection.

Leukemia is still relatively rare, but has become somewhat more common over the past 50 years. Its causes are poorly understood. Exposure to ionizing radiation increases its incidence, but this cannot account for all cases. Viruses can cause leukemia in some animals, although there is no definite evidence of their role in man.

Leukemia is classified as *acute* (short course) or *chronic* (long course), as well as by the type of cells involved: *myeloid, lymphoid* (or *lymphatic*) and *monocytic.*

Acute leukemia occurs most commonly in children and, at any age, is commoner in males than females. Usually the onset of the disease is sudden, with fever, sore throat and often bleeding from the nose or mouth: it quickly becomes apparent that the patient is very ill. Examination of the blood and a bone marrow BIOPSY confirm the diagnosis.

Without treatment death usually occurs within a few days or weeks in all types of acute leukemia. Steady progress in treatment has occurred over the past 20

years, however. It is now possible for a remission of the disease to be induced in most patients, especially in children, by a combination of anticancer drugs and radiation therapy.

Many patients relapse after a period of remission, but further treatment may then be effective. Some patients may be permanently cured by modern treatment, and in the most common leukemia of childhood, *acute lymphoblastic leukemia,* the cure rate is now approaching 50% of all cases.

Chronic myeloid leukemia (CML) occurs most commonly in adult males. Its onset is much more gradual than that of acute leukemia. Symptoms include tiredness caused by anemia and abdominal discomfort associated with massive enlargement of the spleen. Diagnosis is again confirmed from the results of blood tests and a biopsy of the bone marrow. Busulfan is the main drug used for treatment. Patients with CML may survive for several years, but the disease often leads to fatal acute leukemia despite treatment.

Chronic lymphatic leukemia (CLL) occurs particularly in men of late middle age. Symptoms are similar to those of CML, but the spleen is not so large and there is a general enlargement of the lymph nodes. Treatment is with chlorambucil or cyclophosphamide and patients often survive in reasonable health for several years; a few patients have lived for 20 years or more from the time the disease was first diagnosed and treatment begun.

leukoderma

A patchy deficiency of pigmentation of the skin, the patches often being milk-white. Leukoderma is another name for VITILIGO.

leukodystrophy

A group of disorders characterized by progressive degeneration of the white matter of the brain. They are due to an inborn error of metabolism with a breakdown in the enzyme systems concerned with the metabolism of lipids (fats or fatlike substances) in the nerve cells.

There is progressive destruction of the protective and insulating myelin sheaths of the nerve fibers, which usually begins in the back part of the brain and spreads more or less symmetrically throughout the white matter of the cerebral hemispheres.

Some forms of leukodystrophy begin in early childhood; there are also late childhood forms, which usually confine the child to a wheelchair in adolescence.

The symptoms include dementia, paralysis, generalized fits, speech difficulties, disorganization of movement and mental deterioration. There is no known treatment.

leukoplakia

Abnormal thickening and whitening of the tongue, the lining of the mouth, the lips, or the genital area. Affected areas may be yellowish-white and leathery. The lesions may be precancerous. By the time pain is present a lesion is usually advanced.

Leukoplakia is thought to be often caused by chronic irritation in the mouth. This may be due to tobacco, highly seasoned food, alcoholic drinks, excessive heat, trauma, the use of a particularly strong dentifrice (flavored toothpastes and tooth powders), jagged teeth, or dentures. Possible predisposing factors include coexisting syphilis, lack of vitamin A, and gonadal (sex-gland) deficiencies; approximately 65% of cases occur in men.

The first step in treatment is to remove the cause of the irritation. Good oral hygiene should be established. Faulty dentures should be corrected or sharp teeth dealt with. A mild alkaline mouthwash, such as equal parts of water and aluminium hydroxide, four times daily may be useful.

Early thin leukoplakia which fails to respond to conservative measures should be removed completely after a BIOPSY has been obtained. Larger lesions may have to be surgically removed in more than one operation. Regular reexamination of treated areas is advisable in case there is a serious recurrence.

Leukoplakia can also occur in the vulvar or vaginal area in women and on the penis in men. Again conservative measures such as control of any irritating discharge may be sufficient to effect a cure.

leukorrhea

An abnormal whitish discharge from the vagina which may occur at any age. It affects many women at some time.

The amount of normal vaginal secretions varies among women and in the same woman during the menstrual cycle. Excess mucus production may occur normally during pregnancy, as a result of sexual and emotional stimulation, and at the time of ovulation. Secretions are also increased just before and after menstruation.

In leukorrhea the abnormal vaginal discharge may just be excessive or it may be purulent (pus-filled) as the result of an infection by *Trichomonas vaginalis* (a protozoan—see TRICHOMONIASIS), *Candida albicans* (thrush—see CANDIDA), or other pathogens. A purulent discharge may also be due to disease of the cervix or uterus, senile VAGINITIS, or the presence of pessaries or other foreign bodies.

In treatment, hygiene of the genital area is important. A vinegar douche may be helpful. Sulfonamide creams may combat bacterial infections and metronidazole in treating Trichomoniasis. Postmenopausal inflammation of the vagina is usually controlled by local estrogen applications.

leukotomy

Another word for LOBOTOMY.

libido

A drive usually associated with the sexual instinct—that is, for pleasure and the seeking out of a love object. In Jung's original sense of the term, the energy designated "libido" was of a general kind, and applied to any instinctive force.

Freud maintained that in early life instinctive satisfaction is largely obtained from the individual's own body. As development proceeds, instinctive satisfaction is obtained increasingly from without, and the libido is directed toward external objects.

In the early oral and anal craving stages, guilt feelings are said to be established. In the so-called phallic stage, satisfaction is concerned with the genital zone. In the final stage, complete "object-love" is said to be possible.

lice

Three kinds of lice infect man; infestation with lice is known as *pediculosis*. The louse itself is a small wingless flattened insect.

Pediculosis capitis is due to the head louse and affects the scalp, though sometimes involves the eyebrows, eyelashes and beard. Infestation is particularly common in children, especially girls. The lice feed on blood from the scalp and are transmitted by direct contact of hair and by items such as combs, towels and headgear. The bites cause severe persistent itching and the lesions may become infected. The glands of the neck may sometimes enlarge.

Adult lice may be seen particularly around the back of the head and behind the ears. The small ovoid eggs, or nits, are easier to detect, as they are firmly attached to hair shafts. These hatch in 3 to 14 days. They may be removed with a nit comb and the scalp should be treated with benzyl benzoate, gamma benzene hexachloride, or malathion. Members of the same household should also be examined for infestation.

Pediculosis corporis is due to the body louse, which primarily inhabits the seams of clothing worn next to the skin and feeds on the skin. Under good hygienic conditions it is uncommon. The bites of the lice are seen as small red marks and itching leads to severe scratch marks. There may be secondary bacterial infection. Lesions are especially common on the shoulders,

HUMAN LOUSE

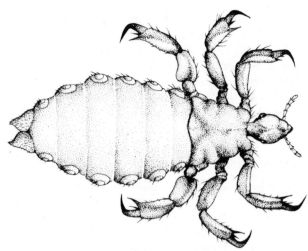

Human lice (length 2–5mm) are small, wingless insects which spend their whole existence on man. They lay their eggs on hair, and spread from person to person by direct contact. The species of louse pictured above lives in hair or underwear and causes itching. More importantly, it transmits the microorganism which causes typhus.

buttocks and abdomen. Both the parasites and nits are easily found in clothing.

Laundering and hot ironing of seams will kill the lice. The skin should be rubbed with gamma benzene hexachloride. Lotions may soothe inflammation.

Nits remain viable in clothing for as long as one month, hatching when they are reexposed to body heat. Dissemination of lice occurs through contact with infested persons, clothing, or bedding.

Pediculosis pubis is caused by the crab louse, which invades the area of the genitals and anus and sometimes other hair regions. Infestation may be venereal or acquired from clothing, bedclothes, or toilet seats. Severe irritation, with scratch marks, occurs. Application of benzyl benzoate or gamma benzene hexachloride is an effective treatment. However, prolonged use of such chemicals should be avoided.

Lice are known to transmit typhus fever, relapsing fever and trench fever, but these infections are rare.

lichen planus

A fairly common benign inflammatory disease of the skin and the lining of the mouth, which often gives rise to itching. There are small discrete raised areas of skin which at times coalesce into rough scaly patches. The raised areas are angular and have a flat shiny surface of pink or violet hue.

Children are rarely affected. Certain drugs may produce an identical eruption. The initial attack persists for weeks or months and may recur intermittently.

The condition frequently affects the wrists, arms, legs and trunk, but is rarely seen on the face. Occasionally the lesions are generalized.

The cause of the disease is unknown. Sedation may be necessary in severe cases, but usually all that is required is the application of a soothing lotion. Hydrocortisone ointment may be administered.

lipodystrophy

A disturbance of fat metabolism in which the subcutaneous fat disappears over some regions of the body, but is unaffected in others.

In progressive lipodystrophy the loss of fat is confined to the upper part of the body above the pelvis. This is a rare disease of unknown origin in which the loss of fat occurs over time and is eventually complete. The subcutaneous fat of the buttocks and lower limbs is unaffected or may be increased. The general health of the patient remains unimpaired. There may be psychological disturbances resulting from the patient's abnormal appearance.

About 80% of cases are female. The onset tends to be early in life—in about half of all cases before the age of 10, and in about three-quarters before the age of 20.

Two endocrine abnormalities have been observed in a significant proportion of cases—HYPOTHYROIDISM and either established DIABETES MELLITUS or a high blood sugar level.

The loss of fat from the face, neck, upper limbs and trunk gives a superficial appearance of emaciation, but closer examination reveals the muscles to be normal in size. Occasionally cases are seen where the fat has left the lower limbs and is normal on the upper part of the body.

There is no treatment for lipodystrophy. Once established, the condition remains more or less stationary, although the life expectation is unaffected.

Localized lipodystrophy may occur in some diabetics where there is loss of fat at the site of repeated insulin injections.

lipoma

A soft round swelling or tumor composed of fat cells, occurring in the dermis or subcutaneous tissue. The fat tissue is enclosed in a fibrous capsule. Usually solitary, but sometimes multiple, lipomas vary in size from minute growths to huge masses weighing several pounds.

They are occasionally associated with endocrine and neurological disturbances, and in these cases probably result from disordered fat metabolism. They may occur from early age to advanced age, but from 40–50%

appear between the ages of 30 and 40, when the body begins to accumulate excess fat—at which time the incidence of these benign tumors is about twice as high in women as in men.

The majority occur on the neck, back, shoulders and abdominal wall; they are seen only rarely on the face, scalp, hands and feet. As a rule such lumps cause few symptoms, but in areas such as the inner surfaces of the thighs they may form pendulous masses.

Lipomas may also be associated with muscles or the larger joints. Internal lipomas, on the intestine for instance, are relatively uncommon.

Microscopically, a typical lipoma is similar to normal fat tissue. As lipomas usually expand without infiltrating adjacent areas, they are easily removed and seldom recur.

liposarcoma

An extremely uncommon malignant tumor composed of mutant fat cells. Liposarcomas rarely arise from lipomas. Unlike lipomas, they arise primarily in deeper structures and have a predilection for certain sites—particularly the thigh, leg and buttock.

Examples of liposarcomas have been recorded in children but they are uncommon in patients under the age of 20 and arise mainly in middle and later life. The frequency in males and females is about equal. Beginning as inconspicuous swellings, they have usually attained an appreciable size before they are diagnosed and treated. Treatment involves surgical removal of the tumor, including removal of sufficient adjacent tissue to discourage recurrence.

lithotomy

The removal of a stone, usually a bladder stone, through an operative incision. Stones (see CALCULUS) may form in the bladder or may enlarge there after being passed from the kidney. The main symptoms are pain, frequent urination and blood in the urine. An x ray usually reveals the presence of the stone. It is removed by the introduction of a crushing instrument via the urethra, or, if too large and hard, by lithotomy—surgical incision into the bladder above the pubis.

The word also describes a position—the *lithotomy position*. The patient lies on the back with the thighs raised and the knees supported and held apart. The position is employed during childbirth, for gynecological procedures, and in operations on the rectum or anus.

livedo

A mottled discoloration of the skin. In *livedo reticularis* (or *marble skin*) there is a blue purplish appearance seen as a constant phenomenon or upon exposure of the skin to cold air.

It is a disorder involving spasm of an artery and is seen most frequently in a "fish net" pattern of the skin on the arms, legs, or trunk. The condition occurs both as a primary disorder and as secondary to an underlying disease.

The condition is benign: those who suffer from it should avoid the cold, and as far as possible avoid emotional stress.

liver disease

In order to understand the consequences of liver disease, it is first necessary to appreciate some of the normal functions of the organ—the largest in the body. They may be considered under three main headings: blood, food, and removal of "poisons."

Red blood cells stay in the circulation for 120 days on average and are then removed by the spleen and other tissues. Most of the HEMOGLOBIN from these cells is converted into bilirubin, which is then transported to the liver. Enzymes in the liver cells modify the chemical structure of bilirubin to make it soluble in water—a process called "conjugation." The conjugated bilirubin is secreted into the bile ducts and eventually passes to the intestines. Here bacteria convert the bilirubin into a number of pigments which form the coloring matter of feces.

The total level of bilirubin in the blood does not normally exceed 10 milligrams per liter; if this concentration doubles for any reason, bilirubin is deposited in the skin and whites of the eyes to produce the characteristic yellow appearance of JAUNDICE. There are numerous causes of jaundice and they do not all originate in the liver itself. Even the purely hepatic (liver) causes interfere with the processing of bilirubin at different stages. *Gilbert's disease* is a common harmless condition which runs in families and is marked by a mild, fluctuating jaundice resulting from the inefficient transportation of bilirubin into the liver cells. Jaundice is almost universally found in newborn babies because their conjugating enzymes have a limited capacity.

HEPATITIS, inflammation of the liver due to viruses, alcohol, or drugs, reduces the number of functioning liver cells and blocks the bile ducts by swelling of the tissues.

The other functions of the liver concerned with blood are the manufacture of plasma proteins (particularly albumin) and factors which are necessary for blood clotting. Both these processes fail in chronic liver diseases such as CIRRHOSIS, when large numbers of cells have been destroyed. The major consequences of these failures are ASCITES (a collection of free fluid in the

THE LIVER

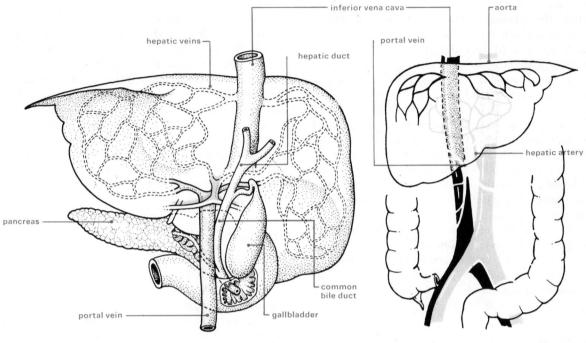

POSTERIOR VIEW OF THE LIVER

BLOOD SUPPLY OF THE LIVER

The liver develops in the embryo as an outgrowth of the intestine and always retains a close link with the digestive system. The portal vein drains blood from the intestine into the liver, where nutrients are utilized and toxic products removed. The liver also secretes bile which is then stored in the gallbladder; after a meal the gallbladder contracts, squeezing bile into the duodenum where it helps to absorb fats.

abdominal cavity) and easy bruising.

The portal vein carries nutrients from their sites of absorption in the small intestine to the liver, where they are extensively processed according to the body's needs. Carbohydrates and other foods are converted into glycogen by the liver. Glycogen is stored in many body cells and can be broken down into glucose (sugar) when energy is needed. GLYCOGEN STORAGE DISEASES are rare conditions in which glycogen stored in the liver or muscles cannot be broken down into glucose. Although the liver controls the level of glucose in the blood, significant disturbances are found only in severe liver disease. This is also true for protein handling—in patients with liver failure the buildup of ammonia and amino acids damages the brain and is an important cause of COMA.

Cirrhosis not only leads to the death of many liver cells but also distorts the "architecture" of the organ, blocking the blood flow through it. This leads to back pressure down the portal vein—*portal hypertension*—and the blood is forced to take alternative routes. The easiest but potentially most dangerous alternative is through the veins around the esophagus. These become dilated and can eventually burst, leading to massive vomiting of blood (HEMATEMESIS). Drastic measures then have to be taken, and if the patient survives there is a great risk of brain damage.

The final major role of the liver is the removal of toxic substances from the blood. As mentioned above, some toxins (for example, ammonia) are derived from proteins in the diet; drugs are the other important group. The liver deals with many drugs in the way it does with bilirubin: it conjugates them into water-soluble substances which can be excreted in the urine. In patients with liver disease, drug therapy presents major problems and common drugs like diuretics (given to reduce the fluid load in ascites) can precipitate coma. Diets too must be strictly controlled with limited amounts of naturally salty foods and no added salt, and protein and fluid restrictions.

Primary cancer of the liver, HEPATOMA, is the most common cancer in Africa and the Orient, but it is relatively rare elsewhere.

lobotomy

A neurosurgical operation (one form of PSYCHOSURGERY) in which association tracts between the prefrontal part of the cerebral cortex and the rest of the brain are destroyed. Also known as *leukotomy*.

The most obvious difference between a monkey's brain and a man's brain is the size of the frontal lobes, but it has proved very difficult to ascribe precise functions to the large areas of brain tissue lying in front of the motor area. Over the years it was noticed that those who had suffered brain injury involving the frontal part of the brain were liable to show less anxiety than normal, and paid less attention to normal social restraints, and in 1935 the Portuguese neurosurgeon Egaz Moniz introduced the operation of lobotomy in cases of extreme anxiety or emotional tension. But the consequent popularity of the operation, which was radical and relatively crude, led to many poor results and indeed tragedies.

With the advent of modern drugs effective in the treatment of anxiety, tension and other psychiatric states, the operation of lobotomy fell into disrepute. It is now performed only as a last resort in cases of intolerable suffering. Such operations are still somewhat unpredictable in their results.

lockjaw

A common name for TETANUS.

lumbago

An old-fashioned term used to describe an acute and severe pain felt in the lower part of the back for which no definite cause can be found. Treatment should be rest in bed, on a hard mattress, analgesics (painkillers, such as aspirin), and the local application of heat.

lung diseases

See PULMONARY DISEASES.

lupus erythematosus

A chronic skin disease, thought to be associated with an immunological disturbance, which manifests itself in two ways: one is confined to the mucous membranes and the skin, the other is a systemic disorder which may affect the skin.

Discoid lupus erythematosus affects patients of middle age, more commonly women than men. It starts as a red patch on the face or on other skin exposed to light, which slowly spreads to become a well-defined disk covered by gray scales. As over months or years the lesions spread the center atrophies and as it scars small blood vessels become prominent (TELANGIECTASIA). It seems that sunlight is an important factor in the development of the disease, and it is therefore important that patients should avoid direct exposure to the sun and use a barrier cream.

About 10% of those affected also develop *systemic lupus erythematosus (SLE)*—also known as *disseminated lupus erythematosus*—a progressive and potentially serious disease. It can affect nearly every organ in the body. Among the complications that may be seen are inflammation of the membrane lining the heart and the smooth membranous sac enveloping the heart, pleurisy, kidney lesions and disorders of the central nervous system.

Treatment recommended is the use of antimalarial drugs by mouth, such as quinacrine or chloroquine, but regular medical supervision is necessary because of toxic effects on the eyes.

lupus vulgaris

Tuberculosis of the skin. It is a slowly developing disease, fortunately now rare. When it does occur it often affects the face or neck. The tubercle bacillus invades the skin directly, or reaches it by spreading from underlying infected glands or joints, or via the lymphatics from a respiratory infection. It is more common in women than in men.

The shape of the lesion is always irregular and the surface may be covered with an adherent crust. The lesion may eventually ulcerate. The mucous membranes of the nose and mouth are frequently affected, and in these cases the ultimate effect (if the condition is left untreated) is serious deformity with scarring. The tongue when attacked has large painful fissures.

Antituberculosis drugs may have to be continued for many months.

lymphadenitis

Inflammation of lymph nodes in the LYMPHATIC SYSTEM.

Acute inflammation of the nodes occurs when there is infection nearby; they may swell to three times their normal size and be very painful. The patient may suffer chills and fever, but can be successfully treated with antibiotics.

Chronic lymphadenitis occurs when there is prolonged or repeated infection of the area from which lymph drains into the node: for example, chronic tonsillar or dental infection may cause chronic lymphadenitis of the neck "glands" and repeated infections of the foot may lead to lymphadenitis of the nodes in the groin. The nodes enlarge but may not be painful or cause fever. Treatment is directed at the chronic or repeated infection.

Sometimes lymphadenitis is caused by direct infection of the lymph nodes themselves, rather than by spread of infection from another site. Among the many conditions that can infect lymph nodes are tuberculosis, typhoid, infectious mononucleosis, measles and several parasitic diseases.

lymphangioma

A malformation—not cancerous—of the lymphatic vessels. It is usually present from birth.

The severity of a lymphangioma ranges from a simple dilatation of a lymph vessel to the formation of groups of thick-walled cysts in the skin. The most common sites are the neck and the limbs.

Diffuse lymphangiomas in the tongue cause *macroglossia* (large tongue) and in the lip *macrocheilia* (large lips). In the limbs they can cause a form of ELEPHANTIASIS (a gross swelling of the tissues of the lower extremities caused by obstruction of the lymphatic vessels).

Treatment of lymphangiomas is difficult. Although they are not malignant they do tend to infiltrate other structures and to recur after surgical removal.

In general, however, lymphangiomas are only a cosmetic problem. They can be more dangerous when they are large and cystic because there is a risk of sudden hemorrhage into the cyst (which would cause it to enlarge and perhaps compress a vital organ or structure, for example, the windpipe).

lymphangitis

Inflammation of a vessel in the LYMPHATIC SYSTEM.

It is caused by the spread of infection from the main site to the lymphatic vessels. Inflamed vessels may throb painfully; in many cases the patient also has a fever and chills. The infection can spread rapidly. Antibiotics are given to avoid the possibility of SEPTICEMIA.

lymphatic system

The vast network of vessels throughout the body (similar to the blood vessels) which transports a watery fluid known as *lymph*.

Lymph is formed from the clear fluid that bathes all tissues of the body and contains material that is too large to enter the blood capillaries. It also carries cells—LYMPHOCYTES—and other substances concerned with the IMMUNE SYSTEM.

The lymphatic system is a network of vessels which drain most of the body's tissues and return excess fluid from between the cells back to the bloodstream. During this journey the lymph fluid filters through lymph nodes, where any foreign particles such as bacteria are trapped.

THE LYMPHATIC SYSTEM

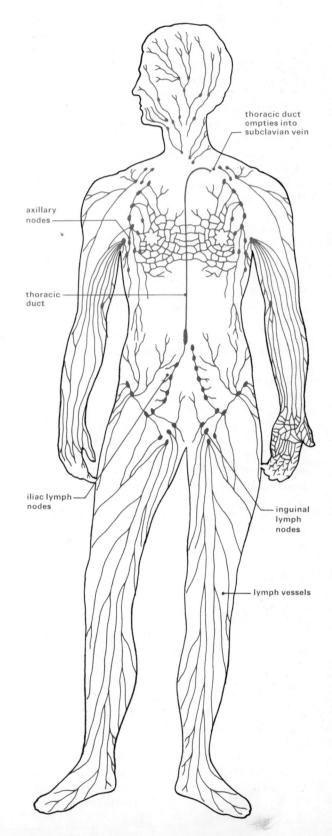

thoracic duct empties into subclavian vein

axillary nodes

thoracic duct

iliac lymph nodes

inguinal lymph nodes

lymph vessels

Tiny lymphatic vessels are found in all organs except the heart and brain. Protein, bacteria and other foreign particles enter the lymphatics, which unite to form larger vessels. Like veins, lymphatic vessels have valves to prevent a backflow of fluid. If for any reason a lymphatic vessel becomes obstructed, the buildup of lymph is called LYMPHEDEMA.

Eventually all the lymphatics drain their contents into two large ducts; from there the lymph reenters the blood circulation through veins at the base of the neck.

Lymphatics draining the small intestine (known as *lacteals*) have a function apart from clearing debris and defending the body: fat is absorbed from the small intestine into the lacteals and so eventually into the bloodstream.

The lymphatic system is interrupted at intervals by groups of glands known as *lymph nodes,* which have two main functions: (1) they have a role in immunity, producing both lymphocytes (defensive white blood cells) and antibodies; and (2) they also act as a second line of defense against infection by bacteria, filtering off and destroying any which bypass the inflammatory response at the site of infection. In the case of cancer cells, the lymph nodes act as a temporary but only partially effective barrier to metastasis (spread of cancer cells from one site to another—see CANCER).

When a lymph node is stimulated into activity, for example by infection, it swells and becomes painful. This swelling may be noticeable even before the infection itself is apparent (swelling of the "glands" in the neck during a throat infection is a common experience).

Apart from those in the back and sides of the neck, the main groups of lymph nodes are in the armpits and groin; either of these groups may be felt to swell and be painful during a limb infection. Other lymph nodes lie at the base of the lungs and around large veins in the abdomen and pelvis.

The tonsils and spleen are also composed of lymphatic tissue and are usually regarded as part of the lymphatic system.

lymphedema

Swelling of a limb, or limbs, caused by blockage of the flow of lymph through the vessels of the LYMPHATIC SYSTEM.

Initially the swollen limb "pits," that is, when pressed with a finger the depression remains—a finding known as *pitting edema.* Later the limb becomes hard and nonpitting and the skin and underlying tissues become thickened.

The condition is occasionally due to congenital abnormalities of the lymphatic vessels. In other cases the blockage of lymph flow is due to inflamed or fibrosed lymph nodes or vessels or to the removal of lymphatics

as part of the treatment of cancer. The lymphatics may also be blocked by parasites (as in some forms of ELEPHANTIASIS). While some relief may be given by elevation of the limb and the use of elastic bandaging or stockings, surgical removal of the thickened tissue from below the skin is the only curative procedure.

lymphocyte

A type of white blood cell. Between 20 and 50% of white blood cells in an adult are lymphocytes.

Lymphocytes play an important role in immunity, in producing antibodies and in recognizing "foreign" tissue. The so-called *B lymphocytes* produce antibodies which they release into the blood. The *T lymphocytes,* on the other hand, are processed in children by the thymus gland; they carry antibodies on their own surface and produce cellular immunity—for instance, in the rejection of transplants.

Large numbers of lymphocytes are found in patients with a chronic infection, both in the blood and commonly at the site of the infection. There may also be excessive numbers of these white cells in LEUKEMIA, but in such cases immunity is depressed because the lymphocytes are abnormal.

In certain rare disorders the number of lymphocytes is decreased, leading to poor immunity.

Normally lymphocytes are produced in the lymphoid tissues of the body (lymph nodes, spleen and tonsils); to a lesser extent they are also produced in the bone marrow.

lymphogranuloma venereum

A sexually transmitted disease caused by virus-like organisms of the genus *Chlamydia*. It is quite rare.

After infection, through sexual contact, there is an incubation period of 5 to 21 days. A blister then forms on the genital area, often unnoticed. It disappears and the infection spreads to the lymph nodes—which enlarge, soften and eventually break down. In women and in homosexual men the rectum may become inflamed. Fistulas (abnormal openings) may form and the rectum and anus may be permanently narrowed.

Elsewhere in the body the infection leads to fever, joint pains, skin eruptions and conjunctivitis.

Early treatment with an appropriate antibiotic (usually tetracycline) cures the condition and prevents the later complications. Pain over the enlarged lymph nodes can be relieved by hot compresses and analgesics.

lymphoma

A cancer of the lymphoid tissue.

There are several types of varying degrees of

malignancy, which can be distinguished by microscopic examination of a sample of tissue.

A technique known as *lymphangiography* may be used to detect the positioning and spread of a lymphoma. Radiopaque material is injected into a lymphatic vessel, which can then be seen on an x ray together with any abnormalities.

Treatment of a lymphoma depends on its type, but is based on the usual anticancer measures of radiotherapy, chemotherapy and surgery.

Common forms of lymphoma are HODGKIN'S DISEASE and LYMPHOSARCOMA.

See also CANCER, LYMPHATIC SYSTEM.

lymphosarcoma

A type of lymphoma (cancer of the LYMPHATIC SYSTEM) mainly affecting middle-aged people and causing symptoms similar to chronic LEUKEMIA.

A lymphosarcoma may arise in any lymph node. Since the cancer spreads rapidly, by the time it is detected more than one site is usually involved. In later stages of the disease, malignant cells spill over into the bloodstream where they are found in large numbers—resembling the blood pattern of chronic lymphatic leukemia. The symptoms are similar: fatigue and loss of energy due to ANEMIA, and abdominal discomfort from the enlarged liver and spleen.

Treatment of a lymphosarcoma is by radiotherapy and chemotherapy, and remissions of the disease often last for several years.

BURKITT'S LYMPHOMA is a type of lymphosarcoma affecting children in tropical countries. There is very strong evidence to suggest that this cancer is caused by a virus (the Epstein-Barr virus which causes infectious mononucleosis). Treatment with a combination of anticancer drugs results in cure in as many as 70–80% of cases.

M

malabsorption

A term applied to a number of conditions in which normal absorption of nutrients is impaired. The consequences are disorders of the body due to deficiencies of substances necessary for health, and disturbed function of the intestines.

Failure to absorb fat from the intestine produces offensive pale stools larger than normal which tend to float in water; sometimes there is diarrhea with colic, sometimes constipation. If the malady involves failure to absorb carbohydrates, the abdomen becomes enlarged and uncomfortable and there is a frothy diarrhea. Various deficiencies may show themselves. In children and infants there is failure to thrive, and perhaps loss of weight.

The patients·are weak and may be anemic. Vitamins are lost: the consequence may be RICKETS, TETANY and a low level of calcium in the blood, or a dry skin and sparse hair, sore mouth and tongue, and various neurological signs. If there is a loss of water and salts there may be a low blood pressure, cramps, thirst and excessive formation of urine, with weakness and abnormalities of sensation.

Malabsorption occurs in many diseases; they range from conditions which block the lymphatic vessels draining the intestine to the operative removal of parts of the intestine or stomach; but the best known are CELIAC DISEASE, TROPICAL SPRUE, CROHN'S DISEASE, liver disease, chronic enteritis, infestation by worms, and the atrophy (wasting away) of the stomach that is part of pernicious ANEMIA. Diseases of the gallbladder and pancreas may produce malabsorption syndromes, as may the effects of radiation. In each case, treatment is directed at the underlying disease.

malaria

A parasitic infection occurring mainly in the tropics and subtropics.

Malaria is caused by a protozoan parasite of the genus *Plasmodium,* which requires two different hosts during its life cycle: man and mosquito. It is transmitted from man to man by the bite of an infected mosquito. The mosquito sucks blood from an infected person, taking in the parasite—which can then continue its life cycle within the mosquito. Later, when the mosquito bites another human, the parasites pass in with the insect's saliva.

Once inside man, the parasites continue to develop in the liver. From there they reenter the bloodstream and multiply inside red blood cells, causing them to rupture within two or three days. This rupture of the red cells is responsible for the characteristic chills, fever and sweating of malaria. Parasites released into the bloodstream when the cells rupture can enter other red cells, and the life cycle is repeated.

Four species of *Plasmodium* cause human malaria. Three of them (*P. vivax, P. falciparum* and *P. ovale*) repeat the cycle every 48 hours and produce symptoms every third day (tertian malaria); *P. malariae* repeats the cycle every 72 hours (quartan malaria).

Among other consequences of the parasitic infestation and rupture of blood cells are anemia, jaundice, an enlarged spleen, congestion of blood vessels in the brain, and kidney failure.

MALARIA

LIFE HISTORY OF *Plasmodium* PARASITE

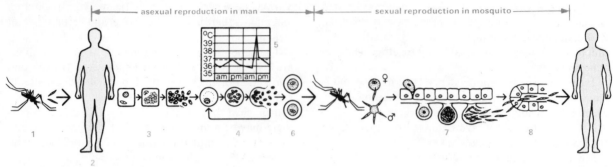

A *female Anopheles mosquito (1) injects
Plasmodium parasites into man (2); they develop
in the liver (3) before reproducing asexually
inside red blood cells (4). These cells periodically
burst, releasing parasites which attack more red
cells, causing fever (5). Some red cells become
filled with sexual forms (6) which reproduce in
the stomach of a mosquito (7) after it has sucked
blood from the man. Infective forms then migrate
to the mosquito's salivary glands (8), ready to
enter the next victim when it bites.*

Quinine was the classic antimalarial drug, but it has
been largely superseded by less toxic drugs such as
chloroquine and primaquine. Other drugs, such as
proguanil and pyrimethamine, can protect against
malaria if taken for two weeks before entering a
malarious area and continued for a month after leaving
it. The inhabitants of malarious regions need to take
regular doses of drugs to protect themselves against the
infection.

At a public health level, eradication of malaria is best
attempted by attacking the mosquito in order to break
the life cycle of the parasites. Partial success has been
achieved by draining swamps and other breeding places
and by the use of special insecticides (unfortunately,
mosquitoes tend to develop resistance to these chemical
agents). Despite prolonged efforts by the World Health
Organization malaria is still a major public health
problem in Africa and Asia.

Malaria may be seen in temperate areas since it can
develop in a traveler after his return from the tropics.
Symptoms may be delayed for weeks or even months.
The parasite can also be transmitted directly from man
to man by the transfusion of contaminated blood.

malignancy

The tendency of a disease to progress relentlessly to a
fatal end. The term is generally used to refer to cancers
as distinct from benign tumors—which, though they
may grow in size, do not invade surrounding tissue,
nor produce "seedlings" which can travel in the circulation and set up secondary growths (*metastases*).

Microscopically, malignant tumors differ from
benign tumors in that their structure is atypical and does
not closely resemble their tissue of origin. There are
varying degrees of imperfect differentiation of tissue; the
poorer the differentiation, the more malignant the
tumor.

The term may also be used to refer to the most
dangerous form of a disease, such as when MALARIA
caused by *Plasmodium falciparum* is called *malignant
tertian malaria* to distinguish it from the benign tertian
forms caused by *Plasmodium vivax* and *Plasmodium
ovale*. *Malignant hypertension* is a severe form of high
blood pressure that is rapidly progressive, usually
accompanied by extensive damage to the blood vessels.

See also CANCER.

malnutrition

The causes of malnutrition, or starvation, fall into two
basic groups: the first includes poverty, famine, natural
disasters and war; the second includes a number of
diseases such as neurological conditions in which the
patient cannot feed himself or cannot swallow food,
cancer, malabsorption syndrome, and psychological
disorders (see ANOREXIA NERVOSA).

The greatest cause of starvation is poverty, present in
all the countries of the world, even the most well-
developed; in less fortunate countries it is from time to
time exacerbated by famine due to the failure of crops.

One of the recognized weapons of war is blockade,
and now herbicides may be used to promote the failure
of crops in hostile lands in order to starve the enemy into
submission. But the last to be affected are the fighting
men, and war means starvation for the women, children
and aged.

A healthy man or woman can go without food for

MALNUTRITION

This child portrays the misery of malnutrition. Although an early case of kwashiorkor—protein deprivation—she displays several characteristic physical changes: muscle wasting, puffy face, protuberant belly and fineness of the hair. The bowed legs are a sign of rickets caused by vitamin D deficiency.

about two weeks with little effect except loss of weight, but he or she needs to have an adequate supply of water. The effects of prolonged undernutrition include swelling of the tissues (edema), most marked in the legs and sometimes in the abdomen, loss of weight and elasticity of the skin, low blood pressure, pulse and temperature, diarrhea, susceptibility to infection, anemia, apathy, and emotional instability.

Recovery depends on the restoration to normal of tissues which have become atrophic, particularly the tissues of the gut and the heart. Those with persisting diarrhea and a systolic blood pressure below 80 mm of mercury may die although there is a plentiful supply of food.

See also CACHEXIA, KWASHIORKOR, MARASMUS.

mammography

X-ray examination of the breast in the diagnosis of the cause of breast lumps; it is used as a screening test for BREAST CANCER.

A picture is obtained of the soft tissues of the breast in which any potentially cancerous areas may be seen. Mammography can detect cysts and tumors in the breast tissue while they are still too small to be readily palpated by a nurse or physician, so that it provides a means for the detection of early cancer.

Like any screening test, its cost has to be weighed against its accuracy, any potential dangers, and the value of detection. Tumors detected by mammography may be either benign or cancerous; further tests and often removal of the tumor may be needed before a firm diagnosis can be made. Breast cancer screening by mammography carries a very small risk since repeated x-ray examinations may themselves induce cancer. For that reason, current policy in the United States is for mammography to be used in screening only for women aged over 50 and for women in high-risk groups, such as those related to women who have had breast cancer. Studies such as the Health Insurance Plan project in New York have shown, however, that in these high-risk groups and in women over the age of 50 mammography can improve the detection rate and lower mortality from breast cancer.

mammoplasty

A cosmetic operation to enlarge or reduce the size of the breast or to restore its shape after a cancer operation.

Reduction mammoplasty consists of removal of tissue from the breasts when they are too large or heavy, followed by their cosmetic "reconstruction."

Augmentation mammoplasty is the opposite: enlargement of the breasts. Surgeons currently prefer to implant a sealed bag containing silicone or saline. The implant is placed into a pocket cut into the breast, and its size can be adjusted up or down after the operation. There is a small long-term risk of scarring and distortion of the shape of the breast, especially if the silicone leaks out of the implant. Mammoplasty is being used increasingly to restore the breast contours after surgical removal of a tumor by partial mastectomy. In such cases the surgeon usually excises most of the breast tissue, leaving the skin and if possible the nipple intact.

The volume of the breast may then be restored to normal either with a silicone implant or with a graft of fat or muscle taken from another part of the body. With such restorative surgery no form of artificial breast or padding is needed, and the fact that surgery has been performed may be unnoticeable even when the patient wears a bikini.

mania

A disordered mental state characterized by a mood change to excitement and elation. Often the mood swings between mania and profound depression—the *manic depressive psychosis.*

The sufferer becomes optimistic, overconfident and has a general feeling of euphoria. He becomes talkative yet flits from subject to subject and is easily distracted. He has little insight into his condition and will rarely admit that he is unwell.

The manic patient often gets into difficulties—for example, overspending, making rash promises or unwise business deals, or becoming violent when thwarted.

The severity of mania varies widely; in mild cases it is necessary to have an idea of the patient's previous personality to be sure of the diagnosis. Mild mania is known as *hypomania* and severe mania as *acute mania.* The extreme form is *delirious mania,* in which mental activity is so "high" that the patient's speech is incoherent and his constant restlessness and failure to sleep can lead to total exhaustion.

Acute mania is a medical emergency needing treatment with large doses of major tranquilizers such as chlorpromazine or haloperidol. The outlook for patients with recurrent attacks of mania (with or without depression) has been transformed by the discovery that regular treatment with *lithium salts* can prevent or reduce the severity of the episodes of mental abnormality. The dose has to be carefully adjusted to avoid toxic side effects (tremor, mental confusion and eventually coma); regular measurement of the blood content of lithium is an essential part of this type of treatment.

Mantoux test

A test for tuberculosis.

The test consists of the injection of tuberculin, a protein derived from the tubercle bacillus, or a purified protein derivative of tuberculin, PPD. If the patient is (or has been) infected with tuberculosis a positive reaction occurs at the site of the injection within 48 to 72 hours. The tuberculin—being a "foreign protein" recognized by the body of a person who has experienced TB—evokes a delayed immune response in the form of a raised, red, itchy swelling.

The reaction may also be positive in a person who has never been infected with TB but who has previously been immunized against the disease by an injection of BCG (BACILLE CALMETTE-GUÉRIN) vaccine. Since a positive reaction may be due to a symptomless infection in the past, it is of little diagnostic help; but a negative response is close to certain proof that the individual concerned has not had TB and has no immunity to it. False negative reactions do occur in persons in poor health and with diseases such as HODGKIN'S DISEASE which affect the body's immune responses.

maple syrup urine disease

An inherited error of metabolism.

As with other metabolic abnormalities the condition is rare, is due to an enzyme defect, and is characterized by excretion of a recognizable substance in the urine—in this case one with a characteristic odor that gives the disease its name.

The patient cannot cope with certain essential amino acids (the "building blocks" of protein); therefore, a special diet is necessary in which these amino acids are contained in the minimum possible quantities. Normal food, especially food rich in protein, cannot be eaten without the risk of severe neurological disease and mental retardation.

The special diet has to be given as early as possible in infancy—as soon as the disease is diagnosed; survival might then be expected for many years.

marasmus (starvation)

Gross undernutrition; the condition caused by a deficiency of both calories and protein.

There is a spectrum of effects of protein-calorie malnutrition: when both are in short supply the result is marasmus; when protein is deficient in a diet adequate in calories, the result is KWASHIORKOR.

Marasmus is most commonly seen in children in the first year of life in Third World countries. There is marked retardation of growth, extreme wasting of muscles and general debility. Although the child remains alert and hungry, there is a risk of long-term mental deficit.

Unlike kwashiorkor, there are no hair changes or swollen abdomen.

Apart from shortage of food, the condition may be caused by poor digestion and absorption (for example, in prematurity), cystic fibrosis, or through mental illness.

Adequate feeding reverses marasmus.

Marburg virus disease

A rare hemorrhagic viral disease first associated with vervet monkeys imported from Africa. Also known as *green monkey disease.*

Marburg virus disease was first identified in an outbreak in laboratory personnel in Germany and Yugoslavia in 1967. Seven people died in this outbreak and a further three in a second episode in Johannesburg. Subsequently there has been a widespread epidemic in Zaire and the Sudan. The first symptoms are fever, headache and muscular pain, followed by nausea, vomiting and diarrhea. Bleeding from the nose and other body orifices may occur. The incubation period is believed to be from 4 to 9 days and the mortality rate in known outbreaks has been about 30%. Transmission of the disease is usually from infected tissues or body fluids, but airborne transmission (by droplet spray from the breath of an infected person) is also suspected. Treatment consists of "barrier nursing" and the administration of serum from a surviving patient.

Marfan's syndrome

A relatively rare inherited disease of connective tissue, in which the patient grows extremely tall and thin and is subject to various other abnormalities.

In addition to the effects on the skeletal system, the main signs of the disease occur in the eyes (the lens often becomes dislocated and the retina may become detached from the underlying tissues). The cardiovascular system may also be affected, manifest especially by the development of a progressive weakness in the wall of the largest artery (aorta).

Patients have exceptionally long bones, including the bones of the hand; this gives rise to an appearance known as *arachnodactyly* ("spider fingers"). The skeletal deformities are the most obvious feature of the condition: long arms and legs, flat feet, a narrow and pointed skull, deformities of the chest and an abnormally wide degree of joint mobility.

Patients who survive to adulthood may pass the disease on to their children.

marijuana

See CANNABIS.

mastectomy

Surgical removal of a breast.

The traditional theory about the progression of BREAST CANCER has been that the tumor arises in a single site, and, at an indeterminate time later, spreads outside the breast to form metastatic deposits. The first metastatic spread is thought to occur via the lymphatic drainage to local lymph nodes in the armpit or beneath the sternum (breastbone). Later spread of cancer cells may be by means of the blood circulation, leading to metastases in the bone, brain and liver. Thus, the logical way to cure breast cancer is to remove the affected breast and any involved lymph nodes in a mastectomy operation.

Around the beginning of the 20th century, Halstead and Meyer independently described their versions of the mastectomy technique. Both employed a *radical* approach in which the breast, the underlying pectoral muscles and the lymph nodes in the corresponding armpit were removed en bloc. Many women found this

to be a mutilating operation; in addition, it produced problems of arm swelling and shoulder immobility. Nevertheless, radical mastectomy is unsurpassed in terms of the number of patients with early breast cancer who survive for five years after operation and has been the mainstay of operative treatment for 75 years.

Although radical mastectomy statistically seems to offer the best chance for survival in early breast cancer, it is only marginally better than other less extensive operations. For this reason and to spare the patient unnecessary psychological suffering, radical mastectomy has been practiced far less in the past few years. A modified radical mastectomy, in which the pectoral muscles and the lymph nodes highest in the armpit are spared, is now probably the most common operation used in the United States. Some surgeons have gone a step further and only perform a *simple mastectomy,* leaving all the lymph nodes in place. The argument advanced for this operation is that the lymph nodes are a powerful natural defense against cancer spread: opponents point out that lymph nodes are often involved when they feel normal and anyway will have to be constantly checked after surgery.

If the breast cancer has already formed distant metastases or large lymph node deposits, mastectomy alone is ineffective. Various combinations of hormones, drugs and radiation therapy are then added to the surgical treatment. Many surgeons now believe that combination therapy should be applied even in early cases because it is likely that microscopic metastases are already present.

MASTECTOMY

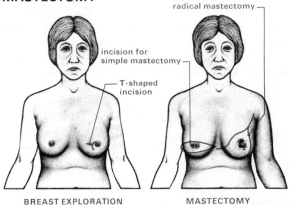

BREAST EXPLORATION   MASTECTOMY

There are many techniques employed in breast surgery. The picture on the left shows the small T-shaped cut used for exploring the nipple region so that any suspicious lumps can be removed and examined microscopically. The right hand figure illustrates two types of mastectomy used in the treatment of breast cancer.

mastitis

Mastitis strictly means inflammation of the breast and its most important manifestations occur in the lactating woman. In one type the woman may have a raised temperature and congested, painful breasts. There is no pus produced and the inflammation is hormonal rather than infective in origin.

By contrast, in *acute suppurative mastitis* the breast becomes infected with *Staphylococcus aureus* or (less commonly) *Streptococcus pyogenes*. The bacteria gain access to the breast either via the ducts or through a crack in the nipple. If appropriate antibiotic treatment is not instigated, an abscess may form, resulting in considerable pain and possibly scarring of the breast.

Chronic mastitis is a term used to describe certain hyperplastic and cystic conditions of the breast. This group of diseases is also referred to as *mammary dysplasia, fibroadenosis* and *mastopathy*. The condition is extremely common and is caused by an imbalance in the hormonal cycle associated with menstruation. As a result the breast tissue feels more nodular than usual and may be tender. Inflammation plays no part in the cause and the major pathological changes are of fibrosis, cystic change, and increase in the number and size of breast lobules.

mastoiditis

A complication of middle ear infection. Infection reaches the middle ear from the throat, via the Eustachian tube. From the middle ear, infection may spread to the *mastoid air cells,* small air-filled cavities in the *mastoid bone* (which forms the bulge in the skull immediately behind the ear). In severe cases an abscess may be formed in the mastoid bone and the infection may then spread, with a danger that it may reach the interior of the skull to cause MENINGITIS (inflammation of the three membranes that cover the brain and spinal cord).

Prompt treatment of middle ear infections with antibiotics is now usually effective in preventing this once common complication but surgery (*mastoidectomy*) may be required if infection becomes established in the bone itself.

measles

A highly contagious viral disease (also known as *morbilli* and, in English-speaking countries, *rubeola*), common in childhood.

Before the introduction of active immunization, epidemics used to occur every two or three years. In affluent countries the illness mainly involves children aged three to five years and is usually mild; in underdeveloped countries, where nutrition is poor, children under two years are predominantly affected and there is a high mortality rate.

The measles virus is 150 millionths of a millimeter in diameter. Infected individuals shed the measles virus in droplet secretions from the nose, mouth, or throat for four to five days before their skin rash appears and for three to five days after the rash disappears—the time during which they can pass the infection to susceptible people.

The incubation period from exposure to the onset of symptoms is usually 10–14 days. The first symptoms are a fever, cough, runny nose, red and watery eyes, and general irritability. During the period just before the rash appears it may be possible to notice what are known as *Koplik's spots,* which resemble coarse grains of salt on a red background; these often appear on the mucous membranes of the mouth opposite the molar teeth.

The rash first emerges behind the ears and along the hairline, and quickly involves the whole face. It then travels downward to reach the feet on about the third day. Initially the rash consists of dusky-red spots, but these coalesce to form irregular blotches. After three days the rash begins to fade, the fever subsides, and the patient's condition rapidly improves.

Complications do occur and mainly involve the respiratory and central nervous systems. Secondary infection with bacteria leading to bronchitis or ear infection is relatively common; it should be suspected if fever persists, and is treated with antibiotics. More seriously, 1 in 1,000 cases develop a postinfectious encephalitis (inflammation of the brain) three to four days after the onset of the rash. It can vary from transient drowsiness to unconsciousness, coma and death.

Active immunity against measles can be induced by giving a live attenuated virus vaccine by injection. Natural immunity due to the disease is lifelong but the duration of immunity conferred by vaccination is unknown.

megacolon, congenital

See HIRSCHSPRUNG'S DISEASE.

Meibomian cyst

Another name for CHALAZION.

melanoma

Malignant melanomas are tumors of pigment cells (melanocytes); they can arise either at the site of preexisting moles (pigmented nevi) or at apparently unblemished sites in the skin. Although such malignant transformation in a mole is very rare (1 in 1 million), any changes in shape, size, or pigmentation, or itching, ulceration or bleeding in a dark spot should arouse strong suspicion.

Early diagnosis and treatment of a malignant melanoma is vital because it spreads cancer cells to other sites and can be fatal. Malignant melanoma is responsible for approximately 800 deaths in England and Wales every year. *Juvenile melanoma* is a term applied to a benign pigmented skin lesion in children; it is not a precursor of malignant melanoma. Factors thought to predispose to malignant melanoma are exposure to excess sunlight in the fair-skinned, x rays, contact with tar and repeated trauma (e.g. shaving or rubbing) to a mole.

A definite diagnosis can only be made after examining a specimen of tissue microscopically. Surgery remains the most effective treatment for the early localized lesion.

During fetal development, melanocytes migrate from the primitive "neuroectoderm" to the eye and meninges (covering membranes of the brain) as well as to the skin. Malignant melanomas occasionally arise in these sites.

melena

The passage of black, tarry stools, indicative of bleeding from the upper gastrointestinal tract. It may occur independently of or in conjunction with hematemesis (the vomiting of blood). The altered color of the blood in melena is due to the action of gastric juice; if the hemorrhage originates below the small intestine, red blood may be passed with the stools.

In patients with melena, two basic questions have to be answered. First, how much blood has been lost? If less than 1 pint, the patient is unlikely to have generalized symptoms of shock, but larger quantities need to be replaced by blood transfusion. Second, what is the source of the bleeding? Melena can be due to swallowed blood from nose bleeds or dental extractions; however, the three most common sources of blood are peptic ulcer, gastritis (inflammation of the stomach lining) and varicose veins around the esophagus.

Other sources of upper gastrointestinal hemorrhage are esophagitis (inflammation of the esophagus) and cancer of the esophagus or stomach. In order to distinguish between these causes, it is usually essential to pass a fiberoptic endoscope through the mouth and into the stomach to visualize any lesions. Once the site of bleeding has been identified, it is possible to initiate the appropriate treatment for the patient.

Finally, it should be remembered that black stools can be caused by ingestion of iron, charcoal or bismuth.

memory

The ability to recall past experiences, ideas, or sensations.

In man, memory is an integral part of the mental processes of learning and thinking, and depends on perception, language, attention and motivation. Thus, memory is not only a complex process in itself, but is extremely difficult to study sensibly in isolation. Nevertheless, the problems of memory have been attacked at various levels by philosophers, psychologists, neurophysiologists and biochemists. In recent years the advent of computer science has led to the analysis of memory in terms of information storage.

The key steps which need to be explained by any theory of memory are: (1) how the information to be remembered is encoded by the brain; (2) how and where this coded information is stored; (3) how the information is retrieved from storage when required. Despite intensive research for many years, any ideas we have about these stages remain largely speculative.

Most psychologists think that human memory has two phases, usually referred to as *short-term memory (STM)* and *long-term memory (LTM)*. STM is operative for a few moments after new information has been received and is of limited capacity. This capacity or memory span was described by Miller (1956) as being of the "magic number 7 plus or minus 2." By this he meant that most people can remember 7 unrelated things, on average, which are presented to them together. The memory span is not limited by information content—7 random digits are remembered for a short time as well as the names of 7 presidents.

Unless the information transiently held in STM is consolidated and transferred to LTM, it is totally lost. However, information which has been properly learned tends to be forgotten bit by bit, over extended periods, if at all. To explain such accurate storage over many years, stable complex molecules such as nucleic acids and proteins have been suggested as the repositories for information in LTM, but this has not been proved. The exact sites of memory storage are also unknown, but lesions in the front part of the temporal lobes of the cerebrum are most often found to impair memory.

menarche

The time of the first menstrual period, at puberty. In temperate climates the average age of a girl at the menarche is about 13 years; it has fallen steadily during the 20th century, perhaps because of the general improvement in nutrition.

The timing of menarche is much influenced by genetic factors and body weight is also important. The natural variation in the age of onset is so wide that menarche is not considered to be abnormally delayed until it has failed to appear by the age of 17.

Normally, estrogen production by the ovaries gradually increases from 8 to 11 years and it becomes cyclical in nature about one year before menarche. Secondary sexual characteristics, such as breast development and pubic hair growth, also often precede the menarche. The initial menstrual periods tend to be irregular and painless (because ovulation does not occur). Nevertheless, their occurrence can be a frightening experience for the girl if she has not been psychologically prepared for her menarche.

In rare cases a girl experiences the symptoms of menstruation, but no menstrual blood is passed. This may indicate a vaginal obstruction due to an imperforate hymen ("maidenhead") which should be corrected surgically. True primary *amenorrhea,* a delay in the menarche beyond the age of 17, may be due to a malfunction or disease of the ovary, the pituitary gland or the hypothalamus. It may also occur in malnutrition anemia or in generalized debilitating disease. Precocious menarche may be a constitutional trait or may result from a hypothalamic disorder.

Ménière's disease

A disorder characterized by vertigo, deafness and tinnitus (ringing in the ears).

In about 50% of cases, unilateral deafness is the first symptom; this may have been present with tinnitus for several years without the patient seeking medical advice. However, the first attack of vertigo is profoundly disturbing to the patient and he feels that either he or his surroundings are spinning. Such an attack may last up to two hours and is often accompanied by vomiting.

The attacks of vertigo recur irregularly, but often every few weeks. During a period of remission the hearing and tinnitus may improve, but they become progressively worse with each attack. Ménière's disease tends to run its course over several years; the attacks tend to decline in severity and finally cease, but the patient is left with severe deafness.

The cause of Ménière's disease is unknown, but the major pathological change is an accumulation of excess fluid in the inner ear *(endolymphatic hydrops)* damaging the delicate nerve endings. Some believe that the chain of events which results in the excess of endolymph is triggered by stress. Treatment for Ménière's disease may be medical or surgical, but there is no definitive cure. Drug treatment largely comprises sedatives and antiemetics (to prevent vomiting) whereas the variety of operations practiced is surprisingly wide. Operation is rare, however; many patients have only mild and occasional attacks of the disease and require relatively little treatment.

meningioma

A tumor of the meninges—the membranes which cover the brain and spinal cord. Meningiomas do not usually occur before middle age and are slightly more common in women than in men.

Characteristically, a meningioma is a single, large, lobulated tumor which is clearly separate from the underlying nerve tissue. They are classified pathologically as benign tumors in that they do not invade the adjacent brain, and do not spread to other parts of the body. However, meningiomas often infiltrate the overlying skull and a bony prominence can sometimes be felt on the head.

Although meningiomas are classed as benign, their presence within the skull or spinal canal displaces the normal tissue and can have serious consequences. *Spinal meningiomas* initially cause sensory symptoms such as pain, but can progress to complete paraplegia. Because meningiomas grow slowly, the brain can often adjust and accommodate tumors 2–3 cm in diameter with little or no evidence of a rise in intracranial pressure. When symptoms do occur they may include paralysis or weakness of limbs, convulsions, headache, impairment of speech, interference with vision and subtle mental changes.

Unless an intracranial meningioma can be removed surgically it may eventually be fatal. The new technique of computerized axial tomography (the CAT scanner) is very effective in displaying small meningiomas, and earlier diagnosis should improve the chances of successful surgery.

meningitis

The brain and spinal cord are covered by three membranes, known technically as the *meninges:* the *dura mater* (the outermost and toughest, in contact with the inner surface of the skull), the *arachnoid* (the middle membrane) and the *pia mater* (the innermost membrane, directly in contact with the surface of the brain). Meningitis means inflammation of these membranes, especially the arachnoid and pia mater.

Meningitis is most commonly caused by a bacterial or viral infection. The microorganisms can reach the meninges from the exterior (such as by means of a severe head wound), from the bloodstream (for example, from another focus of infection such as the upper respiratory tract), or (rarely) directly from the brain itself.

In the United States approximately 70% of all cases of acute pyogenic ("pus-forming") meningitis are caused by infection with any one of three species of bacteria: *Neisseria meningitidis* (or meningococcus), *Diplococcus pneumoniae* (or pneumococcus) or *Hemophilus influenzae* (meningitis caused by the last-named microor-

MENINGITIS

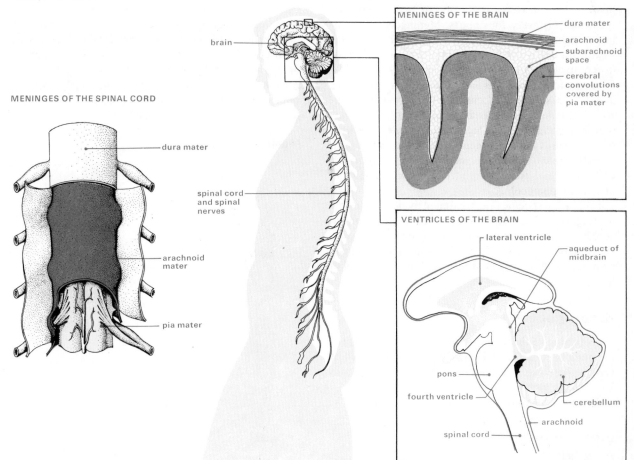

MENINGES OF THE SPINAL CORD

- dura mater
- spinal cord and spinal nerves
- arachnoid mater
- pia mater

brain

MENINGES OF THE BRAIN
- dura mater
- arachnoid
- subarachnoid space
- cerebral convolutions covered by pia mater

VENTRICLES OF THE BRAIN
- lateral ventricle
- aqueduct of midbrain
- pons
- fourth ventricle
- cerebellum
- arachnoid
- spinal cord

The meninges are three layers of protective membranes which cover the brain and spinal cord. The subarachnoid space between the inner two layers contains cerebrospinal fluid (CSF). CSF is produced in the ventricles of the brain and flows into the subarachnoid space through openings in the fourth ventricle. Meningitis, inflammation of the meninges, results from bacteria and viruses multiplying in the CSF.

ganism is more common in children under the age of five). When any of these bacteria infect the lining membranes of the brain the meninges can become quickly inflamed and the space between the two innermost membranes (the "subarachnoid space"), which normally contains clear cerebrospinal fluid, becomes filled with pus. Pus is not usually formed in acute meningitis caused by a viral infection or the causative organism of tuberculosis (*Mycobacterium tuberculosis* or the "tubercle bacillus").

All forms of acute meningitis, regardless of their cause, give rise to a number of common symptoms

(although the symptoms of tuberculous meningitis are insidious rather than dramatic). Headache, increasing in severity, is usually the first symptom. The patient typically has a high fever and pronounced stiffness of the neck. As the disease progresses, the mental state of the patient can change from delirium through drowsiness to coma. Photophobia (extreme sensitivity of the eyes to light) and convulsions are also often experienced. A definitive diagnosis depends largely on a study of the cerebrospinal fluid, obtained by means of a lumbar puncture: insertion of a hollow needle between two of the lumbar vertebrae (in the lower part of the back) to the point where a sample of the fluid can be drawn off. The visual appearance of this fluid (cloudy or clear), its protein and sugar content, and the presence of bacteria—which can be stained and examined under the microscope for specific identification—are all important diagnostic evidence of meningitis. Confirmation of the diagnosis by bacterial culture of the cerebrospinal fluid takes about one or two days, but it is imperative to start treatment immediately.

Both the meningococcus and pneumococcus are

usually sensitive to penicillin; typical initial treatment involves the intravenous injection of benzyl penicillin (penicillin G) every four hours. Meningococcal meningitis responds particularly well to penicillin and this treatment, if it is given sufficiently early, should result in complete cure in the vast majority of cases. Pneumococcal meningitis is typically slower to improve and is occasionally associated with permanent neurological complications (such as impairment of hearing). This condition has a higher fatality rate in patients over the age of about 50. Meningitis caused by infection with *Hemophilus influenzae* can usually be cured in 90% or more of children by prompt treatment with ampicillin or chloramphenicol.

There is no specific drug treatment available for viral meningitis, which comprises the majority of the remaining cases, but fortunately most patients make a complete spontaneous recovery. Tuberculous meningitis usually responds well to specific drugs used in the control of tuberculosis.

meningocele

A protrusion of the covering membranes (meninges) of the brain or spinal cord through a defect in the skull or vertebral column. In the latter case the condition is also known as a *meningomyelocele*.

See also SPINA BIFIDA.

menisectomy

In the knee joint, the medial and lateral cartilages *(menisci;* singular, *meniscus)* are two crescent-shaped wedges of fibrocartilage interposed between the femur and tibia (the thighbone and shinbone, respectively). These menisci compensate for the incongruities in the shapes of the two bones and facilitate smooth movement at the joint. If one or other meniscus should be torn and displaced by injury, or if it is distorted by a cyst, then it is usually removed surgically (a procedure known as menisectomy).

Although the knee is principally a hinge joint, once it has been flexed it is possible for the tibia to be rotated or twisted. When the leg is bearing weight and the flexed knee is violently twisted, the meniscus can be torn. The torn and displaced fragment of cartilage can jam between the femur and tibia, "locking" the knee so that the leg cannot be straightened. Two-thirds of these cases involve the medial meniscus only. Such injuries are often incurred in sports, particularly football.

Initial treatment following injury may be nonsurgical and involve merely splinting the affected joint. However, a true tear does not heal satisfactorily because the cartilage has virtually no blood supply. Therefore, if the symptoms of pain and knee-locking persist, menisectomy is indicated. With appropriate physical therapy, approximately 75% of patients regain complete functional efficiency of the knee joint (a "rim" of fibrocartilage regenerates from the margin of the excised meniscus). In cases where the diagnosis is not clear or where symptoms persist postoperatively, ARTHROSCOPY can be performed—in which a special optical instrument (arthroscope) is inserted into the joint cavity to permit direct inspection of the damage.

MENISECTOMY

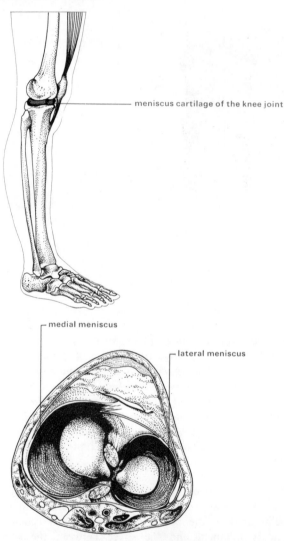

meniscus cartilage of the knee joint

medial meniscus

lateral meniscus

A CROSS SECTION THROUGH THE RIGHT KNEE SEEN FROM ABOVE

The two meniscus cartilages in the knee transmit weight from the thigh to the lower leg. Cartilage injuries result from violent twisting of the knee; torn cartilages do not heal and have to be removed by a menisectomy operation.

menopause

The menopause (or "climacteric") marks the end of a woman's sexual cycle (menstruation) and may occur any time between the ages of 40 to 55 (although the onset is commonly between the ages of 47 and 50).

The precise mechanism underlying the menopause is not fully understood, but it seems that the ovaries become unresponsive to the gonadotropic hormones (GONADOTROPINS) secreted by the pituitary gland. Therefore, the blood level of circulating ESTROGENS falls significantly, resulting in many changes.

In the normal menopause the menstrual periods may be scant and infrequent before the final cessation. Heavy or irregular bleeding should always be investigated. Perhaps up to about 70% of menopausal women experience "hot flushes" (or "hot flashes"). These are produced by vascular disturbances and are characterized by a feeling of warmth in the face, neck and chest; they may be accompanied by blushing or sweating. It has been suggested by some medical experts that the symptoms may be related to increased secretion of FSH (follicle-stimulating hormone) by the pituitary gland, in the absence of the normal inhibitory feedback of ovarian estrogens; however, some physicians dispute this theory. Hot flushes typically last for only a few minutes at a time, but may occur several times a day. Vaginal dryness is also commonly associated with the menopause.

Apart from the physical changes of the menopause, many women experience psychological problems. Nervous tension and irritability are common. Adaptation is often extremely difficult to the idea of approaching old age, the end of childbearing and the diminution of family responsibilities. Some women become severely depressed.

Treatment to relieve some of the more troublesome symptoms of the menopause includes psychotherapy in varying degrees (to allay anxiety and alleviate depression) and hormonal replacement for the suppression of hot flushes. The lowest effective dose of estrogen is frequently prescribed to minimize possible side effects (such as coronary or cerebral thrombosis). Recent evidence has been presented which suggests that estrogen replacement therapy increases the risk of cancer of the uterus.

Postmenopausal bleeding (vaginal bleeding which occurs a year or more following the onset of the menopause) must always be investigated.

menorrhagia

Menorrhagia means excessive or prolonged bleeding at the normal time of menstruation. It may occur in isolation or be associated with other disturbances— such as *polymenorrhea*, where bleeding occurs with abnormal frequency. In menorrhagia, up to 180 ml of blood can be lost during each menstrual cycle and the woman can thus easily become anemic.

Menorrhagia has many possible causes and should always be fully investigated by a gynecologist. Lesions in the pelvis which can give rise to this condition include FIBROIDS, POLYPS and ENDOMETRIOSIS. However, in many cases no specific cause can be found (classified as "dysfunctional bleeding"). This is possibly related to a disorder of the production and release of the hormones which control menstruation.

DILATATION AND CURETTAGE is often the only way to establish the cause of menorrhagia. Besides providing diagnostic information, it is frequently a curative procedure. Hormonal therapy with PROGESTINS (or with the oral contraceptive pill itself) is sometimes successful in controlling dysfunctional bleeding. In severe cases, HYSTERECTOMY may be required.

menstruation

Menstruation is the normal monthly discharge of blood and cellular debris from the vagina which accompanies the periodic shedding of the lining of the uterus in nonpregnant women. By convention, the first day of menstruation is taken as "day 1" of the menstrual cycle (which is an average of 28 days long). It is only human females and other primates who menstruate; other mammals have an "estrous cycle" which is characterized by a period of "heat" when the sexual interest of the mature female is aroused.

In women the time of the first menstrual period (MENARCHE) is generally around the age of 13; the menstrual cycle continues (in the absence of pregnancy or certain other influences) until the MENOPAUSE.

Menstruation normally lasts for about four days, but can vary from approximately two to seven days. On average, 50 ml of blood are lost and at the end of a menstrual cycle all but the deepest layers of the uterine lining have been shed. The lining of the uterus is restored during the "proliferative" phase of the menstrual cycle, which lasts from about the 5th to the 14th day. This "endometrial proliferation" is stimulated by estrogen (secreted by a ripening ovarian follicle). One ovarian follicle develops during each cycle and its progress is controlled by two hormones—FSH (follicle-stimulating hormone) and LH (luteinizing hormone)—from the PITUITARY GLAND in the brain. At about the 14th day there is a burst of LH released from the pituitary gland, which causes the distended ovarian follicle to rupture and release an ovum (egg). This is the process of OVULATION and a simple (although rather unreliable) indicator of its occurrence is a temporary rise in the woman's body temperature. Menstruation without

THE MENSTRUAL CYCLE

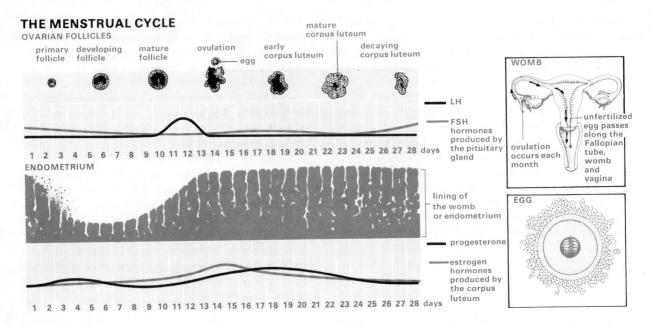

OVARIAN FOLLICLES

primary follicle | developing follicle | mature follicle | ovulation — egg | early corpus luteum | mature corpus luteum | decaying corpus luteum

— LH
— FSH
hormones produced by the pituitary gland

1 2 3 4 5 6 7 8 9 10 11 12 13 14 15 16 17 18 19 20 21 22 23 24 25 26 27 28 days

ENDOMETRIUM

lining of the womb or endometrium

— progesterone
— estrogen
hormones produced by the corpus luteum

1 2 3 4 5 6 7 8 9 10 11 12 13 14 15 16 17 18 19 20 21 22 23 24 25 26 27 28 days

WOMB
ovulation occurs each month
unfertilized egg passes along the Fallopian tube, womb and vagina

EGG

The human menstrual cycle is a monthly fluctuation in the state of the endometrium (lining of the womb), and depends on hormonal changes governed by the pituitary gland in the brain. Day 1 is the first day of menstruation, when the old endometrium starts to slough off. Although the length of the cycle can vary from 23 days to 35 days in normal women, ovulation nearly always occurs 14 days before the end of the cycle.

ovulation is painless and is common in young girls and at the menopause (and for a time following childbirth).

Shortly after ovulation the empty ovarian follicle is transformed into the corpus luteum, which secretes ESTROGENS and PROGESTERONE for the remainder of the menstrual cycle. This period is the "secretory phase" and the glands in the lining of the uterus become tightly coiled. If fertilization of the ovum has not taken place, the corpus luteum begins to decay on about the 24th day. The falling estrogen and progesterone levels lead to certain changes in the blood vessels of the uterine lining and menstruation occurs. If fertilization *does* take place, the corpus luteum enlarges and maintains the uterine lining in a suitable condition for the nourishment of the fertilized egg (and, thus, menstruation does not occur).

mental handicap

An umbrella term used to describe retarded intellectual development resulting in lower intelligence, from whatever cause. It is present at birth as a constitutional trait or develops in childhood as a result of environmental insult, such as trauma or infection.

Although there may be a clear-cut genetic cause for a person's mental handicap, it is always important to provide the optimal environment so that he can maximize his potential, however limited it may be. The deterioration of mental powers later in adult life is normally classified as *dementia* rather than as mental handicap, because a normal level of intelligence has been attained at some stage.

In order to understand the concept of mental handicap, it is first necessary to form a working definition of intelligence and to understand how it can be measured. Psychologists have defined intelligence in many different ways, but most would agree that it involves the individual's ability to adapt successfully to his environment and his capacity to learn and manipulate abstract ideas.

There is much controversy about the worth of intelligence tests, but they do provide a standardized means of comparing one person's mental capacity with that of the general population. Many tests are designed so that if the average intelligence quotient (IQ) is 100, then approximately 68% of the population will have an IQ between 85 and 115, and about 95% will lie between 70 and 130. In fact the distribution of intelligence among the population is not quite symmetrical: there are more people with IQs of less than 70 than there are gifted people with IQs above 130.

As a crude numerical measure, an IQ of less than 70 is often taken as the criterion for mental handicap, although this varies with the type of IQ test used. Obviously there is no clear-cut boundary between high-grade mental handicap and the lower levels of "normal" intelligence. Moreover, while subnormal intelligence is the essential factor in mental handicap, it is often the social incompetence and emotional inadequacy of the individual which present the greatest problems.

In the majority of cases, intellectual deficit is not associated with any known organic disease. However, many mentally handicapped people show physical signs of a brain defect and this is nearly always so in the most severely retarded. The recognized categories of mental handicap are as follows:

Scotland	England and Wales
1. Mild	1. Mild
2. Severe	2. Severe
3. Profound	

However, the medical and psychological professions prefer to use the more accurate I.C.D. (International Classification of Diseases) classification:

Borderline	IQ 68–85	Severe	IQ 20–35
Mild	IQ 52–67	Profound	IQ below 20
Moderate	IQ 36–51		

The Borderline and Mild groups constitute the largest class of mental defectives. They are often the children of parents who themselves are intellectually dull. Their constitutional disadvantage is often compounded by poor living conditions and inadequate parents. As infants they tend to lack curiosity and are quiet and well behaved. For this reason they are often undetected until they go to school, when their performance falls progressively further behind that of their peers. It is especially important to identify these children, because with special training they can be helped to lead independent lives.

By contrast, the Moderate and Severe groups of the handicapped are incapable of independence and are more likely to be diagnosed earlier because of associated physical abnormality. Developmental milestones are delayed and they typically show impulsive, infantile behavior throughout their lives. Their parents usually have normal intelligence, and accept that their child will benefit from special education. Mongolism is by far the most common syndrome associated with this degree of mental subnormality.

The profoundly handicapped constitute the lowest grade and are estimated to have IQs below 20, although this is a largely meaningless figure. They differ from the other groups in that they need to be constantly protected against common physical dangers. The majority have severe brain damage, are stunted in growth and, like all the mentally handicapped – but to a greater extent – may suffer from epileptic fits. Many are bedridden, unable to communicate, and often do not survive childhood.

mental illness

The term "mental illness" covers problems of personality and sexual deviation, NEUROSIS, and the psychotic states classified as SCHIZOPHRENIA and DEPRESSION.

The nature, cause, diagnosis and treatment of mental illnesses are more controversial than is the case with diseases caused by bacteria or due to an obvious physical abnormality such as a tumor. Doctors not only disagree among themselves but also must contend with the theories (helpful or otherwise) of psychologists, philosophers, and even artists (some of whom insist that a mild degree of mental aberration is essential for the creative process).

The major division among psychiatrists concerns the extent to which they regard mental illness as originating primarily in a structural or biochemical disorder in the brain and how much importance they attach to influences in infancy and childhood and to psychological reactions to conscious or unconscious stresses. These two basic approaches are not mutually exclusive— neurological and psychogenic influences may *both* be involved in most mental problems.

When it comes to treatment, psychiatrists tend to fall into one "camp" or the other. Those who believe in an organic cause of mental illness will treat their patients with the use of appropriate physical techniques, including drugs, surgical procedures and electroconvulsive therapy. Those who favor a "psychogenic" cause will lean toward various psychotherapeutic techniques. However, when specific, effective drug treatments are available—such as the use of lithium in manic-depressive psychosis—there is usually a consensus of opinion.

See also MANIA, PSYCHIATRY, PSYCHOANALYSIS, and PSYCHOSES.

mercury poisoning

Mercury and its compounds may cause acute or chronic poisoning. Metallic mercury is not dangerous in very small doses: a child who bites through a clinical thermometer and swallows a few drops of the metal will probably come to no harm. However, mercury salts such as mercuric chloride may cause serious illness; they cause ulceration and burning of the intestinal tract and, after absorption into the bloodstream, may damage the kidneys and nerves. Acute poisoning from a dose of a mercury salt causes vomiting, diarrhea, and kidney failure, which is the usual cause of death in fatal cases of mercury poisoning.

Chronic mercury poisoning is most often due to occupational exposure or to industrial pollution of the environment. It may cause mental disturbances, tremor, nerve damage leading to paralysis, and kidney failure. Mass outbreaks have occurred in the past 20 years:

MINAMATA DISEASE in Japan was due to contamination of fish by industrial effluent, and more recently in the Middle East there have been several epidemics of paralysis, especially in children, from the use for human consumption of chemically treated seed corn.

mesothelioma

A rare malignant tumor of the pleura and peritoneum— the membranous sacs lining the thoracic (chest) and abdominal cavities, respectively.

In 1960 a relation was established between mesothelioma and exposure to asbestos, particularly of the crocidolite or Cape blue fiber type. It was found that exposure to asbestos need only have been for one to two months to account for the development of a mesothelioma 20 to 50 years later. Thus, although protective measures are now taken against environmental pollution with asbestos, new cases of mesothelioma will still be presenting themselves at the end of the 20th century.

While radiation therapy occasionally prolongs survival in cases of *pleural mesothelioma,* most patients die within a year of diagnosis.

metabolism

This term, literally meaning "change," is used to refer to all the chemical and energy transformations that are carried out in an organism or in a single cell.

The first specific function of metabolism is to extract chemical energy from the environment. Higher plants and blue-green algae are photosynthetic: they can extract energy from sunlight and make use of carbon dioxide as their sole source of carbon. The cells of all higher animals cannot make direct use of solar energy or carbon dioxide; they derive energy by the chemical degradation of complex nutrients, principally into carbon dioxide and water. This chemical degradation, carried out in a complex series of individual *oxidation-reduction reactions,* is called *catabolism.*

Beside the complete catabolism of exogenous nutrients to yield energy, the body's metabolic processes have to convert foodstuffs into molecular building blocks and assemble them into the components of cells, such as proteins, nucleic acids and lipids (fats or fatlike substances). This synthesis of cellular macromolecules is called *anabolism.* Finally, some of these macromolecules have to be broken down for use or for excretion, as do drugs administered to the body.

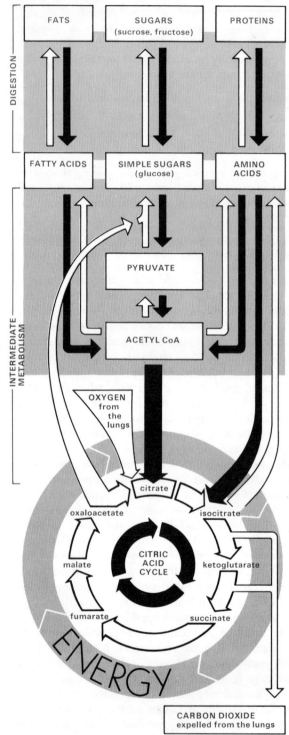

The diagram shows the pathways of metabolism. Sugars, fats, and proteins are broken down into simple chemicals in the stomach and small intestine, absorbed into the blood and transported to the tissues; within each cell they are transformed into a key substance—"acetyl CoA." Then follows the "citric acid cycle," where controlled combustion with oxygen leads to the production of energy; carbon dioxide is released during this process.

The *basal metabolic rate (BMR)* is the amount of energy consumed by a person in a day in order to maintain essential bodily functions. In an average adult under conditions of mental and physical rest, the BMR is about 2,000 kilocalories/day; in order to carry out a sedentary job only about an extra 500 kilocalories are required. (A kilocalorie is also known as a *kilogram calorie, large calorie* or a *Calorie*—spelled with a capital C to distinguish it from the *small calorie* or *gram calorie*.) BMR is raised by anxiety but decreased in depression. Metabolic processes are sensitively regulated by hormones, and increased levels of epinephrine, norepinephrine and thyroid hormone raise the BMR.

The end products of digestion in humans are mainly amino acids, fat derivatives and sugars such as glucose. These digestive products are catabolized to simpler, intermediate molecules which constitute the common "metabolic pool." The intermediate molecules then either undergo anabolism into proteins, fats or carbohydrates or they may be further catabolized into hydrogen atoms and carbon dioxide. This final catabolism is carried out by a biochemical pathway known as the *citric acid cycle* and occurs in the specialized mitochondria of cells. The energy thereby liberated is not used directly by the cell. It is stored in high-energy phosphate compounds, the most important of which is known as adenosine triphosphate (ATP).

metastasis

The spread of cancer cells from one site in the body (especially at the site of a primary cancerous growth) to other parts of the body, where they set up secondary growths.

See CANCER, MALIGNANCY.

migraine

The word migraine is derived from *hemicrania* (literally, "half head") which was introduced into medicine by Galen (A.D. 131–201). Unilateral headache is still regarded as the cardinal feature of migraine, although the diagnosis may be made in the absence of headache.

Classically, a migraine starts with visual disturbances. Jagged brilliant streaks of light (fortification figures) may be seen on one side; bright spots may obscure the vision, which may become blurred or even completely lost. This may be followed by numbness or pins and needles in the hands or face, and possibly transient weakness of a limb or of half the body. After 15 to 30 minutes these symptoms give way to a boring pain on one side of the head, which typically reaches a peak intensity after an hour or so and may persist for days.

The headache becomes throbbing in character and is often accompanied by nausea and vomiting.

The above is a description of "classical" migraine, but there are many variant forms. In "atypical" migraine, which is in fact the most common form, the headache with or without vomiting occurs in the absence of other symptoms. The characteristic feature of all migraine is that it occurs in attacks, separated by intervals of freedom. In addition, the headaches tend to last for several hours and may persist for days.

Migraine usually first appears around the age of puberty and recurs with gradually diminishing frequency through adult life. However, it may begin during early childhood or in middle age. Women are slightly more susceptible than men and it often runs in families. It is popularly believed to occur in intelligent, conscientious individuals and to be triggered by stress, but this view is an oversimplification. Sufferers from migraine are more prone to allergies, and it is not uncommon for attacks to be linked to certain dietary factors, such as red wine, oranges, cheese or chocolate.

An attack of migraine is believed to begin with spasm of the arteries, causing the visual and neurological symptoms, followed by arterial dilation, causing the headache. Ergotamine tartrate, a powerful blood vessel constrictor, is the basis of most antimigraine drugs. It should not be given to patients with vascular disease or during pregnancy (when the attacks usually cease anyway). Mild tranquilizers may reduce the severity and frequency of the attacks, and there are a number of drugs which may prove useful to a varying degree.

miliaria

Miliaria ("heat rash" or "prickly heat") is an acute itching eruption of the skin common among white people in hot summer weather or tropical and subtropical areas. The condition results from excessive sweating and blocked sweat glands.

Prolonged exposure to heat and moisture causes the skin to swell enough to block the openings of the sweat glands. Newly produced sweat is then deposited in the skin and not on it; this results in local irritation and the formation of minute blisters. Pimples may subsequently develop, inflammation leads to an itching sensation, and the affected area may become infected. Sites which tend to be involved are the chest, back, waistline, groin and armpits. The best treatment involves removal of the patient to a cooler, less humid atmosphere. Lotions, cold compresses and cool showers or tub soaks may also help. Any irritants—such as unsuitable clothing, medications and harsh soaps—should be avoided.

If fungal infections develop in the affected areas, they require separate treatment with antifungal ointments or other preparations.

Minamata disease

Another name for MERCURY POISONING; named after Minamata Bay, Japan, where one of the most notorious examples of industrial poisoning occurred between 1953 and 1958. In the outbreak scores of people died and hundreds suffered irreversible brain damage from eating fish containing an organic mercury compound, itself absorbed by the fish from industrial effluent discharged into the sea.

miosis

Constriction of the pupil of the eye. The pupil is controlled by the radial and circular muscle fibers of the iris. The iris is the pigmented, opaque part of the front of the eye; it functions in much the same way as the diaphragm of a camera. Constriction of the pupil (miosis) prevents light from passing through the more peripheral parts of the lens system, cuts down the amount of light reaching the retina and reduces distortion effects of vision known as chromatic and spherical aberration.

Drugs which constrict the pupil are used in the treatment of some eye diseases such as GLAUCOMA. Many drugs acting on the autonomic nervous system cause miosis as a side effect.

miscarriage

In a miscarriage (technically known as a *spontaneous abortion*) the fetus and associated placental membranes are delivered before the 28th week of pregnancy. At this early stage the fetus is not yet sufficiently developed to maintain its life functions outside the womb. The patient undergoes a miniature labor with dilation of the cervix and experiences some pain. The most common time for a miscarriage to occur is about the 12th week.

The cause of spontaneous abortion can often not be determined but the following factors can play a part.

Many early aborted fetuses have abnormalities. Maternal disease may be a cause, such as hypertension, kidney and heart disease, diabetes or thyroid abnormalities. Uterine and placental abnormalities, a "lax" cervix, severe vitamin deficiencies, or possibly violent exercise also tend to interrupt pregnancy.

A threatened miscarriage is indicated by bleeding and a little pain. If it progresses and the cervix becomes dilated, loss of the fetus becomes inevitable. If placental tissue is retained in an incomplete miscarriage there is a danger of hemorrhage and sepsis. Thus, prompt medical attention—including a DILATATION AND CURETTAGE (D & C)—following a miscarriage is essential.

See also ABORTION.

mites

Small organisms (technically known as *arachnids,* the group to which spiders belong), some of which burrow into the skin and cause irritation. They may transmit serious disease, and some varieties may cause allergic reactions such as asthma.

The human parasite *Sarcoptes scabiei* is the cause of SCABIES, an irritative skin disease. Scabies itching is intense, especially at night. The penetration of the mite (smaller than a pinhead) causes linear scratches, small blisters, or pimples. Scabies parasites are transmitted by direct contact and from shared towels and bed linen. The disease is also frequently acquired by sexual contact. Bathing and applications of gamma benzene hexachloride or benzyl benzoate are effective treatments.

House mice are responsible for passing on *rickettsialpox* in North America and Europe. Cases occur annually in New York City, where mice infected with RICKETTSIAE (microorganisms intermediate in size between bacteria and viruses) in apartment houses maintain the infection. Tetracyclines are used in treatment.

Mites living in house dust do not infect man directly, but their presence in the dust is an important cause of hypersensitivity and asthmatic reactions, especially in children. Removal of dust-laden mattresses may cause dramatic relief of symptoms.

mole

A blemish on the skin which may be present at birth or may develop subsequently. Moles are comprised of clusters of nevus cells, which are specialized epithelial cells containing the pigment melanin.

Moles may be small or large, flat or raised, smooth, hairy or warty. They vary in color from yellow-brown to black. A mole is also classified as a type of pigmented NEVUS.

Moles may rarely undergo malignant (cancerous) change to become malignant MELANOMAS. They can be classified according to where they arise and this gives some indication of the likelihood of malignant changes occurring. About a quarter of malignant melanomas do not develop from a preceding mole.

Intradermal or "common" moles—in which the melanin-forming cells are in the lower layer of the skin or dermis—are benign. They are elevated and often have a hair in them. These intradermal nevi need not be removed except for cosmetic purposes as they are not precursors of melanomas.

Another type known as *junctional nevi* arise from nevus cells at the junction between the outer layer of the skin or epidermis and the dermis. They may be flat and are deep brown or black in color. Though more susceptible to activation, only a small percentage become malignant. They do not require removal unless they show a recent change or are situated in the nail matrix, are the site of frequent trauma, or are on surfaces such as the lips, anus, penis or vulva. A sudden increase in size or color, or bleeding or ulceration, is an indication for surgical removal of junctional nevi.

In general, malignant melanomas develop more readily from moles on the lower legs and on mucous membranes than from those elsewhere. Pigmented moles subjected to constant irritation or trauma show a relatively high incidence of malignant changes.

During pregnancy a benign increase in mole size and color is common. Children tend to develop more junctional nevi than intradermal nevi, yet they rarely acquire malignant melanoma. Large speckled, flat, rough lesions on the exposed parts in the elderly resemble junctional nevi and are best removed surgically because of their potential for malignant transformation.

molluscum contagiosum

A viral disease of the skin, characterized by one or more discrete, waxy, dome-shaped nodules or tumors frequently with a central dimple.

The virus is probably transmitted by direct contact or by clothing or other items which have been contaminated with the virus; outbreaks are common in schools.

The condition is of little clinical importance once the diagnosis is known. In many cases the lesions disappear without treatment; if they persist they can be removed by a dermatologist with a curette or by electrodesiccation.

mongolism

Another name for DOWN'S SYNDROME.

Monilia

Another name for CANDIDA.

morning sickness

Nausea and vomiting of varying severity that occurs in pregnancy, usually in the early months. Morning sickness is a common symptom of pregnancy; as the name implies, it tends to occur in the early part of the day. It is seen in about half of pregnancies from about the end of the first month, usually ceasing by the end of the third month.

The symptoms begin with a feeling of nausea on arising. The expectant mother is often unable to retain her breakfast, but by midday the symptoms have disappeared and she feels well until the following morning. In some cases the condition evolves into prolonged bouts of vomiting with a resultant weight loss.

Most women with morning sickness can keep it under control by taking only small meals with generous amounts of fluid between meals. Nausea can sometimes be averted or minimized by getting out of bed slowly. Drugs not prescribed by the doctor should be avoided, if possible, but antinauseants and sedatives may be necessary in the more severe cases.

mosquitoes

Approximately 2,500 different species of mosquitoes have been identified. The bloodsucking habits of the females of a few of these species are responsible for transmitting various disease to man and other mammals. In obtaining their "blood meal," the females use their specially modified mouth parts to pierce the skin of their victims and suck up the blood.

The female mosquito first injects saliva containing an anticoagulant into the skin of its victim to prevent the blood clotting. It also injects a "sensitizing" agent, which may cause severe irritation in some people. Soothing lotions and creams may be applied to alleviate the itching.

As a mosquito feeds it may pass on various disease-causing (pathogenic) microorganisms from one person to another. Several diseases can be spread in this way— including MALARIA, YELLOW FEVER, FILARIASIS and DENGUE FEVER. In some cases the pathogenic microorganisms have evolved a highly complex life cycle using the mosquito as a "vector."

A large number of "arboviruses" are known to produce disease in man. Most of these are examples of a ZOONOSIS, accidentally acquired by man through the bite of an insect such as the mosquito. The diseases can be divided into three basic categories: (1) acute central nervous system diseases, usually with ENCEPHALITIS; (2) acute benign fevers, and (3) hemorrhagic fevers.

Of the mosquito-borne infections in the first category, *Eastern equine encephalitis* carries one of the highest mortality rates. Cases of it are recognized in the eastern and north central parts of the United States and adjacent Canada. Mosquitoes usually acquire the infection from wild birds or rodents.

Dengue fever comes within the second category. During the 20th century, epidemics have occurred in the southeastern and Gulf sections of the United States and elsewhere. The fatality rate is low. Mosquitoes can pick up the pathogenic viruses from patients from the day before the onset of the patient's fever to the fifth day of the disease; 11 days after the mosquito takes its "blood meal" it becomes capable of infecting another person.

In the third category, *hemorrhagic fevers,* comes yellow fever. Except for a few cases in Trinidad, W.I., in 1954 no urban outbreak has been transmitted by mosquitoes since the 1940s. Jungle yellow fever is present from time to time in mainland countries of the Americas from Mexico to South America.

The bite of a mosquito harboring infective larvae of a nematode parasite transmits the tropical condition known as filariasis.

Preventive measures against all these conditions involve keeping the mosquito at bay. They include control of mosquito breeding grounds, the use of residual insecticide sprays in homes and outbuildings, mosquito repellants for personal use, screens on doors and windows in homes or mosquito netting where screens are not practical, and sufficient clothing, particularly after sundown, to protect as much of the skin surface as possible against bites.

motion sickness

See TRAVEL SICKNESS.

multiple myeloma

A malignant growth of certain special cells in the bone marrow. It most commonly occurs in people over 40 and affects men twice as often as women. The condition may be accompanied by anemia, kidney damage and the overproduction of certain proteins and their constituent polypeptides.

The most common initial symptom is bone pain, often in a rib or vertebra. (The bones most frequently affected are the ribs, spine and pelvis.) There are multiple well-defined areas where bone is destroyed and replaced by certain closely packed cells which are active in the formation of antibodies.

Fractures in the ribs and long bones and collapse of the vertebrae may occur. X rays may show general demineralization of the bones or characteristic punched-out lesions.

Anemia, from impaired production of red blood cells, is usual and *hemolytic anemia*—in which there is excessive destruction of red blood cells caused by antibody formation in the blood—may develop. Ultimately a decrease in the platelets in the blood and spontaneous bleeding is to be expected.

The excess plasma cells produce an abnormal protein. The disease gradually disseminates through the body, although a single lesion may be involved initially. The tubules in the kidney may become blocked by coagulated protein.

The drug melphalan may be used in treatment alone or combined with steroids. The pain from local involvement of bone can be relieved by radiotherapy. Transfusion may be required to correct anemia.

multiple sclerosis

A disorder of the brain, spinal cord and nerves, also known as *disseminated sclerosis.* In this condition destruction of the protective myelin sheaths (which insulate nerve fibers) occurs in patches throughout the central nervous system, giving rise to the formation of plaques. The cause is unknown.

The disease has been attributed variously to autoimmune mechanisms (when the body's own immune system turns against the patient—see AUTOIMMUNE DISEASE); to infection by a virus which has a prolonged incubation period before producing symptoms; to toxic agents; metabolic faults; and trauma and blood vessel lesions.

Symptoms of multiple sclerosis usually first appear in late teenage or early adult life. One or more parts of the body may become weak or paralyzed. Among other symptoms, there may be loss of sensation, blurred vision, and loss of control over the bowel and bladder. The patient's speech may be slowed and his or her emotions may be labile. The severity of the symptoms is likely to fluctuate over time with remissions and exacerbations. Onset is usually insidious, and the disease is slowly progressive.

In the early stages there is sometimes complete remission of symptoms, which may last for many years; but with recurrent episodes, remissions are likely to be less complete and the patient may suffer an increasingly permanent disability.

Initially there may be fleeting visual symptoms, or slight stiffness and unusual tiredness in a limb. Far later there is paralysis of the legs and poor coordination of arm movements. In many patients, however, the disorder fortunately remains mild and interferes little with ordinary life.

There is currently no specific cure, but wide claims have been made for a number of treatments. Spontaneous remissions make any treatment difficult to evaluate. Massage of weakened limbs and muscle training are of some benefit.

Prompt treatment of infections and an adequate diet with vitamin supplements, where necessary, are sensible measures. In the later stages of multiple sclerosis, good nursing will help in the prevention of bedsores. Steroids and other drugs are used to alleviate symptoms; for example, vertigo may be treated with chlorpromazine.

There is a definite geographical distribution of incidence; the closer the country is to the Equator, the lower the prevalence of the disease. Statistics show that in Mexico, for instance, the rate is only 1/30 of that in Denmark.

mumps

A contagious viral disease common among children which usually causes painful inflammation and enlargement of the salivary glands, particularly the parotid glands. There is fever, and swelling develops in front of the ears, making the chewing of food difficult. Also called *epidemic parotitis*.

In young children mumps is a relatively trivial illness, but if contracted after puberty it may affect the testicles and have serious complications.

The disease is spread by droplet infection through the respiratory tract. The incubation period is 12 to 28 days, but the great majority of children develop it about 18 days after exposure.

A child with mumps can usually be nursed at home. He is infectious until the swelling subsides. It is said to be impractical and unwise to try to prevent other children in the house from coming into contact with him. A child who has once had the infection is unlikely to contract it again because of the long-term immunity which develops.

The initial symptoms may be a high temperature, headache and sore throat which arise a few days before the characteristic swelling of the parotid glands, but the swelling is often the first symptom. It usually subsides within 7 to 10 days.

The virus occasionally invades tissues other than the salivary glands, notably the testicles, ovaries, pancreas and the meninges (membranes covering the brain and spinal cord). About a quarter of boys over 14 years of age having mumps develop inflammation of the testicles (orchitis) as a complication; this is rare in childhood. Serious consequences of orchitis are not as common as was once believed but may include permanent sterility.

MUMPS

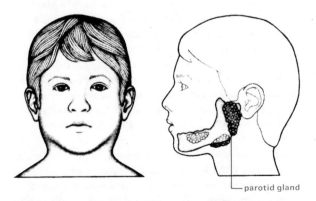

parotid gland

Mumps is one of the common viral diseases of childhood. The virus attacks the parotid gland in front of the ear, producing a painful swollen face.

Live mumps vaccine was introduced in the late 1960s and it may be useful in those who have reached puberty without contracting the illness, or for administration to younger children. The vaccine must not be given to pregnant women, as it endangers the health of the unborn child.

Munchausen's syndrome

A strange type of complaint named after the 16th-century Baron von Munchausen. He was a traveler, served in the Russian army, and was the reputed source of a collection of preposterous stories. The baron has been described as a proverbial liar. (One of the stories attributed to him relates that during a blinding snowstorm he tethered his horse to what he thought was a fence post. On awaking the next morning, he discovered that the horse was dangling from the top of a church steeple.)

His name was first used in the medical context in 1951 by Richard Asher, who described a patient suffering from the syndrome. Such people travel from one hospital or doctor to another telling untruthful stories about their medical condition, describing dramatic but false symptoms, or simulating acute illness. They may happily submit themselves for countless operations (having scars that bear testimony) or undergo what they know to be unnecessary medical investigations.

They often leave a hospital without notice and resume their travels.

muscle

Tissue composed of fibers which have the power to contract. Muscles thus produce movements of the body. *Voluntary* muscle, also known as *striped* or *striated* muscle, is under the direct control of the will. *Involuntary*, or *smooth*, muscle is not under the control of the will. It is to be found in the heart, blood vessels, the walls of the stomach and intestines and in most internal organs. The heart is composed of partially striated muscle.

Voluntary muscles are activated and controlled by motor nerves, which reach them directly from the brain or by way of the spinal cord. If a motor nerve is cut or injured, the muscle or that group of muscles which it supplies is paralyzed, as impulses from the brain are interrupted.

An average fiber in a voluntary muscle is from 2–4 cm long. Under the microscope it has a banded or striped appearance. During contractions one set of filaments (composed of *actin*) pass down between another set (*myosin* filaments), and optically the lighter bands become reduced in size.

The immediate source of energy needed for contraction appears to be a substance known as *adenosine triphosphate*, but the ultimate source is carbohydrate and fat. Oxygen is used in the contraction process and muscle fatigue and rigor are accompanied by the production of lactic acid.

In *muscle strain*, overstretching occurs; there may be a sudden sharp pain at the site of injury, which is followed by swelling.

Cramp (a painful sudden involuntary contraction of a muscle or muscles) is sometimes caused by poor coordination during exercise; by chilling, as in swimming; or by excessive loss of salt and body fluids from severe sweating, diarrhea, or persistent vomiting. Often the cause is not known.

In salt deficiency the patient should be given copious amounts of cold water to which a small quantity of salt has been added.

muscular dystrophy

A group of inherited diseases characterized by progressive weakness due to degeneration of muscles. They are thought to represent inborn errors of metabolism, although precise biochemical abnormalities have yet to be fully identified.

The pathological changes primarily affect the muscles responsible for body movement, but heart muscle may also be involved. There is variation in muscle fiber size, degeneration of fibers and an increase in connective tissue.

Onset is usually in childhood or adolescence. Wasting is symmetrical and slowly progressive. Remissions do not occur in muscular dystrophies. Similar cases frequently occur in the same family (in up to 50% of cases, another member of the direct family line is affected).

The condition usually begins centrally as opposed to in the muscles of the extremities; posture is typically disturbed, with the development of spinal curvature.

Two major variations have been described. In the *Duchenne* or "pseudohypertrophic" form only boys are affected. This form differs from other types in that wasted muscles are replaced by fat, giving the muscles a bulky appearance which contrasts with the weakness present. It usually starts at about the age of four or five. The muscles of the shoulder and pelvic girdle become enlarged, as do the calf muscles. This leads to a waddling gait and frequent falls. The child has a characteristic way of getting up from the lying position; he has to roll over onto his face, and then onto his hands and knees, from which he gradually stands up onto his legs. The shoulders are affected later.

In the other main type, the "facioscapulohumeral" or *Landouzy-Dejerine* form, both sexes are affected. It starts later in adolescence and commences in the face.

Weakness of the shoulder girdle is more prominent than leg weakness. Some patients with the condition are scarcely aware of the symptoms throughout a normal life span: in others, disabilities gradually increase. An affected child may lack normal facial expressions and be unable to raise his arms above his head.

Other forms and intermediate conditions exist. For instance, there is an arm and shoulder variety and a rarer form known as "distal myopathy." In this condition weakness starts in the hands and spreads inward.

There is no specific drug treatment for these diseases. In some cases, muscle-strengthening exercises, corrective surgery and the use of braces may be helpful to patients.

myasthenia gravis

A form of muscle debility which is progressive and characterized by abnormal fatigue of voluntary muscle and rapid recovery after rest. It is a slowly progressive disease, usually encountered in adults and rarely seen before the age of puberty.

Myasthenia gravis affects both sexes. The highest incidence occurs in females between the ages of 18 to 25 and in men over 40. The condition is sometimes associated with HYPERTHYROIDISM as well as with excessive formation of tissue in the thymus gland in a high percentage of cases, or with a thymic tumor.

There is a disorder of conduction at the point where the nerves meet and activate the muscle cells. The muscles thus fail to respond to the signal from the nerve endings. Myasthenia gravis is thought to be caused by the failure of formation of the "neuromuscular transmitter" chemical acetylcholine.

The paralysis produced is normally minimal in the morning and worse at night. The disease most often affects the eyes, facial and shoulder girdle muscles and (less often) the legs.

Paralysis of the eye muscles leads to STRABISMUS (squint) and double vision. Drooping of the eyelids and weakness of the facial muscles cause the typical "myasthenic smile" and lack of expression. Gradual loss of the voice and difficulty in chewing or swallowing during the course of a meal are frequent complaints. Weakness of the arms may also be present.

Symptoms fluctuate in severity from day to day and remissions occur in approximately a quarter of the patients.

For treatment, tablets of neostigmine (a specific antidote), or the longer-acting pyridostigmine may be given. If weakness is severe, an intramuscular injection of neostigmine may be necessary in the morning and before meals.

Removal of the thymus gland is beneficial in about two thirds of cases.

mydriasis

Dilation of the pupil of the eye. Mydriasis occurs when the light falling on the eye decreases in intensity or when the lens focuses from a near object to a distant one. The widening pupil permits more light to fall on the retina and more to be seen in poor light.

Stimulation of sensory nerves may cause a dilation of the pupil. In conditions such as excitement, fear, pain, or asphyxia (which lead to the release of epinephrine from the adrenal glands), the pupils dilate, as they do when the sympathetic nerves to the eyes are stimulated. Certain drugs can produce mydriasis—for example, atropine, homatropine, cocaine and epinephrine. Alcohol intoxication has the same effect.

myelitis

1. A general term that means inflammation of the spinal cord.

Acute transverse myelitis is the name given to a syndrome which may be caused by a viral or bacterial infection; often the cause is undetermined. The symptoms are dramatic, as over the course of 48 hours there is complete loss of muscle power and sensation below the affected section of the spinal cord. Usually there is some recovery as the inflammation subsides; its extent is difficult to predict.

The term *myelitis* is sometimes used imprecisely by members of the medical profession to refer to a lesion of the spinal cord which is not caused by inflammation (in such cases the term *myelopathy* is more correct).

See also POLIOMYELITIS.

2. Inflammation of the bone marrow (see OSTEOMYELITIS).

myelocele

See SPINA BIFIDA.

myeloma

See MULTIPLE MYELOMA.

myiasis

Invasion or infection of a body area or cavity by the larvae (maggots) of flies. Many fly species have been implicated. Some are termed *obligate parasites*—that is, they cannot survive without involving humans in their life cycles. Others, known as *facultative parasites,* are capable of being free-living as well as acting as parasites. In a third category there is only chance invasion of human subjects.

Among those classified as obligate parasites are the human botfly, the rodent botfly and flesh flies. In the second category come the common screwworm fly, the bluebottle, other types of flesh fly and the stable fly. Examples in the final category are houseflies, cheese skippers and fruit flies.

Myiasis usually involves the skin or mucous membranes, especially those of the nasal passages and pharynx. Lesions in the skin may be shallow or deep, leading to "boils" containing the larvae.

In some infestations the larvae burrow deep and reach the membranes or cavities of the nose, pharynx, ear, eye and vagina, where they cause extensive damage.

Gastrointestinal myiasis arises from the accidental swallowing of larvae in contaminated foodstuffs, which may occasionally lead to invasion of the intestinal wall.

Surgical removal of deep-burrowing skin larvae may be necessary, but a more superficial type can be treated with an ethyl chloride spray or the application of ice (which kills the larvae before they are removed).

Larvae in a deep boil are best extracted surgically. Eggs of the screwworm fly, which is found in the southern United States, are laid in an open wound and can invade tissue extensively. The larvae are removed after swabbing the affected area with ether or chloroform in oil. Serious intestinal myiasis may be treated by vermifuges and purges.

myocardial infarction

A technical term for a "heart attack."

See also INFARCT/INFARCTION.

myocarditis

Inflammation of the muscular tissue of the heart. This sometimes serious condition may arise due to an unknown cause or may be a complication of a number of illnesses—such as rheumatic fever, scarlet fever, diphtheria or typhoid fever. Apart from being associated with bacterial, fungal or viral diseases (especially *Coxsackie virus B*), myocarditis may be due to toxic chemicals, alcohol, drugs or to electrical shock or excessive x-ray treatment.

The condition leads to circulatory disturbances and the patient may have a rapid, soft and often irregular pulse. Myocarditis may leave a residual effect on the efficiency of the heart after recovery. Once the condition is suspected, complete bed rest, sedation and continuation of therapy for any underlying illness may help to prevent a sudden exacerbation.

myoclonus

A spasm of muscle. It has been described as a sudden, nonrhythmic, nonpatterned twitching.

Normal individuals often experience an isolated myoclonic jerk or two in drowsiness or light sleep.

The term can be used to refer to such movements in a part of a muscle, a whole muscle or group of muscles, a limb, the trunk or the face. Myoclonus results from a paroxysmal discharge in the central nervous system.

This type of movement can be a characteristic of epilepsy. In such a myoclonic seizure the patient may experience muscular jerks of varying intensity, usually without an evident alteration in the level of consciousness. Myoclonic seizures are often associated with other types of seizure, however, especially those characterized by sudden loss of muscle power and sudden transient lapses of consciousness; they have a tendency to occur more frequently in the mornings or on going to sleep.

Progressive *familial myoclonic epilepsy* is an inherited degenerative disease beginning in childhood or adolescence, characterized by progressively worsening generalized myoclonic seizures and mental disturbances.

In the clonic stage of major general epilepsy there are a series of convulsive movements not only in the trunk and limbs but in the jaw and tongue, so that the tongue may be badly bitten or saliva may be lathered into foam. First aid treatment for a patient undergoing such a seizure is to put a knotted handkerchief or similar soft object between their jaws to protect the tongue. (However, the teeth must *not* be forced apart as serious damage may result.) Keep the patient's airway clear.

myoma

A benign tumor of muscle tissue. They most frequently occur in the smooth muscle wall of the uterus as spherical masses, in which case they are also referred to as *fibromyomas* or *fibroids*. They may arise in any part of the uterus from its top to the cervix (neck of the womb). Uterine myomas occur more frequently in blacks, are more common after the age of 30 and do not develop before the onset of menstruation (menarche) or after the menopause. They most frequently do not cause symptoms, but may be associated with infertility, abnormal menstruation, pain and other symptoms.

If the symptoms warrant, surgical removal of myomas may be performed (myomectomy). When continued fertility is not required, total hysterectomy (surgical removal of the uterus) may be performed.

Myomas may also occur elsewhere in the body—for instance in the stomach and small bowel, where they form masses in the walls. Here they are prone to ulceration and then cause blood in the feces and anemia.

myopia

An optical defect in which the image of distant objects is focused in front of the retina (the light-sensitive "screen" at the back of the eye) rather than directly on the retina. The result of this is that distant objects appear blurred, although near objects can be seen clearly. Also called *near-sightedness*.

In myopia it is an excessive length of the eyeball which gives rise to the focusing defect. This can be corrected for far vision with a concave lens (or a contact lens). Near objects can still be focused on the retina by inhibiting the normal reflex of accommodation of the lens.

MYOPIA

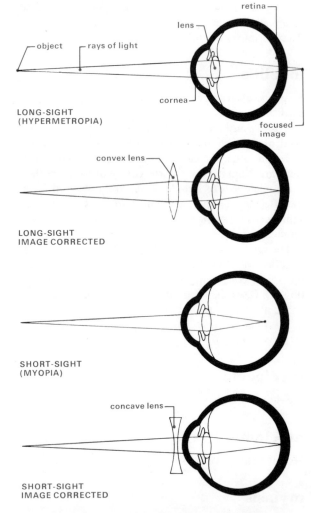

LONG-SIGHT
(HYPERMETROPIA)

LONG-SIGHT
IMAGE CORRECTED

SHORT-SIGHT
(MYOPIA)

SHORT-SIGHT
IMAGE CORRECTED

Myopia, or short-sight, can result either from an elongated eyeball or from a lens which is too powerful. The outcome as shown above is that rays of light are focused in front of the retina so that the image is blurred. Long-sight is the reverse optical error and usually results from the lens weakening with age. Both conditions can be corrected by wearing glasses with lenses of the correct strength.

The normal eye is so shaped that rays of light from distant objects are brought to an exact focus on the retina. Nearer objects are brought into focus by a contraction of the ciliary muscle, allowing the lens to become more spherical.

In the large majority of cases, myopia is simply a variation in the shape of the eyeball. The problem may get no worse after adolescence and a little reduction in the myopia may even take place in late middle-age. In some cases the eyeball may continue to elongate throughout life ("progressive myopia"), leading to a retinal degeneration or even to DETACHED RETINA.

Severely myopic eyeballs may in fact look large and even appear like those of someone suffering from HYPERTHYROIDISM.

Different types of myopia have been outlined by ophthalmologists. In *curvature myopia* the fault is due to excessive curvature of one of the refractive surfaces of the eye where the light path is normally deviated for focusing. The excessive curvature is usually present in the anterior surface of the cornea but sometimes it occurs in the lens.

Index myopia is due to an increase in the refractive index (a unit that indicates the light-refracting properties of a medium). This type of myopia usually refers to change in the lens, which may progress to a future development of CATARACT; but it may also refer to an increase in the refractive index of the aqueous humor of the eye as in IRITIS.

In the myope, then, a concave lens will push the focal point backward toward the backward placed retina, so as to allow clear distant vision. Since the curvature of the cornea is almost never exactly the same in all directions, this associated *astigmatism* (as it is known) may at the same time be corrected by giving the lens the appropriate added convexity or concavity. As a result, the shape of the cornea is adjusted.

myositis

Inflammation of a muscle. The condition usually occurs in a voluntary, or striated, muscle. There is pain, tenderness and stiffness of the muscle and adjacent tissues and joints may also be affected. It may be secondary to trauma, infection, strain, poisons or exposure to damp or cold, but often occurs in older people for no known reason. When connective tissue is also involved the condition is often loosely known by the term "rheumatism." Myositis commonly involves the back, neck, shoulders, chest or thighs. If it affects the neck it may temporarily give rise to wry neck (TORTICOLLIS), in which the head cannot be turned, or may even be drawn downward to the shoulder on one side.

Onset of pain may be sudden and local muscle spasm is present in some cases. Fever is only evident if the condition is part of a general infection.

Fortunately, myositis tends to disappear in a few days, but occasionally it may become chronic or may recur at frequent intervals.

When diagnosing the condition the physician attempts to establish that myositis is not a manifestation of a more serious underlying disease.

Rest, heat, massage, analgesics (painkillers) and application of liniments are simple measures that can be employed to bring relief.

In *myositis ossificans* bone cells deposited in muscle continue to grow and form lumps. It may occur after a fracture—for example, in the elbow region. The type of exercise given to such an arm may affect the development of this condition and only prescribed active exercise should be performed initially.

Passive movements, such as those involved in massage, should be discouraged. With the right kind of exercises and rest the calcified masses usually disappear.

myxedema

A condition caused by malfunction or surgical removal of the thyroid gland. Subsequent lack of circulating thyroid hormone in the body gives rise to a series of signs and symptoms, which represent a severe form of HYPOTHYROIDISM.

There is swelling of the face and limbs because of subcutaneous fluid deposition. This may particularly affect the area around the eyes and the hands and feet. The skin becomes dry and rough and there may be some hair loss. The patient exhibits slowness of action and thought and this mental dullness is accompanied by slow speech, with a voice which may become hoarse. Lethargy and weakness may be associated with slowed reflexes, a slow pulse, lowered metabolism and subnormal body temperature. The patient sometimes experiences poor tolerance to cold and (especially in the elderly) HYPOTHERMIA. The appetite may be poor, yet—in contrast—there is often a mild weight gain. Shortness of breath and constipation are not uncommon. About one third of patients suffer from high blood pressure, ANGINA PECTORIS and palpitations.

The condition may arise through primary disease of the thyroid or following removal of the gland in the treatment of thyrotoxic or malignant goiter. Iodine deficiency or circulating antithyroid antibodies may also be contributory factors.

Recovery is usually excellent with the administration of thyroxin or thyroid extract, which must be continued throughout life. The dose of thyroxin is increased by small amounts about every two weeks, as necessary, until the correct maintenance dose is reached. In older patients with heart disease, the thyroid hormone level is increased slowly, since a rapid rise can precipitate angina pectoris and heart failure.

When thyroid hormone deficiency occurs in infancy it may lead to CRETINISM, characterized by abnormal thickness of the neck, stunted growth and imperfect mental development.

Once diagnosed this condition requires immediate thyroid replacement therapy—ideally within the first three months of life—to avoid long-term damage.

Coma developing in a patient suffering from myxedema represents a medical emergency. It is more likely to occur in the elderly if they are not receiving a satisfactory dose of thyroid extract. Treatment should be intensive but not hasty. The patient is cold to the touch, with a body temperature often below the range of a standard clinical thermometer. Vigorous rewarming of the patient should be avoided, the use of blankets being preferable. In addition, the drug triiodothyronine is given intravenously.

N

naevus

See NEVUS.

naturopathy

A system of health care which suggests that disease is provoked by violation of "Nature's Laws," and that the reparation of physical or psychological disorder depends entirely on the use of diet, massage, or special bathing procedures. The naturopath believes, not incorrectly, that health is the normal state of the human being, and, quite incorrectly, that it can invariably be maintained by "natural" foods alone.

While naturopathy may seem a reasonable philosophy for someone in good health, it may be dangerous in disease; few naturopaths, if any, have formal medical skills and may fail to recognize life-threatening and curable disorders such as tuberculosis.

nausea

A feeling of wanting to vomit, with a characteristic sensation that passes through the upper part of the abdomen.

The stomach normally contracts regularly to empty its contents into the duodenum and the small intestine. If this reflex action temporarily ceases and the duodenum itself contracts to prevent the stomach emptying, the effect on the individual is to experience nausea. Nausea can thus be brought on by virtually anything that affects gastrointestinal function in any way.

necrosis

The death of areas of tissue or bone surrounded by healthy parts.

Necrotic tissue is seen, at the simplest level, in the pustular content of even the smallest septic spot, where the yellow fluid discharged is composed of dead bacteria, the body's dead white blood cells, and skin cells that have failed to survive the ravages of an infective agent. Necrosis takes place even where infective agents are not present when any tissue is deprived of its blood supply: for example, in small areas of the heart muscle after a "heart attack," in the middle of tumors that have outgrown their blood supply and in areas of the body where GANGRENE (which is another name for a wide area of tissue necrosis) has occurred.

Where OSTEOMYELITIS occurs in bone there is necrosis of the bone cells (*sequestrum*) because the inflammation has caused the blockage or thrombosis of the minute arteries supplying these bone cells. In atherosclerosis the blood vessels may be partially blocked by fatty deposits (atheromas) and the blood supply to the peripheral parts of the lower limb may be insufficient to maintain nutrition of the tissues, so that necrosis—or gangrene—may occur in the toes. In frostbite, necrosis of the tissues may occur because the peripheral blood vessels have frozen.

neoplasm

An abnormal new growth of cells or tissues from ordered, original tissue; tumor.

See CANCER.

nephrectomy

Surgical removal of a kidney.

nephritis

Nephritis (inflammation of the kidney) falls into two principal groups: (1) PYELONEPHRITIS, a bacterial infection which spreads from the bladder and ureters and (2) GLOMERULONEPHRITIS, a noninfective disease usually affecting both kidneys.

See also KIDNEY DISEASES.

nephroma

A tumor involving kidney tissue. See KIDNEY DISEASES.

nephrotic syndrome

Many healthy young individuals are found to have protein in their urine at routine medical checks, especially if it is measured after a period of prolonged standing or exercise. However, some people lose an excessive amount of protein in the urine, so that the level of albumin in their blood is greatly reduced (hypoalbuminemia) and excess fluid collects in the tissues as EDEMA.

This triad of signs (heavy proteinuria, hypoalbuminemia, and edema) is known as the *nephrotic syndrome,* and is more common in childhood than in adult life. About 80% of the cases in young children result from "minimal change" pathology in the kidney. Fortunately, the prognosis for children in this group is excellent and nearly all of them make a rapid and complete recovery following treatment with corticosteroid drugs.

When the nephrotic syndrome occurs in a patient over about ten years of age, or if a younger patient shows additional signs such as blood in the urine or high blood pressure, it is necessary to obtain a small piece of kidney by a needle biopsy. When viewed under the microscope, this tissue might reveal changes characteristic of GLOMERULONEPHRITIS, DIABETES MELLITUS, AMYLOIDOSIS, or systemic LUPUS ERYTHEMATOSUS— all possibly associated with the nephrotic syndrome. Nephrotic patients with kidney lesions other than "minimal change" do not respond well to corticosteroid drugs. They are usually maintained on a diet high in protein and low in salt; diuretic drugs ("water pills") are used to control the edema.

See also KIDNEY DISEASES.

neuralgia

A term which implies pain arising along the course of a nerve, which may be severe, dull, or stabbing.

Usually nothing can be seen, but sometimes there is evidence of inflammation or damage to the sensory nerve affected—as in the neuralgia which may follow HERPES ZOSTER (shingles). SCIATICA, which is pain along the course of the sciatic nerve, is associated with interference with the nerve roots making up the nerve by a prolapsed or herniated intervertebral disk ("slipped disk") or by arthritic processes arising in intervertebral joints. Neuralgia in the hands may occur in the CARPAL TUNNEL SYNDROME.

Neuralgia is an imprecise term except when applied to *trigeminal neuralgia,* an affliction of the sensory nerve supplying the face (the Vth cranial nerve, or trigeminal nerve). This is a very severe intermittent pain on one side of the face, coming on in spasms which last less than a minute. During the attack the patient may show agonized contortions of the facial muscles which give the disease its alternative name, *tic douloureux* (see TIC). Treatment involves administration of drugs such as phenytoin sodium or carbamazepine. If these fail, it may be necessary to destroy the ganglion of the nerve inside the skull by injection or by open operation, procedures which are followed by total anesthesia of the face on the affected side. The disease is rare in patients below the age of 50, although it may occur in younger patients in association with multiple sclerosis.

Other patterns of facial neuralgia may occur, usually described as "atypical facial pain," including a neuralgia affecting the IXth cranial nerve (*glossopharyngeal neuralgia*). It is characterized by intermittent attacks of severe pain, usually beginning at the base of the tongue and radiating down the neck or to the ears. It is triggered by movements such as swallowing, chewing, sneezing, or sometimes just by talking. Treatment involves the administration of carbamazepine. Temporary or partial relief is sometimes obtained by the local application of an anesthetic to the throat. In cases that are more severe, however, surgical disruption of the nerve may be necessary.

neurasthenia

An outdated term, neurasthenia (Greek *neuron* = nerve, *asthenia* = weakness) was once commonly used to describe conditions characterized by marked mental and physical irritability with excessive fatigue. An inability to concentrate, impairment of memory and complaints such as "pressure in the head," "eyes ache with reading," palpitations, constipation and impotence would lead to a diagnostic label of neurasthenia.

It was common after a debilitating illness, particularly in the era before antibiotics and was especially applied to professional or intelligently curious patients who required an "explanation" for their symptoms of fatigue. Nowadays it would be considered a normal convalescent stage in which the patient recovers spontaneously and progressively with rest, or where no physical reason was detectable for the complaints—such as a psychoneurotic disorder, anticipating a depressive illness.

neuritis

The general term applied to disease of the peripheral nerves.

Degeneration of the nerve tissue occurs with consequent loss of sensation, impairment of muscular control and symptoms that vary from severe pain to tingling and "pins and needles" brought about by movement of the involved part of the body— particularly if the nerve is stretched. A single nerve or multiple nerves may be involved and the causes may be *infective* (as in diphtheria, tetanus, or leprosy), *mechanical* (as in compression, arthritis, or obstetric injury), *chemical* (as in arsenical poisoning or antibiotic sensitivity), *vascular* (as in arteriosclerosis, diabetes or myxedema), or *nutritional* (as in beriberi, alcoholism or porphyria).

The diagnosis is made by determining the character and distribution of the nerve's impairment. For example, *brachial neuritis* with pains in the whole arm and varied loss of sensation in the skin of the arm (in particular, pain when the muscles are compressed) follows the use of crutches that press on the brachial nerves in the armpit. Generalized neuritis in the diabetic, or the alcoholic, or the patient with malnutrition will affect most peripheral nerves.

Treatment is aimed at relief of the cause, if it is specific, combined with rest, physical therapy and analgesics (painkillers). Correction of dietary inadequacy by the administering of vital nutrients achieves a cure of the neuritis where malnutrition is the cause.

neurofibroma

A tumor of the connective tissue which forms the nerve sheath. It may occur as a single swelling and reach a considerable size; normally benign, the tumor may become malignant, but it usually gives rise to symptoms because it exerts pressure on neighboring structures—for example, the spinal cord or the nerve upon which it lies. A neurofibroma may be evident as a swelling in the skin; treatment of the solitary tumor is surgical removal.

Neurofibromas may occur in considerable numbers as part of VON RECKLINGHAUSEN'S DISEASE (or *multiple neurofibromatosis*). The tumors are associated with irregular brown pigmented patches on the skin (*café au lait* spots), and they represent a defect in the development of the supporting tissue of the nervous system. Where they give rise to symptoms they may require surgical treatment.

neurofibromatosis

Another name for VON RECKLINGHAUSEN'S DISEASE (also known as *multiple neurofibromatosis*).

neuropathy

In medical practice the terms *neuritis* and *neuropathy* are used almost interchangeably, but the implication of neuropathy is that a degenerative change has taken place in the nerve, or nerves, affected by either inflammation, injury, nutritional deprivation or toxic poisoning.

On microscopic examination the nerves show fragmentation of the nerve fibers, but in *generalized neuropathy* the lesions may begin in the nerve roots at the spinal cord. The manifestations are variable but include fluctuating pain that may be deep and aching, sharp, pricking, burning, or any combination of these qualities. Examination of the sensory abilities demonstrates impairment of all sensations but to different degrees; in *peripheral neuropathy* there is often a symmetrical "glove" or "stocking" pattern in the area deprived. Muscular weakness is also variable in severity and the affected muscles are flaccid with loss of the tendon reflexes. The skin of the affected area becomes thin and shiny and there may be excessive sweating in the area. All these manifestations reflect the disordered conduction pathway of the nerve supplying the distinct area.

One of the best examples of generalized neuropathy is that which occurs in the vitamin B_1 (thiamine) deficiency disease of beriberi, but in alcoholics and diabetics the same degrees of peripheral neuropathy are also seen. Metallic poisons—lead, mercury, silver, thallium—and chemicals such as trinitrotoluene, trichlorethylene, and carbon disulfide cause generalized and peripheral neuropathy. Rare inherited diseases may be progressive; but in general, once the cause is identified—if it is specific—correction is possible.

The management of neuropathy is mainly the control of pain and protection of the weakened muscles from stretching and excessive wasting (atrophy). Bed rest is recommended and aspirin or a stronger analgesic is used to control the pain. Heat from infrared lamps or warm baths is helpful. Splints and limb supports may be necessary to prevent deformity; when local muscular tenderness subsides, passive action, massage and other forms of physical therapy are advisable. A well-balanced diet should be maintained and, where undernutrition was responsible for the neuropathy, vitamin supplements may be prescribed. The recovery of a patient from neuropathy depends on the extent of the original damage.

neurosis

A neurosis is a personality disorder. Behavior traits, thought processes, emotional responses and some body functions may all be influenced by the neurosis. It is usually a maladjustment to the ordinary stresses and demands of life, but is often characteristically irrational.

Any neurosis may be traceable in origin to the early learning experiences of life and to childhood in particular, but the individual may suffer great conflict and discomfort in not being able to recognize his or her own failure to adapt to the anxiety that is the cause of their neurosis. Neuroses develop in the predisposed individual from childhood onward, and appear at the particular times of life when society and community living demand adaptation of the personality. For example, in adolescence when a sexual identity is being sought, in adult life when vocational demands or choice provoke stress, and in parenthood when adaptation of the role toward accepting responsibility for the dependence of others is a challenge—in all these common circumstances of life, neurosis is prone to occur in the insecure individual.

Neurosis is seen more commonly in females, particularly as a response to the stress of a career and the responsibilities of marriage and at the menopause, when adjustment to a new life is required. In elderly couples the approach of retirement can sometimes provoke neurosis. It rarely appears anew in the middle-aged individual who has not shown previous neurotic tendencies.

The incidence is estimated at about 3–4% of the normal population, but it is higher in the physically ill; at the University of Chicago Hospital, one survey found what they defined as neurosis present in 30% of patients. Of those rejected on medical grounds from the U.S. Armed Services, 20% had disorders complicated by the presence of neurosis.

Neurosis can commonly take the form of an exaggerated response to physical illness—because it threatens security. In answer to fear, and as a consequence of exposure to anxiety-arousing situations, neurosis can become phobic, obsessive, compulsive, hysteric or psychosomatic in its character. Recent thinking emphasizes the importance, in the development of neurosis, of an individual's feelings of loneliness and the shallowness of his or her interpersonal relations with other individuals. The neurotic person's expectations of helpers and physicians are often immature and demanding of immediate relief; they thus face a lifetime of disappointments and frustrations that compound the neurotic personality.

Acute and severe attacks may provoke psychosomatic symptoms that cause severe distress—*hyperventilation* (overbreathing) is one example; the *panic attack* with an irresistible sense of impending death is another. PHOBIAS with regard to crowds, open spaces, heights, dirt, or insects can be occupationally disabling, as can *compulsive neuroses* that involve ritual hand washing. *Genitourinary neurosis* can produce dyspareunia (pain experienced by a woman during sexual intercourse) or frigidity, dermatological expressions of neurosis may produce chronic skin rashes, gastrointestinal manifestations may include peptic ulcers or colitis, and in particular coronary ischemia (reduced blood supply to the heart muscle) is complicated by a cardiac neurosis that produces invalidism.

Diagnosis involves psychological testing and a careful medical history, which may require analysis to identify the cause. Treatment has to be skilled, prolonged and supportive. Psychotherapy and behavioral techniques can assist in adjustment; medication helps—usually with tranquilizers to resolve the acute phases. Cure is achieved in only about one third of cases, but the considerable success of professional supportive therapy may help the individual to adjust to life's demands, and largely overcome the personality disorder that results in excessive anxiety.

See also PSYCHIATRY and PSYCHOTHERAPY.

neurotransmitters

Chemical substances that transmit nerve impulses between nerve cells.

The basic unit of the human nervous system is the nerve cell (neuron), which has a long extension called an *axon* that comes almost in physical contact with the receiving processes (dendrites) of other nerve cells. Across this microscopic gap (the "synapse") an electrochemical impulse is transmitted from the axon of one neuron to the dendrites of an adjacent neuron, or to a gland cell to cause secretion, or to a muscle to cause contraction. The transmission of the impulse is achieved by the release of neurotransmitters from special parts of the nerve cell membrane.

Neurotransmitters are not all identified chemically, but they include such substances as acetylcholine, norepinephrine, serotonin, glutamine and several other acids. The neurotransmitter is stored on one side of the synapse with the reactive site on the other side. The signal ceases when the neurotransmitter is chemically changed, diffuses away from the synapse, or is reabsorbed.

The neurotransmitter is vulnerable to drugs or toxins which modify its synthesis or action. Anything that interferes with its breakdown will cause prolonged action (as in TETANUS), while substances that delay its release have equally dramatic effects (as in paralysis due to curare poisoning). Many drugs act by their effect on neurotransmitters: for example, certain drugs used to control blood pressure.

nevus

A type of skin discoloration; a "birthmark."

It is due to an anomaly in the embryonic development of the skin, particularly affecting the blood vessels of the subcutaneous layer in small or wide areas. Nevi vary considerably in size and appearance. The most commonly recognized type is the "strawberry" birth mark. Others are the tiny star-shaped discoloration often called the "spider" nevus—commonly seen in adults—and the quite disfiguring "port wine stain" (*nevus flammeus*) that can occupy half the face of the newborn.

Nevi may appear at birth or soon after; occasionally they develop within the first two years of life. They affect all ethnic groups from the "blue" nevus of the Mongolian races to the "pale" nevus of the negroid. There is no known cause and the suggestion that nevi are intrauterine "pressure" marks is untrue. They affect the sexes equally, but are considered cosmetically less acceptable in the female.

Nevi may be single or multiple, faint in discoloration or very obvious. *Pigmented nevi,* containing an excess of melanin making them much darker than normal skin, may grow hairs that are thick, black and profuse. *Vascular nevi*—those containing blood vessels—deepen in color when a child cries or exercises, because the blood vessels are engorged with incomplete blood pathways. Nevi are usually demarcated at the border and rarely increase in size.

The "strawberry" birthmark usually disappears as the child grows, since deposits of subcutaneous fat tend to hide it. Such a nevus therefore requires no treatment.

NEVUS

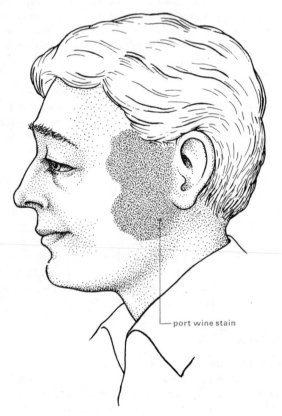

— port wine stain

A nevus, or birthmark, is an area of discolored skin which results from a congenital malformation of surface blood vessels. Certain types of nevus have descriptive names, such as "strawberry nevus" and the "port wine stain" illustrated here.

Pigmented nevi with hairs may also be left, to observe their possible fading or disappearance, but they may occasionally require surgical excision or other treatment—such as electrolysis, diathermy cauterization or "freezing." "Spider" nevi respond to electrolysis. There is no truly effective treatment for a port wine stain, but a cosmetician can prepare a special cream which matches the patient's skin to provide a means of concealing the disfigurement. In all cases the skilled advice of a dermatologist should be sought.

See also MOLE.

Niemann-Pick disease

An extremely rare disease, inherited as a recessive gene. It is characterized by a widespread accumulation of a particular kind of "fat" cells throughout the body, particularly affecting the tissues of the nerves, brain, spleen, liver and lymph glands.

The disease is seen in infants, who rarely survive beyond the sixth month. Mental retardation, spasticity, and convulsions occur and there is progressive wasting of the body with the appearance of jaundice. Diagnosis is confirmed by tissue biopsy. Most common among those of Jewish origin, it is also associated with inbreeding. There is no treatment, and only in a few cases does survival occur to late childhood. It occurs in equal sex distribution.

night blindness

A condition in which vision is fairly normal in good light but defective in dim light. The technical term is *nyctalopia.* It is primarily a symptom of severe vitamin A deficiency but also occurs in RETINITIS PIGMENTOSA, an inherited degenerative disorder of the retina.

The ability of the eye to adapt to varying degrees of light and dark depends on photoreceptors in the retina. One type of photoreceptor, the rods, mediate vision in dim light. They contain pigment known as rhodopsin or "visual purple," which is temporarily bleached by light. The speed of the eye's adaptability to dark depends on the speed with which rhodopsin is re-formed in darkness, which in turn depends on vitamin A.

If night blindness is due to vitamin A deficiency, treatment is by vitamin A replacement; if it is due to retinitis pigmentosa, there is no effective treatment.

See also VISION.

noma

A rare condition of progressive gangrene (necrosis) that affects children in the terminal stages of severe malnutrition. Also known as *cancrum oris* or *gangrenous stomatitis.*

It occurs in Central and South America in areas of starvation and very poor hygiene. Noma may also occur in the genitalia of starving children, particularly in young girls, and may develop in any area of the body that has previously been attacked by infections.

It is caused by the invasion of *fusospirochetal* organisms and other bacteria in children whose resistance is markedly lowered by malnutrition and other infections. A green to black area develops characteristically on the gums and spreads until the ulceration denudes the jaw. The teeth loosen and fall out but pain, surprisingly, is rarely severe—probably because the sensory nerves are deprived of their function. The destruction of local affected areas, mouth, nose and cheek continues unabated unless treatment is initiated; death can result from septicemia and toxemia.

Treatment with penicillin arrests the disease immediately but the malnutrition must be corrected to prevent its recurrence. The damage done by noma is not naturally repaired except by scar tissue, and deformity results.

nonspecific urethritis (NSU)

Urethritis is inflammation of the urethra—the tube through which the bladder discharges urine; it passes from the neck of the bladder to the external genitalia. Urethritis can occur as an inflammation due to various known infective organisms, or as a result of trauma; but when bacteriological investigations fail to yield any positive results the inflammation is said to be *non-specific*. The term is used in the U.K. to imply 'non-venereal'.

The symptoms are pain and a burning sensation on passing urine and urinary frequency. There is a urethral discharge, and the disease is confined to the age of the sexually active.

Nonspecific urethritis is more common in males; but as the urethra is anatomically longer in the male, it may be that it is underdiagnosed in females and many cases of "cystitis" in women may be cases of nonspecific urethritis. It develops 5–30 days after sexual intercourse and varies in the intensity of its symptoms. The condition may last for several weeks and its recurrence rate is high.

The cause, as the name implies, is unknown. Viruses, bacteria, funguses and other genital parasites, as well as allergies, have been blamed but proof of the actual cause is lacking. Diagnosis depends on the medical history and the absence in urine cultures, or urethral swabs—even after massage of the prostate gland in the male—of any positive bacterial growths.

Tetracycline, an antibiotic, is an effective treatment but it may be necessary to take it in prolonged courses.

nosebleed

Bleeding from the nose (known medically as *epistaxis*) is a common experience, usually as a result of trauma to the flexible cartilaginous area of the nose below the nasal bones (i.e., below the "bridge").

If minor trauma is the cause it is of little medical significance—for, with the correct first-aid treatment, it ceases quite quickly. It may occur spontaneously, however; sometimes due to hypertension in an older person, due to allergic rhinitis and excessive sneezing, due to cabin depressurization when flying, or alternatively due to "mountain sickness." When recurrent nosebleeds are experienced, examination may reveal the presence of nasal POLYPS. It is of no danger to the individual unless he is taking anticoagulants; although the quantity of blood lost in a nosebleed may seem to be considerable, it is rarely ever enough to warrant replacement by transfusion.

The correct treatment is to sit the sufferer up with the head held forwards. He is instructed to breathe through the opened mouth, and to grasp the soft part of his nose between his fingers and thumb to close the nostrils down onto the middle septum throughout its length. This pressure should be sustained until the bleeding stops. Thereafter no attempts to sneeze or blow the nose should be made for at least 48 hours so that another nosebleed will not be induced.

Recurrent attacks require referral to a specialist for the affected blood vessel to be cauterized.

nyctalopia

The technical term for NIGHT BLINDNESS.

nystagmus

Rapid, rhythmic flickering movements of the eyeball. The movements may take place in a horizontal, vertical, rotatory, or oblique plane (or rarely in a combination of all planes). There are two main rhythms of movement: a "pendular" variety in which the movements in both directions are equal; and a "jerky" variety consisting of a slow movement in one direction followed by a rapid, jerky movement in the opposite direction.

Normal nystagmus occurs when a person is looking at scenery from a moving vehicle. Otherwise, the causes of abnormal nystagmus fall into three main groups.

The first group consists of defects in vision in which the eye does not receive sufficient visual stimuli for it to fix its gaze. The second group consists of disturbances of the elaborate mechanisms in the ear which help to maintain posture and which have nervous connections to the eye. The third group of causes of abnormal nystagmus consists of diseases of the nervous system.

Nystagmus does not usually produce symptoms but it may sometimes produce vertigo or double vision. Treatment depends on the cause.

O

obesity

The excessive accumulation of body fat. A person is generally considered obese when his weight is more than 20% above the average weight for people of his race and height. In children, age has also to be taken into account. Other causes of overweight, such as accumulation of fluid, or extremely well-developed muscles, should be excluded before an overweight person is said to be obese.

Another simple and commonly used method for assessing obesity is the measurement of *skinfold thickness* using calipers, since a large proportion of the fat stores are found just underneath the skin. There are also a number of sophisticated laboratory methods for measuring obesity which can be used to detect very mild cases of excessive accumulation of fat, or when very accurate measurements are required.

Weight reduction is usually attempted for aesthetic reasons, but there are essential medical reasons why it should be attempted. Obesity predisposes to conditions like diabetes mellitus, atherosclerosis, backache and osteoarthritis.

Most cases of obesity are caused by an energy input (in the form of the caloric value of food eaten) that is greater than energy expenditure. The excessive input is usually one that has gradually built up over a very long time. If such obese patients want to lose weight, this can be achieved only by caloric restriction. Often the excess calories have been taken in the form of carbohydrates, and reducing this aspect of the diet is helpful. Other reducing diets may involve eating small meals throughout the day rather than concentrating the same amount of food into two or three meals a day; yet others recommend avoiding all fat. Whatever the method, the general principle is to reduce the caloric intake below requirements; it is best to ensure that, in doing so, a balanced, nutritious diet is taken. Caloric requirements vary enormously from individual to individual, and the most suitable diet for a person may only be found by trial and error.

The greatest rate of weight loss usually occurs in the first week of a reducing diet, largely because of an accompanying fluid loss. This should be borne in mind, otherwise a person can be extremely disheartened when weight loss slows down after the first week or two. Since the fat has usually accumulated over a long period, it is unrealistic, and indeed unwise, to aim at a sudden weight loss. The rate of weight loss varies between individuals, but a target of an average weekly loss of one pound is reasonable.

The loss of weight achieved by dietary restriction should be accompanied by reeducation in sensible eating habits, so that the weight is not regained. Eating habits are often acquired in childhood, and the possibility of obesity in later life can be minimized by establishing sound eating habits in young children. And since a high proportion (up to 80–90%) of obese children usually remain fat as adults, obesity in childhood should not be dismissed lightly as "puppy fat."

Another way of adjusting the balance between energy input and output is to increase output by exercise. Considerable activity is required: estimates of the amount of exercise required for losing one pound of fat vary from running 50 miles to playing 100 holes of golf! If the increase in activity is sudden and unaccustomed, it may result in increased consumption of food. A moderate, controlled, regular increase in daily activity is helpful in losing weight.

Sometimes additional measures are required to assist in weight reduction. Drugs may be given that depress appetite or increase the utilization of energy. But because some have side effects, such as the possibility of addiction, and others lose their effectiveness in three or four weeks, drugs should be taken only in short courses and only as an adjunct to sustained dietary restriction.

Quite often there is an emotional problem behind the obesity, comfort being found in eating. If so, it is important to try to remove the emotional factor; psychotherapy may be required.

Very rarely surgery may be required. This may consist of removing a portion of the intestine so that absorption of food is impaired. Such extreme procedures are always reserved for serious cases, as they are not without their problems, which include diarrhea, nutritional effects on the liver and disturbances in mineral metabolism.

In a small proportion of cases, obesity may be due to hormonal disturbances or be associated with a number of congenital or hereditary disorders. These are usually accompanied by other symptoms that can be diagnosed by a physician, and treatment should be directed at the underlying cause.

obsession

A repetition of irrational thoughts, doubts, actions, or fears of which the sufferer is aware but which he cannot conquer, however hard he tries. One obsession may lead to another: for example, an obsession with contamination may result in repeated hand washing. The obsession drives the person to wash his hands repeatedly even though he knows they are already clean.

Obsession may be a symptom of several psychiatric disorders or of organic brain disease, or it may exist alone—when it is referred to as an *obsessional state*.

Treatment is essentially by PSYCHOTHERAPY, but if the symptom has led to anxiety, tension, or depression, appropriate drug therapy may be required.

occult blood

Small quantities of blood in feces which are not apparent to the eye and can be detected only by special laboratory tests.

If occult blood is detected it suggests that there is bleeding somewhere along the gastrointestinal tract, which will have to be investigated.

Since the bleeding may be only intermittent, the stools have to be negative for occult blood on several occasions before the physician can be fairly certain that there is no bleeding in the gastrointestinal tract. Blood from ingested meat (even if cooked) can give a positive result to the test; thus, the patient should go on a meat-free diet for about three days before the test to insure an accurate diagnosis.

occupational diseases and disorders

A group of conditions, each of which is more common in people doing certain kinds of work, and is due to repeated exposure to one or more factors in the working environment.

When dealing with occupational disease, the most important aspect is prevention. The law plays a part, for example, by making regulations governing the safety standards of equipment, or specifying the maximum permissible concentrations of different types of dust particles in the work place. Workers themselves should take care to minimize exposure to any factor likely to cause an occupational disease. Those working in very noisy conditions should wear the ear protectors provided, or if they are exposed to irritant chemicals they should take care to wear all the protective clothing necessary, including gloves.

Newer and safer equipment is constantly being designed, and safer substitutes for material such as asbestos are being developed. Unfortunately, new developments often bring new and unforeseen hazards. More and more occupational diseases are being recognized, although many conditions may not be easily recognized as occupational diseases because of the long time they take to develop. A disease may sometimes appear several years after a person has ceased contact with the alleged causal agent.

The two most common types of occupational disease involve the skin and lungs.

Many skin rashes are caused by contact with irritants or are the result of allergic reactions. In both cases the effect is a skin inflammation known as *contact dermatitis*. Those due to allergy are commonly found in people who work with wet cement (the allergy being due to chromate), those who work with epoxy resins, or those in contact with vulcanizing agents in the rubber industry. Irritant dermatitis tends to be more common in certain industries, such as the coal mining industry, metal goods industry, leather industry, chemical and allied industries and the textile industry.

Lung disorders related to occupations (for example, PNEUMOCONIOSIS, SILICOSIS and ASBESTOSIS) occur when very fine dust particles in the environment pass through the body's physical defenses (e.g. hairs in the nostrils or cilia in the bronchi) to reach the air sacs of the lungs. There, over a number of years, they may induce a fibrous reaction which in some cases impairs breathing and produces chronic disability. In other cases they may produce no symptoms and be detected only on x rays. Sometimes the lung may be affected by an allergic reaction with symptoms that resemble those of ASTHMA.

Other well-known occupational diseases include *caisson disease* or *decompression sickness* (the BENDS) which occurs in deep-sea divers and tunnel workers in a compressed-air environment, and RAYNAUD'S DISEASE which has a high incidence in those who handle vibrating tools such as pneumatic drills. People working with animals or handling animal products have to be careful to avoid infections such as BRUCELLOSIS.

Industrial poisoning was once a fairly common occupational disorder. It may be acute in nature, as with a leak of noxious fumes (e.g., ammonia) into the environment; or it may occur insidiously, such as occurs in LEAD POISONING—although this is less common now that many industries in which exposure to lead is likely take blood samples from their workers at regular intervals to test for the possible presence of lead.

Some cancers may be occupational hazards. For example, cancer of the scrotum was recognized more than 200 years ago to be an occupational disease of chimney sweeps. Scrotal cancer is still seen, mainly in those who work with cooling oils in the engineering industry. Cancer of the bladder was at one time quite common in those working with aniline dyes; some of these dyes are no longer produced, but cases have been reported in those working with other amines. There has recently been medical interest in investigating the incidence of liver tumors occurring in those working with vinyl chloride, and MESOTHELIOMA in those exposed to asbestos.

oe-

For words beginning OE- see E-.

Oedipus complex

Excessive love of a boy for his mother, persisting into adolescence and beyond. It is named after the mythical Greek king who killed his father and married his mother.

Freud believed that an individual passes through a series of stages in his psychosexual development. It is in the "genital stage," between the third and sixth years, that an Oedipus situation is said to arise in boys, experiencing sexual desire for the mother but hostile and aggressive feelings toward the father. The corresponding situation for girls, who are said to be sexually attracted to the father, is the *Electra complex*.

Arrest of psychological development or regression to this stage of development is said to be responsible for an Oedipus complex in later life.

oliguria

An abnormal reduction in the amount of urine secreted.

onychia

Inflammation of the nail.

It usually results from PARONYCHIA (inflammation of the tissues surrounding the nail), caused by nutritional disturbances associated with inflammation in the matrix lying just underneath the nail bed.

The most common cause of the inflammation is trauma to the matrix. The nail is often lost but will regrow if the matrix is not permanently injured. If the matrix is chronically inflamed, the nail that forms is discolored and cracked.

Onychia is common among people whose hands have to be immersed in water for long periods. The skin around the nails is red, swollen and painful, while the nails themselves lose their natural gloss, become opaque and—in severe cases—may become loose and drop off.

onychogryphosis

Excessive growth of a nail into the shape of a claw or horn, with a horny texture.

It may occur in any nail but is most common in the toenails, especially on the big toes. The affected nail is thick, elongated, raised, green or black and the surface is irregular and opaque.

Onychogryphosis is usually seen in people who go about barefooted, although it can be caused by tight shoes. Trauma is said to be the usual cause. It may also

be seen in patients with peripheral NEURITIS, congestive HEART FAILURE, LEPROSY, ICHTHYOSIS, some hormonal disturbances, SYPHILIS, and after a STROKE. Sometimes it runs in families.

If there is an underlying cause it must be recognized and treated. Otherwise, attention should be paid to hygiene and shoe fitting. Hot baths and massage with warm olive oil or with hydrogen peroxide may help. Some doctors, though not all, believe that high doses of vitamin A are useful. Another treatment is to remove the nail, but it will grow again.

onychomycosis

Fungal infection of the nail. It is the most common inflammatory nail disorder and may be caused by a number of fungal species which are identified by examining nail scrapings in the laboratory.

Fungal infection is common in people whose resistance to infection is low, such as diabetics, or anyone taking corticosteroid drugs. It is also common in sufferers of PARONYCHIA (inflammation of skin around the nail), usually people whose work involves immersing the hands in water for long periods, or people with ingrowing toenails. (See INGROWING NAILS).

Onychomycosis is chronic but painless. The nail lacks luster and is opaque and brittle. It may show striations, have a "worm-eaten" appearance, or have a surface of heaped-up flakes. Paronychia of the surrounding soft tissues may cause pain and tenderness, with the exudation of serum or pus—especially if there is a superimposed bacterial infection.

Onychomycosis is treated with griseofulvin (an antifungal drug) applied to the nail or given by mouth. The treatment usually has to be continued for months or years and, even then, may not achieve a permanent cure. Filing the affected nails may shorten the course of the disease by removing infected nail. Sometimes the entire nail has to be removed. Any underlying condition should also be treated, as should any superimposed bacterial infection. Patients should keep the nails clean and dry and footwear should never be shared.

oophorectomy

Surgical removal of an ovary.

This operation was first performed in 1809 by Ephraim McDowell (1771–1830) of Danville, Kentucky, on a patient called Jane Crawford who suffered from a large ovarian tumor. It is pleasant to record that she got out of bed on the fifth day and made a complete recovery, despite the fact that the operation had been performed without anesthesia, and that she lived for a further 31 years.

The operation is carried out nowadays mainly (1) on

ovaries which are the seat of malignant disease, usually combined with removal of the Fallopian tubes and the uterus; (2) on ovaries involved in a widespread chronic inflammatory process; or (3) on ovaries almost completely destroyed by a large benign tumor. Usually in the case of a benign tumor every effort is made (especially in the younger patient) to preserve whatever functioning ovarian tissue is left; the ovary has such a good blood supply that it is able to heal quickly and retain normal function. If the ovary has to be removed in an older woman at or near the menopause, the other ovary and the uterus are often removed at the same time although the tumor may be benign, and HYSTERECTOMY in women past the menopause is often accompanied by oophorectomy.

Some malignant tumors of the breast are hormone-dependent, and it may be useful in the management of such a cancer to remove both ovaries. About 30% of patients, particularly those before the menopause, show a degree of remission of symptoms, some for a long time.

Removal of both ovaries may be performed in severe cases of ENDOMETRIOSIS, and is usually accompanied by removal of the uterus and as much of the abnormal endometrial tissue as possible. The operation induces an abrupt menopause, which is the desired effect in endometriosis and cancer of the breast; but in cases of oophorectomy where this effect is unwelcome, patients can be given the ovarian hormone estrogen.

ophthalmia neonatorum

CONJUNCTIVITIS in a newborn baby caused by infection with bacteria or viruses encountered in the mother's vagina during childbirth. The microorganism most commonly responsible is the gonococcus, the bacterium that causes GONORRHEA.

The infection causes a discharge from the eye in the second or third day of life; it rapidly progresses if the infection is not treated. The eyes become puffy, the conjunctiva becomes intensely red and thick, and the discharge runs down the cheeks in a constant stream. The cornea becomes hazy and ulcerated, which can lead to blindness.

Ophthalmia neonatorum was once a very common disease—affecting up to 10% of babies in some urban areas—and was a principal cause of blindness. It was controlled by silver nitrate drops instilled routinely into the eyes of every newborn baby, a practice that became universal and is still used in many places. Modern treatment of the infection, which is quite effective, is the administration of antibiotic injections and eyedrops.

Several organisms apart from the gonococcus can cause ophthalmia neonatorum. The disease is similar, but vaginal scrapings may be necessary to identify the organism and discover its antibiotic sensitivity. Genital

herpes, for example, is considered so dangerous in this respect that experts regard its presence in the mother as a justification or indication for a CESAREAN SECTION.

ophthalmoplegia

Paralysis or weakness of the muscles that control eye movements, together with dilation and contraction of the pupil. If there is only mild weakness, the earliest symptom is double vision. If the muscles are actually paralyzed, it may be obvious that the eye does not move in certain directions.

Ophthalmoplegia can be produced by any condition affecting the muscles themselves or the nerves that supply them. Head injuries, strokes, meningitis, encephalitis, brain tumors and diabetes are the usual causes. The condition also occurs in HYPERTHYROIDISM and MYASTHENIA GRAVIS. The treatment depends on the cause.

opium

Opium, the drug extracted from a particular species of poppy, is the source of morphine, heroin, codeine and other compounds used in medicine. In the past, crude opium was used to relieve pain and opium has been a drug of addiction for many centuries.

Taken by mouth or inhaled from a pipe, opium causes a feeling of contentment or euphoria, relieves pain and hunger, and eventually causes drowsiness and sleep. The dreams of the opium addict may be vivid and sometimes terrifying—as described by poets such as Samuel Taylor Coleridge and writers like Thomas De Quincey. However, the addictive potential of opium is so powerful that most regular users become addicts who are physically and mentally dependent on the drug.

The medicinal use of opium, mainly to relieve pain, led to the purification of its constituent alkaloids and crude opium is no longer used. Nevertheless, its derivatives—especially heroin—retain the powerful addictive properties, and their use is controlled by drug legislation in most countries.

See also ADDICTION, DRUG ABUSE.

orchiopexy

An operation to fix an UNDESCENDED TESTIS in the scrotum.

In the early embryo, the testes lie near the kidneys and usually descend into the scrotum by the time the child is born or a few weeks after (certainly within the first year). A testis that is not in the scrotum by the time a child is six will be most unlikely ever to produce spermatozoa. The operation to correct the undescended testis is therefore generally performed at least by the time the child is five

OPIUM POPPY

Papaver somniferum

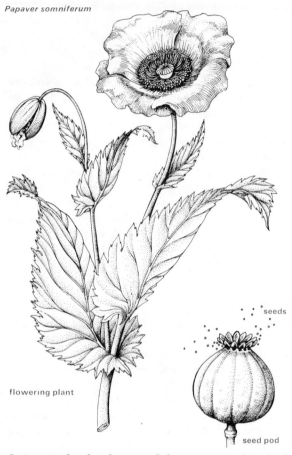

flowering plant

seeds

seed pod

Opium is the dried juice of the unripe seed pod of the poppy Papaver somniferum. *The major constituent of opium is morphine but it also contains lesser amounts of other alkaloids.*

years old and if it is in any way possible much earlier.

If only one testis is undescended, the other should be able to produce enough sperm to maintain fertility; but there are other reasons for orchiopexy. If a testis remains undescended, an inguinal HERNIA is more likely to develop; there is a thirty-fold increase in risk of cancer in that testis; the testis is more likely to be injured or to undergo torsion (in which it twists on its stalk and cuts off its own blood supply—see TORSION OF THE TESTIS); finally, orchiopexy may be performed for cosmetic and psychological reasons.

Sometimes a parent may fear that his boy has an undescended testis when it is, in fact, a "retractile" testis. A retractile testis is one that withdraws up toward the abdomen easily; with careful manipulation it can be brought farther down into the scrotum, and usually stays down by the time of puberty.

The surgical procedure of suturing an undescended testis in the scrotum is also known as *orchiorrhaphy.*

orchitis

Inflammation of the testis.

Acute orchitis is usually the result of a generalized infection such as mumps, scarlet fever, or typhoid. In other cases it may result from the spread of infection from neighboring structures such as the epididymis, the seminal vesicles, or the prostate, or from other distant structures via the bloodstream.

The testis enlarges and there is severe pain in the scrotum, which is tender, red and swollen. The patient usually has a fever and a general feeling of being unwell (malaise). Severe acute orchitis may result in some wasting away of the testis (occasionally enough to cause sterility).

In treatment the scrotum is supported by a suspensory "bridge" and ice packs are applied during the acute phase. Analgesics such as aspirin and codeine will relieve pain; the infection itself is treated with appropriate antibiotics. If there is an abscess the pus has to be drained. Some physicians believe in giving corticosteroid drugs to relieve the inflammation; others make a small incision in the tough, inelastic covering of the testis during the very early stage of the disease. A few doctors prescribe female sex hormones in treating orchitis associated with mumps. If symptoms persist for more than a month, surgical removal of the testis may be necessary.

Chronic orchitis may be caused by syphilis; it is often unnoticed since it is painless. Tuberculosis is another cause of chronic orchitis; here the testis is hard and nodular and may be mistaken for a tumor. Once the diagnosis is confirmed by BIOPSY, an appropriate antibiotic can be given.

orgasm

The climax of sexual activity.

The normal response to sexual stimulation can be divided into four phases: excitement, plateau, orgasm and resolution. In the first two phases a number of physiological changes occur; these include not only changes in the breasts and genitals of both sexes but also flushing of the skin and a rising pulse rate and blood pressure.

During the *orgasmic phase,* which is the shortest of the four phases, there is intense physical activity: involuntary contractions of various muscles, thrusting movements of the pelvis, contraction of the anal sphincter (the muscular ring that controls the opening and closing of the anus), a further quickening of the pulse and breathing rate and a further rise in blood pressure. The female cervix dilates and the male ejaculates semen.

Orgasm is followed by the phase of *resolution* during

which there is a relaxation of sexual tension and a reversal of the physiological processes of sexual excitement. Restimulation of the woman during this phase may induce another orgasm, but in the man there is a variable refractory period during which re-stimulation does not produce another orgasm.

orthodontics

The branch of dentistry concerned with the study of the growth and development of the jaws and teeth and with the correction of irregularities of the teeth (such as abnormal alignment) and associated facial abnor-malities.

Orthodontic treatment may be required for several reasons—in addition to the obvious esthetic and psychological value of regular, symmetrical teeth. Some positions of teeth may result in poor coordination of the chewing muscles, giving rise to symptoms in the joint between the jaw and the rest of the skull. If teeth are overcrowded the teeth and gums cannot be cleaned effectively (naturally or artificially), and the patient may become prone to gum trouble and CARIES ("cavities"). Finally, orthodontics may be required to facilitate other forms of dental treatment—such as the fitting of dentures, bridges or crowns and certain types of oral or dental surgery, or to hold erupted teeth in position so that later teeth can erupt in proper alignment.

The basic principle of orthodontic treatment is to apply pressure to the teeth to direct their growth into the position required. Teeth may be tipped, rotated or moved bodily. Some dentists exert a small pressure continuously, while others prefer stronger pressure with intermittent periods of rest.

Pressure is exerted by a variety of appliances, such as wires, braces, screws, wedges and rubber bands. Some can be attached entirely within the mouth, whereas others need "extra-oral" attachments by bands around the head or neck. Some are fixed, while others have to be removed and replaced by the patient for cleaning. Treatment usually has to be continued for months or even years, and several courses of treatment may be needed as a child grows.

There are limits to what orthodontics can achieve: it is not the solution to every speech defect or to all types of malalignment of the upper and lower jaws. Even so, children should be encouraged to persist with orthodon-tic treatment in spite of any temporary discomfort since good results are more likely while the jaws and teeth are still growing.

orthoptics

The treatment of STRABISMUS (squint or cross-eye) by eye exercises. The treatment is given by an orthoptist, who is medically trained in all aspects of the diagnosis and treatment of strabismus.

The principle behind orthoptic treatment is the retraining of the eye muscles and the brain so that both eyes are used simultaneously to view objects. The brain may have to be retrained because some patients with strabismus overcome their double vision by learning to ignore images coming from one eye. This has to be "unlearned" and the brain taught to appreciate images from the eye it has previously ignored. The orthoptist works with a number of sophisticated instruments which can present pictures separately or together to one or both eyes.

Not all cases of strabismus can be successfully treated by orthoptic methods. Cases which are more suitable are those in which the degree of the cross-eye is not too severe, those in which vision in both eyes is still good, and those which have not appeared suddenly or before the age of two.

Although orthoptic treatment is more likely to be successful the earlier treatment is started, it requires a great deal of cooperation from the patient; thus, young children (under the ages of about five to seven) are not good candidates. Young children can, however, be given "preorthoptic" treatment designed to prevent further deterioration of the squint; occlusion, or covering the unaffected eye, thereby forcing the child to use the affected eye, is the basis of preorthoptic care and may have to be carried out for days or weeks at a time.

When proper orthoptic treatment is begun, the treatments must be frequent and continued for a very long time. The frequency of treatment (usually daily at the beginning) can be reduced over the course of treatment. Treatment is unlikely to be successful if the patient is over the age of about 20.

osteitis

Literally, inflammation of bone.

Inflammatory disease of bone is commonly due to infection and often affects the marrow as well, in which case it is known as OSTEOMYELITIS. The term osteitis tends to be used for a number of other bone disorders, not necessarily inflammatory in nature. Some are the result of biochemical derangements, while others are inherited or of unknown cause.

Osteitis deformans, also known as PAGET'S DISEASE, is of unknown cause. There is excessive bone destruction and subsequent spontaneous repair; the repair takes place in a disorganized fashion leading to deformities. Often there are no symptoms at first, but some patients suffer pain. Later the back may become hunched, the legs bowed and the skull enlarged; a waddling gait may develop and the bones fracture easily.

Complications include kidney stones (the calcium

coming from the destruction of bone) and bone deformities that may press on nerves and cause blindness or deafness. In a few cases, cancer of the bone may develop. A number of drugs are now available to suppress the excessive activity of bone.

Osteitis fibrosa cystica is a bone disease caused by the overactivity of the parathyroid glands (HYPERPARATHYROIDISM). The excessive amounts of parathyroid hormone remove calcium from the bone so that cystic demineralized areas develop throughout the skeleton. Symptoms range from back pain, joint pain and other bone pains to fractures, loss of height and a hunched back. Treatment involves correction of the parathyroid disorder that is often due to benign tumors in the gland. Such tumors can be successfully removed by surgery.

Syphilis, whether congenital or acquired later in life, can cause a type of osteitis. In children, inflammation of the bone, cartilage and periosteum (outer lining of the bone) may pass unnoticed because they produce no symptoms. In some cases, however, fractures may occur and pain may prevent the child from moving the limbs. In adults the bone involvement usually takes the form of localized areas of destruction by "gummata" (the characteristic syphilitic lesions).

Osteitis fibrosa disseminata and *osteitis condensans generalisata* are two rare bone disorders. The former is of unknown cause and is characterized by fibrous overgrowths in bone. The latter is an inherited condition in which the bone becomes very dense.

osteoarthritis

A degenerative disease of the joints, usually accompanied by pain and stiffness.

Radiography shows that over 80% of people between the ages of 55 and 64 show changes characteristic of the disease; of these, about 20% complain of symptoms. It causes a great deal of pain and discomfort to a large number of people of both sexes, although females tend to suffer more severely than males. The cause of the disease is not known, but it may be described as a degenerative disorder developing with age.

Many sufferers give a history of antecedent injury, sometimes many years before; any fracture or joint disease which results in injury to the joint cartilage or misalignment of the joint predisposes a patient to the development of the disease. The large weight-bearing joints of the lower limb are particularly affected, but osteoarthritis can also affect the fingers, elbows, shoulders and the vertebrae. Occupations involving the use of other joints may in time produce signs of the disease in unexpected places.

The basic change in the affected joints is loss of the *articular cartilage*, which normally protects the ends of

the bones and provides a smooth working surface for movement. The exposed ends of the bones become hard and shiny, and at their margins small spurs of bone develop known as *osteophytes*. The changes are evident in radiographs (x rays) which show the osteophytes and narrowing of the joint space where the cartilage has been lost. The membranes lining the joint (synovial membranes) become thickened, and there may be an effusion of fluid into the joint which causes it to swell.

The patient suffers increasing pain on movement of the joint, and the joint becomes stiff. Usually the pain becomes worse as the day progresses, and the affected limb is difficult to use. In advanced cases of the disease, joint function may be lost and the muscles acting on the joint may waste (atrophy). Grating (crepitus) may be felt in the joint on movement. Where the fingers are affected, small swellings (Heberden's nodes) may develop beside the finger joints. As the disease progresses, the hands may become deformed. In the back and neck, degeneration of the intervertebral joints with osteophyte formation may involve the spinal nerves as they leave the spinal cord and produce various neurological symptoms.

The treatment of milder cases includes reduction of body weight in those who are obese. As with all common diseases which are difficult to relieve, a large number of drugs are offered on the market, but most of them have in common an irritant action on the stomach which may provoke the development of a peptic ulcer. They must therefore be used with caution. The most useful drug is aspirin, but it too has undesirable side effects and cannot be used in all cases. Orthopedic surgery has in the last few years improved the treatment of severe cases with the introduction of artificial joints. It is now often possible to replace a painful diseased hip joint with success. In many cases the knee can be replaced, although the operation is not yet as uniformly satisfactory as a hip replacement.

See RHEUMATOID ARTHRITIS.

osteogenesis imperfecta

A condition seen at birth or in infancy in which there is extreme fragility of the skeleton, leading to multiple fractures and deformities. Also known as *brittle bone disease* and *fragilitas ossium*.

The bones are brittle as the result of defective formation in fetal life. The cause is unknown, but the milder form of the disease, seen in infancy, sometimes tends to run in families. Infants with osteogenesis imperfecta may be born with multiple fractures of every bone in the body. The resulting damage to the brain and other organs usually leads to death within a few weeks.

When the disease is less severe, fractures occur after birth and fewer bones are involved. Healing usually occurs readily, but severe deformity may result. The skull is usually flattened and the sclera of the eyes is thin and bluish in color. Deafness due to OTOSCLEROSIS is common later in those who survive.

Diagnosis is made by clinical and x-ray examination. It is important, but sometimes difficult, for the physician to distinguish between osteogenesis imperfecta and the BATTERED CHILD SYNDROME, where fractures in a normal infant result from assault by a parent or guardian.

Osteogenesis imperfecta cannot be prevented, but fractures occurring in infancy can often be minimized by careful attention to the child. When fractures occur, their healing is aided by the usual orthopedic methods in an attempt to prevent deformity.

osteoma

A benign tumor composed of bone.

Osteomas are usually attached to normal bones, but they may also occur in other structures. They are commonly attached to the bones of the skull (including the sinuses) and the lower jaw, but they may occur anywhere in the body.

The cause of osteomas is not known. The common symptom is the presence of a hard, painless lump. Other symptoms may result from pressure of the tumor on nerves or other structures, but these symptoms are quite rare.

Osteomas are not malignant and probably only rarely change into a malignant OSTEOSARCOMA. Treatment of osteomas is surgical removal, but this is necessary only where there are troublesome symptoms, such as pain due to pressure, or for cosmetic reasons.

osteomalacia

A disease of adults, especially women, in which the bones are generally softened, due to the impaired deposition of calcium. The matrix (organic tissue) of the bones is normal or increased in quantity. In childhood, RICKETS leads to a similar softening of the bones and also to characteristic deformities in their development.

Osteomalacia is caused by lack of vitamin D as the result of dietary deficiency, malabsorption from the intestine, abnormal metabolism, or increased requirements for the vitamin during pregnancy. Lack of vitamin D leads, in turn, to decreased absorption of calcium from the intestine and abnormal calcium metabolism in the body.

Vitamin D is lacking from many basic diets, but it is synthesized in the skin (especially in white races) in response to sunlight. Natives of tropical countries who move to temperate climates or who remain indoors are thus particularly liable to osteomalacia. Vitamin D is malabsorbed in conditions such as celiac disease and abnormal metabolism occurs in kidney failure; osteomalacia is fairly common in these circumstances.

Osteomalacia causes bone pain and tenderness. True bone fractures may occur and *pseudofractures*—transverse translucent bands extending across the bones—are commonly seen on x rays. The calcium deficiency causes muscular weakness as well as a loss of appetite and weight. Blood levels of calcium and other substances may help the physician confirm the diagnosis.

Treatment involves the administration of vitamin D or one of its synthetic analogues. Further treatment depends upon the underlying cause and on any complications.

Vitamin D deficiency can be and is prevented in most people by addition of the vitamin to dairy products; but osteomalacia is still quite common in the elderly, the poor and those with disease of the kidneys or small intestine.

osteomyelitis

An infection of bone and bone marrow.

Acute osteomyelitis is fairly uncommon in the Western world, but is still common in areas of poor health and nutrition—especially among children. There is severe pain and tenderness in the affected bone, and the patient rapidly becomes extremely ill with a high fever, drowsiness and dehydration.

Acute osteomyelitis is usually caused by infection with bacteria of the species *Staphylococcus aureus*. The main treatment is the administration of appropriate antibiotics, but in the absence of a rapid response it is also necessary to drain pus from the bone by drilling a hole in it—a surprisingly minor operation.

With rapid diagnosis and antibiotic treatment, most patients with acute osteomyelitis make a full recovery. There is a risk of death due to septicemia (blood poisoning) but this is slight in comparison with the major mortality before antibiotic treatment was available.

Chronic osteomyelitis may be a late result of acute osteomyelitis, it may follow an open fracture of a bone, or it may result from the presence of a foreign body (e.g., a bullet or a surgical plate). Here an area of bone is dead and infected (a *sequestrum*) and infection persists because antibiotics cannot reach the area in adequate amounts. The symptoms fluctuate, but include local pain and the discharge of pus. Deformities may result.

Treatment involves the removal of all dead tissue, surgical drainage, antibiotic treatment and the repair of any resulting bone defect. This treatment is usually lengthy, complicated and hazardous. It is not always successful, and the prognosis of chronic osteomyelitis is correspondingly uncertain. It may cause chronic ill-health and even require amputation of a limb, or it may be totally cured. Fortunately, however, it is a fairly rare disease.

osteoporosis

A disease in which the bones are generally thinned, due to a loss of organic matrix with a corresponding decrease in calcified tissue.

Starting around the age of 20, everyone's bones become progressively thinner with age. When this thinning proceeds faster than normal it leads to osteoporosis. The disease is common in old age, especially in women.

Osteoporosis also occurs in a number of other conditions at any age. These include complications following corticosteroid therapy, Cushing's syndrome, hyperthyroidism, acromegaly, rheumatoid arthritis, and other diseases leading to immobilization.

The disease may be symptomless, or it may cause pain—commonly in the back, ribs or limbs. Vertebrae may collapse suddenly, causing severe back pain; in any case, they contract gradually as the disease progresses, leading to a loss in height and increased curvature of the spine (kyphosis). Osteoporosis of the femur is the underlying cause of most hip fractures in the elderly.

The main treatment for pain is the administration of analgesic drugs. Support of the affected spine by a corset may also help, and physical therapy and exercises may aid the muscles of the spine in supporting the vertebrae and thus minimizing or preventing pain.

Osteoporosis that occurs as the result of another disease demands treatment of the primary disease. Corticosteroid therapy should be avoided or stopped if possible.

Specific therapies for osteoporosis include estrogens in women, androgens in men, calcium by mouth or intravenously, fluoride supplements and a diet high in protein and calcium. The range of treatments used shows that none is entirely satisfactory in dealing with this disease.

Osteoporosis itself does not shorten life expectancy; but fractures, especially of the hip, and underlying diseases may lead to premature death.

osteosarcoma

One of the most common types of malignant bone tumor.

Osteosarcomas may occur at any age, but are more common in children and young adults. They may also occur as a complication of PAGET'S DISEASE, typically in the 60s. They usually occur in the limbs, but may affect any bone.

The usual symptom is pain. Sometimes there is swelling and tenderness; occasionally the diagnosis is made only when the affected bone fractures.

Osteosarcomas are malignant, and the major spread of the cancer cells (metastasis) occurs in the lungs—which is the most frequent cause of death. X rays are helpful in making the diagnosis and in determining whether metastasis has occurred.

Diagnosis demands BIOPSY of the tumor with immediate examination (by frozen section) of the sample. If the diagnosis is confirmed and there is no evidence of metastasis, the affected limb is amputated under the same anesthetic (or the affected part elsewhere in the body is widely excised). An alternative is to give a course of irradiation to the tumor, at the beginning of which it is biopsied. If there is no sign of spread to the lungs or elsewhere after three months the limb is then amputated. This avoids the amputation of a part in a patient who is likely to die from secondary spread in any case, but the results are not quite as good as those from the first approach. There is no effective treatment for metastases, although in some cases, radiation may be palliative.

There is considerable variation in the aggressiveness of the tumors, but on average only 10–15% of patients will survive for five years after diagnosis, even with modern treatment.

See also CANCER.

otitis externa

Inflammation of the outer canal of the ear. It is a common and usually trivial condition.

The ear is composed of four parts: the *pinna* is the part which projects from the head; the *outer ear* includes the opening and the canal to the eardrum; the *middle ear* is the section immediately beyond the eardrum; and the *inner ear* is the part furthest into the head.

Otitis externa affects the outer ear. Sometimes the pinna or the middle ear may be inflamed at the same time, depending on the cause, and the condition may be difficult to distinguish from OTITIS MEDIA (inflammation of the middle ear).

Otitis externa causes pain in the ear and a discharge from it. The pain may be severe and is usually worsened by movements such as chewing and yawning, but hearing is seldom affected.

Causes include foreign bodies in the ear, amateur attempts to remove them by excessive poking, moisture (for instance, if the ears are not dried after swimming), cosmetics, hair sprays, and allergy to drugs contained in eardrops. The ear is often infected with bacteria or fungi, but this infection is frequently a *consequence* of otitis externa and not the primary cause. It may lead to a painful boil in the outer ear.

Most cases of otitis externa resolve spontaneously without treatment, but a doctor should be consulted if the condition persists or grows worse for more than a day or two. The ear may be made more comfortable by moistened gauze or bland eardrops. Antibiotics may be required by mouth for an infected otitis externa. Drops containing antibiotics or other drugs may make the condition worse.

Otitis externa tends to recur, so the sufferer should try to discover the cause and avoid it in the future. Children with otitis externa should not swim until the condition is fully healed, and even then recurrence is common. Otitis externa caused by a fungus infection may take months of treatment to eradicate.

See OTITIS INTERNA.

otitis interna

Inflammation of the inner ear. Also called *labyrinthitis*.

The inner ear, or labyrinth, contains the organs of balance and of hearing, both of which may be affected by the spread of infection from the middle ear (see OTITIS MEDIA). The patient suffers from VERTIGO; if some hearing is retained, the condition is called *diffuse serous labyrinthitis*, but if hearing is totally lost, then the disease is called *diffuse purulent labyrinthitis*. The main danger is spread of infection to the meninges, the membranes covering the brain. Treatment is rest in bed with the administration of appropriate antibiotics, perhaps with the addition of cyclizine or prochlorperazine to relieve the vertigo.

Vertigo of sudden onset may occur without obvious infection or loss of hearing; this condition is called *infective labyrinthitis*, perhaps wrongly, as it is thought to be due to a virus infection of the nerve fibers running from the inner ear to the brain stem. In most cases the disease is self-limiting, with spontaneous recovery, but in a very few the patient later develops signs of MULTIPLE SCLEROSIS.

See also OTITIS EXTERNA.

otitis media

Inflammation of the middle ear (the part just behind the eardrum).

Acute otitis media is most common in infants and young children; about 20% of children under a year of age have at least one attack.

The middle ear is connected to the back of the nose by the Eustachian tube. In children the tube is short and wide and the lower end is easily blocked by enlarged ADENOIDS. Infection spreads freely from the nose and throat to the middle ear.

Acute otitis media can cause severe illness with fever, vomiting, diarrhea and failure to feed; in infants there is

often no reason for the parents to suspect that the ear is the site of infection. Older children usually complain of earache. Deafness may occur during the attacks, but usually resolves with treatment. The infection may give rise to complications such as meningitis or mastoiditis, although this is rare with current therapy.

The doctor examines the patient's ear with a simple instrument called an otoscope. In acute otitis media the eardrum is red, inflamed and swollen. In severe cases it may burst, or the doctor may incise it to relieve pressure ("myringotomy").

Acute otitis media usually responds rapidly to treatment with antibiotics—commonly penicillin—although many cases would resolve spontaneously within 48 hours or so. Analgesics are needed for the pain; soothing eardrops may also be helpful. In children, ephedrine nose drops help to reestablish drainage of the ear through the Eustachian tube. Successfully treated otitis media has no long-term complications. Recurrent attacks may occur, however, and sometimes surgical removal of the adenoids is a helpful measure to take in preventing them.

Chronic otitis media is usually the result of repeated attacks of acute otitis media. The eardrum is scarred. thickened and often perforated. The patient may be partially deaf in the affected ear, which usually scharges. The main risk is the development of a "cholesteatoma," an accumulation of debris which may erode bone and cause further damage to the ear and even to the brain. A cholesteatoma requires skilled surgical treatment.

Secretory otitis media ("glue ear") is a painless condition, most common in children, in which the middle ear fills with viscous fluid. This is usually the result of recurrent or untreated otitis media, but in a few cases the cause may not be known. The condition leads to deafness and there is a risk of permanent ear damage. Treatment involves long-term drainage of the ear by myringotomy or the insertion of tubes ("grommets") through the eardrum to drain the fluid.

otosclerosis

A disease causing deafness which occurs in probably less than 1% of the population.

The disease is due to the abnormal formation of spongy bone in the inner ear which immobilizes the *stapes*, the innermost of the tiny sound-conducting bones in the middle ear. The amplification of sound, normally achieved by these small bones, is ruined.

Otosclerosis often runs in families as part of some rare disease complexes. Otherwise its cause is unknown.

Deafness usually starts in the teens or early twenties and is slowly progressive. It may remain static for many years or it may progress more rapidly for a period, especially in pregnant women. It usually affects one ear before the other, and is accompanied at first by a ringing sensation in the ear (tinnitus). The diagnosis is suggested by the results of hearing tests.

Otosclerosis cannot be prevented, but it can usually be successfully treated by surgery. The stapes is removed and replaced by a Teflon or wire substitute which restores the vibration characteristics of the chain of tiny bones. The operation is extremely delicate—these tiny ear bones are the smallest bones of the body—and carries a 2% risk of causing total deafness in the ear, but the other 98% of patients achieve greatly improved hearing within two to three weeks. It is impossible to predict which patients will become deaf, but most sufferers are prepared to accept the small percentage of risk.

ovarian cyst

A swelling of the ovary, containing fluid.

Ovarian cysts are very common, particularly in women between the ages of 30 to 60. They may be single or multiple and can occur in one or both ovaries. Most are benign, but approximately 15% are malignant.

Some ovarian cysts are related to a persistence of changes which take place in the ovary during every menstrual cycle. They may, for example, result from retention of a Graafian follicle (developing ovum) or a corpus luteum (old ovum)—structures which normally disappear with each cycle. Others, such as *dermoid cysts* or those seen in the STEIN-LEVENTHAL SYNDROME ("polycystic ovary"), are due to developmental abnormalities in the ovary. The cause of most cysts, however, is unknown.

Cysts may grow quietly and cause no symptoms until they are found on routine examination. On the other hand, they may become large enough to cause abdominal distension or even obstruct venous drainage, causing swelling of the legs. Malignant cysts may cause the general symptoms of cancer, such as loss of weight and wasting.

Bleeding may occur in some cysts and others may rupture. Both these complications are painful, as is twisting of a cyst (torsion), which may occur when the cyst is on a "stalk." These diagnoses may all be confused with acute appendicitis and other abdominal emergencies and may only become apparent on LAPAROTOMY (examination through an incision in the abdomen). A further possibility is infection in a cyst, which may cause pain and high fever.

Ovarian cysts are usually removed surgically to prevent further complications. The type of operation depends on the individual case but may include removal of the cyst alone or removal of the entire ovary (oophorectomy). Removal of both ovaries results in sterility and an artificial MENOPAUSE; it is usually performed only in the treatment of ovarian cancer or in postmenopausal women. Ovarian cancer may require follow-up radiation or drug treatment, but surgery alone is sufficient for most ovarian cysts.

ovulation

The release of an ovum from the ovary.

Ovulation occurs around the middle of the menstrual cycle and is followed either by fertilization and pregnancy or, after 14 days, by MENSTRUATION. The ovum travels down the Fallopian tube to the uterus; if it meets and is penetrated by a male sperm cell during its journey down the Fallopian tube, the fertilized ovum becomes implanted in the wall of the uterus. There it

OVULATION

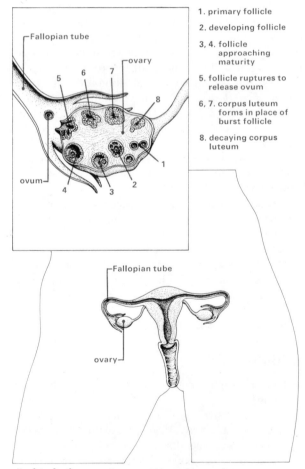

1. primary follicle
2. developing follicle
3, 4. follicle approaching maturity
5. follicle ruptures to release ovum
6, 7. corpus luteum forms in place of burst follicle
8. decaying corpus luteum

At birth the ovaries contain many primary follicles, each containing an immature ovum, or egg. After puberty, one of these follicles ripens and releases an ovum (ovulation) at the midpoint of each menstrual cycle. If the ovum is not fertilized, menstrual bleeding results.

grows and develops into a human embryo.

Ovulation depends on the secretion of hormones by the pituitary gland (at the base of the brain) which is itself under the control of the hypothalamus, the region of the brain concerned with basic sex drives, hunger and sleep. The *hypothalamic releasing factors* stimulate the secretion by the pituitary of follicle-stimulating hormone (FSH), which causes a single ovum to ripen and be released by the ovary. Fertility also depends on other pituitary hormones—luteinizing hormone and prolactin—which interact with the estrogen and progesterone secreted by the ovaries themselves.

Minor impairment of the hormonal cycle may be enough to suppress ovulation while not interfering with menstruation: a woman may have regular periods but be infertile because she does not ovulate. It is for that reason that the investigation of infertility may require careful measurement of hormone levels in the blood and urine and assessment of the woman's response to hormone treatment. When the cause of infertility is shown to be failure of ovulation, there is a good prospect of successful treatment: ovulation may be induced either by drugs such as clomiphene (which alter the hormone balance) or by specific hormone treatment.

oxygen

An odorless, tasteless gas (atomic weight 16) occurring free in the atmosphere, of which it comprises 20% by volume.

Oxygen is essential to most forms of life, including man. Man absorbs it from his lungs into the bloodstream. It is carried in combination with the HEMOGLOBIN in the red cells and discharged from there to the tissues. Oxygen is essential to the metabolism of every living human cell.

The human body can tolerate a lack of oxygen for only a very short time—the brain is the most sensitive organ and it is permanently damaged if its oxygen supply is cut off for more than about three minutes.

Oxygen therapy is necessary in various diseases of the lungs and heart, and "hyperbaric oxygen" (oxygen under pressure) has a role in the treatment of infections such as gas gangrene (see GANGRENE) and some cancers (in combination with radiation therapy).

oxyuriasis

Infestation with PINWORMS.

ozena

A disease of the nose characterized by a foul-smelling discharge of pus and the formation of crusts. Ozena occurs mainly in young adults, especially women.

The lining of the nose starts to waste away or atrophy ("atrophic rhinitis") and the whole cavity becomes larger than normal. The foul-smelling discharge is constantly produced; it cannot easily be removed by blowing the nose.

One cause of ozena is the prolonged abuse of locally applied decongestant drops or sprays, but in many cases the cause is not known.

No specific infection is present and antibiotic treatment is no help. Treatment consists of getting rid of the crusts and discharge by repeated nasal douching and the use of appropriate nose drops. The damage to the lining mucosa is irreversible and treatment may be required for life. Fortunately, the condition is very uncommon.

P

pacemaker

A device which controls the heart rate by the rhythmic discharge of electrical impulses. (This is technically known as an *artificial pacemaker*, since the term "pacemaker" also describes the group of specialized cells in the heart—the "sinoatrial node"—which generates the natural impulses that control the rhythmic beating of the heart.)

Pacemakers are most commonly used for the treatment of "heart block," where the ventricles beat slowly and may stop altogether. In such cases a pacemaker is usually required permanently. They are also used in other cardiac arrhythmias in which the heartbeat is abnormally slow or fast, in some patients after myocardial infarction ("heart attack"), and in some patients after cardiac surgery. Here the pacemaker may be required temporarily or permanently.

Heart muscle has the intrinsic ability to beat and should do so in a controlled way, the beat spreading from a point of stimulus through the whole heart. When heart muscle beats arrhythmically the control has evidently been lost, and the pacemaker is intended to replace it: each pulse of the pacemaker sets off a heartbeat.

The electrodes through which the impulses reach the heart may be on the outside surface of the heart ("external") or on its inside surface ("internal"). External pacemakers require surgical implantation while internal pacemakers can be maneuvered into the right ventricle of the heart via the veins.

Pacemakers are powered by batteries which may be outside the body if the device is temporary but must be implanted beneath the skin of the chest wall (to prevent

CARDIAC PACEMAKER

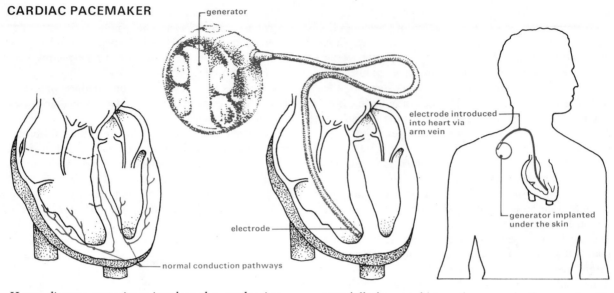

generator

electrode introduced into heart via arm vein

generator implanted under the skin

electrode

normal conduction pathways

Heart disease sometimes involves the conduction pathways so that the pulse becomes dangerously slow or irregular. A cardiac pacemaker may then be inserted, temporarily or permanently, to correct the heartbeat.

infection) if it is permanent. Most permanent pacemakers have batteries which last about two years. Some new models last longer and (in the future) nuclear powered pacemakers may last for 20 years or more. A minor operation is required to change the battery box of the pacemaker.

The main complication of pacemaker therapy is its failure to function—due to battery failure, displacement of the electrode, or fibrosis around the electrode. It is also said that coming into the vicinity of poorly shielded microwave ovens or other microwave devices can interfere with the pacemaker's function. Other complications include infection in the blood or around the battery box, ulceration of the skin above the box and, in rare instances, perforation of the heart by the pacemaker.

Pacemakers are generally safe and effective. Their development during the last 20 years has completely changed the previously poor prognosis of many patients with heart block and other cardiac arrhythmias. Many patients in their 80s and 90s are now equipped with pacemakers.

See also BUNDLE BRANCH BLOCK.

Paget's disease (osteitis deformans)

A bone disease, first described by the English surgeon Sir James Paget in 1877. The affected areas of bone become thickened and soft and there is an increase in the total number of bone cells. It is quite common in old age,

especially in men, but rarely occurs in those under 50. The cause is unknown.

The spine is most commonly affected; other common sites for the disease include the skull, breastbone (sternum), pelvis and thighbones (femurs). The bone enlargement may lead to deformity: for example, bowed legs or an enlarged head (typically discovered by the need for an increased hat size).

The softened bones are often painful and prone to fractures. Enlargement of the skull may compress the nerves which pass through it, leading to deafness or other forms of nerve paralysis (occasionally including blindness). Affected bones have an increased blood flow which may ultimately lead to heart failure. If a patient with Paget's disease is immobilized he may develop increased calcium levels in the blood and urine, which may lead to urinary stones (see CALCULUS). Finally, a risk exists of the development of a type of malignant tumor (OSTEOSARCOMA) in the affected bones.

The pain does not always respond to standard analgesics ("painkillers"), and therapy sometimes requires the use of RADIATION THERAPY and corticosteroids. Although there is no cure for Paget's disease, a number of promising drugs have been used over the past few years which help to relieve pain and may arrest the progress of the disease. (These include the hormones calcitonin and glucagon, the diphosphonate drugs and mithramycin.) Further developments in treatment are likely within the next few years.

pain

A localized feeling of severe discomfort, occurring anywhere in the body and usually caused by disease or injury.

Pain is difficult to define accurately because it means

different things to different people at different times. Its subjective nature makes it hard to identify as an entity requiring treatment. Pain cannot be measured and the physician has to rely mainly on a combination of the patient's medical history and his own experience of pain in assessing its nature and degree and the need for treatment.

The mechanism by which pain is felt is not fully understood despite considerable research. It seems likely that pain results when the balance of nerve impulses entering the central nervous system from a particular area of the body is abnormal in a particular way. It is unlikely that pain is simply the result of the stimulation of specific receptors at nerve endings. The complexity of the origins of pain helps to explain the possible complexity of its treatment.

Pain may be caused by many types of disease, including trauma, infection, cancer, degenerative changes, ischemia (inadequate blood supply to an organ or part) and others. In addition, pain is commonly caused or modified by psychological factors; it may also occur as the result of physical factors which have not caused actual tissue damage—e.g. "gas pain" due to distention of the large intestine. Here it may be considered to be a warning of potential damage rather than a result of that damage.

The doctor evaluates a patient's pain by asking a number of questions relating to its localization, quality, intensity, time relations, modifying factors, physiological relations and any mental changes associated with it. As a result, it is often possible to make a more or less certain diagnosis of, say, ANGINA PECTORIS or MIGRAINE, without the need for further investigations. Many types of pain are not so easy to diagnose; in some cases the cause may never be found. Pain is not always felt at the point from which it arises—for example, pain from the diaphragm is often felt in the shoulder. This phenomenon is known as "referred pain."

Ideally, pain is treated by removal or treatment of its cause. This is not always possible and even when it is it may take time. It is thus frequently necessary to relieve the pain itself. This may be achieved in a large number of ways:

(1) *No treatment*. Most normal people have occasional twinges of pain in one site or another for which they do nothing. Such pain usually has no significance and disappears spontaneously.

(2) *Analgesic drugs* ("painkillers") are the most frequently used and abused treatment for pain. Mild analgesics including aspirin, Paracetamol and many others are taken in large numbers for headaches, menstrual pains, etc. Despite the potential hazards involved in their long-term use, many people take them as a habit. Narcotic analgesics (such as morphine, codeine, etc.) are very effective in the treat-

ment of most severe pain, but they are addictive and their abuse is one of the major medical and social problems in many countries today.

(3) *Local anesthetic drugs* are of value in preventing or relieving local pain where the affected area can be clearly identified and infiltrated or the relevant nerve "blocked" (as in dental surgery).

(4) *Other drugs* may aid specific types of pain—for example, antacids may relieve indigestion and some anti-inflammatory drugs relieve only arthritic pain.

(5) *Surface methods* of pain relief—including heat, cold, vibration, manipulation, electrical stimulation and chemical counterirritants—all have a place in relieving some types of pain.

(6) *Acupuncture* is an ancient Chinese method of pain relief, effective in some circumstances and now fashionable in the West.

(7) *Neurosurgery* on appropriate nerves, the spinal cord or the brain is occasionally necessary and effective for intractable pain.

In additon to the use of these techniques, patients with pain require psychological support and (particularly in rheumatic diseases) physiotherapy and occupational therapy may be helpful.

Where the cause is not clear or the underlying condition cannot be satisfactorily treated, pain relief is probably best achieved with the help of a physician who specializes in solving the problem of intractable pain—since he is likely to be most familiar with the range of possible techniques.

palsy

A less common word for PARALYSIS.

The term survives, however, in the description of particular types of paralysis.

BELL'S PALSY is a paralysis of the muscles of one side of the face, caused by damage to the facial nerve. This is commonly caused by a virus, and complete recovery frequently occurs.

CEREBRAL PALSY is a permanent disorder of movement associated with varying paralysis, caused by a defect or disease of the brain and typically occurring within the first three years of life. Affected patients are called "spastics" and they may also have sensory and mental handicaps. Cerebral palsy may be caused by infection or damage during development in the womb, during birth, or in infancy.

Erb's palsy and *Klumpke's palsy* are two types of paralysis resulting from damage to the nerves of the arm, usually occurring at birth. Also known as *brachial birth palsy*.

Bulbar palsy and *pseudobulbar palsy* both cause weakness of the muscles of the face, throat and tongue due to damage to the brain. They occur in adults and are usually progressive and incurable, with a poor prognosis.

"The Shaking Palsy" was Parkinson's original term for the disease now known as PARKINSON'S DISEASE (or *Parkinsonism*).

pancreas

A large gland situated at the back of the abdominal cavity, behind the stomach and between the duodenum and the spleen.

The pancreas has two main functions. As an *exocrine gland* it produces various enzymes necessary for digestion which flow through the pancreatic duct to the duodenum (the beginning of the small intestine). As an *endocrine gland* it produces hormones which are released into the bloodstream. These include insulin and glucagon, which are essential to normal carbohydrate metabolism, and also more recently discovered hormones related to digestion.

The pancreas may be damaged by infection, injury, tumor or alcoholism and such damage may lead to abnormalities of its endocrine or exocrine functions.

See also INSULIN, ISLET CELL TUMOR, PANCREATECTOMY and PANCREATITIS.

pancreatectomy

Surgical removal of the pancreas.

This is a major operation with considerable risk and it is only appropriate for carefully selected patients. The main reason for the operation is the presence of pancreatic cancer, but it may occasionally be required in the treatment of chronic pancreatitis, pancreatic cysts or following injury to the pancreas.

In some cases of cancer a better operation is pancreaticoduodenectomy, in which only the head of the pancreas is removed, together with a segment of duodenum. In many others the tumor is too far advanced for removal. A major hazard of pancreatic surgery is the leakage of digestive enzymes into the peritoneal cavity, where they can cause severe damage.

Patients who survive total pancreatectomy require insulin therapy for the resulting diabetes and oral therapy with pancreatic extracts to permit the normal digestion of food.

pancreatitis

Inflammation of the pancreas, which may be acute or chronic.

Acute pancreatitis is a disease in which the pancreas appears to "digest itself" due to the liberation of its digestive enzymes into the tissues. It may be provoked by infections (e.g., mumps), trauma, regurgitation of bile up the pancreatic duct, alcoholism and some vascular diseases. Patients have severe abdominal pain and rapidly become seriously ill. Intensive supportive treatment in the hospital is required, although there is no specific treatment.

Chronic pancreatitis may result from repeated attacks of acute pancreatitis or directly from alcoholism or disease of the biliary tract. It causes recurrent abdominal pain and MALABSORPTION, with fatty, offensive stools and, less often, diabetes.

Chronic pancreatitis is common in Western countries, where alcoholism is a widespread problem. Treatment involves prohibition of alcohol, a low-fat diet, pancreatic enzymes by mouth and insulin if necessary, but the disease cannot be cured.

PANCREAS

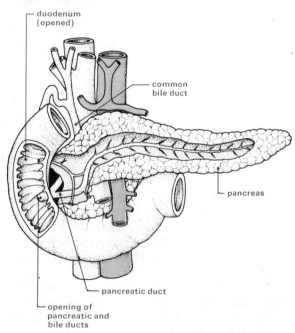

- duodenum (opened)
- common bile duct
- pancreas
- pancreatic duct
- opening of pancreatic and bile ducts

The pancreas is a digestive gland which lies behind the stomach and in front of the major abdominal blood vessels and the left kidney. It secretes digestive enzymes down the pancreatic duct into the duodenum where they break down proteins and fats. In addition it produces two hormones—insulin and glucagon.

papilledema

Swelling and congestion of the "head" of the optic nerve (*optic disk*), at the back of the eye.

The optic nerve, which passes through the "optic foramen" (a tiny hole in the skull), is the pathway along which visual signals from the retina are transmitted to the specialized nerve centers for vision at the back of the brain. If the fluid pressure within the brain is raised above normal, which can result from various disorders within the brain or skull, the pressure change is transmitted along the optic nerve and through the retinal vein to the optic disk. The resulting swelling and pink congestion is visible through an ophthalmoscope (an illuminated instrument for examining the interior of the eye, especially the light-sensitive retina).

Papilledema may occur in one eye or in both, depending upon the extent of pressure change in the brain. It does not usually cause symptoms in itself, but may lead to diminished visual acuity (including blurred vision) when severe. Raised intracranial pressure may lead to headache and vomiting and, ultimately, to unconsciousness; thus, papilledema may provide the doctor with a useful clue in a patient with unconsciousness of unknown cause.

Papilledema is caused most commonly by severe hypertension (high blood pressure) and cerebral tumors. Other masses within the skull, such as an abscess or a hematoma (massive blood clot) may give an identical appearance. Other causes include severe ANEMIA, POLYCYTHEMIA, carbon dioxide poisoning (as in respiratory failure) and a rare but harmless condition of women known as "benign intracranial hypertension."

Papilledema must be distinguished from *papillitis*, in which the optic disk is inflamed and vision severely affected. This is often a complication of MULTIPLE SCLEROSIS. The distinction may require photography of the optic disk following an intravenous injection into a peripheral vein of fluorescein (a fluorescing dye).

Papilledema requires the urgent investigation and treatment of its underlying cause, but no treatment in itself.

papilloma

A basically benign tumor growing on a free surface of epithelium (the outermost layer of cells of the skin or a mucous membrane), commonly as a lobulated mass on a stalk. (Only rarely do they become malignant.) Papillomas, which include growths such as warts and polyps, are most often found on the skin and in the mucous membranes that line the intestinal and urinary tracts.

Papillomas may occur on any part of the skin and are especially common in the elderly. Usually they remain small, but occasionally reach the size of an egg or an orange. Papillomas are normally treated by cautery; the larger ones can be surgically removed by cutting through the supporting stalk.

Intestinal papillomas are most common in the colon and rectum, where they sometimes bleed and are associated with the excess mucus in the patient's stools. They may be single, of unknown cause, or multiple—a condition known as *familial polyposis coli*, which is inherited as a dominant trait. Such forms must be regarded as "premalignant," since malignant change is quite common. Single papillomas can often be removed by using a proctosigmoidoscope—a special instrument inserted into the lower part of the large intestine via the rectum; but multiple polyps are best treated by surgical removal of the affected portion of the bowel.

In the urinary tract, papillomas are most common in the bladder, although they can occur anywhere from the kidney to the urethra (the passage through which urine is voided). The cause is usually not known, but they are particularly common in those who have worked in the rubber industry and in smokers. All are potentially malignant, so all must be removed. In the bladder this is usually done by diathermy (therapeutic use of heat generated by high-frequency current) through a cystoscope (a special instrument for examining the interior of the urinary bladder). Recurrence is common and lifelong regular cystoscopy and diathermy is usually necessary once the diagnosis is made.

See also POLYP.

Pap smear

See CERVICAL SMEAR.

paralysis

The loss of muscular function in a part of the body, caused by damage to the muscles themselves or to a part of the nervous system. Paralysis may vary in severity from affecting a single small muscle or nerve to affecting most of the body.

Disease of the muscles themselves leads more commonly to weakness than the total paralysis. However, the various forms of MUSCULAR DYSTROPHY, most of which occur in childhood, can progress to severe and eventually fatal paralysis. There is no effective treatment for these conditions.

Any block in the transmission of impulses from nerves to muscles may also result in paralysis. This occurs in MYASTHENIA GRAVIS, in BOTULISM and in some other types of poisoning (e.g., with "nerve gas").

The peripheral nerves may be injured directly or damaged by disease, including DIABETES, POLYARTERITIS NODOSA, CANCER, ALCOHOLISM, vitamin deficiencies, LEPROSY, PORPHYRIA and some drug reactions. This damage may lead to weakness or to total paralysis of the muscles supplied by the affected nerves.

The spinal cord may be damaged by a number of diseases, including POLIOMYELITIS, MULTIPLE SCLEROSIS and trauma. The pattern of the resulting paralysis depends on its cause. Complete division of the spinal cord results in PARAPLEGIA—complete paralysis of the legs and the lower part of the body, usually including bladder paralysis. If the spinal cord is damaged in the region of the neck the arms may be paralyzed as well as the legs—*quadriplegia.*

Brain damage may also result in paralysis. The most common cause here is a STROKE, caused by hemorrhage or thrombosis in the brain. The extent of the paralysis is variable, but the most common pattern is partial or complete paralysis of the arm and leg on one side—HEMIPLEGIA. Other causes include MENINGITIS, ENCEPHALITIS, SYPHILIS, brain tumors and impairment of cerebral blood flow. Transient paralysis (*Todd's paralysis*) may occur in part of the body following an epileptic attack.

Paralysis resulting from division of a major nerve tract in the spinal cord or brain is permanent and irreversible, but that resulting from other diseases may have a more variable prognosis. In some diseases, such as "acute infective polyneuritis" (the GUILLAIN-BARRÉ SYNDROME), more or less total paralysis may be followed by complete recovery if the patient survives. In some (e.g., strokes) the extent of recovery is extremely variable and in others (e.g., *motor neuron disease*) recovery is unknown.

Survival in paralysis depends upon the underlying disease and whether or not it affects the respiratory and heart muscles. Artificial ventilation may keep alive patients with some diseases (e.g., poliomyelitis or acute infective polyneuritis) until the paralysis improves or remits; patients may live for years, severely paralyzed, in an "iron lung" respirator.

All paralyzed patients require special care of the affected part of the body to prevent trauma and ulceration, especially if there is also sensory impairment ("sensory paralysis"). Most patients can be taught to overcome their disabilities partially by the clever use of their remaining normal muscles. Physical therapists and other rehabilitation workers have an essential role to play here. The existence of events such as the "Paraplegic Olympics" shows the extent to which many patients can be aided.

paranoia

A chronic personality disorder in which the individual develops systematized, sometimes permanent and mainly persecutory delusions in a setting of otherwise undisturbed thought and personality. Paranoia must be distinguished from *paranoid schizophrenia*, in which the same delusions occur but there is also disturbance of thought processes and personality and the occurrence of hallucinations.

Paranoid reactions are displayed by most people at one time or another in response to severe disappointment or humiliation. The reaction is the mistaken belief that the sufferer is the center of attention and that he is being talked about, usually in a critical way which invades his privacy and embarrasses him.

Paranoia is a state in which the patient experiences constant "paranoid reactions" and where these reactions cannot be dispelled by others. Suspicion and resentment of others arises and the patient takes innocent matters to be a direct attack on himself. He usually feels that his true worth is not recognized by others, and he often has grandiose or exaggerated ideas about what his true worth is.

Temporary paranoid reactions are fairly common and usually harmless—providing they are not associated with other thought disorders or personality changes—although they may be irritating for the family and colleagues of the sufferer. In contrast, true paranoia is relatively rare and can cause considerable annoyance and harm to innocent people outside the sufferer's immediate circle. It is not easy to treat, but is sometimes helped by PSYCHOTHERAPY.

See also PSYCHOSES.

paraplegia

Paralysis of the lower limbs, often accompanied by dysfunction of the rectum and the bladder.

Paraplegia is usually caused by a lesion of the spinal cord; its extent is governed by the position and magnitude of the lesion. Complete severance of the spinal cord will lead to total paralysis of the legs and fecal and urinary INCONTINENCE. Lesser damage may affect the legs and leave the bladder and rectum function unimpaired. Recovery will sometimes take place if the damage to the cord is minimal, but lifelong paralysis is more often the result.

Care of the paraplegic patient should be designed to relieve the symptoms often associated with paralysis, such as pressure sores and urinary infections. As soon as possible a program of physical therapy and retraining should be started—if necessary, in a special center devoted to the care of paraplegics. The provision of special equipment will greatly ease the problems of incontinence and immobility. Many paraplegics, although confined to wheelchairs, live active and useful lives.

parasites

A parasite is an animal or plant which lives inside or upon another living animal or plant without extending any benefit to it in return for the advantages gained.

A large number of organisms find man an ideal place to live. Bacteria, viruses, fungi and protozoa are said to *infect* man, but worms and insects are said to *infest* him and are what is normally meant by the term *parasites*. They may be quite harmless, or may produce symptoms of disease.

In general it may be said that the hotter the country and the worse the standard of hygiene the more parasites flourish. Among the most common in temperate climates are lice, fleas and bedbugs. They are not usually important carriers of disease, but they are disagreeable. They can be controlled by the use of modern insecticides.

More harmful are worms, which range from the pinworm which is more of a nuisance than a threat to life, to the flatworm (trematode) of SCHISTOSOMIASIS which makes life miserable for more than 200 million people in tropical countries and is responsible for untold morbidity and mortality.

Strict attention to personal hygiene will ward off the attentions of most parasites; but those who are not accustomed to the conditions in less developed tropical and subtropical countries may inadvertently lay themselves open to infestation by worms. It is important to avoid uncooked or undercooked food, and to avoid bathing or wading in water which may be the haunt of the freshwater snail that harbors a stage in the development of the parasite which causes schistosomiasis. It is also sensible to wear shoes in wet land in the tropics, and to avoid drinking from village wells and rivers.

The average traveler is in no great danger of becoming infested with parasites, and those whose lives lead them into the remoter parts of the world are usually well informed about such dangers. Nevertheless, it is well to keep the possibility in mind.

The control of parasitic diseases is one of the great tasks of the future for the developing countries; it depends to a large degree on improving the standards of public and private sanitation.

See also FLEAS, FLUKES, LICE, MITES, PINWORMS, ROUNDWORMS, TAPEWORMS, TICKS.

paratyphoid fever

An acute generalized feverish disease caused by bacteria of the genus *Salmonella*.

Paratyphoid fever is so called because it resembles TYPHOID FEVER, but in most cases the symptoms are less severe and the course of the disease is less harmful.

The onset of the disease may be more rapid than in the case of typhoid fever, but the symptoms are much the same. The patient may complain of discomfort, lassitude and headache and suffer from insomnia as well as a high temperature. As in the case of typhoid fever, the fever may be more marked in the morning but the daily peak gradually rises until about the eighth day,

when it levels out. The patient feels restless, hot and uncomfortable; there may be pain in the abdomen which, however, is not as extreme as in typhoid fever. Rose-colored spots are common in typhoid fever, but less common in paratyphoid fever (although they may occur).

Prevention of paratyphoid fever is possible, not only through vaccination but also through the application of measures relating to public hygiene—including a pure water supply—that are common in advanced nations. Travelers to places where paratyphoid fever is still common, such as India, should consult a doctor about vaccination. The TAB vaccine incorporates protection against both typhoid and paratyphoid and is commonly given to children, but the immunity so gained is not permanent. It is prudent to boost the immunity before going to any country where paratyphoid fever exists.

Treatment consists of alleviating the symptoms as far as possible. Drugs such as aspirin to lower the fever may be given under medical supervision and antibiotics may be useful in shortening the period of illness. Caution must be exercised, however, for chloramphenicol—which is used with good effect against typhoid—may have serious side effects and may not be justified for the comparatively trivial paratyphoid. Ampicillin is usually effective.

The diet should be bland and nutritious, with little solid food being given while the gastrointestinal tract is irritated by the bacteria. Convalescence may be prolonged; as in typhoid fever, the attack cannot be regarded as over until six consecutive stool and urine specimens are found to be negative for the presence of the causative bacteria.

Parkinson's disease

A disease, especially of the elderly, characterized by tremor (the head and limbs of the patient shake) and stiffness (muscular rigidity). The patient is unable to initiate movements quickly and has a characteristic bowed posture and immobile face.

Parkinson's disease (also known as *Parkinsonism*) is associated with degeneration of nerve centers deep within the brain (*basal ganglia* and *brain stem nuclei*); these nerve centers are known to be closely linked with the control of posture and movement. The reason for the changes in the brain are now known, although a few cases of Parkinsonism are believed to be related to brain damage caused by toxic substances such as carbon monoxide or high concentrations of manganese. Others arise from the use of certain drugs but in these particular instances the signs and symptoms of the disease are reversible. Some cases follow viral ENCEPHALITIS and Parkinsonism is a feature of the "punch-drunk" syndrome.

Recent research has drawn attention to the importance of *neurotransmitters* in Parkinson's disease. These are chemicals able to facilitate the transmission of impulses across the junctions between nerves. Sufferers from Parkinson's disease show depleted levels of one of these neurotransmitters, *dopamine*, normally found in marked concentrations in the basal ganglia and brain stem nuclei. Since the 1960s, treatment for Parkinson's disease has been concentrated on remedying this deficiency.

The most important drug now used is *levadopa* (or *L-dopa*), which is the immediate chemical precursor to dopamine. As the neurotransmitter itself cannot be administered as a drug, because it cannot penetrate the blood-brain barrier, levadopa must be given to help the body make its own supply of dopamine. About one third of patients shows a great improvement of their condition when given levadopa and another third reports that their symptoms abate. However, levadopa's side effects have caused it to be reserved for more difficult cases.

Some patients cannot take advantage of levadopa

PARKINSON'S DISEASE

Patients with Parkinson's disease are characterized by muscle tremors affecting the head and extremities, staring eyes, an expressionless face, rigidity of some muscle groups and a slow gait marked by short shuffles. Often there is also an involuntary "pill-rolling" movement of the thumb against the first two fingers.

because of severe side effects, including nausea and vomiting. More sophisticated preparations, in which the side effects of the levadopa are countered by other drugs, are now being administered. Some patients, particularly those under the age of 50, who are resistant to drugs can be helped by *stereotaxic* brain operations designed to modify the functions of the basal ganglia. Another important element in the treatment of Parkinson's disease is physiotherapy, since any break in physical activity can be disastrous and lead to immobility.

paronychia

A superficial infection of the epithelium beside a nail, usually a result of tearing a hangnail.

Paronychia is most often caused by infection with staphylococcus. It leads to cellulitis, which can be suppressed by hot applications. There is occasionally a tendency for the infection to burrow under the nail and so form an abscess. This can be painful as well as persistent; it is then necessary to make an incision for the purposes of drainage. The partial or complete removal of the nail may also be necessary. Among nail biters in particular, recurrence is common and it is possible for this comparatively superficial infection to cause severe disability. In diabetes, various fungi can cause chronic paronychial inflammations and similar lesions are sometimes seen in PSORIASIS and some kinds of PEMPHIGUS.

paroxysm

A sudden attack, usually of convulsions or tachycardia, or a sudden exacerbation of disease or a particular symptom, for example the pain in trigeminal neuralgia (see TIC).

pasteurization

The process by which milk and other fluid foods are sterilized.

Unlike boiling, pasteurization does not significantly affect the taste of milk. When Louis Pasteur, the famous 19th-century French scientist, was investigating problems of wine growers, he studied the process of fermentation. Arising from his discoveries, he realized that heating milk to a temperature well below the boiling point would effectively stop fermentation and so prevent milk from being spoiled. It also destroys disease organisms that would otherwise be passed on to human consumers, of which the most important is the tuberculosis bacillus (see TUBERCULOSIS).

Pasteurization is normally achieved by heating the milk for about 40 minutes at 140–160°F (60–70°C).

This destroys some of the vitamin C in the milk, but in a balanced diet this is not an important deficit.

patch test

A test to establish the cause of a contact dermatitis or other sensitivity reaction.

Since sensitivity reactions can be caused by a large number of substances to which the patient's body may be allergic, treatment can be properly planned only when the cause is known. To find out the cause, a small square of gauze is applied to the skin, usually on the upper part of the back. The gauze is impregnated with a purified extract of the suspected substance or substances. If, after about 48 hours, there is an allergic response to the substance under test, it can be safely assumed that the cause of the sensitivity has been correctly identified.

patent ductus arteriosus

A congenital heart defect in which the prenatal circulation of the blood persists after birth.

In a fetus, the blood is oxygenated through the placenta, as the lungs are immersed in fluid and are not used for breathing. In order to bypass the lungs, the circulation is augmented by the *ductus arteriosus*, which connects the left pulmonary artery with the aorta. Occasionally, the ductus arteriosus does not wither away after birth and instead remains *patent* (or open). The result is a mixing of the arterial and venous blood which can lead to failure to thrive, but in the last 25 years surgeons have found that it is possible to cure the condition by means of tying off the duct.

pediculosis

Infestation with LICE.

pellagra

A vitamin deficiency disease, caused by the lack of niacin (or nicotinic acid) in the diet.

Niacin is a substance found in association with the B vitamins that are present in meat, eggs, vegetables and fruit.

Symptoms include digestive upsets, loss of appetite, irritability and headache. Skin involvement leads to redness (similar to a severe sunburn) on the parts exposed to the sun, which later become roughened and brownish. The symptoms recur each year and may eventually lead to paralysis. Treatment involves establishing a balanced diet, with supplements of niacin where necessary.

See also DEFICIENCY DISEASE.

pelvic inflammatory disease

The internal sexual organs of women are liable to be the seat of generalized infection. Although it was long accepted that the main cause of the inflammation was gonorrhea, this is now no longer universally held. It is rare for the gonococcus to be isolated in cases in which an abscess of the Fallopian tubes or ovaries has ruptured and other organisms are known to be involved in the disease, sometimes secondary to gonorrhea. Whether or not it is originally caused by gonorrhea, the inflammation apparently spreads up from the lower genital tract, involving first the Fallopian tubes and then the ovaries.

In most cases the ovaries are turned into a mass several times their original size. Even in cases where they do not have to be removed by surgery the outcome may be infertility. Some cases have been noted following the insertion of an intrauterine contraceptive device (IUD). Death has even resulted in some of these cases.

The symptoms begin with pelvic pain, which may be accompanied by lassitude, chills and low-grade fever. Abdominal and pelvic tenderness will be experienced, and there may be acute pain when an abscess has ruptured. Although the treatment of choice is the administration of appropriate antibiotics, surgery may be necessary to drain abscesses.

pemphigus

A group of diseases of the skin and mucous membranes characterized by the formation of blisters. It is thought that they may be autoimmune disorders, as during the active stages of the disease an immunoglobulin may be found in the circulating serum. (See AUTOIMMUNE DISEASE.)

Pemphigus vulgaris commonly occurs between the ages of 40 and 60. Large blisters suddenly form on the skin, perhaps after blistering has occurred in the mouth. The blisters tend to develop in crops about every three weeks, and may involve the throat, conjunctiva, anal canal and vulva. The natural course of the condition is deterioration after remissions, and the outcome without treatment may be fatal; but the disease responds to the use of corticosteroids.

In *pemphigus vegetans*, the areas of blistering do not tend to heal, but develop outgrowths of wartlike tissue in the armpits, groin, and around the mouth.

Pemphigus foliaceus is rarer; it involves the whole skin, with areas of redness and crusting which looks like exfoliative dermatitis. *Benign familial pemphigus* develops usually in adolescence in the armpits, groins, on the neck and around the anus. It is hereditary and passed on as an autosomal dominant. It tends to heal, but may recur.

peptic ulcer

An ulcer involving those areas of the digestive tract exposed to pepsin—acid gastric juice. The most common are those involving the stomach (GASTRIC ULCER) and the first portion of the duodenum (see DUODENAL ULCER).

See also ULCER.

pericarditis

Inflammation of the pericardium, the membrane surrounding the heart. It is usually secondary to inflammation elsewhere. The causes of this condition include pneumonia, tuberculosis, typhoid fever and, rarely, osteomyelitis; bacteria may gain entry into the body through serious wounds of the chest.

Virus infections may give rise to pericarditis, among which are respiratory infections and infection with echo viruses and the Coxsackie B virus. Underlying infarction of the cardiac muscle may produce aseptic inflammation of the pericardium, and the membrane is affected in the cardiac reaction of rheumatic fever.

The main symptom is pain felt in the center of the chest, which may radiate to the neck, shoulders and upper arms; but the symptoms of the causative disease often predominate. In some cases there is an effusion of fluid into the pericardial sac sufficiently great to affect the action of the heart, and steps must be taken to aspirate the fluid through the chest wall. After some infections scarring may produce a constriction in the pericardium which can disturb the action of the heart.

perifolliculitis

The presence of an inflammatory infiltrate surrounding hair follicles. It frequently occurs in association with FOLLICULITIS.

Pustular perifolliculitis is a disease of the scalp which is not uncommon among business executives and may originate from stress. A few pustules appear on the head and cause intense itching.

Perifolliculitis abscedens et suffodiens is a chronic dissecting folliculitis of the scalp. Another form, *sycosis vulgans* (also known as "barber's itch"), covers the area of the face that is normally shaved.

The various forms of perifolliculitis are caused either by staphylococci or streptococci and may be treated with antibiotics.

periodontics

A branch of dentistry dealing with the study and treatment of diseases of the *periodontium*, the tissues investing (or "embedding") and supporting the teeth.

There are several classes of periodontal diseases. Under the heading of "inflammatory diseases" comes GINGIVITIS, which may be caused by bacteria, nutritional deficiencies, endocrine variations, herpes virus, or by metabolic errors. Also included is *periodontitis*, which may be due to calcified deposits or improper tooth anatomy and position.

"Dystrophic diseases" include *gingivosis*, which involves painful desquamation of the epithelium and degeneration of underlying connective tissue fibers; *periodontosis*, which leads to bone resorption along the side of the tooth; *periodontal atrophy*, which leads to exposure of the root surface on some or all of the teeth; and *hyperplastic periodontal conditions*, in which the periodontium grows in size, because of the side effects of drug therapy or other forms of irritation. Periodontists also treat periodontal trauma.

Much of the work of periodontists involves the removal of calcified deposits from around the teeth and their roots, a feature of several periodontal diseases. In addition, they perform operations for the removal of pockets of pus in the gums and undertake other soft tissue repairs.

Orthodontic aids are used to reposition migrating teeth; it has been shown that stretching and compression of the *periodontal ligament* (connective tissue which attaches a tooth to its bony socket) stimulates new tissue and bone formation. When a tooth is placed under strain by an orthodontic appliance, the periodontal ligament is compressed on the pressure side and

PERIODONTITIS

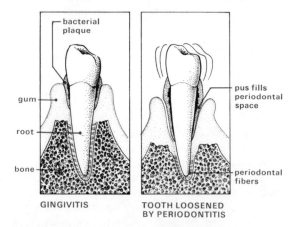

GINGIVITIS   TOOTH LOOSENED BY PERIODONTITIS

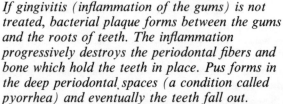

If gingivitis (inflammation of the gums) is not treated, bacterial plaque forms between the gums and the roots of teeth. The inflammation progressively destroys the periodontal fibers and bone which hold the teeth in place. Pus forms in the deep periodontal spaces (a condition called pyorrhea) and eventually the teeth fall out.

stretched on the other. Resorption of bone occurs in the area of compression. Thus, repositioning of the teeth is followed by an improvement in the status of the supporting tissues; the teeth become stable as new bone and periodontal ligament tissues grow.

peritonitis

Inflammation of the peritoneum, the membranes lining the abdominal cavity.

Most acute cases are caused by the perforation of one of the hollow abdominal organs or by infection spreading from an inflamed organ. Occasionally in children no obvious source of infection is found. Peritonitis may remain localized, especially when it arises from inflammation of the gallbladder or the appendix, but in severe perforations—for example of a peptic ulcer or a gangrenous appendix—the whole peritoneal cavity may be involved. Peritonitis resulting from the perforation of a peptic ulcer is at first chemical, but soon bacterial infection spreads and the abdominal cavity becomes full of pus.

The main symptom of peritonitis is severe pain and tenderness of the abdominal wall, which becomes rigid. The patient may experience nausea and vomiting; soon the intestines become paralyzed and the abdomen distends. The pain makes the patient lie still with his legs drawn up. The temperature may be raised or may be subnormal, and the blood pressure may fall. The pulse is quickened and may be weak. In most cases a period of resuscitation with intravenous therapy and the adminis- tration of antibiotics precedes the operation necessary to drain the peritoneal cavity and treat the cause of the peritonitis. The postoperative course is likely to be stormy.

Tuberculosis of the peritoneum is now rare, but at one time it was a cause of chronic peritonitis and the adhesions (see ADHESION) which sometimes form after any case of peritonitis.

Rarely, peritoneal adhesions cause acute or chronic obstruction of the intestine, and may be relieved only by operation; but this in itself may set up further adhesions in patients who are apt to react in this way to disturbance of the peritoneum.

pernicious anemia

See ANEMIA.

personality

The sum total of all the characteristics of a person— including the mental, moral, physical and social qualities—as they are perceived by other people. The word may be used either in a popular sense, in which the meaning is simply linked to the type of person as seen by others, or in a psychological sense, in which the meaning is more complex and sometimes less obvious.

Psychoanalysts regard personality as the result of the interaction between instinct and the environment. Other schools of psychology and psychiatry have more complicated explanations, combining the effects of upbringing, heredity, experience and biochemical factors.

One of the most widely followed divisions is Jung's categories of extroverted and introverted personalities. The distinction in technical terms is that the extrovert directs his LIBIDO and instinctual energy toward the environment, whereas the introvert has weak instinctual energy and directs it inward toward himself. Most people combine aspects of both personality types, and the extreme examples of either can be instantly recognized by their behavior.

Personality may have no medical connotations at all. To describe a person as an "unpleasant" personality or a "miserable" personality is not to suggest that he or she is in any way mentally ill. On the other hand, there are various defects in behavior or lifestyle which are regarded widely as *personality disorders*. These are characterized by pathological trends in personality structure, with minimal subjective anxiety—in most cases manifested by a lifelong pattern of abnormal action or behavior, and not by mental or emotional symptoms.

Sociopathic personality disturbance, for instance, may be a pathological relationship between the patient and the society in which he lives, together with personal discomfort and poor interpersonal relationships. *Personality trait disturbance* is an inability to maintain emotional equilibrium in stressful situations.

Various mental disorders are often expressed in terms of personality. Sufferers will be categorized as *paranoid personalities* or *neurotic personalities* and there are also authenticated cases of *multiple personality*, which most authorities believe are delusional in character. In all these cases personality is distorted into an abnormal type by the underlying mental or emotional disorder.

Perthes' disease

A disease of the growth of ossification centers in children. The child begins to limp and complains of pain, often in the knee. Perthes' disease affects the head of the femur (thigh bone). Technical name: *oesteochondritis deformans juvenilis*.

The disease is of unknown origin and is usually experienced in three stages, each lasting about 9 to 12 months. In the first period, the head of the femur suffers from NECROSIS and degeneration. In the second period, revascularization (the return of blood vessels) takes place; in the final stage the bone is replaced by reossification. Boys between the ages of 4 and 10 are most often affected, and the prognosis may be good or the disease may lead to some permanent disability.

Treatment is usually limited to the avoidance of weight-bearing on the affected leg. It is rarely bilateral.

pertussis

The technical name for WHOOPING COUGH.

pessary

1. Any device placed in the vagina to support the uterus or to provide contraception. 2. Any form of medication (especially a vaginal suppository) placed in the vagina for therapeutic purposes.

petechiae

Minute hemorrhagic spots on the skin, ranging from the size of a pinhead to a pinpoint.

Petechiae are formed by the escape of blood into the skin or mucous membranes. They appear for a variety of reasons when there is a rupture in the junction between capillary and the artery from which it is fed. A large number of conditions and diseases exist which cause these ruptures.

Petechiae are a sign of many illnesses, ranging from Rocky Mountain spotted fever to measles, and from scarlet fever to smallpox. They can also accompany cerebrospinal meningitis and (especially in older people) they may be an external sign of vitamin C deficiency. Their appearance after surgery can be a sign of a fat embolism; the fracture of a long bone may lead to the same sequence of events.

In *hyperglobulinemic purpura*, petechiae appear in "showers" all over the body, but especially on the lower extremities. These attacks may be brought on by prolonged walking or standing, or by wearing constrictive garters or clothing.

Peutz-Jeghers syndrome

An inherited disease characterized by gastrointestinal POLYPS and the appearance of brown lesions on the lips, hands and feet.

The marks, which are not accompanied by any symptoms, usually appear when the patient is a child. The syndrome shows a great deal of variety in its other manifestations. The brown marks, which are pigmented macules, affect the inside of the mouth—including the gums and the palate—and the area around the nose. In addition to the skin symptoms, there are usually polyps in the stomach and intestines, which lead to abdominal

pain and vomiting. In the majority of cases the polyps are most numerous in the small intestine, where they are usually benign; in the large intestine, stomach, duodenum and the rectum they may rarely become malignant.

Inheritance is by an autosomal dominant gene and either sex may be affected.

Peyronie's disease

A painful disease of the penis; also known as *fibrous cavernitis*.

With no known cause, plaques or strands of dense fibrous tissue develop around the *corpus cavernosum* (a cylinder of erectile tissue) of the penis. These cause a deformity, with the penis twisted to one side, and the patient may feel intense pain during an erection. The disease is sometimes associated with DUPUYTREN'S CONTRACTURE, in which there is a profusion of fibrous tissue of the palm, leading to contracture with permanent flexion of the fingers, especially the fourth or fifth. In addition to the unknown form of the disease, cases have been reported in recent years in which the patient had been taking the drug propranolol (Inderal) for heart disease.

The disease is benign and self-limiting, although effective treatment is very difficult.

phagocytosis

The destruction of bacteria by the leukocytes or white blood cells.

Phagocytosis is part of the process of the immune response, by which the body repels or consumes foreign bodies which threaten it. When a bacterium appears in the bloodstream, as long as the immune response is normal in the individual, it is immediately surrounded by leukocytes. The leukocyte is able to absorb the bacterium by smothering it and drawing it through its cell wall.

After digesting the invader, the leukocyte itself will usually die after undergoing a granular fatty degeneration and it is an abundance of dead leukocytes which collect together in an infected wound or an abscess as pus.

It is possible that the leukocytes initiate the process of digestion of the bacteria by secreting substances which are toxic to the invaders.

See also ANTIBODY/ANTIGEN, IMMUNE SYSTEM.

phantom limb syndrome

Following amputation of the whole or part of a limb, it is fairly common for the patient to feel that the part is still there.

The patient may experience feelings of touch, heat, cold and position in the phantom limb, but often the most serious problem is pain. A patient who has lost a hand may, for example, complain of pain in his thumb or at his finger tips.

Most cases of the phantom limb syndrome are mild and disappear within days or weeks of the amputation. Severe persistent pain may be relieved by applying stimuli such as vibration or heat to the amputation stump or by drug treatment. With modern methods of pain relief (see PAIN) the phantom limb syndrome can sometimes be successfully treated.

pharmaceutics/pharmacy/pharmacology

Pharmacy and *pharmaceutics* are alternative terms for the art and science of preparing and dispensing medicines. Pharmacy is also used to describe the place in which drugs are prepared and dispensed; *pharmaceutic* or *pharmaceutical* is used as a term for a medicinal preparation or drug.

Pharmacology is the study of the action of drugs on the living body and its biochemical systems.

Pharmacy is principally concerned with the accurate preparation and presentation of drugs. In the past, most medicines were prepared from their basic ingredients at the point of dispensing—by the physician or in the drugstores. While this is still true of some drugs, the majority are now formulated and prepared in bulk by the pharmaceutical industry. The pharmacist often simply dispenses already prepared drugs in the dosage and form prescribed by the physician or recommended by the manufacturers. However, pharmacists receive a full professional training and are capable of preparing many medicines from their basic ingredients, and of aiding patients in choosing appropriate self-medication.

Pharmacology can be divided into two areas: *basic pharmacology* and *clinical pharmacology*. Basic pharmacology is the study of the basic action of drugs on normal and abnormal living organisms at any level from bacteria to man, or on isolated biochemical pathways from these organisms. Pharmacologists working in this field may not be medically qualified—often a training in biochemistry and physiology is more relevant than a full medical training.

Clinical pharmacologists have a special expertise and interest in the action of drugs in man. They have become increasingly important as the number of potent drugs available has multiplied over the past 30 years. All doctors must understand much about clinical pharmacology, but those with a special interest study details of drug actions and interactions with diseases and with each other.

"Polypharmacy," the prescription of multiple drugs to the individual patient, while sometimes essential, runs the risk of causing interactions between drugs which may endanger the patient. These risks have become increasingly publicized and are a major field of current study for clinical pharmacologists.

pharyngitis

Inflammation of the pharynx, the common cause of sore throat. The pharynx is the passageway that connects the back of the mouth and nose with the larynx and esophagus and contains the tonsils.

Pharyngitis is a common component of upper respiratory infection, usually caused by viruses such as those of the common cold or bacterial infections (especially with *Streptococci*).

Chronic pharyngitis may be caused by heavy smoking or by the "postnasal drip" associated with allergic or other diseases of the nose. In debilitated patients, pharyngitis may be caused by thrush (*candidiasis*—see CANDIDA) or by several species of microorganisms that ordinarily cause no problems in those who are otherwise healthy. Some blood diseases (including leukemia) may sometimes cause pharyngitis.

Viral pharyngitis usually resolves spontaneously within a few days. No curative treatment is possible, but the sore throat may sometimes be relieved by gargles containing aspirin. Penicillin or other antibiotics are of no value in viral infections (but are necessary in streptococcal and other bacterial infections).

TONSILLECTOMY may be required for severe recurrent pharyngitis involving the tonsils.

Culture of microorganisms obtained by means of a throat swab can identify most of the dangerous causes of pharyngitis. A drawback to this technique, however, is that it is impracticable to perform this test on all patients with sore throats.

phenylketonuria

A disease characterized by an inborn error of metabolism of the amino acid phenylalanine.

The disease is present from birth in affected individuals, although it is not clinically recognizable at first. Progressive mental retardation occurs from the age of a few weeks, and irritability and vomiting are early features. Dermatitis may occur at five or six months of age. Affected children are usually of fairer complexion than unaffected siblings. Untreated patients become so retarded that institutional care is usually required, and they frequently develop epilepsy.

The disease is inherited on a recessive basis: both parents are unaffected but carry the trait, and they have a one in four chance of producing an affected infant in each pregnancy. The incidence of phenylketonuria (PKU) in Scotland is 1 in 8,000 births, and in SE England 1 in 30,000.

The diagnosis can often be made by urine testing, but the most reliable method is to test a drop of the baby's blood within a few days of birth (Guthrie Test). This test is used routinely on all newborn babies in Scotland, and the Scriver technique is used in some other areas. Testing for PKU on about the fifth day is now performed routinely in the U.K.

Treatment involves strict adherence to a low phenylalanine diet. A small amount of phenylalanine is required for normal growth, but no more than this must be consumed. Most normal foods contain phenylalanine, so the special diet involves considerable modifications. The diet should probably be continued for life, but this is not yet certain as it has only been in use for about the past 20 years.

In the future it is possible that "enzyme transplantation" from a normal individual (e.g., by partial liver transplantation) may be used to give normal phenylalanine metabolism to affected individuals.

pheochromocytoma

A tumor of the adrenal gland which causes hypertension.

Pheochromocytoma is rare, accounting for less than 0.1% of all cases of hypertension, but it is important because it causes potentially lethal hypertension—which can usually be completely cured by surgery.

Some pheochromocytomas cause a persistent increase in blood pressure, but many lead to sudden attacks associated with the release of epinephrine and norepinephrine from the tumor. The hypertensive attacks may be associated with sweating, palpitations, headaches, anxiety and facial pallor or flushing.

A screening test for pheochromocytoma is performed on the urine of most patients with hypertension; positive results are confirmed by special blood, urine and radiographic tests. Treatment is by removal of the tumor, preceded by appropriate drug therapy.

Very few pheochromocytomas are malignant, but multiple tumors may occur. Removal of all tumor tissue usually cures the hypertension.

phimosis

Tightness of the foreskin of the penis, which prevents it from being drawn down over the glans.

Until the age of five it may be quite normal for the foreskin not to retract. Forcible attempts to retract the foreskin at this age may cause damage and even lead to true phimosis in later life. Above the age of five the

PHIMOSIS

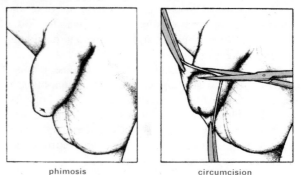

phimosis   circumcision

Phimosis is a tight foreskin which cannot be pulled back over the head of the penis. In boys under the age of 4 years, the foreskin normally adheres to the penis and should not be forced back during washing. Such attempts are likely to cause a true phimosis by scarring the foreskin. Phimosis is relieved by circumcision.

foreskin normally will retract; if it does not, true phimosis exists.

If phimosis at any age causes obstruction to the flow of urine, with "ballooning" of the foreskin, or if after puberty it interferes with normal erection of the penis, then CIRCUMCISION is required.

phlebitis

Inflammation of the wall of a vein, commonly associated with THROMBOSIS within the vein.

Phlebitis occurs most frequently in varicose veins in the leg, where it may be spontaneous or may follow trauma or infection. It may also occur elsewhere in the body in abnormal veins (e.g., hemorrhoids) or in normal veins. It may occur at the site of an intravenous infusion or injection or may be deliberately induced by "sclerosing agents" to cure varicose veins or hemorrhoids.

Symptoms vary from mild discomfort over the affected vein to severe pain associated with tenderness and swelling of the surrounding tissue and sometimes a high fever.

Treatment involves supporting and elevating the affected part to prevent painful swelling and movement. Elevation of the leg helps to drain blood efficiently through the deep veins, but a similar effect can often be obtained in the ambulant patient by the use of supportive elastic stockings or dressings. Infection may require antibiotic treatment. Aspirin-like drugs may help to suppress both the inflammation and the pain.

Most cases of phlebitis are harmless and resolve spontaneously. Pulmonary EMBOLISM occurs very rarely following *superficial venous phlebitis* in contrast to the high risk of this complication following *deep vein thrombosis.* Where phlebitis is associated with infection there is a risk of septicemia (blood poisoning), but this should be rare with adequate treatment.

phlebothrombosis

Thrombosis (clotting) in veins which are not inflamed. Compare THROMBOPHLEBITIS.

phlebotomy

Another name for VENESECTION—incision into a vein for the purpose of drawing blood; bloodletting.

phobia

A persistent excessive fear of an object or situation which is not of real danger. Examples include CLAUSTROPHOBIA (fear of confined spaces), AGORAPHOBIA (fear of being in the open), specific phobias (e.g., for spiders, mice, thunder or darkness) and social phobias (e.g., excessive anxiety in the presence of other people).

Phobias, especially specific phobias, may be isolated abnormalities in an otherwise normal person, or they may sometimes be a manifestation of underlying anxiety or depression of a more general nature. It is likely that many phobias may represent a prolonged response to an unpleasant experience in childhood, but the original stimulus is usually forgotten.

Phobias of all kinds are more common in women than in men, but most individuals have some degree of phobia for some situation.

Phobias produce three main kinds of response: (1) a subjective experience of fear for the object or situation; (2) physiological changes such as palpitations or blushing in response to it; and (3) behavioral tendencies to avoid or escape from it. Some truly phobic patients experience symptoms rarely because they avoid the feared situation, but most patients with a severe phobia ultimately seek treatment.

Patients with underlying anxiety or depressive states often benefit from drug therapy or psychotherapy, but most other phobias are resistant to these techniques. Here the most effective therapy is often "desensitization," a form of behavior therapy in which the patient is gradually taught to relax while imagining the feared object. An alternative technique is "flooding" or "implosion" therapy, in which the patient is confronted by the feared object or situation at once and encouraged to remain in contact with it until his anxiety disappears.

Therapy for phobias is not always successful, and "cures" are not always permanent, but most sufferers can be helped by current treatment. The understanding and patience of family and friends is essential in dealing with all kinds of phobias.

photophobia

1. Abnormal sensitivity of the eyes to light.

It is a feature of various conditions, including MIGRAINE, MEASLES, MENINGITIS, CONJUNCTIVITIS, IRITIS and KERATITIS. Photophobia may also be experienced by persons taking or addicted to certain drugs.

2. A morbid or irrational fear of light or of being in well-lit places.

physiotherapy

The treatment of patients by physical methods and agents to treat or prevent disease, or to assist in rehabilitation and restoration of normal function following a disease or surgical operation.

Physiotherapy is practiced to some extent by all people who are involved in the care of patients, but those paramedical personnel who are specially trained in this particular field are known as physiotherapists.

Physiotherapy is usually carried out under medical supervision and prescribed by a doctor. The methods used include the following:

Therapeutic exercises for the limbs, abdominal muscles, chest muscles, etc. These are of value before and after any significant operation, in prenatal and postnatal care, in any patient who has been confined to bed by illness and (more specifically) in those with disabilities resulting from injury or disease. "Active" exercises are those carried out by the patient, but "passive movements"—made on the patient's body by the therapist—are of value in unconscious patients and some others, especially to prevent the development of muscle contractures.

Massage and *manipulation*, properly carried out, may be of value in a number of musculoskeletal diseases.

Movement in a pool of water (*hydrotherapy*) is easier for patients with many kinds of arthritis than movement in air, and this may help to strengthen muscles.

Heat therapy may aid in the restoration of joint and muscle function. Heat may be applied in a number of ways including lamps, pads, hot water and hot wax.

A number of other techniques including *ultrasound, electrotherapy*, etc., have special applications in different areas of medicine and may be administered by physiotherapists. Many of these forms of therapy can be carried out anywhere, but some need the facilities of a well-equipped hospital department.

pica

The habit of eating substances which are not normally taken as food, particularly clay, earth, charcoal, ashes, feces, or paint off cots, windowsills, etc.

Pica derives its name from the scientific name for one species of magpie, *Pica pica*—a bird which is traditionally believed to sample all available substances. The reason for the human habit is not known, but it is widespread—particularly in pregnant women and in children. It is linked to the cravings which pregnant women sometimes exhibit for inappropriate foods at inappropriate times (such as pickles and ice cream at midnight!).

Some work has been done to investigate the theory that the craving for clay and earth may be a sign of a lack of various nutrients. It is possible that pica is characteristic of individuals lacking iron and potassium; in some parts of India the habit (and perhaps this form of malnutrition) is so common that cakes of clay are sold in markets.

pinworms

The most common worm PARASITES of man, particularly among schoolchildren. The worm is also known as the "threadworm" (scientific name: *Enterobius vermicularis*, formerly known as *Oxyuris vermicularis*). The infestation they cause is known as *enterobiasis* or *oxyuriasis*.

The adult worms live within the human intestine. Females are about half an inch long; males are much smaller. Mature females crawl through the anus to the perianal skinfolds where they lay up to 10,000 eggs each, typically at night. This process usually causes intense itching at the anus (*pruritus ani*). Within six hours the eggs turn into infectious larvae. If swallowed by man these develop into adult worms in the small intestine and the cycle starts again.

The severe itching at the anus causes great discomfort and scratching, and it may lead to irritability and insomnia, but other symptoms are unlikely to be due to pinworms. In particular it is doubtful if they ever cause the abdominal pain or weight loss so often blamed on them. In females they may wander into the vagina, uterus, and Fallopian tubes, but serious consequences are very rare.

Transmission of the parasites occurs by self-infection from anus to mouth as a result of scratching in sleep or poor hygiene, by cross-infection from anus to hand to the hand of another individual, or by taking in eggs from dust in homes or classrooms.

The worms may be seen in the stools, or swabs may be taken from around the anus, using Scotch Tape which is then examined under the microscope.

Pinworms can be killed by drugs such as piperazine taken by mouth, but reinfection is extremely common and repeated treatment is often necessary. Although irritating, the infection is harmless; complications of

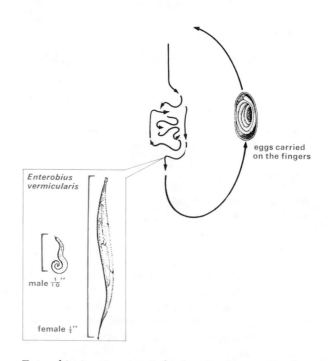

PINWORM (THREADWORM)

Enterobius vermicularis

male $\frac{1}{10}$"

female $\frac{1}{4}$"

eggs carried on the fingers

Enterobiasis, pinworm infection, is characterized by intense itching around the anus. This is due to the female worm migrating down the gut at night and laying eggs on the anal skin. Scratching contaminates the fingers with eggs, which are then carried to the mouth and ingested.

infection and treatment are very rare. When one member of a family is infected, all members of the family should be treated at the same time.

pituitary gland

A pea-sized endocrine gland at the base of the brain, which is enclosed within a bony cavity in the skull (the pituitary fossa) situated just above and behind the nasal cavity. The gland is connected to the hypothalamus of the brain by a thin stalk and divided into two parts, the *anterior* and *posterior* divisions (or lobes) of the pituitary gland.

The pituitary gland produces a number of hormones which influence the function of other endocrine glands and organs throughout the body. It was once described as "the conductor of the endocrine orchestra" of the body, but it has become clear in recent years that the anterior pituitary is itself strongly influenced by hormones released by the hypothalamus, which travel directly to it through special blood vessels. The hypothalamus in turn is influenced by a complex of factors including the rest of the nervous system and the concentration of various substances in the blood.

The anterior division of the pituitary gland (*adeno-hypophysis*) releases a number of hormones into the blood:

Growth hormone (SOMATOTROPIN) is necessary for normal growth, and has other metabolic actions. Deficiency in childhood leads to dwarfism; excessive production, usually caused by a tumor of the pituitary, leads to gigantism in childhood and ACROMEGALY in adult life.

Thyroid-stimulating hormone (*TSH*) stimulates the thyroid gland to produce thyroxine and triiodothyronine. The level of TSH in the blood is usually raised in MYXEDEMA and lowered in thyrotoxicosis (see HYPERTHYROIDISM) by a feedback effect of thyroid hormones on the pituitary.

Adrenocorticotropic hormone (ACTH) maintains normal activity in the cortex (outer portion) of the adrenal gland, stimulating the normal secretion of cortico-steroid hormones.

Luteinizing hormone (also known as *interstitial cell-stimulating hormone*) and *follicle-stimulating hormone* regulate the secretion and activity of the testes and ovaries. Abnormalities of secretion may result in abnormal sexual characteristics and infertility.

Prolactin regulates milk production and breast development in pregnancy. Recently high levels of secretion have been recognized as a factor in some women with infertility, but the output from the pituitary can be diminished by drugs such as bromocriptine.

The posterior division of the pituitary gland (*neuro-hypophysis*) releases two hormones into the blood. Both are produced in nerve cells in the hypothalamus and pass through the stalk to the far end of the cells in the neurohypophysis:

Antidiuretic hormone (or *vasopressin*) acts on the kidneys to prevent excessive water loss in the urine. If the secretion is low due to hypothalamic or pituitary disease, DIABETES INSIPIDUS develops.

Oxytocin makes the uterine muscle contract in labor. Its role in men and at other times in women is less well defined.

The pituitary gland may be damaged by trauma to the head, by infections of various kinds and by tumors. Where deficiencies of hormones occur as a result, those produced by the "target organs" may often be used in treatment, rather than those produced by the pituitary gland itself, which are difficult to obtain in large amounts.

ACTH is available in large amounts, however, and human growth hormone is used for the treatment of pituitary dwarfism. Oxytocin and antidiuretic hormone are synthesized and generally available.

See also HORMONES.

PITUITARY GLAND

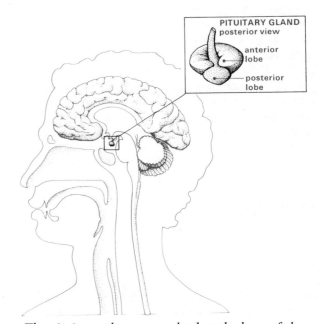

The pituitary, the master gland at the base of the brain, regulates much of the body's hormonal system. Its anterior lobe secretes hormones which stimulate many other glands to produce hormones of their own. Occasionally benign tumors grow in this anterior lobe and disturb the body's growth, its response to stress and other functions. The posterior lobe secretes only two hormones; the first acts on the kidney to retain body water and the second makes the womb contract in labor.

pityriasis rosea

A mild inflammatory skin disease, probably caused by a virus. It produces a characteristic skin rash and there are rarely any other symptoms. The disease is quite common in the United States, especially in winter.

The rash starts with a single flat red spot, an oval area about 1 inch across with a ring of tiny scales near its edge, usually on the front of the chest. After a few days smaller but similar oval patches appear, mainly on the chest and abdomen, but also sometimes on the back, upper arms and thighs. The number of patches ranges from a few to hundreds.

The patches increase in number for two or three weeks and the disease then resolves spontaneously over six to ten weeks. Itching is occasionally troublesome and may require treatment with a lotion such as calamine, but there are no other symptoms. Recovery is complete within ten weeks; there are no long-term effects and relapses or second attacks are very rare.

placenta

The afterbirth—the fleshy round pancake-like organ which is delivered shortly after the birth of the baby, and which is connected to the child by the umbilical cord. The child's blood flows through it until a few minutes after the birth.

When the baby is in the womb it receives all its nutrients and oxygen from the mother via the umbilical cord. It is the placenta which makes this possible. It develops on the inner wall of the womb at a very early stage of pregnancy, and remains firmly attached to the womb until just after the child has been born. The mother's blood passes through the wall of the womb and transfers its precious cargo of oxygen and food into the placenta, where the baby's blood picks it up before returning to the child via the umbilical cord.

There is ordinarily no actual mixing of the mother's blood with the baby's, but simply a transfer of oxygen and nutrients through the wall of the placenta (which lies in intimate contact with the wall of the womb).

The placenta is usually about 8 in. (20 cm) across and 1½ in. (4 cm) thick. It weighs about one sixth of the weight of the baby—ordinarily about 1 to 1½ lb. (450 to 700 grams). Because of its relatively small mass, it causes the mother little or no discomfort during its expulsion. After the umbilical cord has been tied off and cut by the obstetrician, the placenta is usually disposed of, unless there is some good reason to examine it for evidence of disease.

See also CHILDBIRTH.

PLACENTA

The placenta develops early in pregnancy and normally occupies an area high in the uterus. The maternal and fetal circulations do not mix, but are able to exchange nutrients and waste products across the placenta. Maternal blood is pumped into "lakes" which surround the villi containing delicate fetal blood vessels. The placenta also secretes hormones.

placental insufficiency

The situation in which a fetus fails to grow normally and becomes "small-for-date"—traditionally ascribed to inadequacy of the PLACENTA for the needs of the fetus. Such presumed *placental insufficiency* has been supported by the finding of a "gritty," calcified and sometimes partly damaged placenta at birth, and by studies on levels of hormones produced in part by the placenta.

In recent years, however, it has become clear that the state of the placenta at birth does not necessarily bear any relation to the state of the baby. Many normal and healthy babies are born with apparently "unhealthy" placentas and vice versa.

"Placental insufficiency" is thus often a misnomer for more complex problems affecting the mother or fetus, or both, rather than the placenta alone.

placenta previa

A PLACENTA positioned in the lower segment of the uterus, bridging or on the edge of the opening from the uterus into the vagina. The consequence is complication of late pregnancy and labor.

The major complication is bleeding, which occurs as the lower segment of the uterus dilates in late pregnancy—the placenta cannot stretch with it, so some degree of separation from the uterus occurs by tearing.

Placenta previa causes no symptoms until the bleeding begins, but this may be severe and of sudden onset. Placenta previa may be suspected earlier on clinical examination and confirmed by a number of radiologic, ultrasonic and isotopic techniques.

Bleeding is treated by rest and blood transfusion if necessary. If it persists or recurs, or if the fetus is in danger, immediate Cesarean section is required (see

CHILDBIRTH); otherwise, this may be delayed until 38 weeks of pregnancy. Normal delivery is rarely possible—the placenta would be delivered first and the baby would be in danger.

Placenta previa usually results from chance; subsequent pregnancies are very rarely affected.

plague

An infectious disease caused by the bacterium *Pasteurella pestis*. The disease is endemic in the western United States and in South America, China and parts of Africa.

The causative bacteria normally infect rodents and are carried by the rat flea. These may bite humans, especially when the host rats are dying of plague.

There are three forms of plague: *bubonic plague*, with general enlargement of lymph glands and a rash; *pneumonic plague*, with pneumonia due to organisms in the lungs which can be spread to others by coughing; and *septicemic plague*, where there is rapid spread of the organisms throughout the body in the blood.

The "Black Death" in the 14th century in Europe was due to plague. Epidemics are now fortunately rare and precautions can be taken to limit their spread, but the disease is still extremely dangerous and antimicrobial treatment is usually only effective if started within a few hours of onset. Treatment involves the administration of sulfonamides, streptomycin, chloramphenicol or tetracyclines.

plantar reflex

A reflex movement of the toes, especially the big toe, elicited by scratching the outside of the sole of the foot.

The normal reflex is downward movement of the big toe (flexion). An abnormal response is upward movement (extension) followed usually by flexion. Except in young babies the abnormal response (BABINSKI'S REFLEX) is an indication of neurological abnormality (upper motor neuron damage).

plantar wart

A wart occurring on the sole of the foot.

Like other WARTS, plantar warts are caused by a virus. They are common and contagious and are spread particularly by close contact with bare feet, e.g., in swimming pools and school locker rooms. Some individuals seem completely immune while others may develop large numbers of warts. Plantar warts, unlike most warts, are usually painful because pressure forces them into the foot.

There is no reliable treatment, but many are used. Warts can usually be removed by cautery, curettage or the application of liquid nitrogen, and regular soaking of the feet in formalin. Special plasters and a number of other techniques are sometimes effective. In all cases of these kinds of warts recurrence is common; but, it is also rather mystifyingly true that the warts may disappear suddenly and permanently for no obvious reason.

plastic surgery

See COSMETIC SURGERY.

platelets

A component of the blood. Platelets (also known as *thrombocytes*) are colorless disks, much smaller than the red and white cells; there are approximately 300,000 per cubic millimeter of blood. They are not cells but cellular fragments, produced by large cells (*megakaryocytes*) in the bone marrow. They have a normal lifespan in the blood of about ten days.

The best understood function of platelets is their role in the formation of blood clots. They stick to the walls of damaged blood vessels and release substances which initiate the formation of a clot. They are not essential for all blood clotting, but a deficiency of platelets may lead to abnormal bleeding, especially in the skin (*thrombocytopenic purpura*).

Several diseases lead to a fall in the number of platelets in the blood. These include leukemia, aplastic anemia, cancer which has spread to the bone marrow, severe infections, collagen diseases and some cases of heart and kidney failure. In addition, some conditions (such as kidney failure) may impair the function of the platelets which do remain. Some patients develop a low platelet count for no obvious reason—a condition known as *idiopathic thrombocytopenic purpura*.

In POLYCYTHEMIA the platelet count can be greatly increased and add to the risk of thrombosis.

Platelets can be separated from blood and transfused into patients with a deficiency. The effect is temporary but may be of value if such a patient is bleeding or requires surgery.

Platelets are also involved in the formation of abnormal and dangerous venous thromboses and are also implicated in the formation of the fatty plaques ATHEROSCLEROSIS. Platelet function can be suppressed by drugs such as aspirin.

See also THROMBOCYTOPENIA.

pleural effusion

An abnormal collection of fluid in the pleural space.

The pleural space separates the membranes (pleura) covering the lungs, the chest wall and the diaphragm; it normally contains only a small amount of fluid which lubricates the surface of the lungs as they move with respiration. An abnormally large amount of fluid may accumulate in a number of conditions including cancer of the lung, breast or ovary, tuberculosis, pneumonia, pulmonary embolism, heart failure, cirrhosis and collagen diseases.

Small effusions may cause no symptoms. Large effusions, however, may cause severe shortness of breath and pain, especially if associated with PLEURISY.

Where possible treatment is directed at the underlying condition; but it is also often necessary to relieve breathlessness by aspirating the fluid through a needle. Examination of this fluid may also help to diagnose the cause.

The prognosis of pleural effusions depends upon the cause, but they are often recurrent and repeated aspiration may be necessary.

pleurisy

Inflammation of the pleura. The pleura is the membrane which covers the outer surface of the lungs and the inner surface of the thorax (chest). These two surfaces normally move on one another with respiration, being lubricated by a small amount of pleural fluid.

Pleurisy may occur in a number of conditions and in two forms: "dry pleurisy" and "pleurisy with effusion." (The causes of pleurisy with effusion are listed under PLEURAL EFFUSION). Dry pleurisy is pleural inflammation without significant effusion. It may be caused by a number of serious conditions including tuberculosis, pneumonia, pulmonary infarction, chest injury, chronic kidney failure and primary viral infections.

The main symptom of pleurisy is sharp, stabbing chest pain, which is usually made worse by coughing or deep breathing. The patient often takes only short, grunting breaths; he usually has a fever and a painful cough. The physician can usually hear a characteristic sound—a "pleural rub"—when he listens with a stethoscope. If there is also a pleural effusion there may be additional findings and the patient may be severely breathless.

The immediate treatment of pleurisy usually involves bed rest and painkilling drugs.

The prognosis depends largely on the underlying cause. Pleurisy due to viral infection is usually benign and responds to supportive treatment, but recurrent attacks are quite common.

See also LUNG DISEASES, PULMONARY DISEASES.

pleurodynia

See EPIDEMIC PLEURODYNIA.

PLEURISY

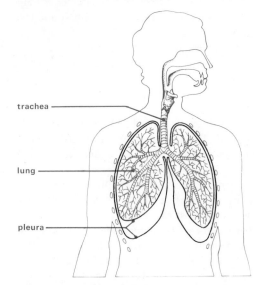

The outer surface of the lungs and the inner surface of the chest wall are covered with shiny, lubricated membranes—the pleura. Pleurisy is the condition where the pleura are inflamed and no longer slide over each other smoothly.

pneumoconiosis

The inhalation of particular forms of dust, over long periods, can lead to changes in the lungs that are non-reversible. This disease is called pneumoconiosis. Mineral dusts, notably silica and asbestos, are the most common causes. Vegetable fiber dusts from sources such as hay and grass may cause what is known as "farmers' lung." Similar dusts to which workers are exposed during many years in the sugar cane and cotton industries can also lead to pneumoconiosis. In the U.S. the most common form is SILICOSIS.

The nasal passages and the lining of the respiratory passages usually prevent the absorption by the lungs of most dust particles. Minute particles inhaled over a period of at least five years may be constantly deposited in the smallest bronchial passages; silica, in particular, sets up an acidic response that leads to scar formation or FIBROSIS. The thickened lung tissue is then deprived of its distensibility and the symptoms of DYSPNEA (shortness of breath) coughing and wheezing on exertion and impaired respiratory function develop. X-ray studies confirm the diagnosis of mottling of the lungs with formation of scar tissue. There is no treatment.

Prevention of the disease requires effective ventilation in the industries of mining, stone-cutting, and sandblasting and the wearing of respirators and the suppression of dust by every means possible.

See also PULMONARY DISEASES.

pneumonia

Inflammation of the lungs from bacterial, fungal, or viral infection or from chemical damage. The outflow of fluid and cells from the inflamed lung tissue fills the airspaces, causing difficulty in breathing and in severe cases the disease may be fatal.

The lungs are unusually open to infection, since the air inhaled with each breath always contains micro-organisms. Their defenses include the filtration of air by the nose, the mucous lining of the air passages that traps dust particles and bacteria, and the IMMUNE SYSTEM operating within the lung tissues—the combination of antibodies and protective white blood cells (phago-cytes). If these defenses are impaired by old age, by a virus infection such as measles, or by *immunosuppressive* drugs (given to prevent rejection of a transplanted organ) then pneumonia is more likely.

Before the antibiotic era the most common type of pneumonia was *lobar pneumonia*, due to one species of bacterium, the pneumococcus. Pneumococcal pneu-monia is usually confined to one lung or one lobe of a lung, which is so heavily inflamed that it changes from a normal spongy, air-filled consistency to a heavy, "consolidated" state. Lobar pneumonia causes a high fever, often with delirium; if it is extensive, the lack of normal lung tissue means that oxygenation is in-adequate and the patient becomes very short of breath and cyanosed and may lose consciousness. There may be associated inflammation of the membrane covering the lung and chest wall—PLEURISY—causing a sharp pain in the chest with each breath. The sputum coughed up may be bloodstained.

Before antibiotics lobar pneumonia was often fatal, especially when it affected both lungs (*double pneu-monia*). Nowadays, however, penicillin typically pro-duces a dramatic cure in up to 95% of cases.

In *bronchopneumonia* patches of inflammation and consolidation are scattered through the lungs. The symptoms are usually less dramatic than in lobar pneumonia, but again there will be cough, difficulty in breathing and fever. Bronchopneumonia may be fatal, especially in the elderly and in anyone weakened by another illness such as advanced cancer, and it is indeed a common cause of death in such diseases.

Bronchopneumonia may be due to bacteria such as Hemophilus, to mycoplasma, and to viruses. It is a common complication of influenza. Treatment with antibiotics is usually effective in the bacterial pneu-monias, but there is still no effective specific treatment for viral pneumonias. However, the symptoms may be relieved by oxygen therapy and drugs to lower the temperature and relieve chest pain.

Pneumonia may also be due to chemical damage to the lungs from inhalation of gases such as sulfur dioxide

PNEUMONIA

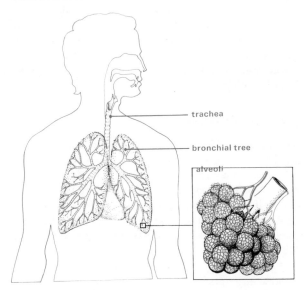

Pneumonia is inflammation of lung tissue usually caused by bacteria or viruses. Fluid and cells pour into the alveoli (air sacs) so that the air is excluded. Thus breathing is impaired, and pneumonia can be life-threatening in the very young and very old.

in industrial accidents, or from inhalation of vomit by an unconscious or semiconscious person. The treatment of chemical pneumonias depends on the removal of inflammatory fluid from the lungs by suction, anti-inflammatory drugs and oxygen therapy.

Some forms of pneumonia may be prevented by vaccination against the virus or bacterium responsible. Vaccines against influenza and the pneumococcus are available, and their use may be recommended in the elderly and patients with debilitating illness.

See also PULMONARY DISEASES.

pneumonitis

Literally meaning inflammation of the lung tissue, pneumonitis occurs in the development of any infective invasion of the lower respiratory tract (such as PNEUMONIA). It is the initial stage where the cells of the lung in the alveoli (the air sacs or terminal passages) are swollen and infected and where the lining cells of the smaller respiratory passages leading to the alveoli are being attacked by infective organisms. In the absence of infection, pneumonitis can occur as a result of inhaling noxious gases or markedly subzero atmosphere (as in Arctic conditions) which paralyze the respiratory cilia (the hairlike processes that project from the lining of the larger air passages and propel mucus, dust particles, etc., away from the lungs). The symptoms are a painful cough which is initially dry and unproductive (no mucus or phlegm is coughed up) with pain on inhalation.

Treatment is directed at the underlying cause, if this is known. For example, antibiotics are usually effective in controlling a primary or secondary bacterial infection (although they have no effect on viral pneumonitis).

pneumothorax

The presence of free air or gas in the *pleural cavity*. (The pleural cavity is a narrow space between two layers of the *pleura*, the serous membrane that lines the chest cavity—*thorax*—and surrounds each lung.) When this occurs it may cause the lung to retract from the thoracic wall and provoke a collapse of the lung. The condition may be barely detectable or massive and threatening to life.

A superficial "blister" of the lung tissue may accidentally burst and allow the escape of inhaled air from within the lung (forceful increases in lung pressure may provoke this, as in blowing a trumpet or filling a balloon). Among the healthy it is most common in young adult life due to profound respiratory exertions and occurs more frequently in males. In those over 45, *spontaneous pneumothorax* (as this type is called) is usually associated with chronic EMPHYSEMA, ASTHMA, FIBROSIS, SILICOSIS and other chronic lung disease. *Traumatic pneumothorax* may occur when air enters the pleural cavity through a penetrating wound of the chest (e.g., a stabbing or gunshot wound).

The onset of a pneumothorax is painful on the affected side, with shortness of breath and a sense of tightness in the chest. No special treatment is necessary in less serious cases, apart from rest, as the air is absorbed into the tissues over a period of a week or more. In more severe cases of pneumothorax, surgical aspiration through a puncture of the chest wall may be immediately necessary. Full recovery is usual.

See also PULMONARY DISEASES.

podiatry

The skills of foot care are practiced by those trained in podiatry (also known as *chiropody*.) Special schools conduct training, examination and licencing in the United Kingdom.

The skills are sought by those who have particular problems associated with the feet. PLANTAR WARTS (warts on the sole of the foot) may require attention by the careful removal of the hardened skin over the surface of the wart or scraping (curretting) it out followed by DIATHERMY to the base. Calluses (areas of hardened skin) may require similar but more gentle treatment. INGROWING NAILS frequently require prolonged atten-

tion to overcome the infection at the side of the nail until the nail grows correctly; surgical treatment may be required if other measures fail to overcome the problem.

Flat foot (technically known as *pes planus*), or reduction of the longitudinal arch of the foot, is another common cause of podiatric attention. It is often associated with some partial twisting or rotation of the foot. All children for the first two years after walking have "flat" feet, where the middle of the arch almost presses on the ground; but the choice of correct footwear with a heel and arch support in the shoe overcomes this. *Foot strain* in the middle-aged is commonly caused by stress on the longitudinal arch ligaments and sometimes by muscle weakening of the foot due to lack of adequate exercise. Foot-strengthening exercises and electrical stimulation of the affected muscles can overcome this, in addition to the use of appropriate arch supports in the shoe.

For the elderly person deprived (by arthritis, fragility or dizziness on bending) of the opportunity to maintain normal foot care, podiatric attention can be essential to prevent deformities occurring in uncut nails. Similarly, foot deformities due to OSTEOARTHRITIS, hallux valgus (inturning big toe) BUNIONS (thickened bursa on the big toe joint) are common in the elderly; podiatry becomes necessary for foot comfort and to permit normal physical activity and mobility. Diabetic patients require similar attention and care because of the hazard of foot infections in the elderly diabetic.

poisoning

The accidental (or deliberate) ingestion of substances that may be poisonous—in small or large doses—is an occurrence of increasing frequency. The incidence of poisoning in one form or another is rising annually throughout the developed world because of the availability of potent medicines and the cultural phenomenon of "overdosing," because of the frequency of the illicit use of drugs, and because of the ever-increasing number of toxic chemicals, gases and liquids employed in modern industry. Fortunately, because of the increase in sophistication in medical techniques for supporting life's vital functions during hospitalization, death from poisoning is not as common as it once was.

Poisoning can produce abdominal pains, vomiting, delirium, loss of consciousness, suppression of respiration and death. A multitude of other symptoms can also occur during this progression that are specific or characteristic to the noxious substance. The effects of some poisons (e.g., alcohol) are reversible; given time, the human body is capable of excreting them or biochemically changing them to substances that are less toxic. Others (e.g., lead) are accumulative in small doses and permanently stored by the body until they destroy vital functions. Still others (e.g., the toxic elements of FOOD POISONING) may be rapidly evacuated from the body, although survival and prompt recovery depends on the initial state of health of the individual.

In all cases the finding of an unconscious person must initiate the same "first aid" procedures; because of the danger to the unconscious victim of choking to death on inhaled vomit, he must be turned to the *recovery position*—lying prone, the head resting on a raised arm, the knees bent, and the mouth and face pointing sideways and down—while transport to the hospital emergency room is arranged. Should breathing cease, artificial "mouth to mouth" resuscitation should be undertaken. Providing the physician knows what has recently been ingested, the conscious patient may be encouraged to vomit, after which he should also be transferred to the hospital in the recovery position.

Identification of the poison may depend on finding medicine bottles or other substances near the victim, retaining a specimen of vomit for hospital laboratory analysis, or the questioning of relatives and friends. The physician can be greatly aided in the treatment of the poisoned patient by such information. Barbiturates (sleeping pills), opiates (morphine, cocaine, heroin), tranquilizers and antidepressants are the most common pharmaceutical agents used in deliberate overdosage or poisoning. The danger from these is *respiratory suppression*. Thus, delay in hospitalization can prove fatal—for only with the proper facilities can respiration be maintained until full recovery occurs.

Metallic poisons (such as cadmium, lead, mercury and other substances) are an industrial risk even though their effects may take many months or years before they are noted. Appropriate legislation can prevent or minimize these industrial hazards by requiring proper safeguards for worker protection. Herbicides and pesticides can be accidentally inhaled or absorbed through the skin in crop-spraying; the use of respirators and protective clothing prevent poisoning for those handling these substances. Poisoning by gas inhalation, (e.g., *carbon monoxide* car exhaust fumes) may be deliberate or accidental; it requires oxygen administration for recovery plus respiratory support. Children are particularly prone to accidental poisoning from medicines found in the home, the eating of poisonous berries, contact with household cleaners or other household or agricultural chemicals that are unguarded or unsafely stored. In all circumstances, if it is suspected that the child has ingested or come into contact with poisonous substances, he must receive immediate hospital care. Small doses of poisonous substances that might not harm an adult may be lethal to a small child.

The prognosis for many cases is good. Some antidotes may be specific (as in barbiturate poisoning), but in general the prevention of death depends on maintaining respiration and sometimes on "washing out" the poison by DIALYSIS (the artificial kidney)—thus ensuring the victim's survival until the poison is excreted. In some more serious instances, ingestion of caustic materials by children may require prolonged medical or surgical treatment.

See also LEAD POISONING, MERCURY POISONING.

poliomyelitis

Once called "infantile paralysis," poliomyelitis is an acute viral infection of the gastrointestinal tract that may attack the central nervous system to produce motor nerve paralysis. It has a worldwide distribution and in temperate zones occurs in epidemics in the summer months, being transmitted by dust and fecal contact—especially in areas of poor sanitation and hygiene. Artificial immunity can be provoked by the injection of the "killed virus" developed by Dr. Jonas Salk or by the oral administration of a "live attenuated (weakened)" virus vaccine developed by Dr. Albert Sabin. In the unvaccinated, susceptible person, the virus of poliomyelitis can be inhaled or ingested. The first symptoms may fall into any of three patterns: sore throat and fever, diarrhea, or aching in the limbs and back. These symptoms may resolve within three to five days (*nonparalytic polio*) or the virus may spread through the bloodstream to invade the central nervous system.

Signs of irritation of the covering membranes of the brain develop (stiff neck, PHOTOPHOBIA, headache) as well as painful muscular cramps and spasms. The virus causes most damage to the nerve cells controlling the muscles (the motor neurons) and within 48 hours there is obvious paralysis of the muscles. This may be limited to the muscles of the limbs or (bulbar polio) it may affect respiration and swallowing. Diagnosis is made clinically and by virus culture or determination of increases in the specific antibodies. Treatment involves hospitalization and nursing care to rest the affected muscles, and (if necessary) artificial maintenance of respiratory function (the "iron lung" machine). No medication is effective against the polio virus. The overall mortality rate is around 5%. Many patients recover with a return of some degree of muscle function, but a few remain severely or even totally paralyzed.

Prevention depends entirely on immunization. The live oral vaccine confers 100% gastrointestinal immunity to attack and by "boosters" prevents spread. A policy of infant immunization has virtually eradicated the disease from the United States and other developed countries, but booster doses are recommended every eight years in childhood and before foreign travel for adults, since polio is still a major public health problem in much of Africa, Asia, and Southern Europe.

polyarteritis nodosa

This rare disease is characterized by areas of inflammation that develop in the walls of blood vessels—both arteries and veins—which may be segmental, diffuse or discrete. The "node" of inflammation may result in NECROSIS of the blood vessel wall and the extent of the damage may vary from the ANEURYSM (blister) or rupture, to healing with FIBROSIS or THROMBOSIS. The cause is unknown for this disease of connective tissue, although allergic, infective, toxic, rheumatic and neurogenic causes have all, at times, been implicated. It more commonly attacks males, of all ethnic groups, in their 40s. Any blood vessel in the body may be affected.

Since the area of attack, the extent of the damage, and even the onset in stages may all vary there are no "typical" symptoms. Fever with drenching sweats, complaints of weakness, muscular pains and general fatigue are experienced while the disease is active; but the diagnosis can be made if minute but sore nodules are detected along visible blood vessels in the skin, tongue, retina or conjunctiva. Any organ in the body may be affected with consequent symptoms or disturbed function; in particular, NEURITIS (inflammation of a nerve or nerves) may occur. BIOPSY of skin or muscle may be necessary for the diagnosis; treatment is by administration of steroids (for example, prednisolone). The likelihood of recurrence is high.

polycystic kidney

This inherited disease, passed as a dominant gene to either male or female, causes dilation of the tubules in the kidney and leads to obstruction, infection, cysts and kidney failure (see KIDNEY DISEASES). Its manifestations may appear in infancy, or be delayed until adult life. The extent of the disease may vary, with the more severely affected cases occurring early in life. Cysts may also occur on blood vessels in other parts of the body. Progressive kidney failure occurs but may be delayed by continuous medical care that reduces infection, and death from UREMIA is prevented by DIALYSIS ("artificial kidney" machine) or a kidney transplant, when the disease has not seriously affected other organs.

polycythemia

Literally, an increase in the number of circulating red blood cells. Polycythemia may occur as a result of a demand on the body to produce more hemoglobin, in order to absorb more oxygen, in environments where the atmospheric oxygen is reduced—such as at high altitudes. Thus, healthy people living in the Andes, Rockies or other high mountainous areas may show "relative polycythemia" which is normal. New residents may develop *acute polycythemia* and initially experience "mountain sickness" with DYSPNEA, CYANOSIS, headache, vomiting and lethargy. But on their return to lower altitudes the symptoms disappear.

As a disease that is *not* an environmental adaption, it may occur in CUSHING'S SYNDROME, brain, liver and uterine tumors and in kidney disease, or spontaneously (*polycythemia vera*) as an overproduction of red cells by the bone marrow. This latter type of the disease is of high incidence in Jews, low in blacks, and men in middle or later life are more frequently affected than women. A ruddy engorged complexion, abdominal pain due to spleen and liver enlargement, headaches and bleeding from mucous membranes may occur. The diagnosis is made by blood tests and a biopsy of the bone marrow. Complications of the disease include THROMBOSIS and hemorrhages in the gastrointestinal tract. Treatment is by blood removal (phlebotomy) to balance the overproduction, and radioactive chemicals or cytotoxic drugs to suppress the bone marrow. Prognosis is a chronic recurrence over many years with ultimate anemia and cardiovascular or kidney complications which may lead to death.

polymyalgia rheumatica

Muscular pains throughout the body—appearing abruptly in the neck and shoulder muscles and spreading down the back to the buttocks and thighs—with stiffness, headache, fever, and loss of appetite and weight. Characteristically it attacks middle-aged and elderly persons and is more common in women over 60.

Laboratory tests such as ESR (ERYTHROCYTE SEDIMENTATION RATE) are helpful: a very high ESR is virtual confirmation of the diagnosis.

The course fluctuates with remissions and exacerbations but is usually self-limiting, with relief after a few months. The disability may be severe but bed rest and medication with anti-inflammatory agents or steroids will usually produce rapid relief. The symptoms may recur when treatment is stopped, but the prognosis (with treatment) is good and there is no long-lasting disability.

polyp

A polyp is an overgrowth of the "submucous" tissue, which pushes up its covering of mucous membrane to project (often from a stalklike connection) into the anatomical cavity or passage. Multiple polyps frequently occur in the nose, cervix and uterus; they are rarely malignant in these sites but cause symptoms due to obstruction or deformation of the anatomical cavity and excessive stretching of the mucous membrane. Chronic superficial infections predispose to their development and they are usually only seen in adults.

Patients with allergies or chronic RHINITIS are more prone to develop nasal polyps. Excess mucous formation, nose bleeds and loss of the sense of smell may occur, and the polyps are easily recognized on examination as glistening extrusions of the nasal lining. In the cervix or uterus, bleeding between menstrual periods is a possible sign of polyp development; some FIBROIDS of the uterus may resemble polyps in shape. Polyps may occur in the colon and rectum as a rare genetic trait (*familial adenomatous polyposis*) and appear in hundreds. Lower abdominal pain, loss of weight, diarrhea and the passage of mucus and blood in the stools may signal their development. This rare familial disease does show malignant change in a significant number of cases.

Polyps are mainly removed by surgery, cautery or dissection. Periodic medical examinations are necessary because polyps tend to recur. In the rare genetic disease of *colonic polyps*, surgical removal of the affected portion of the large intestine may be necessary.

porphyrias

The porphyrias are a group of very rare disorders usually caused by an "inborn error" of metabolism.

POLYPS

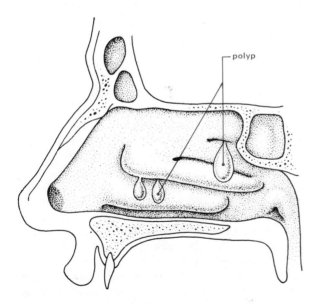

— polyp

MULTIPLE POLYPS IN THE NASAL CAVITY

Nasal polyps are areas of the membrane lining the nose which become distended with excess tissue fluid and hang down into the nasal cavity. They are usually due to an allergy. Since they can cause nasal obstruction, they may have to be removed.

Porphyrins are complex chemical compounds which are normally produced as steps in the formation of *heme*, the red pigment which contributes its color to the hemoglobin in the red blood cells. In the porphyrias, a "block" is present at one of several sites in this chain of chemical reactions—resulting in an abnormal accumulation in the tissues of various types of porphyrin pigment. Their presence in excess in the tissues leads to their excretion in increased amounts in the urine and feces.

Symptoms of the porphyrias include excessive sensitivity to sunlight with blistering, pigmentation, and various types of skin eruption. Discoloration of the teeth and bones also typically occurs. Nerve damage from the toxic effects of the porphyrins on nerve fibers may occur with muscular weakness and paralysis, severe abdominal pain and other neurological symptoms. Psychological disturbances may occur with MANIA, delirium or coma; death may sometimes occur. Some cases, however, are very mild with only slight sensitivity to sunlight and no other symptoms.

The disease is familial and has, for example, been traced with some certainty in the British Royal Family from James I to his living descendants through the Hanoverian line.

Diagnosis is confirmed by the presence of porphyrins in the urine, which is often reddish ("port wine urine") or darkens on standing in the light. Excessive amounts are also present in the feces, where they can be identified by means of chemical tests.

Treatment is unsatisfactory, but patients must be protected from sunlight. Certain drugs may be used to control the psychological manifestations.

However, drugs such as barbiturate "sleeping tablets," which can precipitate an attack, must be avoided.

post mortem

See AUTOPSY.

postnasal drip

A trickling of mucus from the posterior portion of the nasal cavity onto the surface of the throat, usually caused by a common cold or an allergy (allergic rhinitis).

postpartum depression

Depressive reactions are fairly common in the first week after childbirth, with some 90% of women experiencing "fourth day blues." True depressive illness—with insomnia, tearfulness, irrational fears, irritability, guilt and psychic disturbances (which may include rejection of the baby and even infanticide in extremely severe cases)—is much more rare. But at least 15% of women experience some symptoms of depression within the first six months after labor.

Hormonal origins are suspected and menstrual irregularity is a frequent accompaniment; but environmental, social and sexual difficulties also predispose the woman to the development of postpartum depression. In addition, any emotional disorder prior to pregnancy is frequently magnified or exacerbated in the postpartum stage. (Depression following miscarriage or abortion is similar in its pattern.)

Suicide is extremely rare, but neglect of or physical harm to the baby is a common manifestation. The diagnosis is made by psychiatric specialists when family problems emerge that cannot be overcome by support from husbands, relatives and close friends. Treatment is essential; antidepressant medication is usually effective if administered in the early stages. Admission to a psychiatric hospital may be necessary in a very few cases; the woman is often advised to avoid further pregnancies. In addition, in severe cases, sterilization may be considered. Fortunately, however, most cases of postpartum depression are mild and transient.

posture

Modern man (*Homo sapiens*) evolved from primates who learned to walk on two feet (*Homo erectus*). Problems with posture have been a consequence ever since, for the human spine is not yet perfectly adapted to what is required of it. The multiple vertebrae of the spinal column are maintained in position, flexibly, by what are normally strong ligaments over which the spinal muscles lie.

Disease of the spinal column, congenital or acquired disorders of the spinal bones, and injury or weakness of the spinal ligaments or muscles can all result in compensatory postures—often leading to curvatures, pains or lack of flexibility. Normally, with the shoulders held back and the head upright looking forward, there are two natural curves in the spine (the sacrolumbar and the cervicothoracic) which look roughly like an "S" bend when viewed from the side and straight when viewed from the front or rear. If there is hip disease or leg shortening, then the pelvis tilts and the spinal column will curve laterally to compensate—a condition known as *scoliosis*. *Kyphosis* ("humpback" or "hunchback") is an excessive curvature due to disease, abnormal development, or injuries of the upper spine. *Lordosis* is exaggeration of the normal curve in the lower part of the back (the lumbar region) due to obesity, a heavy abdomen and lax muscles. Minor degrees of spinal deformity and postural abnormality are quite common.

Encouragement of habits of good posture in children is important, not only for a pleasing physical appearance but also to prevent the possible development

POSTURE

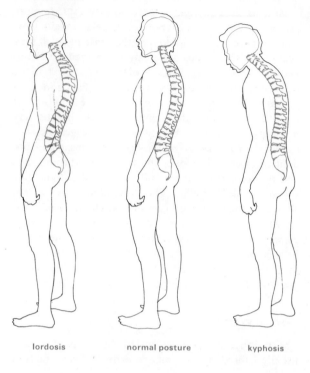

lordosis   normal posture   kyphosis

The illustration shows how the curvature of the spinal column determines posture, whether correct or incorrect. Abnormal postures such as lordosis and kyphosis are usually the result of laziness, and can interfere with the body's mechanisms for supporting weight. This can cause symptoms, for example, low back pain.

of permanent deformities. In the adult, *postural backache* due to lifting injuries, strain and sitting slouched (especially in poorly designed furniture) is the most common single reason for referral to an orthopedist (a medical expert on disorders of the bones and joints). The spinal ligaments loosen with childbirth, debilitating illness and obesity—particularly in tall individuals, who become prone to pain in the lower part of the back. Postural backache, which is worse on stooping, causes great and often recurrent distress. Treatment typically involves physical therapy (heat, massage and special exercises), manipulation of the lower parts of the spine, or the wearing of an external support (corset).

See also SPINAL CURVATURE.

Pott's fracture

A fracture-dislocation of the ankle first described in 1769 by Percival Pott (1713–1788), a London surgeon.

(Pott had sustained such a fracture himself in 1756.) The fracture usually results from the foot being caught while the body is moving forward (for example, during walking or skiing). As a result the foot is twisted outwards, producing a spiral fracture at the lower end of the *fibula* (the bony prominence felt on the outer side of the ankle).

This type of fracture is treated by immobilization in a plaster cast from below the knee to the base of the toes; the cast is usually left in position for about three weeks. However, more severe torsion can pull a flake of bone from the inner side of the ankle and also fracture the bottom of the *tibia,* or "shin bone." In such cases, the bones have to be realigned under anesthesia and sometimes held in place with screws; the plaster cast is then left in position for up to three months.

preeclampsia

A rise in blood pressure during pregnancy, with PROTEINURIA (the abnormal presence of protein in the urine), weight gain and EDEMA. It occurs in some 10% of women, most commonly in young women during their first pregnancies, anytime after the 12th week up to and including labor and the immediate postpartum period.

Placental causes—by secretion or an excess of hormones that provoke hypertension; *immune response causes*—with antibody formation against the fetus or the placenta, thus affecting the kidney; *dietary causes; hormonal causes*, due to excess adrenal gland secretions, and *alterations in blood coagulability* have all been variously blamed; but the underlying mechanism remains unexplained.

Early detection is essential. Routine prenatal care with regular surveillance is the only way to detect and correct the abnormality. Untreated, the progressive rise in blood pressure threatens thrombosis of the placenta, which can lead to its premature separation, death of the fetus, and subsequent hypertensive coma in the mother.

Bed rest is required, in addition to a restriction of salt; antihypertensive drugs may be administered to counteract the rise in blood pressure. In the majority of cases this is successful, preventing *eclampsia* (the flagrant untreated condition); but, in some, premature labor by induction or Cesarean section is necessary. Recurrence in future pregnancies is less than 20%.

pregnancy

Conception, the fertilization of an ovum by a sperm, can occur in a woman from the menarche to the menopause, and takes place in one of the Fallopian tubes. Pregnancy occurs when the fertilized ovum moves down and implants on the wall of the uterine cavity—usually four or five days later; it lasts until labor takes place—on average, 40 weeks later. The initial signs of pregnancy are breast engorgement, blueness of the vagina and absence of the expected period. The early symptoms are nausea and frequency of urination. Tests to confirm the diagnosis are undertaken on a sample of urine to detect the excess of hormones that are only present from the second week after the expected period.

In the first three months the breast signs are the most obvious with enlargement of the areola (the dark ring of tissue surrounding the nipple) and prominence of the sebaceous glands around it. In the fourth month the uterus enlarges to be palpable above the pubis; thereafter the abdominal swelling is plainly visible. Fetal movements are felt at this time by a woman experiencing her first pregnancy (20 weeks), a little earlier by those who have previously experienced childbirth. In the eighth month there is a "lightening" as the fetal head descends into the pelvic brim. The onset of labor in the ninth month is announced by a "show" as the mucous plug of the cervix is discharged into the vagina, after contractions of the uterine muscle have been experienced as regular cramplike pains.

The incidence of miscarriage (spontaneous abortion) is high, with as many as 20% of conceptions failing to implant, sustain their growth beyond the next menstrual period, or survive beyond the eighth week. The complications of any pregnancy after the 12th week include PREECLAMPSIA, anemia, premature delivery, and labor abnormalities. Congenital abnormalities have an incidence of one in every hundred live births.

The essence of medical care is the prevention of problems in pregnancy by ensuring, initially, good health in women of reproductive age and their immunization (if required) against diseases such as rubella and polio which can cause fetal abnormality. Antenatal care must be regular, commencing from the first month and involving periodic supervision, comparison of blood pressure, weight, hemoglobin and urinalysis to maintain maternal health. Surveillance of fetal health includes the detection of maternal antibodies to blood-group incompatibility, ultrasound visualization to monitor fetal growth rate, and AMNIOCENTESIS in the event of suspicion of certain fetal abnormalities. Medication for all pregnant women includes iron, vitamins and extra calcium as required, to prevent anemia and maternal deficiency diseases. The normal diet must be rich in protein, fat and vitamins, but controlled in carbohydrate to prevent excessive weight increase.

An average weight gain of 20 lbs. is associated with minimal complications; most of this is put on after the 20th week, but many women experience appetite variations in pregnancy—in particular, bizarre or obsessional tastes in the first three months. Constipation is a frequent problem in the later months, and hemorrhoids may be a complication; both need to be dealt with by dietary advice and appropriate medication.

Fetal position changes frequently in the last three months of pregnancy, but after the 32nd week the head should be entering the pelvis, the body uppermost (*vertex presentation*); safe delivery is compatible with other presentations but more liable to hazards in labor. Backache due to loosening of the ligaments in the last three months is also commonly experienced; but correct posture, exercise and antenatal relaxation goes far to avoid such problems and to prepare the woman for effective labor.

Pregnant women should avoid taking any drugs except under medical supervision, particularly during the first three months.

See also CHILDBIRTH.

PREGNANCY

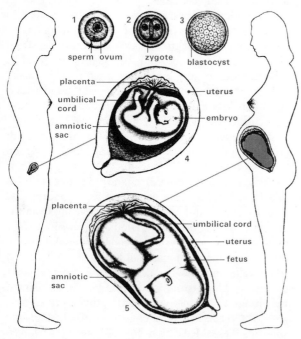

Conception occurs when a sperm fertilizes an ovum (1), and a zygote (2) forms. The zygote divides into many identical cells and becomes a blastocyst (3) which embeds itself in the lining of the uterus. During the first three months the embryo takes shape (4) with the appearance of all its major organs. In the last six months the fetus increases in size dramatically (5).

premature ejaculation

This is a common condition, on occasions, in perfectly normal males who are relatively inexperienced, or have had infrequent coitus and who are excessively stimulated—by accident or design—by their sexual partner.

It is the ejaculation of seminal fluid from the penis prior to the time at which it would have been desired. As such it may be a subjective judgment that it occurs prematurely, for if the achievement of the partner's orgasm is the criterion, then retention and delay of ejaculation will depend on the sexual partner's level of excitation (which is obviously variable).

Control over ejaculation is acquired with experience, though frequently denied initially to the young and inexperienced; but the level of psychic control varies with fatigue, fantasy and drugs such as alcohol. In middle age infrequency of coitus may cause the return of premature ejaculation and lead to sexual difficulties, particularly since with age the male becomes relatively less sexually demanding and the female often more. Masters and Johnson reported premature ejaculation as a problem, at some time, in at least 60% of marriages, and an experience that was common at least on some occasions in all men.

Treatment is necessary when it provokes marital problems and occurs with greater frequency after relative control over ejaculation had been established for some time. Isolated occurrences are compensated for by resumption of intercourse after a period of delay, to achieve a second orgasm; repeated occurrence may lead to *psychic impotence* as a compensation that prevents exposure to the risk, and so treatment becomes essential.

Medication has little to offer. Sexual counseling of both partners is recommended—in particular, instruction in the "squeeze" technique. After erection and just prior to the overwhelming desire to ejaculate the tip of the penis (glans) is firmly compressed—more effectively by the female—by fingers and thumb placed above and below the coronal ridge. This counteracts the reflex of ejaculation and may be repeated periodically when the desire to achieve orgasm returns. Effective control over ejaculation is reestablished in a high percentage of cases where this technique is mutually employed.

premenstrual tension

The condition of mental tension, irritability, headache, depression and a feeling of "bloatedness," with some evidence of EDEMA, that begins in the week prior to menstruation and resolves completely the day after a menstrual period's flow has begun.

It is a common condition which causes a good deal of

distress to those affected by it—which includes women of all ethnic groups. It is *cyclical* in that it may occur before the menarche, after the menopause and even after a hysterectomy. Hormonal origins are the obvious cause, with water and salt retention as the consequence of a hormonal imbalance; but psychogenic causes play their part in initiating a behavioral response to physical changes in the body.

Conditions described as *psychosomatic* have been reported as being exacerbated in the premenstrual period—such as eczema, migraine and allergic responses. Various conditions not in themselves clearly associated with the menstrual cycle can also occur, such as admissions to psychiatric hospitals, suicides, accidents and misbehavior in school—which are found to be present more frequently in the premenstrual period.

In severe cases, treatment is often effective with hormonal supplements of the progesterone type, with the initiation of anovulatory cycles by use of the oral contraceptive pill and with diuretics ("water pills") taken for the immediate premenstrual period.

pressure sore

An area of local tissue death due to pressure on the blood vessels supplying the area, usually found in patients confined to bed or to a chair.

Pressure sores are most likely to occur in an elderly, debilitated, paralyzed and/or incontinent patient. Good nursing techniques should always anticipate the occurrence of a pressure sore and be directed towards prevention in the first place.

Pressure sores can be avoided by frequent changes of position—passive change if active change is impossible—and by attention to the skin, such as washing, drying and massage at frequent intervals. An even pressure is essential—a wrinkled sheet can be enough to start a sore in an immobile patient.

Treatment of an established sore varies from relief of pressure by encouraging the patient to move and allowing him to get up if possible, to excision of the ulcer and suturing, and to skin-grafting in extensive cases. A high-protein diet to counteract the serum loss helps, and the services of a physiotherapist can be invaluable.

priapism

When the penis remains erect, is painful, and despite the conclusion of sexual excitement does not subside, priapism exists. The erection may have occurred and been sustained without sexual excitement. The cause of priapism is most often THROMBOSIS in the veins of the prostate gland. It may occur as a result of leukemia or sickle cell anemia, and secondary deposits of cancer in the corpora cavernosa of the penis—leading to obstruction and thus unrelieved venous engorgement—may be responsible. Spinal injury and brain injury may lead to priapism because of interference with neurological control.

Anticoagulant therapy and sedation will often resolve the condition.

prickly heat

Another name for MILIARIA.

proctitis

Inflammation in the region of the anus or rectum.

There are a variety of causes of proctitis, but one which is causing particular concern to public health officials is that arising from GONORRHEA. This is a self-limited inflammatory disease of the rectum caused by infection with the gonococcus, leading to severe rectal burning and itching; it usually lasts less than a month. The condition is now more common than it used to be among male homosexuals, but it is also found in women with gonorrhea.

Treatment is aimed at relief of symptoms such as pain and itching. The gonorrheal form does not appear to respond to treatment, naturally regressing in most cases, but forms due to other organisms will be affected by antibiotic or steroid treatment in varying degrees. Constipation should be avoided as far as possible in patients with any form of proctitis. The affected area should be washed regularly and care taken to avoid harsh abrasion.

progesterone

Of the two major types of female sex hormones secreted by the ovary, progesterone is the main one of the progestogen group.

During the menstrual cycle, progesterone—in combination with estrogens—is secreted by the corpus luteum, which develops in the ovarian follicle after *ovulation*, and the decline of both hormones is associated with the onset of menstruation. Progesterone, like estrogen, thus has the effect of maintaining the uterus in a state of receptivity for the implantation of a fertilized ovum.

In early pregnancy the corpus luteum secretes progesterone, as does the developing placenta. Initially the greatest quantity comes from the corpus luteum, but by the tenth week of pregnancy placental secretion is fully established and rises steadily as pregnancy advances.

See also HORMONES.

progestin

The name originally given to the crude hormone of the corpus luteum (which develops in the empty ovarian follicle after OVULATION) now known as progesterone. The function of this hormone is to prepare the uterus for the reception and development of the fertilized ovum by inducing secretion in proliferated glands.

The term progestin is now applied generally to *progestational agents*, a group of hormones secreted by the corpora lutea and the placenta. It is the synthetic analogues of these hormones that are the basis of the ovulation-inhibiting effect of the oral contraceptives.

Progestational agents are combined with estrogen to give the best protection from conception, together with the minimum of side effects such as breakthrough bleeding.

prognosis

A prediction regarding the likely course and outcome of a disease, disorder, etc., especially one based on the judgment of the attending physician.

prolapse

The "falling down" of any organ: usually applied to the uterus (womb) and the rectum.

Prolapse of the uterus is relatively common, particularly in elderly women. It is associated with the increasing lack of tone of the muscles and other supportive structures in the pelvic area in later life. This is often caused by injury to or overstretching of the pelvic floor in childbirth. Injury to the perineum (the bottom of the trunk of the body) and the vagina may contribute to the prolapse.

Prolapse of the "first degree' implies the presence of the cervix (neck of the womb) at the vaginal opening. In "second degree" prolapse the cervix protrudes through the vaginal opening; in "third degree" prolapse the entire uterus protrudes through the vaginal opening. In some cases no symptoms exist apart from the mechanical discomfort of the movement of the uterus; but there may be some feeling of "bearing down" or heaviness in the lower part of the abdomen and back.

Treatment is ideally by surgery in many cases. The laxness in the ligaments and muscles is taken up and the uterus replaced in its proper position. In women past childbearing age the more radical operation of removal of the uterus (hysterectomy) may be preferred. Another form of treatment in elderly women or those who are poor operative risks is the insertion of a hard rubber ring to take up the slack in the vagina and to support the neck of the womb.

In *prolapse of the rectum*, all the layers of the rectal wall may protrude through the anal opening, in which case it is called "complete prolapse." If only the mucous membrane protrudes it is known as a "partial prolapse." The latter is much more common, especially in old age. The protrusion is rarely more than one inch long.

Complete prolapse, which may contain coils of small intestine, is approximately six times more common in women than in men and is associated with repeated pregnancies and consequent weakening of the pelvic floor. Any condition that leads to straining at stool may lead to prolapse; these include chronic constipation and threadworm infection, but the most common cause is hemorrhoids ("piles"). Again, surgical treatment is necessary if the prolapse is not to recur. Attention must also be given to the predisposing causes.

prophylaxis

Prevention of disease or various measures which prevent the development and spread of disease.

proptosis

Abnormal protrusion of the eyeball. It may be bilateral or unilateral.

One-sided proptosis may be caused by inflammation within the orbit (the bony cavity that houses the eye), usually consequent upon infection of the air sinuses or puncture wounds of the tissue around the eye. There is pain, paralysis of the eye muscles, protrusion of the eyeball, malaise (a general feeling of being unwell) and fever. Treatment involves the administration of appropriate antibiotics.

Another cause of unilateral proptosis is the development of a tumor in the orbit. Dermoid cysts, meningiomas and tumors of the optic nerve may be implicated, as may tumors arising in the nasopharynx.

Proptosis is a feature of *thyrotoxicosis;* it may be present on one side or both. In this form of exophthalmos the white of the eye is exposed above the pupil, especially on looking downward. The cause is not known, but microscopy shows the tissues behind the eye to be edematous and fatty, often infiltrated by lymphocytes and leukocytes. In most cases of exophthalmos associated with thyrotoxicosis (*exophthalmic goiter*) the condition develops slowly and is relatively mild, but there are cases of sudden onset and rapid progression—known as *malignant exophthalmos*. This is accompanied by paralysis of the extrinsic muscles of the eye giving rise to double vision, with inflammation and swelling of the conjunctiva and swelling of the tissues around the orbit. It may become impossible to close the eyelids properly, so that the cornea is liable to become damaged and scarred. Treatment of the thryotoxicosis in cases of exophthalmic goiter does not necessarily improve the condition; it may be advisable to close the eyelids by surgical operation in order to protect the cornea.

In all cases of exophthalmos of any degree of severity the operation of *orbital decompression*, in which the bone of the orbit is removed, may be necessary in order to preserve the eyeball and restore eye movement.

prostaglandins

Seminal fluid (semen) contains lipid-soluble substances which cause smooth muscle fibers to contract. When they were first isolated the active principles were called prostaglandins, from their origin. Since that time they have been found in many other tissues in the body, so that the name is to a certain extent misleading.

Prostaglandins stimulate smooth muscle, change the heart rate, affect the motility of the intestine, influence blood pressure, and cause the uterus to contract. They have been used to promote abortion in the first weeks of pregnancy. They also act upon hormones, antagonizing the action of epinephrine, glucagon, vasopressin and ACTH; it seems that they play a part in metabolic processes. They alter the stickiness of the blood platelets and prevent clotting in arteries.

So far over 20 different prostaglandins have been isolated, and research in the field is active. Among their possible uses, beside their use to induce abortion or labor at term, may be an application in depressing male fertility which could make a male contraceptive pill practical.

prostatectomy

Surgical removal of part or the whole of the prostate gland, which in men surrounds the urethra as it leaves the bladder.

Because of its position, enlargement of the prostate leads to difficulty in passing urine and ultimately to complete urinary obstruction. There are two common causes of prostatic enlargement; simple hypertrophy (or overgrowth) of the gland and the development of cancer.

Simple hypertrophy of the prostate is a complication of later life, which most commonly develops between the ages of 60 to 90. About 80% of men over the age of 80 suffer from its effects to some degree. The cause is unknown, but it never occurs in those who have been castrated. At first there may be difficulty in starting to urinate and increased frequency; later, as a result of congestion, the urethra may be completely blocked and urination becomes impossible. This is the state of acute retention. In some cases the process stops short of complete blockage, but as the patient finds it progressively harder to empty the bladder completely, it gradually distends and more urine remains in it after the

patient urinates—thus producing the state of chronic urinary retention.

Similar symptoms are caused by cancer of the prostate. Diagnosis between the two is made by physical examination and by blood tests. Both causes of obstruction are dealt with first by catheterization.

If the enlargement of the prostate is benign, the surgeon will (if the physical state of the patient permits) proceed to remove the gland—either through the abdominal wall, which makes it easier to be sure that the gland has been removed entirely, or through an instrument passed into the urethra.

In cases of cancer many surgeons prefer to try to reduce the enlargement by the administration of estrogens, for the tumor is hormone-dependent. If difficulty in urination persists it may be necessary to performs a *transurethral prostatectomy*.

Cancer of the prostate is the third most common cancer in men, exceeded only by cancer of the lung and cancer of the large intestine.

prostatitis

Inflammation of the prostate gland.

The prostate can become inflamed for a variety of reasons, sometimes in association with the hyperplasia (excessive proliferation of normal cells) of the gland

PROSTATE GLAND

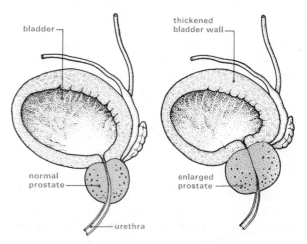

bladder

thickened bladder wall

normal prostate

enlarged prostate

urethra

Some degree of prostatic enlargement is extremely common in men over the age of 45. In most cases it causes either no or only minor symptoms, but urination may be difficult because the urethra is obstructed. The bladder wall becomes thickened in its attempts to force urine past the obstruction, and there is also damaging back-pressure on the kidneys.

which occurs with increasing frequency among men over the age of 40. Many cases are nonspecific in the sense that there is no known cause although some follow infection with gonorrhea. Patients complain of slight fever and pain in the perineum (the area between the thighs) and in the lower part of the back.

While the probable infecting organism may be identified, the success rate for eliminating prostatic bacteria is low because antibiotics have difficulty in reaching the tissues of the gland.

Nonspecific granulomatous prostatitis is thought to be a severe reaction to the gland's own secretion which is retained. *Eosinophilic prostatitis* is a rare variation of the disease which is associated with bronchial asthma. A disease known as *malacoplakia* (often associated with a bacterial infection) is usually found in the urinary tract but also in the prostate. Other forms of prostatitis are associated with tuberculosis of the urinary tract, schistosomiasis (bilharziasis) and malignant disease.

Treatment involves drinking large quantities of liquids and emptying the bladder frequently and completely. For complete recovery it may be necessary for the patient to follow a course of antibiotics for many months to neutralize the organisms as they escape into the urethra.

prosthesis

Any device used to replace a part, organ, or limb, usually taking over all or part of its function.

The most common prosthetic device (and the only one which most people are likely to need) is the *artificial denture* ("false teeth" or a "false tooth"). One-third of the total population of the U.K. over the age of 40 has no teeth, and 50% of post-teenagers wear some form of dental prosthesis.

The design of *artificial limbs* has been much improved in recent years. At one time an artificial leg was little better than the old-fashioned wooden leg; but the use of lightweight materials and improvements in articulation (joint movement) have now made it possible for amputees to pass undetected in company. The most recent advance is the development of artificial limbs which are controlled by nerve impulses fed from the stump of the natural arm. These prostheses look like a normal limb, and their internal power systems enable the user to pick up and manipulate objects.

A third common use of prostheses is in the treatment of ARTHRITIS. Replacement of the hip joint in cases of both rheumatoid arthritis and osteoarthritis is now commonplace, using stainless steel and plastic materials. As a result of the success of this type of operation, surgeons have gone on to design elbow, knee, shoulder, and finger joints which are now implanted in the hands of many patients with severe arthritis.

One of the most common reasons for open-heart surgery is the implantation of artificial valves in the hearts of patients whose valves are distorted or damaged from conditions such as RHEUMATIC HEART DISEASE.

Other prostheses in current use include acrylic lenses to replace those affected by CATARACT and artificial eyes, whose purpose is entirely cosmetic. An artificial larynx ("voice-box") is still under trial, and attempts are being made to miniaturize an artificial pancreas for use by diabetics. In the case of many complex internal organs, however, TRANSPLANTATION has so far proved more practicable than the development of mechanical prostheses.

proteinuria

A condition in which protein is present in the urine. Proteinuria is sometimes also known as ALBUMINURIA. This is not exactly correct, however, since both the blood proteins (globulin as well as albumin) may be present in the urine in this condition.

Presence of the proteins is often a symptom of serious disease of the kidney or heart. The detection of albumin in the urine may, in fact, be the earliest and most conclusive evidence of kidney disease. Heart failure leads to proteinuria as a result of the accompanying congestion of the kidneys. Patients are treated for the underlying disease.

prothrombin

A constituent of normal blood plasma which is essential for the clotting of blood.

prurigo

A chronic inflammatory eruption of the skin which is usually characterized by the formation of small whitish papules (small, solid, circumscribed elevations of the skin) accompanied by severe itching.

The eruptions characteristically begin early in life. There are two main forms: *prurigo mitis* (which is comparatively mild) and *prurigo agria* (which is severe). The condition may be permanent or it may come and go. In young children the nonpermanent form may be associated with problems of teething. The papules, which are deeply seated, are most prominent on the extensor surfaces of the limbs.

Summer prurigo is another name for *hydroa vacciniforme*, a skin disease usually affecting adolescent boys and young men; it appears in the summer on exposed parts of the body and fades in the winter. It is characterized by the formation of ulcers (on which crust may appear) and by vesicles. Following the onset of puberty, this disease gradually disappears.

pruritus ani/pruritus vulvae

An intractable itching in the region of the anus (*pruritus ani*) or the vulva (*pruritus vulvae*).

Pruritus ani is usually found in men and is quite common. It can be intensely irritating and should be treated if it reaches the point of acute discomfort. The first line of treatment is to find the cause of the pruritus and if possible remove it. One common cause is parasites, particularly PINWORMS, which lay their eggs around the anus and so cause itching. CANDIDA (thrush) infections also cause itching and invasion by yeasts can be another cause.

Both lack of cleanliness and excessive sweating can contribute, and the latter may be due to unsuitable underclothes which prevent proper evaporation. In the past woolen underwear was to blame, but now in many cases it is nylon and other synthetic fibers which are the cause of pruritus. A patient may also be sitting for long periods on plastic seats, either at home or at work, which would not give sufficient ventilation.

Some pruritus is undoubtedly caused by garments having been washed in harsh detergents; the enzyme detergents have been said to have been involved in some cases.

Discharges from the anus or the vagina, as in HEMORRHOIDS (piles) or VAGINITIS, can be a potent cause of itching.

Pruritus vulvae has similar causes, complicated by the fungus and yeast infections that the vagina is prone to, while the modern habit of wearing panty hose made of nylon has exacerbated the problem.

Patients should pay particular attention to personal hygiene. After the use of the toilet the perianal region should be cleaned with damp cotton wool and then dried. It is advisable for patients to avoid the use of detergents in washing their clothes, taking care to wash them only in soap powder. Underwear of synthetic material should be avoided, and cellular cotton garments substituted. Panty hose should be ruled out and patients should be encouraged to avoid plastic seats and sit on a sheepskin rug or something similar.

Calamine lotion is effective in soothing the itching and keeping the area dry. In cases of thrush infections, special ointments can be used. Some cases of pruritus ani and pruritus vulvae are psychological in origin and tranquilizers may be effective.

psittacosis

A disease (also known as *ornithosis* or *parrot fever*) caused by a strain of the microorganism known as *Chlamydia psittaci*, transmitted to humans by a variety of birds. It was first detected in parrots, thus the name—which is based on the Greek word for parrot. But it is now known that there are several species of birds that harbor the microorganisms and can pass them on to man.

In man the disease usually takes the form of a pneumonia, with fever, cough and perhaps an enlarged spleen. It has been compared with typhoid in its manifestations, and may cause hepatitis, myocarditis, delirium and coma.

Domestic fowl have been implicated in outbreaks, and other birds involved include pigeons, parakeets, budgerigars, ducks, turkeys, pheasants and chickens. The organism is sensitive to tetracycline.

psoriasis

A skin disease, believed to result from a disturbance in skin enzymes, which affects between 1–2% of the population. The disease is associated with an increased turnover of epidermal cells and a dilation of the dermal capillaries. Some sufferers also have a form of arthritis and the skin lesions may be precipitated by mental stress.

Psoriasis is not contagious and the skin lesions can vary enormously. They can include chronic scaling plaques, ringed lesions, smooth red areas, acute pustules and droplike (guttate) lesions. Most often the condition becomes apparent for the first time in adolescence, but it is sometimes delayed until old age.

Oral corticosteroids are used to treat only two forms of the disease, those of severe *erythrodermic* or *generalized pustular* types. These should be treated in the hospital. In ordinary cases, a powerful peeling agent can be used to remove encrusted scales; the same agents,

PSORIASIS

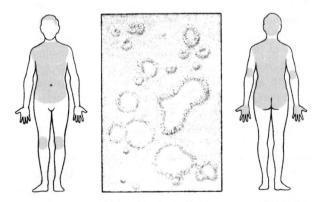

The center picture shows the characteristic skin changes in psoriasis—a clearly defined, red, raised plaque topped by silvery scales. These plaques are usually present over the elbows, knees and scalp, but may spread more extensively to involve the trunk and hands as illustrated here.

used with ultraviolet light and tar baths, can remove chronic thickened psoriatic plaques. Topical steroid creams and ointments can also be used to relieve the skin lesions, and antifungal agents applied if fungal infection supervenes.

Special therapy involving a mixture of coal tar and oils may be necessary to deal with thick psoriatic crusts on the scalp and betamethason lotion is useful. The face may be treated with an ointment of coal tar and salicyclic acid, coal tar treatment sometimes being combined with exposure to ultraviolet light or sunlight. The drug methotrexate has been used by mouth to control exacerbations of the disease.

Psoriatic patients often need support from their families and their family physicians, as the chronic nature and unsightly appearance of their lesions can cause depression. There is now some ground for encouraging patients with the idea that although the cause of psoriasis is still unknown, many of the symptoms can be alleviated by new methods of treatment. The complex biochemistry of the reaction may yield up its secrets to concentrated research in due course.

psychiatry

The study and treatment of mental disturbances of all kinds.

At least 1% of any population is suffering at any one time from some form of mental disorder, and an estimated 10% will need treatment at some time in their lives. During the 20th century, classification of mental abnormalities has become more scientific and psychiatry has developed methods of treating them—ranging from chemotherapy to psychosurgery and from psychotherapy and psychoanalysis to electroconvulsive therapy.

Nowadays, although psychiatry set out in the modern era to deal with the psychoses (such as schizophrenia and manic-depressive illness), psychiatrists spend a great amount of their time dealing with neurotic patients, together with addicts and other "deviants." The environmental stresses of life are great enough in a significant minority of any population to cause anxiety, depression and behavioral disorders in patients who are not psychotic (that is, who do not suffer from serious mental disturbances).

Psychiatry has evolved into many groups whose rationale and methods are often mutually contradictory. It can be said in general that at one extreme are the psychiatrists who try to modify the behavior of their patients by altering their body chemistry, while at the other it is postulated that psychotherapy without drugs is the most likely course to be successful. In practice, few psychiatrists adopt an extreme position; a psycho-

therapist, for example, will often prescribe tranquilizers to lower a patient's level of anxiety.

Psychiatrists are all medically qualified doctors, although there is nowadays a school of thought that maintains that a full medical training is not really necessary.

See PSYCHOANALYSIS, PSYCHOTHERAPY.

psychoanalysis

The system of analyzing emotional patterns and developments in patients devised by Sigmund Freud (1856–1939), used to bring out valuable information from the unconscious mind and so make it available to manipulation by the conscious mind.

Psychoanalysis is now a widely accepted method of treating emotional disorders such as neuroses. Essentially, it consists of allowing the patient, usually lying on a couch to relax mind and body, to give free expression to his thoughts, ideas and fantasies. The analyst meanwhile adopts a neutral attitude, not making any judgment on anything that he is told, but encouraging the flow of words.

The object is to persuade the patient to go further and further back into his childhood and reenact his early emotional attitudes. It is hoped in this phase to release various infantile emotional tensions which, according to Freud's theories, can affect the whole of one's emotional development.

Theoretically, once enlightenment about the cause of one's mental symptoms has been reached (such as hatred of one's father or guilt about sex), the symptoms should be relieved. Freud's theories were based on the concept that much of our later development is based on the experience of the first five years of life, thus the interest in the earliest memories.

The psychoanalytic theory is based on a threefold division of the human personality: the *id*, the *ego* and the *superego*. The *id* is the "instinctual self" which is concerned with the immediate discharge of energy or tension; the *ego* regulates the interactions of the person with his environment; and the *superego* is the "superior being" representing the moral aspects of personality or "conscience."

Freud postulated that there are two great groups of instincts that provide energy for the id. The first, serving the purposes of life, provide the energy known as *libido*. According to Freud, all activities of the mind are driven by the need to reduce or eliminate the tension caused by the painful impact of the life instincts. The second group of instincts, such as aggression, sadism, masochism and the urge to suicide, are in the service of *death*.

To protect itself from anxiety, the Freudian ego develops many defense mechanisms and it is the task of psychoanalysis to break down the barriers that conceal these mechanisms, which often cripple the personality. However, one should point out that treatment is lengthy and very expensive, and overall results have not been particularly good—especially in comparison with the therapeutic usefulness of several new psychoactive drugs.

Finally, it should also be noted that whereas Freud got the ball rolling, his theories have been greatly modified, and a whole subsequent superstructure of analytic theory is now in use.

See PSYCHIATRY.

psychoses

Mental disorders of a severe kind in which there is an extensive disorder of the personality. They are usually more severe and more disabling than other psychiatric syndromes and are often accompanied by an inability to cope with reality.

One of the main psychoses is SCHIZOPHRENIA, a description given to a group of illnesses which are marked mainly by disordered thought processes. By-products of this disorder include difficulty in communication and in relationship with other people.

Affective disorders are those psychoses in which the main symptom is a severe disorder of mood. They include *involutional melancholia*, which is a major mental illness usually having its onset in women aged 45 to 55 and men aged 50 to 65. The main symptom is agitated depression and suicide is a real risk. Therapy commonly involves electric shock treatment and the administration of monoamine oxidase (MAO) inhibitors.

Outgoing, sociable people are at risk from *manic-depressive illness*, in which severe depression alternates with elation. PARANOIA is a term applied to a group of psychoses in which there are delusions of grandeur or of persecution, and which often respond favorably to psychotherapy.

See PSYCHIATRY, PSYCHOANALYSIS.

psychosomatic illnesses

Disorders with physical symptoms that are thought to be caused by emotional factors. When modern medicine first began to evolve, developments led to an early belief that illness was mainly, if not entirely, physical in origin. With greater understanding of disease processes, it is now realized that the body (or *soma*) and the mind (or *psyche*) are intimately linked in ways that can lead to a wide variety of illnesses.

When a person is put under stress he may react *normally*, *neurotically* (when his defense against the stress becomes ineffective), or *psychotically* (when the alarm is misconceived or ignored). The fourth possi-

bility is that he may react in a "psychophysiologic" way—the alert is translated into an effect on somatic systems, causing changes in body tissues (*blushing* is a simple example of how the emotions can have a physical manifestation). What is happening is that the physical changes are normal for the emotional states involved, but they are either too sustained or too intense. The individual may not be consciously aware of his emotional state.

An example which is widely known is the peptic ulcer. Tension in work or home can produce or exacerbate ulcers, although it is now believed that ulcer patients may also be genetically predisposed to the complaint by a chromosomal fault (which gives them too little of an enzyme which is necessary for a healthy stomach). Stress can be caused by such opposites as success and failure, puberty and aging, parenthood and conflict. Suppression of anxiety or rage may lead to cardiovascular problems and to the so-called "vascular headache."

Irritable colon (see IRRITABLE BOWEL SYNDROME) is now regarded as psychosomatic, but in these cases as well there may be a congenitally high sensitivity to parasympathetic stimulation. ULCERATIVE COLITIS, too, is a disease triggered by "psychic insult" in people who are often described as neat, orderly, punctual, conscientious and conforming. Asthma is the general description applied to a group of respiratory disorders, some of which are certainly psychosomatic in origin.

In general it may be said that some individuals seem to be predisposed by the nature of their personality structure to react to a difficult life situation which threatens their security not by adequate action but by emotional conflict. If the conflict is not discharged either by action or speech, it persists and can create a state of either acute or chronic emotional tension which seeks another outlet and leads to physical symptoms.

psychosurgery

Surgery of the brain designed to cure or alleviate symptoms of severe mental illness.

While "psychosurgery" is the generic term it is in effect a synonym for the main operation, *lobotomy*, in which the surgeon severs the connection between the frontal lobes and the rest of the brain.

There has been a great deal of controversy on the subject of psychosurgery. Some authorities maintain that it is unnecessary, ineffective and inimical to the civil rights of the patient. Advocates of psychosurgery maintain that in cases of very severe incapacitation lobotomy is the only treatment which can possibly bring relief.

On average, patients who undergo lobotomy have been incapacitated for ten years with intractable depression, anxiety and obsessional neurosis. Some have made suicide attempts. Psychosurgery is employed according to the supporters of the procedure only after other methods of treatment have failed to bring about any improvement over a long period, and only with the full and informed consent of the patient.

At one time the operation was done "freehand" by the surgeon, which had the disadvantage that the lesions which were produced were not always the same. Therefore the outcome could not be predicted on any organized basis.

Nowadays the *stereotactic* approach is employed. Orderly measurements of the connexions between the frontal lobes and the rest of the brain are taken by means of x rays, thus locating the "target" area in three dimensions. Electrocoagulation is then brought about by the introduction of a thin probe into the brain, or radioactive "seeds" are planted to produce the same effect.

Except for removing brain tumors that are responsible for some forms of epileptic attacks (e.g. *temporal lobe epilepsy*), psychosurgery in any form is becoming an outmoded therapeutic approach.

psychotherapy

A method of treating a psychiatric disorder based mainly on verbal communication between the therapist and his patient.

The object is to cure or alleviate the symptoms of the disorder by making the emotionally disturbed patient feel better or helping him to learn to live more effectively. A feature of many types of psychotherapy is the patient's relief at being able to talk to a noncritical listener. Apart from being able to obtain relief through "confession," the patient may be able to experience the emotional discharge known as *abreaction* by recalling significant incidents and sensations that had been forgotten or repressed. It is also possible through psychotherapy to "desensitize" a patient by referring repeatedly to a disturbing topic and to clarify his own feelings by exploring them. Psychotherapy also relieves many patients of the burden of loneliness.

The role of the therapist is often to interpret and explain to the patient reasons for recurring patterns of behavior and so clear the way for an improvement in the patient's interactions with the environment and with others. Psychotherapy, which is normally carried out on the basis of weekly interviews, embraces PSYCHO-ANALYSIS, HYPNOSIS, hypnotherapy, conditioning and aversion therapy. *Group therapy*, while enabling patients to develop skills in interacting with others, and overcoming feelings of isolation and alienation, has the disadvantage of lack of confidentiality. It also leads to less individual attention being given to patients; but it is, nevertheless, a popular and growing form of psychotherapy. It has one sterling advantage—it is within the financial means of many patients.

See PSYCHIATRY, PSYCHOANALYSIS.

pterygium

A degenerative condition of the eye in which a triangular area of fleshy conjunctiva, usually on the nasal side, extends across the eye and on to the cornea. The base is toward the nose and the apex of the triangle toward the pupil. The apex is immovably united to the cornea, while it is firmly attached to the sclera throughout its middle portion, and merges with the conjunctiva at its base.

Pterygium is particularly common in windy, dusty climates, and it is believed that the degeneration takes place as a result of continual bombardment of the eye by dust particles.

The condition causes no known medical problems, but eye surgeons often remove the pterygium for cosmetic reasons as it is unsightly.

ptosis

Prolapse or drooping of an organ, often used to describe the drooping of an upper eyelid.

Paralysis of the third cranial nerve causes this condition in many cases, which may be congenital or acquired.

Ptosis adiposa is drooping of the eyelid caused by orbital fat coming forward into the lid owing to its atrophic (wasting) condition. In young children, *congenital ptosis* is due to malformation of the levator palpebrae superioris muscle, or to a defective nerve supply to the muscle. *Hysterical ptosis* is a drooping of the eyelid caused by a spasm of the orbicularis oculi muscle. *Mechanical ptosis* is due to the thickening and consequent increase of the weight of the upper eyelid which arises in diseases such as trachoma.

A fairly common experience is *waking* (or *morning*) *ptosis*, in which difficulty is found in raising an upper eyelid. This may be due to an early stage of *keratoconjunctivitis sicca*. In elderly people the condition is often caused by loss of orbital fat and lack of tone in the levator palpebrae superioris muscle. In some cases of trauma, particularly where the skull is fractured (as in automobile accidents), the levator muscle may be damaged and subsequently be unable to control the eyelid correctly. It is possible to correct the condition surgically, to some extent, by resecting the levator muscle; but the eye surgeon has to be careful not to raise the eyelid so high that the eye cannot be closed, and also to make it match the other lid as closely as possible.

puerperal fever

Blood poisoning (septicemia) caused by bacterial infection of the genital tract shortly after childbirth. The disease is also known as *puerperal sepsis* or *childbed fever*.

In the mid-19th century, deaths from puerperal fever were so common that women were afraid to have their babies in the hospital. The high death rates dropped sharply when doctors realized that they were caused by attendants carrying the infection from one patient to another. Strict observance of the rules of hygiene and the use of antiseptics greatly improved survival rates, but childbed fever remained a source of anxiety until the discovery of sulfonamides.

The raw surface of the womb left after separation of the placenta provides ideal circumstances for the growth of bacteria, and in puerperal fever the wound is colonized by *streptococci*, bacteria commonly found in the nose and throat of healthy persons. Nowadays any woman whose temperature rises above 100°F (38°C) in the 14 days after delivery will be treated with appropriate antibiotics. Septicemia after childbirth has become extremely rare.

pulmonary diseases

The exchange of gases between the air and the blood occurs in the lungs; oxygen is absorbed and carbon dioxide excreted. The process is essential for life.

Inspired air passes down into the lungs through the windpipe (trachea), which branches into right and left main bronchi and then divides into even smaller branches until the smallest (bronchioles) end in minute air sacs (alveoli), whose walls are one cell thick and in direct contact with the capillary blood vessels. Through the walls of the alveoli gaseous exchange takes place.

Disease can affect any of these structures and interfere with their vital functions.

An early sign of a lung problem is persistent coughing, which may be dry and irritating in the early stages and later produce sputum. The sputum may be stained with blood (hemoptysis), or may be clear, yellow, or greenish—according to the nature of the disease. Pain may occur on breathing because the membranes covering the lungs (the pleura) may be inflamed. Interference with the respiratory function of the lungs may produce breathlessness.

Diseases affecting the lungs are usually inflammatory infections or new growths. Infections may be viral or bacterial; not infrequently, virus infections such as influenza or measles are followed by a secondary bacterial infection. Inflammation of the air passages (bronchi) is called BRONCHITIS; inflammation of the substance of the lung is PNEUMONIA.

Because the air we breathe in cities is far from clean, the bronchi are subjected to continual irritation—which is worse in those who work in dusty surroundings or who smoke. It would appear that the worse the pollution of the air becomes the greater is the incidence of lung cancer.

Certain substances are more likely to produce malignant growths than others, among them being the tar contained in cigarette smoke. Continual smoking or exposure to polluted air, combined with liability to virus infections, often causes chronic bronchitis, which may proceed in time to EMPHYSEMA—a condition in which there is dilation and loss of function of the alveoli (air sacs of the lungs). This may also be found in association with ASTHMA, a disease of complex causation producing spasm of the air passages.

THE LUNGS

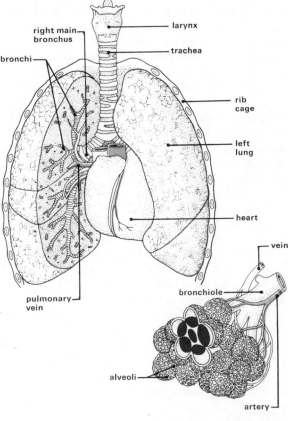

RESPIRATORY UNIT OF LUNG

The lungs are delicate and complex organs; their function is to allow oxygen to enter the bloodstream and to remove carbon dioxide. Respiration is impaired either when the bronchi are obstructed (for example by foreign bodies, cancer or inflammation) or the alveoli are diseased (emphysema, pneumonia or fibrosis).

Although cancer of the lung has become the most common form of cancer in men, two other lung diseases are now far less dangerous than formerly; pneumonia is usually susceptible to treatment with antibiotics, and so is tuberculosis.

pulmonary embolism

Blockage of one of the pulmonary arteries (those which take blood from the heart to the lungs) by a clot of blood, a clump of fat, or any other solid object. If one of the main pulmonary arteries is blocked the result may be collapse and sudden death. Less severe episodes of pulmonary embolism commonly cause chest pain associated with shortness of breath and the coughing up of bloodstained sputum.

By far the most common cause of pulmonary embolism is a blood clot carried by the bloodstream into the lungs from one of the veins in the legs. Blood clots are most likely to form in these veins as a result of prolonged bed rest or immobility; *venous thrombosis* in the calves and thighs occurs in as many as one third of all patients who have an operation under general anesthesia. The thrombus or clot goes unnoticed by the patient and eventually dissolves, but it may remain in the legs, causing localized pain and swelling, or (very occasionally) a fragment of the clot may become detached (at which point it is known as an *embolus*) and be swept up through the veins into the heart and so into the lungs.

Other sources of pulmonary embolism include fat globules after injuries causing bone fractures, and the formation of blood clots inside the heart after a coronary thrombosis ("heart attack").

Major pulmonary embolism is a medical emergency. Sometimes an immediate operation may be performed to remove the blood clot; more commonly treatment is given with anticoagulant drugs to prevent extension of the clot. The most effective treatment is preventive, and many surgeons now use anticoagulant drugs such as heparin as a routine to reduce the risk of venous thrombosis and pulmonary embolism in the postoperative period.

See also EMBOLISM/EMBOLUS.

pulpitis

Inflammation of the dental pulp (the soft vascular part in the center of a tooth). It may be *open* or *closed*, and there may be a number of causes, but in the main it is associated with dental caries ("cavities"). In *closed pulpitis*, where there is no break in the surrounding dentin, considerable pain may be experienced. *Open pulpitis* occurs when dental caries leads to a break in the

dentin and exposure of the pulp, to which bacteria are attracted by local irritation.

Hyperplastic pulpitis is distinguished by exuberant proliferation of chronically inflamed dental pulp. It appears as a soft pink insensitive mass, which pushes through an aperture in the wall of the pulp cavity into a carious cavity.

The acknowledged treatment for pulpitis involves the proper correction of the underlying caries after first controlling any infection by administering the appropriate antibiotics.

pulse

The palpable and sometimes visible change in arterial pressure caused by the pumping action of the heart.

When the heart contracts, pumping blood through the arterial system, the arteries expand slightly during the increased blood flow. It is this periodic expansion which is felt when a finger is placed on an artery close to the skin surface. Normally, the *radial artery* (in the wrist) is used to take the pulse, but several others in the body and the limbs may also be used.

The pulse is a useful indicator of several aspects of health, disease and injury. It is usually said that the "normal" pulse rate is about 72 per minute, but in healthy individuals at rest it can vary anywhere between 50 and 100. While undergoing severe exercise, or while under mental stress, the pulse rate can go far above this range (even above 200) without harm.

The pulse rate is quicker in children than in adults and slows down progressively throughout life. When a patient is suffering from a fever the pulse rate is usually elevated. The absence of perceptible pulse is not a definite sign of death; a person suffering from disease or injuries may exhibit no pulse, and this startling fact does not always mean that the heart has stopped beating. Patients with heart disease often exhibit irregular pulse rhythms; irregularities and variations are a diagnostic aid in diseases of the heart and the arteries.

See also BLOOD PRESSURE.

purpura

A condition in which tiny red or purple spots appear on the surface of the skin, in mucous membranes and elsewhere, due to the escape of blood from the vessels.

Purpura appears either when the capillaries become more permeable or when there is a shortage of blood platelets, which normally seal off damage to the walls of the capillaries.

A variety of diseases and conditions cause purpura. It may follow an infection such as scarlet fever; it sometimes appears in wasting diseases; and it can be caused by toxic drugs or malnutrition. In addition, the signs and symptoms occur in what is known as *thrombocytopenic purpura*, when there is a shortage of platelets (THROMBOCYTOPENIA), and in *anaphylactoid purpura*, which is thought to be associated with an allergic reaction. *Henoch's purpura* is a form of allergic reaction in the walls of the intestine, and *Schönlein's purpura* is a form that affects the joints of young adults.

The symptoms of purpura are usually feverishness and lassitude, followed by characteristic spots on the trunk and limbs. The spots may change color from red to purple until they are nearly black, and finally disappear in much the same way as a bruise. The most serious form is *purpura hemorrhagica*, in which bleeding occurs from mucous surfaces in the nose and also in the mouth, digestive organs and womb, and may be fatal. Thrombocytopenic purpura responds to steroid drugs, but in some cases surgical removal of the spleen (splenectomy) may be necessary. Where purpura follows infection or other disease, treatment is directed at the underlying condition.

pus

A yellowish or creamy white collection of viscid fluid that often forms at the site of a wound or infection. It contains normal and damaged white blood cells and other cellular debris.

pyelitis

Inflammation of the pelvis of a kidney—the funnel-shaped expansion which collects urine formed in the nephrons and conveys it to the ureter (the passage from each kidney leading to the bladder).

Pyelitis alone is extremely uncommon, since almost invariably the main body (or *parenchyma*) of the kidney is also infected.

Inflammation of both the pelvis and the parenchyma of the kidney is known as PYELONEPHRITIS. The term pyelitis is sometimes used loosely to mean pyelonephritis.

See also KIDNEY DISEASES.

pyelonephritis

Inflammation of the main substance (parenchyma) and pelvis of the kidney due to infection. It is a very common condition, females being more commonly affected than males. (Compare PYELITIS.)

The infecting microorganisms may reach the kidneys by means of the bloodstream or may travel upward from the bladder via the ureter and the lymphatic vessels around the ureters. The organisms which most commonly cause pyelonephritis are those found in the gastrointestinal tract.

Stasis or collection of urine in the bladder is an important factor which invariably predisposes to infection. This is why there are three peaks at which acute pyelonephritis is most common—in childhood, during pregnancy, and in the elderly. In childhood, major or minor degrees of urinary tract abnormalities may cause some degree of reflux of urine up the ureter when the bladder contracts to expel urine, and an attack of acute pyelonephritis may be the first sign that an abnormality exists. In pregnancy, the uterus compresses the ureters and causes stasis of urine. In the elderly, stasis is often caused by PROLAPSE of the uterus in the female and by enlargement of the prostate in men.

Other conditions which predispose to pyelonephritis include DIABETES MELLITUS, kidney stones and surgical procedures which require instruments to be passed into the urinary tract.

Pyelonephritis can be acute or chronic. An attack of pyelonephritis is characterized by fever accompanied by chills, pain in the loin, the need to pass urine very frequently and urgently, and burning pain at the urethra (the urinary outlet from the bladder) on passing urine. The last two symptoms on their own usually suggest infection of the bladder and infection of the urethra respectively.

Treatment consists of the administration of antibiotics. The urine will have to be examined in the laboratory to determine which microorganisms are responsible for the infection, so that the appropriate antibiotic can be given. Repeated laboratory examinations of the urine will have to be carried out on one or two occasions in the first few months after completion of a full course of antibiotics to ensure that the infection has been completely eradicated or that reinfection has not taken place. If the infection recurs, or another infection occurs, a predisposing cause for the infection must be sought.

Before kidney failure develops, the steps taken to prevent or delay further damage include vigorous treatment of any low-grade urinary tract infection (determined by laboratory examination of the urine) and thorough investigation to discover treatable conditions which predispose to pyelonephritis.

Compare GLOMERULONEPHRITIS. See also KIDNEY DISEASES.

pyoderma

Any of various pus-forming skin infections. The group of conditions known collectively as the pyodermas include: (1) IMPETIGO—a common, contagious, superficial, bacterial infection seen most often in children. The lesions vary from small to large blisters that rupture and release a honey-colored liquid. New lesions can develop very rapidly (within hours). Crusts form from the discharge. (2) *Ecthyma*—similar to impetigo, but it affects slightly deeper layers of the skin. (3) *Folliculitis*—which affects hair follicles anywhere on the body, including the eyelashes (to form a STY). (4) *Furuncle* (or boil)—a more extensive infection of the hair follicle involving deeper underlying tissues. (5) CARBUNCLE—an extensive infection of several adjoining hair follicles; the carbuncle drains with multiple openings on to the skin surface. (6) *Sweat gland infections*—not a common condition. (7) ERYSIPELAS—an uncommon infection caused by streptococcal bacteria; it results in a characteristic type of CELLULITIS (inflammation of the loose connective tissue under the skin) which appears as a red, warm, raised, well-defined plaque; blisters may form on the skin.

The general principles of treatment include: (a) administration of the appropriate antibiotic; (b) general isolation of the patient, with frequent change of clothing and bedding (towels should not be shared) and strict hygiene. (c) if the furuncle or carbuncle comes to a "head"—that is, when an abscess has formed with a definite point—the pus should be drained by an incision. (d) if pyodermas recur, investigations should be carried out to exclude diabetes (which makes a person prone to infections).

pyorrhea

Literally, "a copious discharge of pus." But the term is usually used to mean *pyorrhea alveolaris*—inflammation or degeneration of tissues which surround and support the teeth, including the gums, the bone surrounding the tooth socket, the ligaments around the bone and the *cementum* (the bonelike connective tissue covering the root of the tooth and assisting in its support).

Pyorrhea usually begins as gingivitis (inflammation of the gums) and progresses to periodontitis. The most common source of the infecting organism which causes gingivitis is bacterial plaque (microbial colonies found on the tooth surface). Gingivitis need not be infective in origin. It may be a sign of: (1) vitamin deficiency, (2) an allergic reaction, (3) a reaction to heavy-metal poisoning, (4) a reaction to drugs, or (5) leukemia. In addition, it may accompany pregnancy. Whatever the cause, inflamed gums often become secondarily infected.

The symptoms of gingivitis consist of redness, swelling, changes of contour, and bleeding of the gum. A cleft may form between the gum and the tooth in which food debris collects and the infection may become chronic. Treatment is by correction of the underlying cause, proper hygiene of the mouth, antibiotics, and sometimes extensive dental surgery.

When gingivitis spreads to produce periodontitis, there is deepening of the pockets between the gums and the teeth, loss of the supporting bone, loosening of teeth

and recession of gums. Dental treatment is required to eliminate local irritating factors, reconstruct gingival (gum) tissues, splint loose teeth or extract hopelessly decayed teeth.

See also ABSCESS.

pyrexia

The technical name for FEVER. The condition of an exceptionally high fever is known as *hyperpyrexia*.

Q

Q fever

An infection caused by the microorganism (rickettsia) *Coxiella burneti*, a parasite of cattle in which it produces mild or subclinical infections. These animals excrete the microorganisms in the milk or feces. Man becomes infected usually by inhaling dusts which have become contaminated by infected animal material; sometimes infection occurs by drinking infected milk, as the rickettsiae are relatively resistant to pasteurization.

After an incubation period of two to four weeks, symptoms may appear. These consist of fever, headaches, prostration and cough. X rays usually show an inflammation of the lung, although the cough may be slight. Occasionally the heart may be affected, sometimes months after the original infection. The disease may be acute, or chronic and relapsing. Even in untreated patients, the infection is rarely fatal.

Prevention is by avoiding contact with infected cattle. If the disease develops, symptoms may be suppressed by the administration of tetracyclines, although the infection may not necessarily be eradicated.

See also RICKETTSIAE.

quarantine

The detention or limitation of freedom of movement of man (or domestic animals) who are apparently well but who have been in contact with a serious communicable disease (one that can be transmitted directly or indirectly from one individual to another). The reason for this is that such persons or animals may have become infected, although they have not yet shown signs or symptoms of the disease—that is, they are in the *incubation* stage of the disease, during which time they may be able to pass the disease on to unaffected others. To prevent this they are quarantined for the longest usual incubation period of the disease in question, by the end of which time it should have become clearer who are the ones who have been infected and who need to be isolated or nursed by *isolation* techniques.

Quarantine need not be carried out in the hospital. The person can be quarantined anywhere as long as he does not have unlimited contact with unaffected persons.

There are various degrees of quarantine. *Complete quarantine* means the quarantine of all persons who have been in contact with the communicable disease. With *modified quarantine*, it may be that only those who are likely to pass the disease on to particularly susceptible people are held in quarantine. For example, if children are particularly susceptible to the disease, child contacts of the case may be asked to stay away from school; or perhaps only those contacts who have no immunity to the disease have to stay away from school, since they are the ones most likely to have caught the infection and be "incubating" it.

The least strict form of quarantine is personal surveillance in which the contact's movements are not limited—except for the fact that health officials should be able to get in touch with him daily or at frequent intervals to ensure that he has not fallen ill.

The type of quarantine applied varies depending on the seriousness of the disease, the closeness of the contact with the disease, and the state of immunity of the susceptible people within the community.

quinsy

An abscess forming in the space around the tonsils (peritonsillar abscess). It is a complication of acute tonsillitis.

When a peritonsillar abscess forms, the sore throat of acute tonsillitis suddenly becomes severe on one side, there is an acute increase in the difficulty in swallowing and there may be spasm of the muscles around the jaw.

Treatment consists of antibiotics, bed rest, a light diet, plenty of fluids, and analgesics (such as aspirin). When the abscess is fully formed it may discharge itself, or it may require surgical incision and drainage. After the infection has subsided a TONSILLECTOMY may be considered to prevent recurrence.

R

rabies

A viral disease affecting animals (especially carnivores) characterized by irritation of the nervous system followed by paralysis and (in virtually every case) death.

The virus is found in the saliva of infected animals, which transmit the disease by their bites. The disease may also be spread if open wounds are contaminated by infected saliva. Also called *hydrophobia*.

At present there is no rabies in the U.K., largely because of the strict quarantining of animals being imported. Vaccination of dogs in the United States has controlled canine rabies. Most cases are the result of bites of infected wild animals such as skunks, foxes and bats. Infected animals may have the "furious" form of the disease (in which they become very agitated and aggressive) or the "dumb" form (in which change of habits or paralysis predominate). The diagnosis may require laboratory tests and examination of the nervous tissue of the animal.

In man the incubation period varies from approximately ten days to over a year, but most often it is from 30 to 60 days. The incubation period is shorter the more extensive the bite or the nearer the bite to the head. Once the first symptoms of rabies appear, the disease is inevitably fatal.

The initial symptom in man consists of sensitivity of the area around the wound to changes in temperature. This is typically followed by a period of mental depression, restlessness and fever. The restlessness may increase to states of rage and violent convulsions. Attempts to drink result in spasm of the larynx ("voicebox") so that the patient eventually refuses to drink (becomes "hydrophobic"). Spasm of the larynx is also easily precipitated by mild stimuli such as a gentle breeze. The attacks of asphyxia produced by laryngeal spasm can lead to death. Death may also result from exhaustion and paralysis of the muscles that control respiration.

Vaccination should be started after a person is bitten by an animal suspected to be rabid. The animal should be confined and observed for symptoms of rabies so that the diagnosis can be confirmed and permit a prompt vaccination of the victim—a painful and prolonged procedure which is not always successful. The local wound should be thoroughly washed with soft medicinal soap.

No cure currently exists once the first symptoms are experienced. Supportive treatment is the best that can be offered.

radiation therapy

Treatment of disease by ionizing radiation or high-energy radiation. The radiation may be given in the form of a beam, or a radioactive material (such as radium or cobalt) may be contained in various devices which can be inserted directly into the tissues or into a body cavity. The radioactive material may also be given by injection into a vein or as a drink (radioactive phosphorus is usually given by injection or as a drink, and radioactive iodine given as a drink).

The most common condition for which radiation is used is CANCER. Some cancers respond well to radiation therapy alone; others are best treated with radiation therapy in conjunction with surgery or anticancer drugs (or both). When a cancer is too far advanced for surgery, radiation therapy can often help to relieve symptoms.

Radiation kills not only cancer cells, it can also have harmful effects on normal cells. But cancer cells are more susceptible because radiation acts best on cells that are dividing (multiplying) rapidly. The normal cells most commonly affected are those which are dividing rapidly—such as the skin cells, those lining the gastrointestinal tract and the bone marrow cells. Side effects of radiation are known as *radiation sickness*. Symptoms usually consist of diarrhea and vomiting, mouth ulcers, temporary loss of hair and anemia. The treatment is simply to reduce the dose of radiation (or to stop treatment). Recovery may be rapid, but in some cases recurrences occur even after the treatment has been stopped. Sometimes the inflammation that is produced around the site of treatment becomes chronic and causes symptoms later. Radiation to the abdomen, for example, may cause fibrotic reactions which lead to intermittent abdominal pains. Chronic inflammation of the LYMPHATIC SYSTEM produced by radiation to lymph nodes may impede the flow of lymph from the area drained and result in a form of ELEPHANTIASIS.

However, improvements in technique—which allow doses to be more accurately calculated, and which enable the radiation to be directed more specifically to the small area of tissues to be treated—have considerably reduced the frequency of side effects.

The other conditions for which radiation therapy is used include ANKYLOSING SPONDYLITIS, polycythemia vera (see POLYCYTHEMIA) and thyrotoxic goiter (see HYPERTHYROIDISM).

rash

A skin eruption which typically takes the form of red patches or spots and is often accompanied by itching. The rash may be localized in one part of the body or involve extensive areas. A rash may be the result of a number of conditions, including certain communicable diseases (such as measles or chickenpox).

Nappy rash is the dermatitis (skin inflammation) which occurs in infants on the areas covered by nappies and is due to irritation by wet or soiled nappies. A fungal infection (candidiasis or moniliasis) may be superimposed in nappy rash; if it develops, antifungal treatment is required. In most cases, however, rash can be controlled by keeping the nappy area dry and clean and by prompt changing of wet nappies.

MILIARIA ("heat rash" or "prickly heat") is a form of rash due to blockage of sweat ducts. The function of the sweat glands is to flood the skin surface with water for cooling. They become very active in hot weather. The constant maceration of the skin because of the moist environment around the sweat pores blocks the ducts, so that the part of the duct behind the blockage swells up.

An *allergic rash* usually appears as weals, which are well-defined elevated lesions caused by local accumulation of fluid in the tissues. It is the type of rash seen with insect bites or STINGS, allergies to food or drugs, or URTICARIA ("hives"). Drug eruptions, however, may take on a number of other forms ranging from a measles-like rash to sloughing off of the skin. The treatment for allergic rash is to stop contact with the agent causing the rash; if the eruption does not clear up, antiallergic agents such as antihistamines and corticosteroids may be required.

Many *viral infections* produce a rash, which in some infections are fairly characteristic of the particular infection. In MEASLES and GERMAN MEASLES the rash usually starts around the ears or on the face and neck before spreading to the trunk and limbs. In mild cases, the limbs may be unaffected. In CHICKENPOX, the rash usually starts on the trunk and later spreads to the face and extremities; blisters soon form. In SMALLPOX, the rash first appears on the face and quickly spreads to the trunk and hands, forming fluid-filled blisters (pustules), or "spots." The fluid within the center of the spots turns to pus (which dries and forms scabs). In INFECTIOUS MONONUCLEOSIS, the rash is most prominent over the trunk.

Bacterial infections may also produce rashes; for example, secondary SYPHILIS is characterized by a transient skin eruption.

A rash may also be seen in the group of conditions known as the AUTOIMMUNE DISEASES. With lupus erythematosus, a "butterfly rash" may form (so named because of the typical "butterfly" pattern it forms across the bridge of the nose and over the adjacent areas of the cheeks).

Raynaud's phenomenon

First described by Maurice Raynaud in 1862, Raynaud's phenomenon is most common in young women: first the fingertips (then the rest of the fingers) go white and cold, the fingers feel numb and may become stiff, and it is evident that their blood supply has temporarily been cut off. On recovery the blood comes slowly back to the fingers, which turn bright red and become painful.

The condition may be slight or severe; in severe cases small ulcers may form on the fingertips and the nails may be affected. If there is no underlying cause, the cond.tion usually improves and in the end subsides. But in some cases the phenomenon is a complication of more widespread disease such as atheroma, scleroderma, or systemic lupus erythematosus; the "cervical rib syndrome" may include Raynaud's phenomenon, or it may be precipitated by the use of vibrating tools. It may also be an occupational disease (e.g., of butchers).

All sufferers should avoid cold hands, and they should avoid handling cold metal with bare hands. Attacks may be made worse by emotional disturbances, particularly anxiety. Treatment includes keeping the whole body warm as well as the hands and feet, and the relief of pain with analgesics. In severe cases it may be useful to block the sympathetic nervous supply to the affected limb, or to interrupt it by surgical operation. Patients may have to change their employment.

Recklinghausen's disease

See VON RECKLINGHAUSEN'S DISEASE.

rectal cancer

The most common cancer of the gastrointestinal tract, generally occurring in middle age but sometimes in the young. It may arise more often in those who have a family history of multiple polyposis, chronic ulcerative colitis, or simple rectal tumors, and the incidence increases with age.

The onset is often insidious, and the first sign may be bleeding from the anus or bloodstained stools which may lead the patient to think he has hemorrhoids (piles). The bowel habits change, constipation alternating with attacks of diarrhea. It may feel that the rectum is never entirely empty, and there may be a dragging dull discomfort. Pain develops with the growth of the tumor—which may reach a considerable size, filling the lower part of the abdomen. If the growth is neglected, partial obstruction occurs which leads to offensive diarrhea.

Providing that the condition is recognized early, surgical removal of the tumor offers a considerable hope of cure; it is therefore of the utmost importance that rectal bleeding should never be dismissed as being due to hemorrhoids without a proper medical examination by a physician. This will include a rectal examination and, possibly, endoscopy.

rectocele

A pouch formed when part of the rectum protrudes into the vagina. It is the result of rupture (during childbirth) of the fibrous connective tissue that separates the rectum from the vagina. It may be due to a rapid delivery or to a difficult one. Sometimes the diagnosis is made soon after delivery, but usually symptoms do not appear until a woman is aged about 35 to 40.

Factors which affect the development of a rectocele include the condition of the tissues, the degree of damage, and persistent straining at stool. There is a vicious cycle here because one of the signs of a rectocele is constipation due to collection of feces in the pouch; this leads to straining, which further aggravates the herniation. Patients may complain of a sense of rectal or vaginal fullness and the constant urge for a bowel movement.

Treatment consists of good dietary habits to avoid constipation or straining at stool. Laxatives or suppositories may be necessary. Surgery is required to achieve a cure, the chances for which are good if subsequent vaginal delivery and straining at stool can be avoided.

reflex

A reflex is an involuntary action or movement which occurs in response to a stimulus. Examples of reflex actions are the quick closure of the eye when an object approaches it or when the eyelash is touched, or the sharp recovery of balance when a person begins to slip. There are also reflexes of which one may not be conscious; for example, the secretion of gastric juices at the sight of food, or the movement of the pupil in response to change in the intensity of light.

A reflex is brought about by the activity of the *reflex arc*. In its simplest form, the reflex arc consists of a nerve cell which acts as a "receptor" for the stimulus, and a nerve cell which acts as an "effector" for the reflex action. In addition there is a *reflex center* (the brain or the spinal cord). The nerve from the receptor brings the message from the receptor to the reflex center where it meets the nerve leading to the effector and passes the message on. Thus nerve cells in the retina (receptors) receive light (the stimulus) and pass the message on to the effectors (muscles which control the movement of the pupil).

Some reflexes can be conditioned—that is learned or modified. The classic example is the experiments with dogs conducted by the Russian physician and physiologist Ian Pavlov (1849–1936). A bell was rung whenever the dog was served food. The normal response to food is salivation. After a number of times, the dog salivated when the bell was rung without food being served at the same time.

Many reflexes may be tested during a general medical examination. When an appropriate stimulus is provided by the doctor, the reflex response is involuntary; any disturbance in the expected reflex thus affords an objective sign of disturbed neural function. One common test is the "knee jerk" reflex. This is commonly elicited by a firm tap with a rubber-headed mallet on the tendon just below the kneecap (a test with which many people are familiar). The normal response is for the lower leg to jerk outward suddenly and then return to its former position.

Another fairly common test of neurological function is BABINSKI'S REFLEX, which is elicited by stimulating the sole of the foot (as by firmly stroking the sole with the blunt end of a key). In adults, the normal response is for the large toe and usually the other toes to "clench" or be drawn down; if the large toe extends instead of flexes, and the other toes fan out, it is a sign of some disorder of the nerve tract from the spinal cord to the brain (corticospinal tract).

Reiter's syndrome

A group of three conditions (also known as *Reiter's disease*): nongonococcal urethritis, arthritis and conjunctivitis. In addition to these three main disorders, the disease may include a number of other features such as balanitis, anterior uveitis, stomatitis, or thrombophlebitis. Sometimes the disease appears in a less complete form—that is, with one or two of the three main features, plus one or more of the other features.

The cause of the disease is unknown. Most cases are preceded either by an attack of dysentery or by sexual contact. The nondysenteric cases are thought to be of venereal origin. Although some organisms have been isolated from urethral or conjunctival discharges and from joint fluids in Reiter's disease, it is still not certain what their role is in causing the disease, which most commonly affects young men.

The arthritis usually appears about 10 to 14 days after the manifestation of dysentery or urethritis and affects mainly the large joints, often the knees and ankles. It may persist for months, whereas most of the other symptoms usually disappear within a few days or weeks.

The condition usually resolves on its own, but recurrences are common. The recurrent attacks tend to be milder than the first attack. Recurrent involvement, however, may lead to permanent changes.

There is no specific treatment, only treatment to relieve symptoms.

relaxation therapy

A form of behavior therapy which is used as a preliminary to "desensitization"—a technique of getting patients to overcome irrational fears which can lead to NEUROSIS. Desensitization works best when a subject is not anxious and tense. When a person is able to relax his muscles voluntarily, certain physiological changes occur (such as a slight reduction in the rate of the heartbeat, a slowed rate of breathing and a detectable

diminution in the resistance of the skin to an electrical current). These changes are the opposite of those found in an *anxious* person. The voluntary relaxation of muscles has an overall calming effect which makes desensitization easier. The muscle relaxation has to be achieved voluntarily; paralyzing the muscles by using drugs does not produce the same effect.

The therapist first gets the patient to *contract* a group of muscles—for example, the muscles of the upper limbs—and then gradually trains the patient to *relax* these muscles. The patient is then taught how to relax other muscle groups—for example, the lower limbs, the neck, the face, the eye muscles, and so on—until he is able to relax all muscles in the body. There need not be a strict order in which one learns to relax muscle groups; the order varies with the therapist.

If a person has difficulty in relaxing muscles at will, HYPNOSIS or tranquilizing drugs may help.

See also DESENSITIZATION.

renal failure

See KIDNEY DISEASES.

resection

The surgical procedure of cutting out, especially the surgical removal of a segment or section of an organ.

respiration

The exchange of oxygen and carbon dioxide between the atmosphere and body cells. Oxygen combines with carbon and hydrogen furnished by food. These reactions generate heat and provide the living organism with energy for physical work as well as for the many other processes essential for life, such as digestion, growth and brain function. The carbon dioxide that is produced during respiration has to be eliminated; accumulation of carbon dioxide in the body disturbs body function by causing the tissue fluids to be too acid.

In an adult at rest the frequency of respiration is about 14 to 20 breaths per minute; children tend to breathe at a faster rate. Atmospheric air breathed in contains approximately 21% oxygen and 0.03% carbon dioxide. Air breathed out of the lungs contains approximately 14% oxygen and 5.6% carbon dioxide.

All the air in the lungs is not expelled with each breath. The amount of inspired air that actually reaches the lungs with each breath (during normal quiet breathing) is known as the *tidal volume;* it represents only about 1/18 of the total capacity of the lungs. The *vital capacity* is the amount of air the lungs can hold after trying to force out as much air from the lungs as possible and then taking the deepest possible breath.

The *residual volume* is the amount of air the lungs hold after trying to breathe out as hard as possible; it is impossible to empty the lungs of all their air in this manner, and approximately 1,200 cubic centimeters (cc) remain—compared with approximately 500 cc of air drawn into the lungs with each breath during normal breathing.

The act of breathing is accomplished by the action of the diaphragm (which moves down) and the muscles between the ribs (which expand the chest upward, outward and sideways). As air is drawn into the lungs (*inspiration*) the pleural cavity—the airless space between the lungs and the chest wall—becomes larger; this creates a suction effect on the lungs and causes them to expand. As the volume of the lungs increases, it creates a partial vacuum within the lungs; air rushes in through the nose, mouth (if open) and air passages to fill this space. Breathing out (*expiration*) is a passive action caused by the escape of air temporarily held in the lungs at a slightly higher pressure than the atmospheric air.

There are three components involved in the transport of oxygen and carbon dioxide between the cells and the external environment. Exchange of the two gases between the body cells and the atmosphere takes place in the lungs. Breathing consists of alternate acts of inspiration and expiration; during inspiration, atmospheric air is taken into the lungs while during expiration the air which is relatively poor in oxygen and rich in carbon dioxide is expelled into the atmosphere.

In the lungs, exchange of gases takes place by diffusion across the walls of the air sacs (alveoli); oxygen from inspired air diffuses across the lining of the air sacs and enters the circulation, while carbon dioxide moves in the opposite direction. The gases are transported between cells and the lung by the blood circulation.

Any disorder that affects transport of the gases can impair respiration and, if the impairment is severe enough, death occurs; death may be of the whole organism or localized, such as occurs in heart attacks (myocardial infarction) or STROKES when the blood supply to specific tissues is cut off. Other disorders which can affect transport of gases include nervous or muscular disorders which impair the movement of chest and abdominal muscles required for breathing, or disorders which affect the lining of the air sacs, such as PNEUMONIA or collapse of the lung (ATELECTASIS).

See also PULMONARY DISEASES.

respiratory distress syndrome

Another name for HYALINE MEMBRANE DISEASE.

respiratory tract infection

The respiratory tract extends from the nostrils down to

RESPIRATION

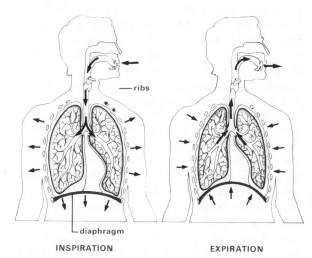

INSPIRATION   EXPIRATION

At rest, a normal adult breathes about 14 times per minute; oxygen enters the blood in the capillaries of the lungs and carbon dioxide is carried away in the expired air. Muscle action lifts the ribs and pulls down the diaphragm, so increasing the volume of the chest: the lungs expand, drawing in air through the nose or mouth. When these muscles relax, the lungs recoil, and air is expelled.

the air sacs in the lungs (pulmonary alveoli). Broadly speaking, the respiratory tract can be divided into the *upper respiratory tract* (above the larynx) and the *lower respiratory tract* (below the larynx). Infections (producing inflammation) of specific parts of the respiratory tract are known as RHINITIS (inflammation of the nasal passages); PHARYNGITIS (inflammation of the pharynx, or throat); LARYNGITIS (inflammation of the larynx, or "voice-box"); TRACHEITIS (inflammation of the trachea, or "windpipe"); and BRONCHITIS (inflammation of the bronchi or major air passages below the trachea). When the air sacs are affected the infection is known as PNEUMONITIS. Untreated infection of any part can spread readily to other parts.

The infecting microorganisms—usually bacteria or viruses—most commonly enter the respiratory tract by inhalation of infected droplets exhaled (or coughed or sneezed out) by someone with an existing respiratory tract infection. Sometimes a respiratory tract infection spreads from a previously localized infection in the mouth or is introduced from other parts of the body by means of the bloodstream.

The body has a number of defense mechanisms specifically designed to ward off or attack respiratory tract infections. The nostrils have lining hairs which act as filters for the air breathed in. There are also a number of "turbinates" in the nasal passages which have mucus-covered surfaces that act very much like "fly-paper" to trap irritants and infective organisms. (The turbinates—or *nasal conchae*—are intricately shaped and roughly parallel and horizontal bony ridges that separate the deeper airways on either side of the nose into three drainage channels—each of which is known as a *meatus*.) Furthermore, nasal secretions contain enzymes and antibodies which can kill or interfere with the growth and multiplication of some bacteria and viruses. Irritation of the nose and nasopharynx (the part behind the nose just above the roof of the mouth) also initiates sneezing, which expels irritants; similarly, irritation of the larynx or upper part of the trachea triggers the cough reflex. Lower down, the diameter of the air passages progressively diminishes so that the velocity of air is gradually reduced as it passes down the respiratory tract, allowing particles to fall out of the airstream and stick to the mucus-covered walls; these walls bear cilia (hair-like structures) on their surface. The cilia move in such a way as to sweep the mucus upward and out of the respiratory tract. Obstruction of the respiratory tract by a foreign body or by a tumor will prevent the mucus from being effectively swept upward. The action of cilia is also impaired by chronic inflammation, such as that associated with chronic bronchitis, the common

RESPIRATORY TRACT INFECTION

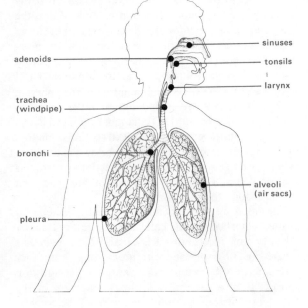

Infections of the respiratory tract cover anything from the common cold to pneumonia. The illustration shows the possible sites of infection; symptoms may include cough, excess phlegm, chest pain and breathing difficulties.

cold and by some anesthetics. When the mucus is abnormally thick, and thus unable to flow easily, infection is common.

A number of factors make a person more susceptible to respiratory tract infection; these include the extremes of age, debilitation by chronic illness, and DIABETES MELLITUS.

Symptoms of an infection of the respiratory tract depend primarily on the severity of the attack and on the site affected.

Treatment is primarily the administration of the appropriate antibiotic.

See also PULMONARY DISEASES.

restless legs syndrome

A relatively common condition (of unknown cause) characterized by aching or burning sensations in the muscles of the lower limbs, accompanied by a desire to move the legs. Also known as *jittery legs syndrome* or *Ekbom's syndrome*.

The onset of symptoms typically occurs when the patient is resting, especially when in bed. After a period of restless shuffling, the patient may be compelled to get up and walk about to obtain relief. Except for occasional muscular cramps, there is usually no associated pain or any sign of disease in the muscles or nerves of the legs. Although no specific medical treatment exists to relieve the condition, many patients benefit from the administration of an appropriate tranquilizer just before bedtime.

resuscitation

The emergency measures performed to attempt to restore breathing and the heartbeat in someone who has apparently just died. There are three essential measures in resuscitation, most easily remembered by the letters *A* (keep the *airways* clear), *B* (restore *breathing*), and *C* (restore the *circulation*).

To prevent blockage of the airway by the tongue (which may have fallen back and obstructed the upper part of the airway), the patient's head should be tilted right back. If the airway is blocked by vomit, mucus, mud, or dentures it should be "hooked out" very rapidly with a finger.

If the patient is not breathing spontaneously, mouth-to-mouth breathing should be initiated at once. This consists of the first-aider taking a deep breath of air which is then immediately blown out into the patient's mouth, taking care to pinch the patient's nostrils at the same time so that the air blown in does not escape through the nostrils. This should be repeated about 12 times per minute.

If after the first three or four breaths the victim's color

has not improved, the pupils of his eyes remain very wide, and there is no detectable pulse or heartbeat, then CARDIAC MASSAGE is indicated. This procedure is also known as *external cardiac compression*.

External cardiac compression carried out by inexperienced people can fracture ribs and cause damage to internal organs.

Sometimes the heart will start after a sharp thump on the chest and this should be attempted before external cardiac compression. When cardiac compression is given it must be accompanied by the continuation of artificial respiration.

retention of urine

Inability to empty the bladder may be caused by obstruction of the urinary passages or by neurological disorders which disturb the neuromuscular mechanisms of urination. Retention of urine may be acute or chronic.

Obstruction to the outlet of the bladder may be caused by enlargement of the prostate gland in men, by benign or malignant tumors, fibrosis of the bladder neck, stones, blood clots, or pressure from outside by fibroids of the uterus or a pregnant uterus. The urethra may be obstructed by strictures (usually the result of previous infection or injury), stones, foreign bodies, or acute inflammation.

One of the most common causes of acute urinary retention is postoperative pain; other conditions disturbing neuromuscular reflexes are diseases of the spinal cord such as multiple sclerosis and tabes dorsalis (locomotor ataxia), tumors, injuries and inflammations. It is possible for hysteria to produce acute or chronic urinary retention, and in the elderly the bladder may not be emptied because of confusion and loss of awareness.

Acute retention is painful except in neurological disorders. The pain is felt above the pubis at the lower part of the abdomen; chronic retention is usually painless.

Treatment includes the use of catheters and operative relief of obstructions. In chronic conditions it may be necessary to introduce a catheter permanently; in some cases permanent drainage may be carried out through the lower part of the abdominal wall.

retinitis

Inflammation of the retina, the light-sensitive lining at the back of the eyeball.

The retina forms the innermost of the three coats (tunics) of the eye. True inflammation of the retina rarely occurs on its own, but usually together with inflammation of the *choroid* (the middle coat)—a condition known as *chorioretinitis*. This may be caused by infections such as TUBERCULOSIS or SYPHILIS, or by parasitic infestations. Symptoms include blurring of vision, distortion of the size and shape of the image, and extreme sensitivity of the eye to bright light (photophobia). If the cause is known, specific treatment is administered; if not, corticosteroids may help.

All three coats of the eye may sometimes become infected with pus-forming (pyogenic) microorganisms. This can occur after injury, when a corneal ulcer perforates, or when the infection spreads from other parts of the body. This serious condition is characterized by intense pain and rapid loss of vision. Treatment is the administration of appropriate antibiotics.

Two degenerative (not inflammatory) conditions are also known as retinitis—RETINITIS PIGMENTOSA, and *retinitis proliferans*. The latter is a complication of diabetes mellitus and is characterized by the formation of masses of new blood vessels in the retina.

retinitis pigmentosa

An inherited disorder characterized by a slowly progressive degeneration of the retina of both eyes.

Symptoms may be noticed from early childhood, the earliest signs usually being defective night vision since the degeneration first affects the *rods*, which are receptors that mediate vision in dim light. Later the central field of vision becomes lost; this gradually progresses until (in some cases) total blindness occurs.

There is no effective treatment for retinitis pigmentosa. Genetic counseling may help to prevent the disease. About 90% of cases are inherited as an "autosomal recessive" feature, 9% as an "autosomal dominant" feature and the rest as "sex-linked."

retinopathy

Damage to the retina (the light-sensitive layer at the back of the eye) caused by disease of the blood vessels.

In advancing age the blood vessels in general become hardened and narrow (arteriosclerosis). In some people the condition may be severe enough to lead to small hemorrhages into the retina, but usually hemorrhages occur if the blood pressure is above normal and undue strain is put upon the aging blood vessels. These hemorrhages may produce defects in vision.

Malignant hypertension can bring about similar changes in younger people, for it produces widespread damage to the smaller arteries (arterioles) which leads to the formation of exudates and hemorrhages.

Retinopathy is one of the most serious complications of advanced diabetes mellitus; it is present in about 90% of cases of over 25 years duration, and is dependent on the duration rather than the severity of the disease. It can result in complete bilateral blindness in early adult life, but if the condition is diagnosed early enough it can be treated. It is therefore extremely important that all people with a diabetic condition have the retina examined at least once a year by an ophthalmologist.

Rh (Rhesus) factor

Prior to 1940, it was thought that the ABO BLOOD GROUPS were the only groups of clinical importance, particularly in the area of blood transfusion. However, unexplained reactions occurred in patients when transfused with blood of their own ABO group. There had also been interest for many years in the fact that certain women were prone to bear children who were born jaundiced and anemic, who sometimes died soon after birth, or, in severe cases, who were stillborn.

Some parallel work with red cells from Rhesus monkeys involved the preparation of antibodies (agglutinins) capable of clumping or agglutinating Rhesus monkey cells. It was a surprising discovery that such agglutinins would react with 85% of human red cells (*Rhesus positive*) but not with the remaining 15% (*Rhesus negative*). Furthermore, women who had produced jaundiced or dead infants, as described above, were found to be invariably Rhesus negative while their husbands were Rhesus positive.

The conclusion from this work was that incompatibility within the Rhesus system was responsible for the abnormalities in these "Rhesus babies" suffering from *erythroblastosis fetalis* (a "hemolytic" disease of the newborn, characterized by enlargement of the liver and spleen, anemia and jaundice) and that transfusion of Rhesus negative patients with Rhesus positive blood was responsible for subsequent incompatibility reactions when further Rhesus positive blood was given. Understanding of the nature of the problem has led to good control of both transfusion reactions and Rh disorders of pregnancy and the salvage of many babies.

rheumatic fever

A once common disease of childhood and adolescence which today is less frequent. It occurs as a delayed complication of infection of the throat by bacteria known as *Group A hemolytic streptococci*. It is now known to be an example of an AUTOIMMUNE DISEASE, resulting from an allergic reaction following the release of poisonous substances (toxins) by the bacteria.

It occurs in about 1 in 50,000 children and affects the joints, heart, skin and (sometimes) the brain. The acute attack produces painful swollen joints, skin rashes, nodules in the tissues just beneath the skin, and fever. The effect on the heart is variable. There may be a persistently raised heart rate, minor irregularities in the heartbeat, or even acute congestive heart failure, but recovery is the rule. Damage to the heart valves may reveal itself many years later in RHEUMATIC HEART DISEASE with serious disturbance of cardiac function.

Treatment involves the administration of penicillin to clear up the streptococcal infection; cortisone-like drugs (steroids) and aspirin are used to relieve symptoms. Better and earlier treatment of streptococcal infections (and of rheumatic fever itself) has reduced the chance of subsequent heart problems.

rheumatic heart disease

A complication or end result of an attack of RHEUMATIC FEVER.

The interval between the original rheumatic fever (usually occurring in childhood or adolescence), and the appearance of symptoms of rheumatic heart disease may vary from a few years to many decades. Rheumatic fever attacks the heart muscle and the heart valves; while the damage to the heart muscle is usually repairable, changes in the heart valves may subsequently cause the cusps of the valves to become deformed or stick together at their margins.

The heart valves most affected are the *mitral* and *aortic* valves. Two main types of defect can be produced: (1) narrowing of the valve opening with obstruction to the flow of blood (*stenosis*) or (2) *incompetence* and *regurgitation,* in which the valve fails to close properly and allows a reverse flow of blood.

Symptoms depend largely on the type of defect present and its severity. For many years the heart may continue to compensate for a defectively functioning valve; but shortness of breath on fairly severe exertion, occurring in a patient in his 20s or 30s, is characteristic of *mitral stenosis* in particular. *Aortic stenosis* is typically a complication seen later in life. *Incompetence* of the valves will also eventually produce symptoms; these may include increasing shortness of breath on exercise, palpitations, angina pectoris, attacks of shortness of breath on lying down at night, or fainting attacks.

Treatment involves first increasing the strength of the heartbeat with suitable drugs and the avoidance of overexertion. If the problem is severe, surgical repair of the valve or its replacement by a grafted or plastic valve may be required.

rheumatism

A general term that indicates any of the various diseases of the musculoskeletal system characterized by pain and stiffness of the joints.

See ARTHRITIS, RHEUMATOID ARTHRITIS, OSTEO-ARTHRITIS.

rheumatoid arthritis

A chronic inflammatory disease affecting the connective tissue of the joints. It has been found all over the world, although the incidence is considerably higher in temperate climates, and the symptoms are more pronounced in cold damp places.

Women are affected more often than men, and the usual age of onset is between 25 and 55. There is a slight genetic factor. The cause of the disease is not known; both autoimmune and infective factors have been implicated. It has been suggested that a "slow virus" infection may be a cause, and in many cases a rheumatoid factor (RF) is detected in the blood. It is an immunoglobulin, but is not thought to be the cause of the disease but rather to develop as a consequence of the disease.

The onset of rheumatoid arthritis is usually insidious, but in some cases it may be acute and accompanied by fever and loss of weight. In others, there may be malaise (a general feeling of being unwell) and fatigue for some weeks with pains and stiffness in the joints. In time arthritis appears, often beginning in the joints of the fingers and spreading to involve the wrists and elbows; less commonly the feet are first affected, with the disease spreading to the ankles and knees. The shoulders and hips may be involved. The joints become swollen, tender and hot, and all movement is painful. The joints are stiff, particularly in the morning and after rest. When the large joints of the shoulder and hip are affected, the resulting disability may be serious.

The joints of the spinal column may be affected, especially in the neck, and the patient may have pain and tenderness in the joint of the lower jaw just in front of the ear; this interferes with eating. Nodules may develop under the skin, and disturbances of the circulation are common in which the hands may sweat to an abnormal extent or may become cold and blue. Complications sometimes involve the chest, with the development of an effusion in the pleural cavity and even acute pneumonia. The lymph nodes draining the affected joints are often enlarged, and in about 5% of patients the spleen is also enlarged. Anemia is common, its severity being proportional to the severity of the disease; the eye may be inflamed or dry.

Diagnosis of the disease may be difficult, as the presence of rheumatoid factor is not entirely specific. The ERYTHROCYTE SEDIMENTATION RATE of the blood is raised, but again the finding is not specific. In a typical case, radiographic examination will show characteristic changes in the joints; these, with the polyarthritis and a positive test for rheumatoid factor, will make the diagnosis certain.

Treatment begins with rest, initially in bed (if necessary, with sedation). Anemia must be treated; as it responds poorly to iron given by mouth, a blood transfusion may be recommended. The diet must be good, possibly with vitamin supplements. In the acute phase of the disease the inflamed joints are fixed in light splints to prevent the development of deformity, but they must be put through a full range of movement at least twice a day, and the patient must try to prevent wasting of the muscles by carrying out isometric contractions at least 12 times an hour. As soon as active movement of the affected joints is possible, they must be exercised by graded movement; active exercises are then started, designed to rebuild wasted muscles.

A number of drugs may be used in treatment. The least expensive and most effective is aspirin, given daily in divided doses. About one-third of patients find that they develop indigestion, in which case it is possible to use special preparations of the drug. Other anti-inflammatory drugs are used such as indomethacin, phenylbutazone, flufenamic acid and ibuprofen, but they sometimes have adverse effects on the blood and the digestive system. Gold salts have been shown to produce symptomatic relief, but they have a number of serious adverse effects which mean that they must be used with caution under close medical supervision. Chloroquine is useful in chronic cases, but corticosteroids are not advised for long-term treatment and are not used in short-term treatment except under special circumstances. They may be injected locally into inflamed joints to relieve pain. Penicillamine has proved useful in severe cases, but its place in treatment is not yet fully determined.

Surgery has a considerable part to play in the treatment both of acute cases and of the deformity that may result in chronic disease. In the acute stages where there is much pain and thickening of the synovial membranes, excision of the affected membrane may be most beneficial; in chronic disease, ARTHROPLASTY and tendon surgery may be employed in selected cases.

See also OSTEOARTHRITIS.

rhinitis

Inflammation of the mucous membrane that lines the nose (nasal mucosa). Rhinitis may be caused by the common cold virus (of which there are over 100 species) or by an allergic reaction to substances such as grass pollens, in which case it is a symptom of hay fever. Repeated attacks of acute rhinitis may lead to a chronic form.

The symptoms of allergic rhinitis (hay fever) include nasal congestion, runny nose, sneezing, and itching of the nose, eyes and, sometimes, the throat

ribonucleic acid

See DNA/RNA.

rickets

A disease of childhood resulting from deficiency of vitamin D, which leads to faulty or inadequate bone growth.

Vitamin D is essential to health because it aids the absorption of calcium from food and is also important for the incorporation of minerals into bone. Vitamin D is formed in the skin after exposure to sunlight and is also found in small amounts in milk and dairy products. Fish oils are rich in vitamin D. Many margarines are fortified with vitamin D, and so are most milks on the market, including dried milk. Cheap, monotonous diets often contain too little of the vitamin, particularly among the poorer sections of the community. A contributory factor to the development of rickets, especially in high altitudes, is that there is often insufficient winter sunlight to assist the natural formation of vitamin D in the skin.

Children suffering from vitamin D deficiency typically have softening and irregular growth of bones, swollen joints, distorted limbs, deformities of the chest and similar malformations. Many "cripples" of the past were actually people who had suffered as children from bone disease due to vitamin D deficiency and were grossly handicapped as a result. Although rickets is much less common in developed countries than it used to be, it is still seen in poorer areas—especially in inner cities where children see little sunlight.

When milk or margarine is fortified with vitamin D there is usually little need to supplement the diet with vitamin D. Synthetic forms of the vitamin are many times more effective in preventing rickets than the natural oils.

rickettsiae

Microorganisms intermediate in size between bacteria and viruses; like viruses, they grow within the cells, but like bacteria are sensitive to appropriate antibiotics. They are transmitted to man by the bites of certain arthropods—lice, fleas, ticks and mites.

In addition to infecting humans rickettsiae can infect small mammals such as rats, rabbits and squirrels—who may form a reservoir of infection. They produce the Typhus group of fevers including trench fever, murine typhus, louse-borne typhus, scrub typhus (TSUTSUGAMUSHI DISEASE), Q FEVER and ROCKY MOUNTAIN SPOTTED FEVER.

rigor mortis

The stiffening of the muscles that occurs after death as a result of changes in substances in the blood. It begins four to ten hours after death in the muscles at the back of the neck, spreads to the rest of the body in a few hours and lasts approximately two to four days.

ringworm

See TINEA.

RNA

See DNA/RNA.

Rocky Mountain spotted fever

A tick-borne typhus fever. There are a number of typhus fevers caused by infection with various species of RICKETTSIAE, which vary in the manner of their occurrence according to the nature of the insects spreading the infection and the mammals which form a reservoir for the rickettsiae. Rabbits, chipmunks, squirrels, rats and mice as well as dogs harbor the organisms responsible for Rocky Mountain spotted fever; the disease is spread to man by *Ixodes* ticks.

The disease shows a seasonal incidence, being prevalent from May to September, and occurs not only in the Rocky Mountains but in other parts of the United States and in other countries.

About 12 days after the tick bite the patient develops fever, with pains in the muscles and joints. The fever may rise high enough to produce delirium; there is a cough, and on the fourth or fifth day a rash appears. Between the 12th and 14th day the condition improves.

The disease is treated by the administration of chloramphenicol and tetracyclines.

rodent ulcer

A chronic, "gnawing" ulcer arising from a tumor known as a *basal-cell epithelioma*. The ulcer, usually on the face or nose of elderly people, is locally malignant but the cancer cells do not (like most cancers) spread to other parts of the body.

It may be excised by surgery, or may be treated by RADIATION THERAPY: the ulcer will often heal completely after a few exposures to radium.

rosacea

A chronic disease (formerly known as *acne rosacea*) affecting the skin of the nose, forehead, cheeks and chin. The skin is colored red or pink as a result of the dilation of capillaries (tiny blood vessels near the surface) and papules and pustules frequently develop.

In severe cases the condition may progress to *rhinophyma*, in which the nose is hugely swollen and deformed. A great deal of debate exists over the cause of rosacea. There is some evidence to link it with the excessive consumption of stimulants such as coffee, tea and alcohol; but it is more common in women over 40, so hormonal influences may be important.

Treatment typically involves the administration of oral tetracycline and application of cortisone ointments; more recently, the drug metronidazole has been found to be effective.

roundworms

The roundworm *Ascaris lumbricoides* is a human parasite found all over the world, especially in the tropics. Its life cycle is bizarre.

The human host swallows the eggs; larvae hatch out in the small intestine, make their way through the intestinal wall into the bloodstream and become lodged in the lungs. Here they pass through the walls of the capillary blood vessels into the air spaces of the lungs and wriggle up through the air passages into the throat (pharynx). They then make for the intestine again via the esophagus and on reaching the small intestine develop into adults. They may live in the intestine for a year.

ROUNDWORM

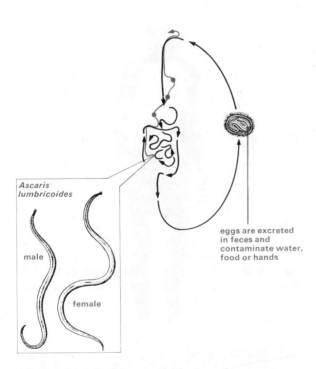

*Ascaris
lumbricoides*

male

female

eggs are excreted
in feces and
contaminate water,
food or hands

Ascariasis, infestation with the roundworm pictured above, is due to poor hygiene and is estimated to affect one quarter of the world's population.

If their numbers are few they may produce no symptoms; but if they are present as a heavy infection they produce a cough and spasm of the air passages as they pass through the lungs, and interfere with the absorption of food from the intestine. They may wander up the esophagus to emerge at the mouth or the nose, or may be vomited up, or passed from the rectum. They may entwine to form a ball of worms which obstructs the small intestine.

The most effective treatment is piperazine, given as piperazine citrate in a single dose from 500 mg for a child 1 year old to 3 gm for an adult. Thiabendazole may also be used.

rubella

Another name for GERMAN MEASLES.

rupture

See HERNIA.

S

salpingitis

Inflammation of a FALLOPIAN TUBE. The inflammation often arises from GONORRHEA, either immediately or months or years after the infection. Another kind of salpingitis is caused by streptococci or staphylococci bacteria, which may reach the Fallopian tubes following childbirth or abortion. The infection typically produces EDEMA in the mucous membrane which lines the tubes and a discharge of pus may leave the tubes and cause PERITONITIS or an abscess.

Among the consequences of salpingitis are sterility, as a result of the tubes becoming blocked so that ova can no longer reach the womb; and ECTOPIC PREGNANCY, in which the fertilized ovum does not reach the uterus but grows in the tube itself, eventually causing it to rupture—requiring emergency surgery.

Most early cases of salpingitis can be controlled by the administration of an appropriate antibiotic. However, in advanced or long-term cases, surgical incision and drainage or removal of the Fallopian tube may be needed.

sarcoidosis

A disease of unknown cause mainly affecting young adults; in many ways it resembles tuberculosis, but there is no evidence of any infective element. Many organs of the body can be affected by the disease; on examination they are seen to contain *granulomas* (tumor-like masses of granular tissue).

The lungs, eyes and skin may be involved as well as the lymphatic system, liver, spleen, heart, muscles and nervous system. In many cases there are no symptoms and the disease is discovered only by routine x-ray examination.

There is often no need for treatment in these cases and spontaneous remissions are common; steroid drugs may be effective in relieving any troublesome symptoms. Sufferers have a normal expectation of life.

sarcoma

A malignant tumor originating in connective tissues, bone or muscle.

Sarcoma is distinguished from the other main type of malignant tumor, *carcinoma* (which is composed mainly of cells similar to skin or mucous membrane). There are about 20 cases of carcinoma to every one of sarcoma. The most common sarcomas are the malignant bone tumors, some of which (such as *osteogenic sarcoma*) are especially common in childhood. A combination of radiation therapy and anticancer drugs may arrest the disease for long periods. In some cases surgery is needed.

See also CANCER.

scabies

A skin disease caused by infestation with the parasitic "itch mite" (*Sarcoptes scabiei*). The disease is spread by close contact with infested persons.

The female of the parasite burrows into the skin, particularly on the front of the wrist, the sides and webs of the fingers, the buttocks, the genitals and the feet. Eggs are deposited in the small tunnels she makes, while the male remains on the surface of the skin.

The burrowing activities of the parasites cause intense itching and the original small blister-like lesions may be made much worse by scratching. Treatment will be successful only if all of the patient's close contacts and his family are treated for the disease. Various effective applications are now available to people with this condition, including benzyl benzoate emulsion, gamma benzene hexachloride cream, and monosulfiram in alcohol.

scar

The mark (also known technically as a *cicatrix*) in the skin or an internal organ left by a healed wound, ulcer or other lesion.

Scar tissue consists essentially of fibers which, in the case of scars on the skin surface, are covered by an imperfect formation of cuticle. The fibrous tissue is produced by cells of connective tissue brought to the lesion by the bloodstream.

At first the scar is soft because the fibrous tissue is supplied with ample blood vessels, so that the scar appears more red than the surrounding skin. As fibers contract and harden, the scar loses its blood vessels and becomes whitish.

There is wide variation in the amount of scar tissue which appears, depending on the extent to which the wound is allowed to gape during the healing process. The smaller the distance between the edges of the wound, the less will be the amount of scar tissue. That is one of the reasons why it is considered essential to close a wound (either surgical or traumatic) with stitches to make the resulting scar as thin and as faint as possible.

In general, scars do not regenerate specialized tissue, such as the hair follicles and sweat glands of skin, although damaged muscles and nerves do regenerate specialized fibers in scars.

When large areas of skin have been damaged, as in burning, the resulting scars may contract so much that movement becomes restricted. In such cases plastic surgery is indicated, as it is for disfiguring facial scars.

scarlet fever

Some of the streptococci which cause sore throats produce a toxin (poison) which brings the skin out in a characteristic scarlet rash. This is most commonly seen in children of school age, who develop fever, a rapid pulse, headache, sore throat and perhaps abdominal pain and vomiting. After one or two days a rash starts on the neck, spreads to the chest and then covers the abdomen and the limbs. It leaves a pale area around the mouth which lasts for a few days, after which it fades. The skin becomes scaly, and the scales flake off. While the rash is present the tongue is covered with a white "fur" which peels off to leave the tongue red, with prominent papillae ("strawberry tongue").

In the last century scarlet fever (or *scarlatina*) was a serious disease, complicated by infection of the middle ear, rheumatic fever and inflammation of the kidneys. But with the advent of drugs such as sulfonamides and penicillin, its importance has declined. The streptococcus involved may be found in the throat or nose of healthy carriers.

schistosomiasis

A chronic illness caused by parasitic worms which live in the blood vessels around the liver and bladder. Schistosomiasis is one of the most important causes of ill health, lethargy and premature death in tropical

SCHISTOSOMIASIS

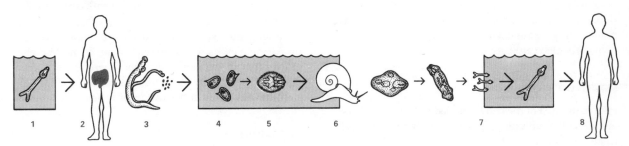

LIFE CYCLE OF *Schistosomatidae* FLUKES

Schistosomiasis affects 200 million people throughout the world. Infective larvae (1) abound in freshwater in many countries and penetrate the skin of bathers (2). They develop into flukes which enter the bloodstream and damage many organs. Adult flukes lay eggs (3) which are excreted into water (4) and hatch into miracidia *(5). These penetrate a snail host (6) and change into thousands of larvae which are released into the water (7), where they can reinfect humans.*

countries: worldwide more than 200 million people are infected.

The complex life cycle of the parasite starts with an infected person discharging eggs in the urine or feces. If the eggs reach fresh water in a lake, canal or irrigation ditch they hatch into *miracidia*, which may infect a particular form of snail. After multiplication inside the snail the *schistosomes* are released into the water as *cercariae*, and this larval form is highly infectious. The cercariae readily penetrate the skin of anyone swimming or wading in contaminated water for even a few minutes.

Once in the bloodstream, the cercariae migrate to the lungs; then, depending on their subtype, they move either to the veins leading to the liver or to veins around the bladder. Having reached the network of veins, the cercariae mature into adult worms: the male is about 2 cm long and the thinner, longer female lives in a cleft in the male's body. Schistosome worms may live for as long as 30 years and some varieties lay up to 3,000 eggs daily. The eggs penetrate the lining of the bowel and bladder and so are passed out of the body with the excreta.

Schistosomiasis may cause few or no symptoms, but when the infection is heavy the patient may pass blood in the urine or have repeated attacks of diarrhea. Weakness, lack of energy and repeated attacks of abdominal pain cause chronic ill health, eventually leading to failure of either the liver or kidneys.

Schistosomiasis can be treated by drugs which destroy the worms, but long-term control depends on public health measures supported by individuals and communities—the life cycle of the parasite can be interrupted by providing safe disposal of sewage, backed up by the elimination of the snails from irrigation channels and watercourses.

schizophrenia

A mental illness characterized by false beliefs, irrational thinking and a retreat from contact with the normal world. Over half the long-term patients in mental institutions have schizophrenia, which affects about 1% of the adult population of all countries.

The illness typically begins in adolescence; the onset may be abrupt or gradual. Early symptoms include hallucinations—especially the hearing of voices critical of current actions, with the patient discussed in the third person; *delusions*, typically of persecution (PARANOIA); and *flight of ideas*—rapid and apparently meaningless changes in the topic of conversation. Often the schizophrenic withdraws from his family and friends to spend hours and days on end in solitary silence. He may become convinced that his thoughts and actions are being controlled by outside influences. Among other common variants of schizophrenia are CATATONIA, in which the patient spends minutes or hours motionless and mute, often in a bizarre posture; and *hebephrenia*, with rapid swings in the emotional mood, incoherent speech, and outbursts of laughing and crying.

The cause of schizophrenia is unknown, but there is a genetic factor; the disease is found in 5% of brothers or sisters of schizophrenic patients and even more often in twins. There also seems to be an environmental factor—the first attack of schizophrenia may be provoked by emotional conflicts within the family. Despite enormous research efforts no one has yet found convincing evidence of an underlying chemical disturbance in the brain of schizophrenics.

Even so, there is an effective treatment; drugs of the phenothiazine group, such as chlorpromazine (Largactil) or trifluoperazine (Stelazine), reduce the length and severity of attacks of schizophrenia. Many patients with chronic schizophrenia are able to live in the community or with their families as long as they have regular drug treatment.

See also PSYCHOSES.

sciatica

Pain in the area of the body supplied by the sciatic nerve, including the buttocks, hip, back and outer part of the thigh, leg, ankle and foot.

It is caused by irritation of the spinal nerve roots which go to make up the sciatic nerve. The most common reason for the irritation is disease of the joint between the 4th and 5th lumbar vertebrae. The intervertebral disk—a cushion of cartilage between the vertebrae—may protrude and encroach on the space through which the nerve root passes (SLIPPED DISK), or the space may become narrowed by arthritic changes in the bones and ligaments of the joint. Rarely, sciatica is a symptom of a more serious disease of the lumbar part of the spine.

The pain down the leg is aggravated by straining, coughing, sneezing or bending and the part of the leg affected may become numb. The ankle reflex disappears, and the sensation produced by a pin prick is blunted. The muscles may be weakened and, in consequence, the foot may drop in severe cases. The lower part of the back is stiff and loses its normal contour (it becomes flat), while the muscles along each side of the spine go into spasm. Sciatica is usually accompanied by lower back pain, and raising the leg straight makes the pain in the back and the leg more intense.

The first line of treatment is rest in bed: the bed must be firm, and in most cases this is best assured by putting boards under the mattress. Analgesics (painkillers, such as aspirin) are useful, as may be the local application of heat. Resistant cases may need physical therapy followed by special exercises and perhaps manipulation of the back.

Only in severe cases of demonstrable disk protrusion (slipped disk) is an operation advisable; but when the protruded disk is removed in a well-chosen case, the relief is usually immediate and lasting.

scleroderma

A rare disease which produces hardening of the skin, which becomes smooth, shiny and tight. The skin of the face may shrink so much that it becomes difficult to open the mouth widely; movement of the fingers is hampered and they may develop contractures.

The skin manifestations are part of a general systemic disturbance which affects the connective tissue of the intestine, lungs and kidneys, and may affect the heart. The cause of the disease is not known with certainty, but it is thought to be an immunological disorder.

Patients may survive for 20 years or more after the disease makes its appearance, usually in middle age, more often in women than men. There is no known effective treatment, but administration of cortico-steroids may bring subjective improvement.

scoliosis

Scoliosis refers to an abnormal side-to-side curvature of the spine. It may involve the neck (*cervical scoliosis*), the chest region (*dorsal scoliosis*) or the small of the back (*lumbar scoliosis*). The main area of curvature will have secondary curvatures above and below it as a result of the body's attempt to maintain a more or less upright posture.

Scoliosis may be congenital, in which case it is associated with malformation of one or more vertebrae. Acquired forms of the condition occurring in later life are more common, however, and may result from disease of the bones of the spine or paralysis of the muscles which support the spinal column (*paralytic scoliosis*).

Paralysis of the muscles as a result of a disease such as poliomyelitis results in a loss of support to the spine from the muscles of the trunk. Scoliosis affecting one or the other side will then occur; if allowed to persist, it may result in secondary bony deformities.

The most common type of scoliosis has no detectable cause and the bones and muscles appear normal. The deformity is not usually severe in cases such as these, which are probably the result of prolonged habits of incorrect posture.

Special exercises are important in the treatment of the simpler types of postural scoliosis; but if bony deformity or muscle weakness is involved, surgical treatment or the use of various types of spinal supports may be necessary.

The prognosis for the simpler types is good but in more severe cases complete correction of the deformity may be impossible.

scotoma

A defect in the visual field that may be caused by a variety of disorders affecting the optic nerves. A "blind spot" may be one-sided or bilateral and sometimes not appreciated until full visual field testing is performed by an eye specialist.

Color scotoma may occur where certain areas of the retina are insensitive to color vision. They may be congenital, or acquired through damage to the nerve fibers brought about by optic neuritis—itself caused by a large number of conditions from anemia, disseminated sclerosis and diabetes, to tobacco, alcohol, chemical toxic agents and vitamin deficiencies. The treatment of the neuritis is directed toward the cause, and recovery from its effects is possible if the condition is not progressive.

screening

The periodic examination of the body to determine the general state of health and to discover the development of any early signs or symptoms of disease.

A screening program may involve individuals or entire communities exposed to special risks. It may be devoted to looking for one disorder of one part of the body—as in routine "Pap smears" of the cervix to assess any cellular change that may indicate early signs of cancer of the cervix, or routine chest x rays of miners to detect early signs of silicosis. It may be devoted to an assessment of as many of the body's organs or systems as are amenable to standardized tests—sometimes called *multiphasic screening*—and be done as part of an annual or periodic physical. Presymptomatic testing, as in multiphasic screening, is thus a routine of some health care systems for communities, and for others may perhaps only be offered as a preemployment examination by the employer's medical service. Most physicians nevertheless nowadays do some screening of their patients, although—because of the cost of the more complicated tests—in most cases the screening will be undertaken only in the presence of preexisting symptoms (in order to help obtain accurate diagnosis).

In a complete screening program, much of the testing may be done by specially trained nursing staff or technicians. It may involve all or any of the standard measurements of height, weight, skinfold thickness, chest expansion and abdominal girth. The vision will be tested, and a hearing test and dental examination may be included. Respiratory efficiency will be measured by a flow-meter and the blood pressure will be noted lying and standing. An electrocardiogram (ECG) will be taken at rest and after exercise, as well as a chest x ray and perhaps a sputum analysis. The female's breasts will be palpated and MAMMOGRAPHY may be undertaken. In the man a rectal examination may be included to check for enlargement of the prostate gland; in a female the physician will perform a pelvic examination (vagina and uterus) and take a cervical smear. A urine specimen will be analyzed for the presence of sugar, protein or bacteria, and perhaps a specimen of stool will be examined for the presence of intestinal parasites or contagious organisms, where the medical history indicates a possible risk. Blood tests are given which indicate the hemoglobin level (abnormally low in

anemia) and reveal the concentration of many chemical constituents of the blood (for example, an abnormal elevation in uric acid is diagnostic of gout). A blood count to determine the relative number of white cells, red cells and platelets per unit of blood, is also diagnostically useful—characteristic changes occur in various diseases, while a normal count is a good sign. Tests of liver and kidney function may also be performed.

In some community screening services, questionnaires have been used to gain some insight into individual psychological makeup and to attempt to identify those in need of follow-up. The value of screening is considerable, particularly if it is directed to those with special need or known vulnerability. Economically, however, it may be both expensive and time-consuming and may give a low yield of abnormality in well-cared for patients and communities as a whole.

scurvy

A condition caused by prolonged dietary deficiency of vitamin C (ascorbic acid), which man cannot synthesize. It is characterized by bruising of the dry scaly skin, bleeding gums (which are swollen and spongy), and delayed wound repair. Lassitude and weakness, anemia, loss of appetite, and internal bleeding may also occur. It was once an extremely common disease in seafarers deprived of fresh fruit and vegetables, but full-blown scurvy is rare today.

An average person needs 75 mg of ascorbic acid a day, and a normal diet contains an excess; but elderly persons may frequently suffer from deficiencies due to inadequate diet. Infant feeding with cow's milk alone may lead to scurvy.

Scurvy can be cured by the administration of ascorbic acid (100 mg/day) within two weeks; a balanced diet must thereafter be maintained.

sebaceous cyst

The sebaceous glands of the skin, which secrete *sebum*— a lubricant which helps maintain the health of the epidermis—are present throughout the surface of the body except for the palms and soles. They are most common on the head, shoulders and trunk. If the gland's outlet on the skin surface becomes blocked, the gland may continue to secrete and thus form a *retention cyst*, distended with sebum. Typically, it is a hemispherical swelling, firm and discrete. The cyst may proceed, if uninfected, to reach a considerable size.

Sebaceous cysts frequently become infected, discharge and collapse. If a cyst remains or poses a problem it can be surgically removed.

seizures

Sudden convulsions, usually caused by epilepsy, high fever (in children), poisoning, or hysteria.

Hysterical fits have a purpose, very often to gain sympathy, and never occur without an audience. The patient is not incontinent, never hurts himself, and "wakes up" quickly if painful stimuli are applied. The true epileptic fit (see EPILEPSY) is usually a very different matter.

The patient with *petit mal* (a form of epileptic attack) experiences a very quick and short loss of consciousness, which may amount to no more than a momentary silence or loss of attention. The patient is typically anxious to conceal what has happened—or may not realize anything has happened.

The patient with *grand mal* (the typical epileptic attack) often becomes unconscious, falls, shakes, is incontinent and may hurt himself—perhaps biting his tongue during the attack. He recovers consciousness slowly and cannot be aroused during the attack, even by painful stimuli. There are several different variations on this pattern, with epileptic attacks ranging in duration and seriousness.

In *focal* or *Jacksonian epilepsy* only a part of the body shakes and the patient may remain conscious, although such a seizure often goes on to a full-blown generalized convulsion. In *temporal lobe epilepsy* the features of the attack are varied and can be bizarre: the patient may suffer a dramatic change of mood, talk nonsense and experience hallucinations or feelings of DEJA VU (the sensation that what are in reality new experiences have happened to the patient before). After the seizure has passed he may embark on acts at variance with his usual personality for which he afterward has no recollection.

Children may develop convulsions as the result of a high fever; such seizures do not necessarily mean that the child is epileptic. They are rare in the first six months of life and after the age of five years are always generalized.

Simple fainting may be confused with epilepsy, for the patient may show minor twitching movements, and there are diseases such as diabetes mellitus which may produce loss of consciousness. Some middle-aged women suffer from a condition described as "benign episodic falling" in which the legs suddenly give way, possibly as a result of momentary interruption of the blood supply to the brain; such patients do not usually lose consciousness.

While a patient with known epilepsy has no need of medical attention each time he has a seizure, attacks occurring for the first time should always be referred to a doctor, who will be very grateful for a full and accurate description of the seizure.

senility

Progressive impairment of mental and physical functions, brought about by aging, may lead to a state of senility—characterized by mental deterioration.

In the early stages, mental versatility and the ability to maintain adequate intellectual performance during stress are reduced. Mental fatigue, anxiety and irritability increase with time. Speech becomes slower and impairment is noted in concentration, memory and time orientation. Dress and personal appearance are less tidy and appetite diminished. Alcohol and sedatives have an increased effect. Senile persons become increasingly self-absorbed and insensitive to the feelings and reactions of others; recall is delayed, calculation labored and there may be incomprehensible speech.

Some senile persons show restless overactive behavior and impulsive or inappropriate activity that can prove dangerous or hazardous to themselves. In the final stages, skills in performing even routine domestic tasks are lost, apathetic demeanor and behavior indicate an inability to communicate; there may be repetition of old familiar phrases that conceal the emptiness of the personality. The last intellectual function to disappear is loss of personal identity, manifested by the inability to recall one's own name. Progressive impairment of mental ability and other functions often leads to fecal and urinary incontinence, an inability to walk and ultimately stupor and coma.

Senility is basically caused by diminished circulation of blood to the brain, in most cases as the consequence of progressive arteriosclerosis. Because the onset of this is variable, senility may occur over a wide age range. It must not be confused with depression, a condition common in old age, which may produce similar symptoms.

septal defect

See HOLE IN THE HEART.

septicemia

The presence and persistence in the bloodstream of pathogenic (disease-causing) bacteria. If the bacteria are not destroyed with the administration of an appropriate antibiotic, they can multiply and cause a massive infection of the body (systemic infection) possibly leading to death.

The signs and symptoms of septicemia usually include chills, fever, and the formation of pustules and abscesses.

The most commonly encountered bacteria that can cause septicemia are: *Enterobacter* species, *Escherichia coli*, *Klebsiella* species, *Meningococcus*, *Pneumococcus*,

Proteus species and *Staphylococcus aureus*. Less commonly encountered bacteria that can cause septicemia include *Pseudomonas aeruginosa, Staphylococcus epidermidis* and *ß-Hemolytic streptococcus*.

Also called *blood poisoning*.

serum sickness

When sera were widely used for the treatment of microbial disease, a number of patients developed reactions to the injections. These were usually reactions to foreign proteins from the animals in whom the sera had been prepared—the horse in particular—and often appeared days or weeks after the injection had been given.

Serum sickness produces swelling of the face, itching of the skin and severe joint pains and there may be nausea, vomiting and fever. It should be noted that very similar allergic reactions may occur in some patients given drugs or receiving blood transfusions.

The condition is now rare since most microbial diseases are now treated with antibiotics; sera prepared from human sources, less likely to cause allergic reactions, are widely available when their use is unavoidable.

The best treatment for serum sickness is the use of cortisone-like drugs (steroids), though antihistamines may also help. Response is usually rapid.

sex hormones

Chemical substances, secreted by the testis in the male and the ovary in the female, which determine sexual characteristics and function.

In the male the secretion of *androgens* (the most potent of which is *testosterone*) from the testis aid the development of the male sex organs, stimulate the secretion of semen, and are responsible for the masculine sexual characteristics.

In the female the secretion of *estrogen* and *progesterone* from the ovary stimulates the development of the breasts, the uterus and the external genitals, and maintains the menstrual cycle and the capacity of the woman for reproduction through pregnancy. In both sexes the sex organs (gonads) are under the control of the PITUITARY GLAND, which initiates their development at puberty and maintains their function in adult life.

Deficiencies of the sex hormones may occur where the glands themselves are abnormal, or where pituitary secretions are insufficient. In contrast, sexual precocity may be associated in either sex with tumors of the gonads, pituitary gland, or ADRENAL GLANDS.

Treatment with sex hormones is effective for identified deficiencies, but the tailoring of the dosage to the

individual is essential and requires complicated biochemical analysis. Moderate supplementation is used in treating infertility, in either sex, and the menopause in the female; sex hormones are also sometimes used in the treatment of certain types of maglignant disease. For example, some hormones have antitumor effects on breast and womb cancers.

See also HORMONES.

sexually transmitted diseases

See VENEREAL DISEASE.

shock (cardiovascular)

Shock is the medical term for collapse due to inadequate circulation of the blood. Whatever the cause, the symptoms include pallor, sweating, nausea, restlessness, confusion, weakness and finally loss of consciousness. Shock may be caused by failure of the heart to pump sufficient blood through the body—because of, say, a CORONARY THROMBOSIS—by loss of blood as the result of hemorrhage (internal or external), by the plasma loss associated with severe burns, or by loss of body fluids from excessive vomiting or diarrhea (as in CHOLERA). Primary shock, or a faint, may be caused by the blood pooling in some veins and arteries which have suddenly lost their reflex tone; the consequent loss of consciousness is caused by impaired circulation to the brain.

When shock occurs the patient should be placed at rest, kept warm with light coverings, and the legs raised slightly to encourage the return of blood to the brain. Shock due to diminished circulatory volume—as in hemorrhage, trauma or dehydration—requires restoration of the volume to normal by the intravenous administration of fluids.

The prevention of shock depends on the proper evaluation of the factors causing circulatory failure. The prompt initiation of therapy in cases of trauma, by teams of medical or paramedical personnel, has done much to save lives that would otherwise have been lost through irreversible damage to the heart, brain, or kidneys brought about through sustained circulatory collapse.

sickle cell anemia

Red blood cells contain the red pigment HEMOGLOBIN. In the majority of people, hemoglobin has a characteristic and unvarying structure and is referred to as *hemoglobin A* (or *adult hemoglobin*).

In certain people, a minute abnormality occurs in the chemical structure of the hemoglobin molecule, resulting in what is referred to as a *mutant hemoglobin*. These abnormal hemoglobin pigments are inherited from parent to child. Two forms of inheritance occur. The abnormal hemoglobin may be present in only one of the parents and the child can then only inherit a single dose and its cells will contain only a small proportion of the abnormal pigment. In such cases little harm will result. If both parents carry the abnormality, however, the child may inherit a double dose, causing the red blood cells to contain a large amount of the abnormal pigment. Serious illness may follow.

In many cases, fortunately, the clinical effects of even a double type of inheritance are minimal. In the case of the abnormal pigment referred to as *hemoglobin S* (or *sickle hemoglobin*)—which is common in persons from Africa or of African descent—the chemical abnormality present results in a tendency for the red blood cells to become distorted in a crescent shape ("sickle cells") if the level of oxygen in the arterial blood falls. This "sickling trait" can be identified by microscopic examination of the blood.

Sickle cell anemia refers to the double inheritance of hemoglobin S from both parents with large amounts of sickle hemoglobin in the cells. Even slight degrees of oxygen lack will result in a marked "sickling" change in the blood and consequent obstruction to the circulation in various parts of the body by masses of sickled cells ("sickle cell crisis"). During a sickle cell crisis (and, to a lesser extent, at other times as well), the sickle cells hemolyze (are destroyed and liberate hemoglobin into the surrounding fluid) in great numbers—sometimes enough to produce jaundice and to lower the red cell count seriously. Severe pain, dangerous organ damage and even death may result. In addition, sickle cell anemia creates a predisposition to stroke. Recovery is possible, however; with good medical care the patient may live a normal life, though crises may recur.

The single type of inheritance usually presents no symptoms.

See also ANEMIA.

siderosis

A disease caused by the excessive inhalation of iron oxide dust. It is comparable initially to the effects of inhaling silica dust (which produces SILICOSIS).

Iron-ore miners and workers in the iron and steel industries are at special risk if they are unprotected by respirators. The condition causes less progressive lung damage than silicosis because the iron oxide particles do not provoke such an extensive fibrotic reaction (abnormal formation of fibrous tissue) in the lungs. The patient experiences breathlessness (DYSPNEA) and may cough up phlegm that is stained a dark color. Recovery, though with some permanent dyspnea that is not progressive, occurs when exposure to the dust-inhaling occupation ceases. There is no effective specific

treatment of the established case. Eradication depends on prevention.

Pulmonary siderosis is a rarity. More important is *hemosiderosis*, in which damage to the heart, liver and other internal organs is caused by an excess of iron in the body. It occurs most commonly as a complication of repeated blood transfusions for chronic anemias such as THALASSEMIA. The symptoms are similar to those of HEMOCHROMATOSIS, in which the accumulation of iron in the body is due to an inherited abnormality of iron metabolism.

See also PULMONARY DISEASES, ASBESTOSIS, PNEUMOCONIOSIS.

sigmoidectomy

Surgical removal of the final descending part of the large intestine (colon), which joins on to the rectum. It is usually performed because of cancer (sometimes because of ULCERATIVE COLITIS) in that part of the colon.

See also COLOSTOMY.

silicosis

A disease of the lungs caused by the prolonged inhalation of fine particles of silica, which provoke a response of FIBROSIS (or permanent scarring) in the pulmonary tissues.

The most common form of silica is quartz, which is abundantly distributed in the earth's surface. Thus, miners, rock-cutters, sand-blasters and those who work in the ceramic and glass industries are especially exposed to the risk of silicosis. In the areas in the lung in which the particles accumulate, nodules of fibrosis develop; in advanced cases, both lungs may be heavily scarred. The mechanical and chemical irritant effects of silica are responsible. The characteristic feature of silicosis is loss of the normal elasticity of the lungs, so that breathing requires more effort.

The earliest symptom is shortness of breath on exertion (DYSPNEA); this may be followed by coughing, wheezing, and other features similar to bronchitis. There is a particular proneness to tuberculosis. Diagnosis is made by chest x rays, which reveal the characteristic changes, although exposure to the dust over a period of 10 to 20 years may occur before symptoms are experienced. The changes in the lungs are irreversible and treatment is limited to the relief of symptoms. Methods by which the disease may be prevented include the use of efficient ventilation in modern industry, the regular use of respirators, and techniques of dust control.

See also PULMONARY DISEASES, ASBESTOSIS, PNEUMOCONIOSIS.

sinusitis

The sinuses are cavities in the bones of the face and skull. They reduce the weight of the skull and add resonance to the voice. The largest are the *frontal sinuses* in the forehead and the *maxillary sinuses* in the cheeks. The maxillary sinuses communicate with the nasal cavity; because of extension of infections from the nose, these are the most liable to infection. The symptoms of pain and tenderness over them (frequently with a thick nasal discharge) are the classical signs of sinusitis.

Because the floor of the maxillary sinus lies directly above the first and second upper molars on either side of the upper jaw, abscess of the roots of these teeth can also extend upward and may drain into the sinus to cause a spread of infection. However, a complication arising from the common cold is the most frequent cause of sinusitis; obstruction of the normal sinus drainage by thickened mucus produces intense pain in the sinus itself as the fluid level rises. The affected side of the face may swell, as well as the lower eyelid. X rays of the skull may reveal fluid that requires drainage.

Acute sinusitis may resolve rapidly with the administration of antibiotics and steam inhalations, which reduce the viscosity of the obstructive fluid. Chronic recurrent sinusitis may require surgical drainage and "sinus washout" to remove the accumulated pus. To achieve a permanent cure, it may be necessary to remove the lining membrane of the affected sinus surgically.

SINUSITIS

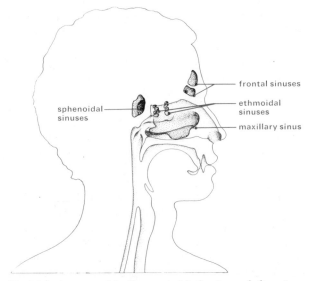

Sinusitis is caused by bacterial infection of the air sinuses which connect with the nose. It usually follows a head cold and causes a heavy feeling in the face and a blocked nose.

STRUCTURE OF THE SKIN

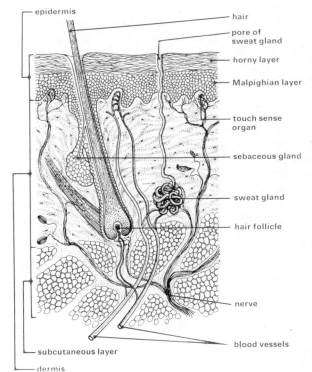

Skin encloses our entire body and provides a barrier against the entry of infection and the loss of tissue fluid. Although we think of skin as being extremely thin, the magnified section shown here reveals that it has many layers.

skin diseases

The skin may be affected by diseases which involve the whole body, but it is also especially vulnerable to external factors such as heat, radiation, and contact with chemicals and other irritants.

Structurally, the skin is divided into three rather distinct layers. The innermost (*subcutaneous*) layer serves as the receptacle for the formation and storage of fat and as a support for blood vessels and nerves which pass to the more superficial parts of the skin. It is also the layer in which the deeper hair follicles and the sweat glands originate.

The middle layer (*dermis*) consists of connective tissue which contributes to the support and elasticity of the skin. It is made up of a variety of cells which each have their own function—some to produce connective tissue, some to fight infection and so on. The dermis is also the layer in which sebaceous (oil-secreting) glands and the shorter hair follicles originate.

The *epidermis* is made up of layers of cells which form keratin (a tough protein substance which is found in hair, nails and other "horny" tissues), and cells which produce the pigment responsible for skin color (melanin). The epidermis constantly renews itself by shedding old layers as new ones are formed.

Any structure of the skin may be the primary structure affected by a particular disease; a malignant MELANOMA, for example, arises from the melanin-producing cells.

Exposure of the skin to the sun may cause burning and in pale-skinned persons prolonged exposure to strong sunlight increases the risk of skin cancer. Soap powders, solvents, dyes and cosmetics may all damage the skin, causing DERMATITIS. Some people develop an allergic sensitivity to metal (especially nickel) or other substances and are affected by a localized inflammation where the skin is in contact with the sensitizing agent (*contact dermatitis*).

Among the more common diseases are ECZEMA, in which the skin is reddened, weeping and intensely itchy; PSORIASIS, in which patches of silvery gray scales appear on the knees, elbows, and sometimes affect the whole body; thickening and roughening of the skin, as in LICHEN PLANUS; infection with bacteria and funguses, such as TINEA ("ringworm"); and a large spectrum of rashes associated with generalized infections, from measles to typhoid fever.

Identification of the cause of a skin disease often allows the irritant or the cause of an allergy to be removed. But even when the cause remains unknown (as in psoriasis), the symptoms can often be relieved by treatment with creams containing corticosteroid drugs, such as prednisolone or betamethasone. Sometimes the disease can be suppressed and symptoms eased by drugs taken by mouth.

See also ACNE, ALLERGY, BLACKHEADS, BLISTER, BOIL, BURNS, CARBUNCLE, CELLULITIS, CHILBLAIN, CORNS, DERMATOFIBROMA, DERMATOMYOSITIS, DERMATOSIS, ERYTHEMA, EXANTHEMA, FROSTBITE, HERPES SIMPLEX, HERPES ZOSTER, ICHTHYOSIS, INTERTRIGO, JAUNDICE, KERATITIS, KERATOSIS, KERATOSIS FOLLICULARIS, NEVUS, PAPILLOMA, PATCH TEST, PETECHIAE, PRURIGO, PRURITUS, RASH, RODENT ULCER, ROSACEA, SCABIES, SCAR, SCLERODERMA, SEBACEOUS CYST, STINGS, TATTOOING, TELANGIECTASIA, URTICARIA, WARTS, VITILIGO, XERODERMA.

sleep

A recurring state of inactivity accompanied by loss of awareness and a reduction in responsiveness to the environment. Unlike a coma, or unconsciousness caused by general anesthesia, a sleeping person can be easily aroused. Sleep is not a single state; electroencephalographic (EEG) studies, which measure the

electrical activity in the brain, show that there are two basic alternating states.

The first is known as *nonrapid eye movement (NREM) sleep*, during which the heart and respiratory rates slow down, the muscles are greatly but not completely relaxed, and the eyelids remain quite still. This can be divided into four general states of increasing depth of sleep. If awakened during the NREM sleep, the individual may say that he was "thinking" at the time of waking up.

During *rapid eye movement (REM) sleep*, the eyeballs move jerkily under closed lids, the heart and respiratory rates quicken (but this is variable), and the muscles (especially the neck muscles) are completely relaxed. This is the stage during which dreams occur, and dreams are more likely to be remembered if the individual wakes up or is awakened during REM sleep. (See DREAMING).

On going to bed, drowsiness is followed by NREM sleep of progressively increasing depth. After about 90 minutes, REM sleep takes over; during this first cycle of sleep, the REM stage may last only about 5 to 10 minutes. There are also fewer eye movements in the first cycle. During a night's sleep there may be 4 to 6 cycles of sleep, each lasting 80 to 100 minutes; the duration of REM sleep increases with each successive cycle and may make up about 30 minutes of the later cycles.

The amount of sleep required by an individual and the pattern of cycles varies according to age. The young adult who has about 6 to 8 hours of sleep spends about 20–25% of the night in REM sleep. The baby, whose sleep cycle is short (about 40 to 45 minutes) spends about 50% of the sleep in REM sleep. In the elderly—in whom the total sleep time required gradually diminishes—the proportion spent in REM sleep also reduces gradually toward 20%.

Despite these general patterns of sleep, the amount required varies a great deal from person to person. The function of sleep is not entirely clear, but is thought to be a time which the body uses to catch up with the growth processes and repair. Some sleep is certainly required, but how much is difficult to say. Extreme sleep deprivation (used as one method of "brainwashing") can lead to hallucinations and paranoia. However, most people manage to adapt to smaller amounts of sleep deprivation; they may complain of irritability and loss of efficiency (but again it is difficult to quantify how much of this is caused by the loss of sleep and how much to *worry* about loss of sleep and lack of efficiency). When they do get a chance to catch up on the lost sleep, they do so not only by longer hours of sleep but also by spending a greater proportion of it in REM sleep.

Sleep disorders may be *primary*—the inability to fall asleep or stay asleep for very long (insomnia) or the abnormal tendency to fall asleep or have uncontrollable

SLEEP

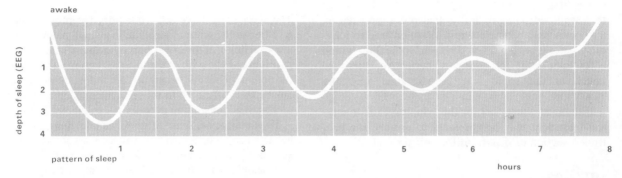

This diagram shows the fluctuations in the depth of sleep during a typical night as reflected by an EEG recording of brain waves. These waves change through stages 1 to 4 as the person becomes more deeply asleep. About every 90 minutes, the sleeper makes rapid eye movements (REMs); it is generally accepted that these coincide with periods of dreaming.

attacks of drowsiness in the daytime (narcolepsy)—or they may be *secondary* to various emotional or mental disturbances, chronic alcoholism, disease of the thyroid gland (hyperthyroidism), or brain disease.

The treatment of primary sleep disorders is the administration of the appropriate drug: stimulants (such as amphetamines) to control narcolepsy and sedatives or *hypnotics* (drugs that induce sleep) to control insomnia. It should be remembered, however, that it is unwise to take hypnotics for prolonged periods. Most of these drugs lose their effectiveness when used excessively and they may make the person psychologically and physically dependent on them. Withdrawal of most of these drugs may cause the individual to react by having more than usual amounts of REM sleep; this leads to vivid dreams, which then make the individual even more reluctant to stop taking hypnotics, creating a vicious cycle. Because of this, most doctors have become more selective in prescribing sleeping pills.

sleeping sickness

1. Short for *African sleeping sickness* (see AFRICAN TRYPANOSOMIASIS). 2. Another name for ENCEPHALITIS LETHARGICA.

slipped disk

The intervertebral disks—which act largely as "shock absorbers" between the vertebral bodies and convey flexibility of the spine—may herniate, or "slip" forward or sideways, as the result of trauma (80% of cases), weakness of the retaining ligaments, or changes

occurring in the fibrous consistency of the disk's outer wall. Typically, the disk "slips" while lifting a heavy weight with the body bent. The risk of a disk injury can be reduced by keeping the back straight while lifting. The condition is also known technically as *herniated disk*, *ruptured disk*, or *prolapsed disk*.

Protrusions of the lumbar disks (in the lower part of the back) are approximately 15 times more common than cervical (in the neck); thoracic disks (in the chest region) are rarely affected. Protrusion forward may impinge on the spinal cord or the nerves leading from it, so causing pain (SCIATICA), weakness, and numbness.

X rays of the spinal area will usually show loss of disk space between particular vertebral bodies (but will not show the disk itself, which is not opaque to x rays). Injection of a radiopaque dye (a myelogram) is required to define the precise extent of a disk's protrusion forward. Treatment depends largely on the severity of

SLIPPED DISK

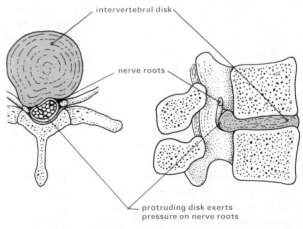

VERTEBRA SEEN FROM ABOVE   VERTEBRAE SEEN FROM SIDE

The picture shows a "slipped disk" where the fluid center of the disk herniates into the spinal canal. Such herniation results from excess strain or degeneration of the disk, and it presses on nearby nerves causing backache and pain in the legs.

the symptoms and the nature of the injury.

The first treatment for slipped disk is for the patient to rest in bed, lying on a firm mattress supported on a wooden base. Complete rest will often lead to relief of symptoms within a few days and to healing within a few weeks. If rest alone is ineffective, then the bones of the spine may be stretched apart by TRACTION.

If these measures fail, or the symptoms recur surgical treatment may be necessary to remove the protruded section of disk from the spinal canal.

smallpox

A highly contagious viral disease of man (also known as *variola* or *variola major*). At one time it was a major cause of death throughout the world.

Smallpox is characterized by a high fever of three or four days duration followed by a generalized skin eruption—consisting of crops of pink-red spots (1–2 mm in diameter) which typically appear first on the face and about the mouth. Within a few hours they begin to spread to the neck, arms and trunk. After a day or so the clear fluid in the center of the spots turns to pus, and this later dries to form scabs. The pustules (pus-filled sores) involve the deeper layers of the skin and after the crusty scabs fall off may leave pockmarks on the face or neck.

In people unprotected by vaccination, the mortality rate in epidemics has been as high as 20–40%. The disease is prevented by vaccination.

No specific treatment exists for smallpox, although some relatively new antiviral agents have been tried with variable success. Only by means of vaccination against smallpox—which establishes artificial immunity—is protection ensured. Revaccination is necessary at intervals of three years or less to maintain a high level of immunity.

Some countries require medical evidence of a smallpox vaccination before entry is permitted. Children with eczema are usually not vaccinated against smallpox, since there is a danger of the disease spreading from the vaccination site.

In 1921 there were over 100,000 cases in the United States; since 1953 no new cases have been reported. In 1958 over 250,000 cases were reported throughout the world—the majority on the Indian subcontinent. In 1977, for the first time, there were no reported cases of *variola major* anywhere in the world. However, cases of a less severe variant of smallpox (*variola minor*) continued to occur up to the late 1970s among the nomads in the remote desert regions of Somalia and near the borders of Ethiopia and Kenya. The last recorded case of endemic smallpox was in October 1977, and the World Health Organization firmly believes that the disease has been eradicated.

smell

The specialized nerve cells (olfactory receptors) which give rise to the sense of smell lie in a small patch of the mucosal lining of the upper part of the nasal cavity. This part is above the path of the main air currents that enter the nose with normal breathing, and odorous molecules must either diffuse up to the receptor cells or be drawn up by the act of sniffing in order to be detected.

To stimulate the sense of smell, an odorous molecule has to dissolve in the mucus which covers the receptor and set up a particular chemical change; this, in turn, electrically excites the nerve fibers of the main olfactory nerve.

Sensitivity to smell varies with the state of the nasal mucosa. It decreases during the common cold (especially if the nose is stuffy or runny), is impaired by smoking, and is increased in conditions of hunger. In general, females appear to have a slightly more acute sense of smell than males. Damage to nasal bones—in particular, fractures of the frontal base of the skull—may permanently impair the efficiency of the olfactory nerve; in some cases the sense of smell may be totally lost.

Discrimination between tens of thousands of different odor qualities is possible in the trained individual (for example, those who blend tea or prepare new types of

SMELL

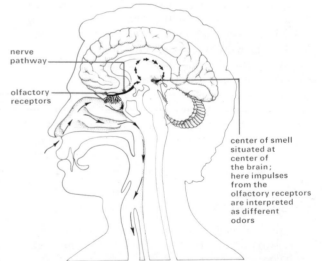

nerve pathway

olfactory receptors

center of smell situated at center of the brain; here impulses from the olfactory receptors are interpreted as different odors

Although our sense of smell is poorly developed compared with that of most animals, we are capable of distinguishing thousands of different aromas. Without it, our appreciation of food, our ability to enjoy numerous pleasant odors and our capacity to react to important signals from the environment—including dangerous fumes—would be lost.

perfumes). Physiological perception of smell may be based on the recognition of a limited number of *primary odors* (as is similarly true with the senses of taste and sight); varying intensities of stimuli from different combinations of odor molecules simultaneously and differentially excite large numbers of receptors in the nasal cavity.

smoking

Smoking affects health in three basic ways: (1) nicotine and other chemical constituents of tobacco smoke have an immediate effect on the body; (2) repeated exposure to smoke damages the lungs; and (3) regular smokers have a heightened susceptibility to heart disease and several common forms of cancer.

Nicotine is a brain stimulant, although habitual smokers often find it also has a calming effect. It speeds the heart, raises the blood pressure and reduces the appetite. (Many people find that they can skip a meal and have a cigarette instead. Therefore, when they stop smoking their appetite increases.)

The irritants in tobacco smoke narrow the air passages in the lungs. Smoke slows down the action of the hair-like cilia lining these passages, and so reduces the efficiency of the natural process of removal of inhaled dust from the lungs. Smoking also accentuates the normal loss of lung elasticity with age. These two effects account for the frequency of BRONCHITIS in smokers, who often accept a chronic cough as inevitable. In fact smokers are six times more likely than nonsmokers to die of bronchitis.

Smoking is a major factor in death from coronary thrombosis ("heart attack"). In men aged 40 to 55 who smoke, coronary attacks are three times as common as in male nonsmokers in the same age range—and sudden death from coronary disease is five times as common. As yet the mechanism by which smoking increases the risk of heart disease is not understood by modern science—so that claims that some cigarettes are "safer" than others cannot be justified.

Lung cancer is the best known disease associated with smoking: it is extremely rare in those who have never smoked; many studies have shown that the risk of the disease is proportional to the amount smoked. Smoking cigarettes carries a higher risk than smoking cigars or a pipe. Smokers also have a higher than average risk of other diseases, such as bladder cancer, laryngeal cancer and stomach ulcers.

Taken together, the associations of smoking and disease make tobacco the single most important cause of death so far identified in Western society—which is why doctors in the United States and Britain smoke less than any other occupational or social group, and why their mortality rate from lung cancer has fallen.

sneeze

The respiratory tract, including the passages of the nose, is lined with specially adapted nerve cells (receptors) which are exposed on the surface of the mucous membrane. Stimulation of these receptors by noxious gases, irritant fumes, particles, microorganisms, or dust can result in an urgent stimulation of the brain's respiratory center. This produces a deep inspiration and a violent expiration so that particles can be literally exploded out of the respiratory tract. The sneeze is thus a protective mechanism.

somatotropin

The growth hormone; it is released by the anterior lobe of the PITUITARY GLAND.

The physiological effects of this hormone are numerous; they are associated not only with bone growth and cartilage extension, but the release of stored body fat and its conversion to energy, an increased rate in protein absorption by muscle cells—thus muscle development and growth—and an accelerated use of the body's glucose (sugar). The hormone itself is inextricably linked with the release and the effect of thyroid, adrenal and sex hormones.

Where pituitary disease or damage has occurred and somatotropin is deficient, growth is defective. Children born with a pituitary defect may grow very slowly (*pituitary dwarfs*), but if the condition is recognized early enough treatment with the hormone will permit them to reach a normal height. Excess growth hormone production during childhood causes *gigantism*: most of the famous giants had pituitary tumors. Excess growth hormone secretion caused by a tumor in later life produces ACROMEGALY, a disorder characterized by an increase in the size of hands, feet, and head; the condition can often be cured by treatment of the pituitary tumor.

See also HORMONES.

South American trypanosomiasis

Another name for CHAGAS' DISEASE.

spasticity

The special type of paralysis associated with damage to the nerve cells in the cerebral cortex (the upper motor neurones). Spastic paralysis occurs in stroke, cerebral tumors, and in multiple sclerosis, but the term is most often used in connection with the birth handicap spastic diplegia, cerebral palsy, or simply spastic paralysis. The neurological damage responsible for this type of paralysis is first noted in infancy, is nonprogressive and therefore assumed to be due either to birth trauma or defective development, being more common in prematurely born babies or in babies who sustain a cerebral hemorrhage. In particular, spasticity involves increased resistance to passive movement, exaggerated reflexes, spasms of the limbs and uncontrolled movements (ATHETOSIS). There is considerable variation in severity and in the defects (and, therefore, of muscular control), but it is important to remember that intellectual function and intelligence may not be impaired.

Approximately 25% of the infantile cases are mildly involved; another estimated 25% are severely affected, with loss of speech control and the development of seizures. There is no cure for what is essentially an irreversible defect of neurological control; but with physical therapy, bracing of limbs and the use of other appliances, considerable benefits can be achieved. Surgical intervention can be helpful to minimize deformities, and tendons can be transplanted so that the controllable muscles can achieve voluntary movement and overcome involuntary spasm. Drugs to overcome reflex spasticity are occasionally helpful but frequently sedate the intellect excessively. Survival prospects are nowadays excellent, provided the respiratory (breathing) mechanisms are not involved.

speculum

An instrument for examining body passages or canals.

The cone attachment of the *otoscope*, which is inserted in the ear to examine the eardrum, is a speculum. A *nasal speculum* is frequently a small flat-edged springed device that gently expands the nostrils so that the nasal passages can be examined. A *rectal speculum* is an illuminated cylindrical instrument with a removable tip which is withdrawn after insertion, so that the inside of the rectal canal can be examined in the diagnosis of disease of the rectum and nearby areas of the lower part of the large intestine. *Vaginal specula* are designed in various types and sizes. Some are single-bladed to pull the lower wall of the vagina downward to reveal the inside of the orifice, the upper wall and the front, or the cervix (neck of the womb); others are dual-bladed and open the vagina to reveal the deepest recesses and a larger area of the cervix. These are frequently used to obtain a "Pap smear" in diagnosing cervical cancer.

speech

The use of sounds made by the mouth, tongue, and respiratory system to communicate specific thoughts from one person either to another or to many others.

The development of a spoken language is the most obvious difference between man and animals. Chimpanzees and other primates can be taught a language based on signs or pictures, but so far no animal has been taught to speak.

Speech develops slowly in the normal child. Between the age of 9 months and 5 years he learns a simple vocabulary and the basic elements of sentence construction, but the acquisition of full language skills takes the whole of childhood. Even in normal children there is great variation in the pace at which speech develops, but a child may be slow to speak because of low intelligence, extraordinary shyness, a physical defect such as deafness, or lack of stimulation in a deprived social environment. Speech defects such as stammering are more often due to psychological than to physical causes.

Once speech has been developed it may be lost again due to physical injury or disease of the larynx or tongue, or more commonly due to damage to the brain from a stroke, a tumor, or any other lesion.

When the loss of difficulty in speech is due to impairment of the control of the muscles used in forming the sounds the defect is termed *dysarthria*. One common example is the difficulty in speech associated with BELL'S PALSY, a paralysis of the nerve supplying the muscles of the face. When the defect is in the brain centers concerned with language, the condition is termed *dysphasia* or *aphasia*. Loss of speech after a stroke may be due to either or both of these mechanisms; some recovery is usual and speech therapy may be helpful. Loss of speech in adult life may also be due to psychiatric disorders such as hysteria.

spermatocele

A cystic dilatation in the epididymis (the sperm-store of the testis), filled with a milky fluid. Rupture into the tunica vaginalis of the testis produces spermatic hydrocele.

If spermatoceles become large or painful they should be removed.

spherocytosis

A condition in which red blood cells change in shape and become thick and almost spherical. It is a rare inherited disorder, found in northern Europe, with an incidence of 20 to 30 per 100,000 of the population.

The abnormal cells are unusually fragile, so that their life span is reduced, and the spleen usually enlarges owing to its role in destroying the defective cells. There may be no symptoms, or the high rate of cell destruction may cause a chronic anemia. Diagnosis of the condition, which is not usually obvious until adulthood, is made by a blood test. Treatment is by surgical removal of the spleen—which does not prevent spherocytes from still being made, but reduces the anemia and the incidence of complications from the increased rate of destruction of red blood cells (hemolysis).

SPEECH

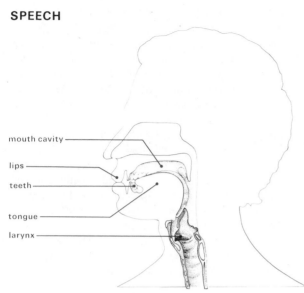

mouth cavity

lips

teeth

tongue

larynx

VOICE PRODUCTION

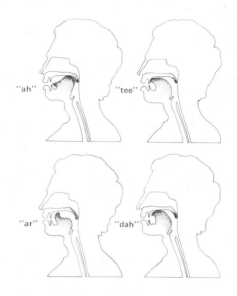

"ah"   "tee"

"ar"   "dah"

Vibrations of the vocal cords in the larynx produce the basic sound of the voice. The different elements of speech are produced by modifying the shape of the mouth cavity, position of the tongue, and the use of the teeth and lips.

sphygmomanometer

A device for measuring the BLOOD PRESSURE. Many types are in use, often bearing the names of their originators.

The most common instrument consists of an upright glass column filled with mercury and calibrated in millimeters. To this is attached, by a length of plastic or rubber tubing, an inflatable cuff designed to be wrapped around the patient's upper arm. Inflation of the cuff by compression of a rubber bulb applies pressure to the arm and the pressure in the cuff is recorded by the height to which the mercury rises up the calibrated glass tube (manometer).

When a STETHOSCOPE is applied over the main artery of the arm just below the cuff, the pulsation of the vessel can be heard. If the pressure in the cuff exceeds the highest pressure generated in the arteries with each heartbeat, no blood will pass through the artery and no sound will be heard. Lowering the pressure slowly, a point is reached at which the blood begins to flow through the vessel with each heartbeat but the vessel collapses again between beats and the flow ceases. The coming together of the vessel walls results in a sharp tapping noise, heard by the examining doctor, and the point at which this is first heard is described as the *systolic pressure*—the highest pressure generated by each heartbeat (see SYSTOLE).

Lowering the pressure still further, a point is reached

SPHYGMOMANOMETER

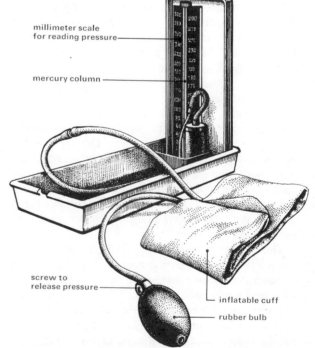

millimeter scale for reading pressure

mercury column

screw to release pressure

inflatable cuff

rubber bulb

The familiar sphygmomanometer is a simple but accurate device for measuring blood pressure. The cuff is wrapped tightly around the patient's arm and inflated to a high pressure by pumping the rubber bulb; this stops blood flow through the arm. The operator then slowly reduces the pressure and listens with a stethoscope over the artery for the sounds of the pulse. He records the levels of the mercury at which these sounds appear and then disappear.

where the blood flow becomes continuous but the individual heartbeats can still be heard as a softer tapping sound. The point at which this is first heard is described as the *diastolic pressure* (see DIASTOLE) and represents the steady pressure remaining in the arteries between heartbeats. Further reduction of the pressure results in the loss of all sounds in the stethoscope.

The final result of the measurement is recorded in millimeters of mercury pressure—often expressed, for example, as 120/80 (indicating a systolic pressure of 120 millimeters of mercury and a diastolic pressure of 80).

Modern variants of the instrument use direct-reading manometers or the pressure may be electrically recorded, but the underlying principle remains the same.

spina bifida

During the third and fourth weeks of embryonic life, the *neural groove*, which runs along the back of the embryo, fuses to form the *neural tube*. This tube is the forerunner of the central nervous system (the brain and spinal cord). Spina bifida results when closure of the neural tube is incomplete and is accompanied by a similar defect in the closure of the bony vertebral canal. The site most frequently involved is the lumbosacral region (at the bottom of the back), although higher regions are occasionally affected. Three varieties of spina bifida are recognized: *spina bifida occulta*, meningocele, and meningomyelocele.

Spina bifida occulta, the least severe form, results from incomplete fusion of the bony vertebral arch and is usually of no medical significance. The site may be marked externally by a tuft of hair, but often is detected only by chance on x-ray examination. Rarely, spina bifida occulta is accompanied by another spinal cord lesion such as a benign fat tumor, cyst or fibrous band. These may give rise to symptoms which can be relieved surgically.

The other two varieties of spina bifida are far more serious and involve the protrusion of a sac through the vertebral defect. In *meningocele*, the sac contains only the membranes which cover the spinal cord (the *meninges* or meningeal membranes); in the more common *meningomyelocele*, the sac contains spinal cord tissues or nerve roots as well as meningeal membranes. These forms frequently coexist with other congenital abnormalities, especially HYDROCEPHALUS (accumulation of fluid within the brain). Severe degrees of spina bifida may be incompatible with life, the baby being stillborn or only surviving a few hours. Neurological defects commonly found in those who survive include mental handicap, variable motor and sensory loss in the limbs, and impaired control of the muscular ring which controls the opening of the anus (anal sphincter).

The cause of spina bifida is unknown, but a woman who has had one affected child stands an increased risk of having another. It has recently become possible to diagnose meningocele and meningomyelocele before birth, by detecting increased levels of ALPHA-FETOPROTEIN in the amniotic fluid (which surrounds the fetus) so that the mother can be offered a therapeutic termination of pregnancy. A blood test for screening purposes is also available; at present its use is limited to women known to have a higher than average risk of giving birth to an abnormal child.

By 1954 it became possible to decompress hydrocephalus surgically, which dramatically cut the mortality rate in meningomyelocele. In addition, early repair of spinal defects was found to reduce MENINGITIS (inflammation of the meningeal membranes) and neurologic damage. Application of these new techniques has led to the survival of many severely handicapped children, while benefiting others enormously.

However, neurosurgeons have been placed in a considerable ethical dilemma by the development of improved surgical techniques; many do not now operate on children with the most severe defects who would not have an acceptable quality of life despite surgery.

spinal curvature

The human spine normally curves outward in the thoracic region, inward in the lumbar region and like an elongated "S" curves again in the sacrum to finish at the coccyx pointing downward and forward. Vertically, in correct posture, the uppermost cervical vertebra is directly in a gravitational line above the end of the sacrum. Abnormal curvature may be an exaggeration of the normal curves (KYPHOSIS), or extend laterally on either side of the vertical (SCOLIOSIS), or be a combination of both *kyphoscoliosis*.

Lateral curvature—scoliosis—is often associated with a compensatory twisting of the spine and may be due to congenital abnormalities of the vertebrae, bad posture in the child, paralytic disease affecting the muscles (such as POLIOMYELITIS) or pulmonary disease, particularly where the effects on one lung have caused contraction of the chest wall on that side. Cases which develop in puberty are recognized as more common in girls and require constant supervision involving serial x-ray examinations, physical therapy, exercises, spinal jackets and (if necessary) spinal fusion to prevent the development of permanent deformities.

Excessive convexity of the spine—kyphosis—may result from trauma (particularly mild compression fracture of a dorsal vertebra), from TUBERCULOSIS (now rare, but formerly known as Pott's disease of the spine) which erodes the vertebral bodies, and from secondary growths of a tumor.

ABNORMAL SPINAL CURVATURES

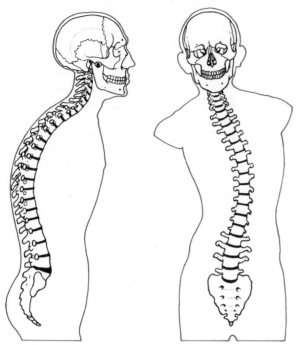

kyphosis—exaggerated convexity
of the spine

scoliosis—lateral curvature
of the spine

Illustrated above are two of the most common spinal deformities. Kyphosis, or "humpback," may result from poor posture (in which case it is often reversible) or from structural abnormalities in the vertebrae. Likewise, scoliosis may be postural, a congenital deformity or the result of a neurological disease such as poliomyelitis. The two deformities are sometimes combined in a condition called kyphoscoliosis.

ANKYLOSING SPONDYLITIS, by its production of rigidity in the lower spine, may cause an excessive curvature (as a compensation) in the cervical region. Paget's disease (see OSTEITIS) leads to a slow bending of the vertebra which, in the elderly, can also be a cause of kyphotic deformity. In the postmenopausal and the elderly, OSTEOPOROSIS can cause excessive spinal curvature as the result of weakening of the vertebral bodies. These disorders are less amenable to successful correction than those which first appear in the developing young.

See also POSTURE, SPINE.

The spinal column (right) consists of 24 separate vertebrae plus two composite bones—the sacrum and coccyx. Our upright posture has led to the characteristic curvature of the column seen from the side, and means that the skull sits supported on a springlike structure.

SPINAL COLUMN

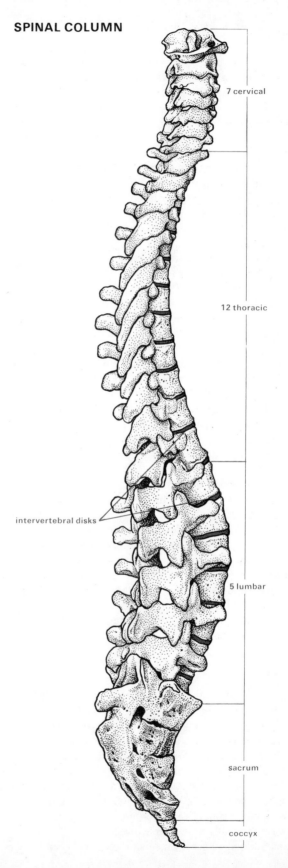

7 cervical

12 thoracic

intervertebral disks

5 lumbar

sacrum

coccyx

spine

The human spine consists of 29 bones (the vertebrae) which provide a stiff but flexible "backbone" for upright locomotion, and which encase the spinal cord and its nerve roots.

There are seven *cervical vertebrae* (supporting the skull and the neck), twelve *thoracic vertebrae* (providing anchorage for the rib case) five *lumbar vertebrae*—which are the largest—and five *sacral vertebrae* fused together (supporting the pelvis). The *coccyx* at the end of the sacrum is a small triangular bone; it is formed by fused and vestigial vertebrae, like a "tail." The two uppermost cervical vertebrae, which permit movement of the head, are called the *atlas* and the *axis*.

The spinal vertebrae are separated from each other by a disk of cartilage tissue (*intervertebral disk*). From the second cervical bone (axis) to the first sacral the vertebrae are held in close proximity by ligaments and muscles, which permit a limited range of bending and twisting while also protecting the spinal cord. Although the range of movements between the spinal bones is small, the somewhat elastic nature of the disks also permits them to be compressed. This ability to absorb compression stresses, aided also by the natural curvatures of the spine, means that the effects of the weight of the upright body and the impact of the feet—whether light (as in walking) or more heavy (as in running or jumping)—are smoothed out by this system of "shock absorption."

The anatomy of the spine is complicated in that each vertebral bone is different from another, but each has a thick and substantial *body* with extensions outward that form the protective arch for the nerves. Injury to the spine may be direct, causing fracture of one or other of these vertebral bodies, or excessive bending may cause a *compression fracture* of a vertebral body—in either case the pressure on the spinal cord can result in paralysis below that site. Deformities associated with disease, chronic bad posture or malignancy may occur and treatment is required at the first sign of abnormality.

spleen

An organ lying within the abdominal cavity, situated under the margin of the ribs on the left side. In shape and size it roughly resembles its owner's cupped hand.

The spleen resembles a large lymph gland in structure, similar to the glands found in the neck, armpits, groins and elsewhere in the body. It is, however, the largest of these structures and has special features not seen in the lymph glands. It is a vascular organ, having a large arterial blood supply. On entering the spleen, the blood flow slows greatly as it enters a meshwork of "sinuses" (dilated blood vessels). These sinuses lie between large

masses of lymphocytes, one of the more common types of circulating white blood cells. Their walls contain other cells (known as *phagocytes*) capable of engulfing certain cells and foreign particles in the blood and removing them from the circulation.

After its slow passage through the spleen, the relatively large volume of arterial blood which enters the spleen leaves it by the *splenic vein* and passes to the liver via the *portal vein*.

Like the lymph glands, the spleen plays an important part in the production of the antibodies, which are part of the body's resistance to infection (see ANTIBODY). To a greater extent than the lymph nodes, however, the spleen is concerned with the removal of abnormal or normally worn out ("dying") blood cells from the circulation. Its function in antibody formation can be

SPLEEN

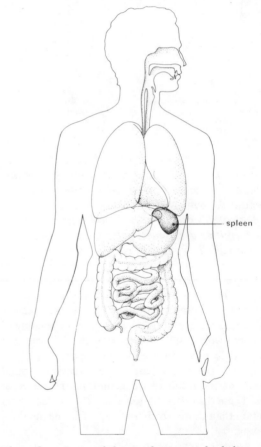

spleen

The spleen is an abdominal organ which lies underneath the lower ribs on the left of the body. It cannot be felt during a physical examination unless it has become enlarged by disease. It is frequently traumatized in automobile accidents and a splenectomy then has to be performed; removal of the spleen does not lead to any permanent disabilities in an adult.

readily taken over by the lymph nodes and removal of the spleen (following an injury, for example) is without serious effects except in very small children. In certain blood diseases, however, the spleen enlarges and removes blood cells more rapidly than usual from the blood; its removal may then be beneficial (SPLENECTOMY).

Enlargement of the spleen (SPLENOMEGALY) also occurs in a number of other conditions, including some infections, parasitic disorders, diseases of the liver and malignant tumors affecting the LYMPHATIC SYSTEM.

splenectomy

Surgical removal of the spleen. This organ lies under the margin of the ribs on the left side of the abdomen. The surgeon will approach it either by an incision made vertically on the front of the abdomen or by an oblique incision below the margin of the left rib.

The most common reason for removal of the spleen is accidental damage to the organ. This can occur on impact with the steering wheel in automobile accidents, as a result of blows to the abdomen, or as part of more widespread injuries received in a fall or other accident. Damage to the spleen—an extremely vascular organ—leads to a tear in its enclosing capsule; being soft and "friable," it does not lend itself to surgical repair and it is safer to remove it. Failure to do so may lead to dangerous hemorrhage within the abdomen.

The spleen may also have to be removed because it is diseased. This occurs commonly in malignant tumors of the LYMPHATIC SYSTEM and in HODGKIN'S DISEASE. It may then be removed as part of an exploratory operation on the abdomen designed to determine the extent of the disease before starting treatment. In certain blood diseases the spleen may remove red and white cells and platelets from the circulation at a sharply increased rate; surgical removal of the spleen may greatly alleviate these conditions. In other conditions, the spleen becomes abnormally enlarged (SPLENOMEGALY) and may cause the patient much discomfort, in addition to producing adverse effects on the number of circulating blood cells, and it may be removed for this reason.

Removal of a normal spleen is not considered to be a particularly dangerous operation, although if the organ is diseased or greatly enlarged the operation may be technically difficult and the risk increased. Except in very small children, removal of the spleen is not accompanied by an undue risk of adverse effects.

splenomegaly

Abnormal enlargement of the spleen, an organ lying in the abdominal cavity under the margin of the left rib and forming part of the LYMPHATIC SYSTEM.

A spleen of normal size cannot be felt by the doctor when examining the abdomen since it lies wholly beneath the rib margin. When checking for an enlarged spleen it can be felt more easily if the patient lies on his right side and takes a deep breath; descent of the diaphragm will then displace the spleen downward so that (if enlarged) it can then be felt protruding below the left rib margin.

Many different conditions may cause enlargement of the spleen. Enlargement occurs in some blood disorders (including the chronic leukemias) and a grossly enlarged organ may occupy much of the abdominal cavity. More common causes of enlargement, however, are certain infectious diseases; the detection of an enlarged spleen may be an important diagnostic finding in such conditions as INFECTIOUS MONONUCLEOSIS, TYPHOID FEVER and MALARIA.

splint

A rigid appliance for the immobilization of a part of the body's musculoskeletal system, or for the correction of a deformity.

It may thus be a simple slab of plaster of Paris, or acrylic, on the lower forearm and wrist to protect against excessive movements of an injured wrist bone or tendon—or a whole-body plaster jacket, also encasing part of the head, to secure immobility of a fractured spine. Following the correction of some bone injuries or joint disorders, plaster-impregnated bandages can be applied after wetting. They can be molded to the individual's needs, they set quickly and can be left on as long as necessary to secure healing. X rays can be taken through them and they are easily removed by cutting, using special plaster shears or saws that oscillate and do not cut the skin.

When a plaster splint has been applied over a fresh fracture, a careful watch is necessary in case swelling of the limb in a close-fitting splint impairs the blood circulation. The period of greatest potential danger is from about 12 to 36 hours after injury; severe pain or swelling of the exposed limb beyond the splint is a sign for reassessment and perhaps splint removal and replacement, or merely splitting open the splint. In emergencies a splint can be made from any material—a piece of wood or a tree branch, or one injured limb can be splinted to another part of the body by binding (for example, the legs can be bound together or an arm can be bound across the chest). Inflatable splints—fitting like gloves over an injured limb, which then stiffen when inflated—are a relatively recent invention of great benefit to emergency services. Specialized splints (such as supports for the legs, back braces, or cervical collars) are "tailor-made," frequently from steel or inflexible plastic. Internal splints for fractures and deformities are achieved with metal plates and screws, or rods and nails; this method is used where external splintage would be unsatisfactory.

spondylosis

A degenerative disorder of the spine which leads to narrowing of the spinal canal. It can occur in the cervical or lumbar area and leads to pressure on the spinal nerves or spinal cord.

Initially the cause can be trauma, which shows itself in middle life and old age to produce symptoms chiefly in those between the ages of 50 to 60. Degeneration of the nucleus of the intervertebral disk and the surrounding fibrous tissue leads to a reaction of the adjacent areas of vertebra. Variable calcified outgrowths from the vertebra may then protrude to press on the spinal cord, or occlude the spinal nerve's exit from the cord and so cause considerable neurological discomfort. This slow progression of disk degeneration followed by bony overgrowth of the spine may take place over many years and be the result of former sporting injuries, whiplash or trauma.

Commonly pain is the initial symptom, with some loss of comfortable spinal movement. Muscular weakness may occur in the specific areas supplied by the spinal nerves and, where spinal cord compression occurs, sensory deprivation over wide areas of the body (below the affected level) is experienced.

Diagnosis is by x ray of the spine and myelography. Treatment consists primarily of rest by immobilization

CERVICAL SPONDYLOSIS

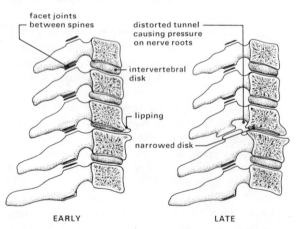

facet joints
between spines

distorted tunnel
causing pressure
on nerve roots

intervertebral
disk

lipping

narrowed disk

EARLY   LATE

Cervical spondylosis is simply osteoarthrosis of the spine in the neck and results from years of wear and tear. The intervertebral disks become narrowed and extra spurs of bone encroach into the spinal canal and nerve tunnels.

of the affected area of the spine, in a plaster or plastic jacket or collar. Surgery to relieve compression may be necessary in cases where paralysis is severe.

See also OSTEOARTHRITIS.

sporotrichosis

A fungus infection that may gain entry to the body through inhalation, ingestion or inoculation from a contaminated environment. The fungus exists in soil, peat moss, and decaying vegetation, and the disease is contracted mainly by laborers, farmers and florists. Outbreaks commonly occur in Mexico and Florida.

Pustules on the exposed skin enlarge and lead to involvement of the lymph glands, which themselves may ulcerate. Internal absorption of the organism produces the same lymph gland response and the disease, if untreated, may be fatal.

Diagnosis is made by blood tests and culture of the organism from the gland or pustule. Treatment is usually effective with antifungal medication, which may need to be continued for several weeks.

sprain

The incomplete tear of a ligament. Sprains are not serious injuries, but it is important to distinguish between sprains and complete disruption of a ligament, which may lead to subsequent instability of the affected joint. Complete tears are recognized by abnormal mobility of the joint, and the diagnosis may rest on radiological (x-ray) appearances. A severe sprain may be difficult to distinguish from a fracture.

The ligaments of the knee and ankle are most commonly sprained (the ankles more often than the knee), although it is not uncommon for the wrist to be sprained in a fall. The injury is often very painful and is accompanied by considerable swelling and bruising. Movement is painful.

At first the joint will probably be more comfortable if it is bandaged to limit movement and help keep the swelling down, but as soon as possible the joint should be moved and used.

sprue

1. See TROPICAL SPRUE.
2. A term used to describe the adult form of CELIAC DISEASE; also known as *nontropical sprue*.

sputum

An adult in normal health secretes about 100 milliliters (ml) of mucus from the cells lining the respiratory tract each day. This is removed from the air passages by the action of the ciliated cells which line the trachea (windpipe), bronchi and bronchioles, and is not noticed.

Sputum is the word used to describe excess secretions which cannot be removed by ciliary action; it stimulates the nerve endings in the mucous membrane and sets up a cough reflex. It is the result of irritation or inflammation of the air passages, and may be classified under six headings; (1) *mucoid*, which is clear; (2) *black*, which contains dust, or cigarette and atmospheric smoke; (3) *purulent*, which contains pus; (4) *mucopurulent*, with mixed pus and mucus; (5) *bloodstained*, with streaks of clots of blood (hemoptysis); and (6) *rusty*, which is mucus mixed with small amounts of altered blood and is found mainly in association with pneumonia.

The appearance of blood in the sputum always requires medical investigation to rule out a potentially serious condition.

squint

Another name for STRABISMUS.

stammering

Stammering or stuttering is a disturbance of speech in which it is abruptly interrupted or certain sounds or syllables are rapidly repeated.

It is much more common in men than women and more common in left-handed or ambidextrous persons as well as in those who have attempted to become ambidextrous though originally left-handed. It occurs in up to 1% of schoolchildren, usually before the age of 10, and tends to run in families.

Whether speech is disturbed by repetition of sounds or syllables, or is interrupted completely because the patient "cannot get the word out," a degree of shame or embarrassment is usually present. Patients may thus often appear to have psychological problems or to be shy or withdrawn; but these features may be the *result* of the condition rather than its *cause*. Most patients who stammer or stutter do not have an underlying psychological disturbance.

Treatment involves speech training, the restoration of confidence and the overcoming of any psychological problems which may have arisen as a result of the disorder. A skilled speech therapist (or speech pathologist) will employ relaxation exercises, breathing exercises and carefully controlled speech exercises. A slow, "syllable-by-syllable" type of speech may be cultivated and confidence restored by singing or shouting words over which difficulty is experienced. Stressful situations are avoided until confidence returns. Tranquilizing or sedative drugs may be helpful. The enthusiastic encouragement of therapist and family plays an essential role.

Prognosis is good with proper treatment; the less the patient is disturbed by his speech problem, the better the outlook.

stapedectomy

A surgical procedure to correct one form of hearing loss.

Sound waves entering the outer ear cause the eardrum, between the outer and middle ear cavities, to vibrate. These vibrations are conducted across the middle ear cavity to the inner ear (where they are transformed into nerve impulses and sent to the brain) by a chain of three tiny bones (*ossicles*) which bridge the cavity of the middle ear.

In the condition of OTOSCLEROSIS there is formation of new bone at the point where the innermost ossicle (the *stapes*) fits into the *oval window*—a minute aperture between the middle and inner ears. The "footplate" of the stapes, normally free to move in the aperture and thus to transmit the vibrations to the inner ear, becomes fixed in position and sound-conduction deafness results.

STAPEDECTOMY

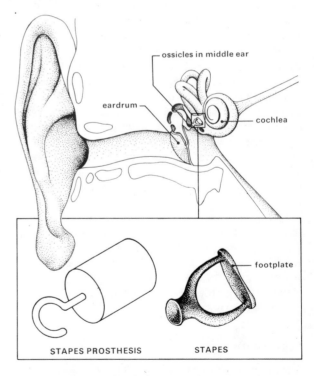

ossicles in middle ear

eardrum

cochlea

footplate

STAPES PROSTHESIS   STAPES

Hearing depends on the ability of the ossicles (little bones) of the middle ear to transmit sound. Occasionally, the footplate of the stapes becomes fused to the cochlea in a disease called otosclerosis. The resulting deafness can be cured by a stapedectomy operation, where the stapes is replaced a tiny stainless-steel piston.

Surgical removal of the stapes—*stapedectomy*—performed through an incision into the middle ear, is followed by re-establishment of the chain of conduction for the vibrations of the eardrum by means of a plastic or metal prosthesis (replacement part). The success rate of this operation in restoring a useful degree of hearing is about 80%.

The operation is not without potential complications, including total loss of function of the organ of hearing itself in the inner ear, perforation of the eardrum and damage to nerves in the vicinity of the middle ear. Dizziness may also occur, but usually, it is only temporary.

starvation

In *acute starvation* the patient's intake of calories falls seriously below his normal energy requirements. Unless reduction in his physical activity can reduce these requirements to bring them within the calorie intake available, he must draw on his own tissues as an energy source.

Fat is the obvious energy storage tissue, having a high calorific value, but some protein must be mobilized as well to provide essential nutrients for certain tissues that require them. Loss of body weight occurs both from loss of fat and of muscle protein. There may be swelling of the tissues as the result of an accumulation of fluid in them, especially in the legs and feet, when standing.

When the last reserves of fat have been mobilized, the patient's condition deteriorates rapidly—since only essential protein-containing tissues can now be drawn on for energy supplies. Lassitude, weakness, a fall in blood pressure and death will soon follow. In some cases, dehydration due to water deprivation is also present; complete lack of water is much more rapidly fatal than starvation alone.

In *chronic starvation* the condition may be complicated by the symptoms of multiple deficiencies of vitamins, minerals and protein. Deficiency diseases which may then be seen include BERIBERI, PELLAGRA, SCURVY, RICKETS and the protein deficiency disease KWASHIORKOR. (See also MARASMUS.)

See also ANOREXIA NERVOSA.

steatoma

A term used to describe either a SEBACEOUS CYST or a LIPOMA.

steatorrhea

The condition of having an excessive amount of fat in the stools. It is common in most conditions that cause MALABSORPTION.

Stein-Leventhal syndrome

Abnormally large cystic ovaries with fibrosed capsules are found in about 1% of women; in some cases these findings are associated with AMENORRHEA, abnormal growth of hair, obesity and infertility, and the pattern is known as the Stein-Leventhal syndrome.

The disturbances are thought to be the effect of disordered steroid production in the ovaries, possibly following disturbed function of the pituitary gland and the hypothalamus.

It has been found that surgical removal of part of the enlarged ovaries is followed by renewal of menstrual flow, reversal of the masculinizing changes and restored fertility, but it is also possible to treat the condition with clomiphene (Clomid).

stenosis

The abnormal narrowing or constriction of a hollow passage or orifice (the entrance to a cavity or tube).

sterilization

Any surgical procedure which makes a man or woman infertile while leaving sexual desire and capacity unaffected. In men the operation is *vasectomy*, a simple procedure done under local anesthesia. The surgeon makes a small opening in the scrotum and cuts through each of the two *vas deferens* (the tubes connecting the testes to the base of the penis). After vasectomy there is no apparent change in sexual performance, but the ejaculated semen no longer contains spermatozoa (once the stores are used up, which takes a few weeks). There are no long-term effects on general health or on sexuality.

In women the most usual sterilization procedure is cutting or blocking the Fallopian tubes which connect the ovaries to the uterus. Only a minor operation is needed, for the surgeon can locate and divide the tubes through an incision only half an inch or so long, using an operating "laparascope"—a thin tube through which the interior of the abdominal cavity can be examined. Division of the Fallopian tubes does not have any apparent effect on the menstrual periods or on sexuality.

Sterilization is being used increasingly as an alternative to contraception by couples who have completed their families: it is safe and reliable and (unlike the use of oral contraceptives) carries no risk to general health. The procedures are not readily reversible: a man or woman who has been sterilized has only a small chance of being restored to normal fertility if the surgeon reconnects the separated tubes. However, successful techniques for reversal of sterilization are currently being developed.

STETHOSCOPE

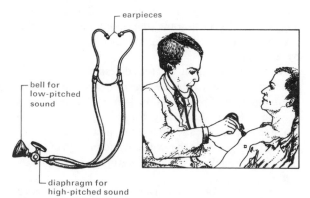

earpieces

bell for
low-pitched
sound

diaphragm for
high-pitched sound

*The stethoscope is a very simple instrument which
has been in use for many years, but still retains
an important place as a diagnostic tool in modern
medicine. Doctors use it to listen to the sounds
from our hearts and lungs.*

stethoscope

The common instrument used by a doctor to listen to the
sounds made by a patient's heart or lungs
(AUSCULTATION). It can also be used to listen to sounds
produced in blood vessels in the limbs and the sounds
produced by the movements of the intestines during
digestion. Together with a SPHYGMOMANOMETER, it is
an essential piece of equipment for taking the blood
pressure.

The general shape of the stethoscope will be familiar.
The chest piece, which is applied to the patient's chest
wall, may be of two types. One is bell-shaped and open,
the other (Bowles type) is flat and covered with a plastic
or metal diaphragm. The chest piece is attached to a Y-
shaped connector which transmits the sounds by means
of two lengths of thick-walled rubber tubing to the ear
pieces.

Modern variants include electronic detection and
amplification of the sounds. A simpler type of instrument using only one ear piece is more efficient and
convenient for obstetric use.

stings

Two major groups of stinging creatures exist, fish and
other types of marine life and the venomous or biting
arthropods (a phylum of invertebrate animals containing over 700,000 species, including the insects, spiders
and crustaceans).

Among the marine group are the venomous fish that
carry poisonous spines. These include the stone fish,
scorpion fish, lion fish and the weever fish. These all
inhabit shallow waters and lie concealed in sand or
among rocks. Swimmers and skin divers may be stung

by them and fishermen may be injured while removing
them from nets and lines. Pain from their stings may be
very severe, constitutional symptoms may occur and
death may occasionally result. In the case of the
stingrays, the fish carries the sting in its tail and drives it
into the victim when disturbed.

Jellyfish can cause painful stings and both the
Portuguese man-of-war group and the true jellyfish may
produce severe pain, extensive rashes or even death.
Jellyfish cannot of course "attack" man; contact with
them occurs accidentally among swimmers and skin
divers.

The stinging insects include the many varieties of
wasps and bees. The effect of stings from bees and wasps
depend on the patient's personal sensitivity. Lethal
reactions are relatively rare. In the case of the potentially
dangerous scorpion sting, the mortality rate may be as
high as 5%.

In serious cases immediate medical aid should be
urgently sought to combat shock; specific *antisera* are
available in most cases. Symptoms of milder stings may
be relieved by the administration of antihistamines
smoothed gently into the skin, steroids, and painkilling
drugs.

Stokes-Adams syndrome

See ADAMS-STOKES SYNDROME.

stoma

1. A small opening, pore, or mouth.
2. An opening created artificially between two body
cavities or passages and the surface of the body (such as
the surgical opening created by a COLOSTOMY).

stomach

The stomach lies centrally in the upper part of the
abdomen and provides a receptacle for the immediate
reception of food after it has been chewed and
swallowed. Food enters the stomach at the *cardiac
sphincter*, a valve-like ring of muscle at the lower end of
the esophagus ("gullet") and leaves it by the *pylorus* (a
similar structure at the lower end of the stomach) to pass
to the duodenum and small intestine.

Between the cardiac sphincter and the pylorus, the
upper and lower borders of the stomach (as it lies in the
abdomen when the subject is erect) are referred to as the
lesser and greater curvatures, respectively. The organ is
also subdivided into an upper portion (above the entry
of the esophagus at the cardiac sphincter) called the
fundus and a lower portion (close to the pylorus) called
the *antrum*. Between these lies the *body* of the stomach.

The stomach has a thick muscular coat and can

STOMACH

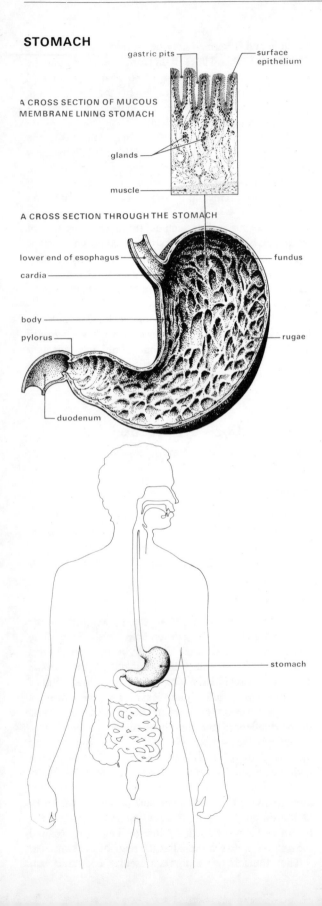

A CROSS SECTION OF MUCOUS MEMBRANE LINING STOMACH

gastric pits

surface epithelium

glands

muscle

A CROSS SECTION THROUGH THE STOMACH

lower end of esophagus

cardia

body

pylorus

duodenum

fundus

rugae

stomach

contract to force food through the pylorus or, in vomiting, up through the esophagus. It is lined by a mucus-secreting membrane (the *gastric mucosa*), which is also responsible for the digestive secretions produced by the organ.

As its contribution to the digestive process, the stomach produces *hydrochloric acid* and an enzyme, *pepsin*, capable of breaking down protein in the presence of acid. The food, already broken up and partially digested by chewing and mixture with saliva, mixes with the acid and pepsin in the stomach and protein digestion begins—although no major absorption occurs in the organ.

Contractions of the stomach wall, while the pylorus remains closed, mix the food thoroughly with the digestive juices. When digestion with pepsin is completed, the pylorus opens and allows the food to pass on into the duodenum—where it meets other digestive juices from the liver and pancreas.

Another very important secretion produced by the stomach wall is known as *intrinsic factor*. This substance is required for the normal absorption of vitamin B_{12} from the diet. In "pernicious anemia," thinning and degeneration of the mucosa occurs with loss of intrinsic factor secretion, failure of vitamin B_{12} absorption and the development of a characteristic type of ANEMIA as the result of lack of the vitamin.

stomatitis

Inflammation of the lining membrane of the mouth (*oral mucosa*). It often involves the tongue as well and the patient complains of a sore mouth.

Many conditions can produce a sore and inflamed mouth. Scalding by hot fluids or burning by caustic ones, hot or spicy foods and damage from jagged teeth or ill-fitting dentures can all cause stomatitis.

Local infections which produce a sore mouth include CANDIDIASIS ("thrush") and infections with bacteria known as "Vincent's organisms." Some virus infections—including HERPES ZOSTER ("shingles"), CHICKENPOX and MEASLES—may involve the mouth. Prolonged antibiotic therapy, by altering the balance of normal bacteria which inhabit the mouth, can also produce stomatitis.

The stomach acts as both a reservoir for food and a site for its digestion. The interior of an empty stomach is marked by prominent folds (rugae) which are flattened out as the stomach expands after a meal. The surface of the body and fundus when seen under a microscope is marked by numerous small openings, the gastric pits. Digestive juices well up from these pits when the stomach is stimulated by food.

Certain vitamin deficiencies cause stomatitis. A prolonged lack of riboflavin and nicotinamide (in the vitamin B group) produces a characteristic clinical picture; SCURVY, the result of a lack of vitamin C, can produce swelling and hemorrhage in the gums. Vitamin B deficiency in "pernicious anemia" is accompanied by a sore mouth and tongue, which is also the case in patients with folic acid deficiency and iron-deficiency anemia. (See ANEMIA.)

Other blood disorders—including leukemia, agranulocytosis (loss of circulating white blood cells, sometimes as a side effect of drug therapy) and "aplastic anemia" (failure of production of all blood cells by the bone marrow)—may be accompanied by severe stomatitis, often with ulceration of the oral mucosa. A condition of unknown cause is *aphthous ulceration* (or *aphthous stomatitis*), in which recurrent crops of small ulcers ("canker sores") appear spontaneously on the oral mucosa.

Treatment of stomatitis is directed toward the underlying cause. Milder cases clear up spontaneously with antiseptic mouth washes or good dental hygiene and aphthous ulcers usually disappear spontaneously within a few days.

stones

See CALCULUS.

strabismus

The medical term for a "squint." The condition is most common in young children and several types are found.

In a patient with a squint the eyes do not (as in normal persons) remain parallel; one or the other eye diverges from the direction in which the gaze is directed. A tendency exists for one eye to become the "master eye" and, when the patient looks at an object, it is fixed by the master eye and the other is seen to be directed in a slightly different direction. Squints may thus be *divergent* if the squinting eye looks away from the line of the master eye ("wall-eye") and *convergent* if it looks toward the master eye ("cross-eye").

Squints may also be divided into the *concomitant* squints (commonly seen in childhood), in which an imbalance exists in the strengths of the paired muscles which move the eyeball, and the rarer *paralytic* squints, in which there is a complete or partial paralysis of one or more muscles in the affected eye.

The appearance of a squint may lead the patient to seek medical advice; double vision may occur, especially in paralytic squint. Squint in young children is an important condition, since the brain suppresses the image seen by the squinting eye; if correction of the squint is delayed the eye may become functionally blind (AMBLYOPIA), either temporarily or permanently. In such circumstances the child will never develop binocular vision.

Treatment of concomitant squint is either by eye exercises designed to strengthen the muscles whose power is deficient (*orthoptics*) or by surgery. Orthoptic treatment requires a long period of therapy and much cooperation from the patient, but may be helpful. Operative treatment involves the shortening of the affected muscles so that their contractions are able to balance the pull of their opponents.

stress

Stress is a term used medically to describe pressure or physical force such as the compression of the lower teeth against the upper teeth during chewing or the forces acting on a joint during weight-bearing or during physical exercise. It is also used to refer to any influence that disturbs the natural equilibrium or internal environment of the body.

Such stress may be produced by physical injury, temperature changes, disease, emotional disturbances, or prolonged demands on physical or mental endurance. If the stress persists for too long or is too intense for the body's regulating mechanisms, one or more of the *stress diseases* may develop: these include mental disorders such as schizophrenia and physical conditions such as peptic ulcer, ulcerative colitis, hypertension, eczema, or asthma.

The most stressful life events are loss of a job or change in working conditions, marital conflicts, and death of a family member.

The ADRENAL GLANDS, which are two small endocrine glands situated on top of the kidneys, play a key role in regulating the body's response to stress by releasing their hormones into the blood circulation.

Epinephrine and *norepinephrine* (two hormones secreted by the adrenal glands) increase the heart rate and blood pressure, constrict the blood vessels in the skin and digestive system (thus diverting blood to the muscles), and encourage the release of glucose (sugar) from the liver stores to supply the body's energy demands. In other words, they induce changes in the body which prepare the animal for "fight" or "flight."

The adrenal glands also secrete the *corticosteroid hormones*, which play a major role in the body's response to infections and other diseases. They control the internal balance of sugars, fats and minerals and the incorporation of protein into the muscles. The interaction between the external stresses and the internal response by the adrenal glands help to determine whether the individual concerned remains healthy; prolonged stress will eventually exhaust the internal reserves and precipitate some form of mental or physical ill health.

stridor

Any harsh, high-pitched, rattling or "snoring" sound produced during respiration—either while awake or during sleep. It is fairly common in babies and young infants, in whom it may have no medical significance. Such prolonged (chronic) noisy breathing is frequently caused by the "floppiness" of the epiglottis, which may vibrate during breathing. (The epiglottis is a fleshy structure that covers the entrance to the larynx, or "voice-box," during swallowing to prevent food or liquid from entering the air passages.) In such cases there is rarely a danger of any obstruction of the baby's airways. In older children or adults, however, such breathing may be a sign of a serious disorder and requires prompt medical attention.

There are many causes of stridor, including the presence of an inhaled foreign body (see FOREIGN BODIES) or spasm of the vocal cords following the inhalation of irritant material or vomit. Acute infection can produce obstruction to the airway. Simple LARYNGITIS in a small child—in whom the airway is smaller and therefore more easily obstructed by swelling of its lining membrane—can produce the type of stridor commonly known as CROUP. DIPHTHERIA can also obstruct the airway.

In older patients, tumors of the larynx, windpipe or lungs may cause stridor. Treatment depends on the underlying cause. If the obstruction is severe and cannot otherwise be rapidly relieved, a temporary opening must be made into the windpipe below the obstruction (TRACHEOSTOMY) to provide an artificial airway. Croup in children often responds well to simple procedures such as increasing the amount of water vapor in the air of the child's room through the use of a vaporizer.

stroke

The common name for a sudden paralysis or loss of sensation resulting from THROMBOSIS in or bleeding from one of the arteries supplying the brain (CERE-BRAL HEMORRHAGE). Each year there are approximately 40,000 deaths from this cause in Great Britain. The severity of strokes is variable; sometimes the

A stroke results from damage to brain cells, following a prolonged interruption to their blood supply. Each artery in the brain is responsible for nourishing a particular territory and the severity of a stroke depends on which vessel is involved. The general arrangement of nerve fibers means that when the right side of the brain is damaged, symptoms of paralysis and numbness affect the left side of the body and vice versa.

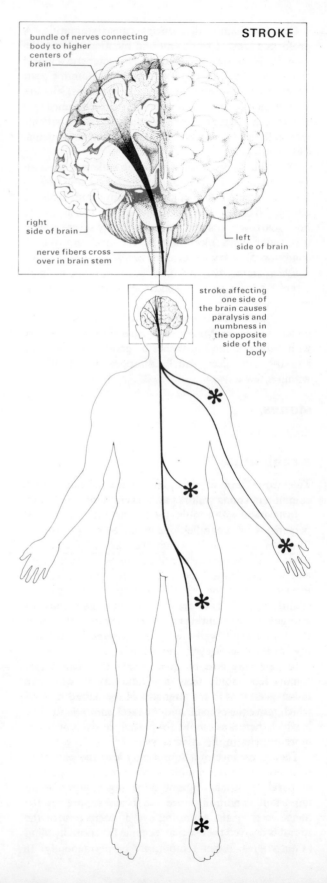

STROKE

bundle of nerves connecting body to higher centers of brain

right side of brain

left side of brain

nerve fibers cross over in brain stem

stroke affecting one side of the brain causes paralysis and numbness in the opposite side of the body

episode lasts only for a few minutes, or for less than 24 hours, with complete recovery afterwards (a "transient ischemic attack"). At the other extreme there may be sudden loss of consciousness progressing to death within a few hours. More typically, the onset of symptoms takes a few minutes, with gradual loss of power and feeling in an arm or leg.

The most common form of stroke is caused by thrombosis in one of the main blood vessels of the brain (the middle cerebral artery). The resultant partial or total paralysis affects one arm and leg (HEMIPLEGIA) and the facial muscles on the same side. If the right side is affected there may be loss of speech (*aphasia*) as an added disability. Other equally distinctive stroke syndromes, due to thrombosis in different arteries, may affect balance, vision, sensation, memory, or any other brain function. Loss of muscular control may occur without any effect on mental alertness or intelligence, and a stroke patient who has difficulty in speaking may retain normal understanding.

About 20–25% of patients who have a stroke die within hours or days. The outlook is worse with patients over 70 years of age and in cases in which there is loss of consciousness and profound paralysis. For those who survive the initial episode, however, there is a good chance of substantial recovery in the weeks that follow, especially in patients whose general health is otherwise good. There is no specific curative treatment for the common forms of stroke, but physical therapy can be very helpful in speeding the recovery of muscular power and control. More specific help may be needed with the functions of walking and speech, and the relearning of day-to-day tasks.

Little is known of the cause of stroke, except that there is a strong association with raised blood pressure (hypertension). Other predisposing factors are diabetes and any condition that makes thrombosis more likely (including use of oral contraceptives and POLYCYTHEMIA). The best prospects of reducing the ill-health due to stroke lies in the detection and treatment of the conditions which increase the risk.

sty (hordeolum)

A common type of inflammation of the eyelid, often the upper lid. Each eyelash follicle is accompanied by a sebaceous gland, which secretes an oily material (sebum) that keeps the skin of the lids soft and pliable. Infection (usually with staphylococcal bacteria) starts in a sebaceous gland and spreads to the follicle of the eyelash. Swelling and redness are evident and considerable pain is felt at the margin of the lid. The infection may "come to a head" with a spontaneous discharge of pus.

Special treatment is not often required. If the

STY

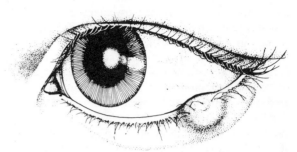

A sty is a bacterial abscess in the follicle of an eyelash. It appears as a localized red swelling on the upper or lower lid. The main symptom is pain, which can be helped by warm compresses.

condition is severe, however, treatment may include removal of the affected eyelash, the local application of penicillin ointment and hot fomentations to the eye. Administration of antibiotics by mouth or injection are rarely required.

In recurrent cases, a local source of infection (such as boils on the neck or face) should be sought (see BOIL). Inadequate personal hygiene may predispose to infection and certain general diseases such as diabetes (in which there is a special susceptibility to infection) must be excluded.

sudden infant death syndrome

The sudden and unexplained death of an infant during sleep. See COT DEATH.

suicide

The deliberate taking of one's own life, which accounts for less than 1% of all deaths in most Western countries. In contrast, so-called attempted suicide from an overdose of sleeping pills or tranquilizers is now one of the most common causes of hospital admission.

Most successful suicides are in persons suffering from severe DEPRESSION, in which the thoughts become dominated by irrational feelings of guilt and unworthiness. The high suicide rate in severely depressed patients justifies the opinion that the condition is a potentially life-threatening medical emergency warranting urgent treatment. Patients who refuse treatment may need close supervision if the risk of suicide is to be minimized. The belief that people who talk about suicide do not carry out their threats is false. Men are more likely to use violent means such as shooting, drowning or hanging; women commonly take an overdose of drugs, often combined with alcohol.

However, most people who take an overdose of drugs

are not suffering from depression and have no real determination to die. Indeed psychiatrists distinguish two separate conditions: *attempted suicide* and *para-suicide*, in which the suicidal gesture is a means of seeking attention at a time of emotional conflict. Parasuicide is most common in teenagers and young adults, women more than men, usually with some personality disorder and a past history of behavioral problems. In contrast, suicide occurs more commonly in middle-aged and elderly persons, with a preponderance of men. Many countries now have organizations (such as the Samaritans) which offer a 24-hour telephone counseling service for anyone contemplating suicide; many individual communities have "crisis lines" for the same purpose. The growth of these services has coincided with a fall in the numbers of deaths.

Anyone found having recently taken an overdose of pills should be taken to a hospital emergency room; loss of consciousness may develop quite suddenly in such circumstances, when immediate treatment may be needed.

sunburn

A reaction of susceptible skin to exposure to the ultraviolet rays of the sun. It can range from slight redness and tenderness to severe blistering. Sunburn is common among swimmers, skiers and outdoor workers (if unprotected).

Blonds are more susceptible than brunettes, although previous exposure and tanning of the skin gives some protection. The effect of exposure to sunlight is greatest when the sun is high in the sky (between about 10 am and 2 pm) and in midsummer. Reflection will also increase the effect—snow, water and sand reflect much of the burning wavelengths of sunlight. Scattered rays may also produce sunburn, even in the presence of haze or thin fog.

The symptoms of simple sunburn need no description; when sunburn is severe, however, there may be a marked constitutional disturbance with nausea, chills and fever and the symptoms may be mixed with those of heat stroke and HEAT EXHAUSTION. Sunburn may also bring on or aggravate other conditions, notably cold sores on the lips and a variety of skin disorders. However, ACNE and some other skin conditions may actually be improved by cautious exposure to the ultraviolet rays of the sun.

Treatment is usually limited to the application of cold compresses to the skin and the administration of emollient lotions to counteract dryness and painkilling drugs to relieve the discomfort. In severe cases, medical advice should be sought and admission to the hospital may even be necessary if the patient becomes ill.

Prevention is by avoidance of exposure to the sun when it is directly overhead or by graduated exposure so that protection is obtained by prior tanning of the skin. Certain drugs may increase the rate of tanning. "Sunscreen" lotions are available which may provide some degree of protection by helping to obstruct the ultraviolet rays responsible for sunburns.

sympathectomy

Surgical removal of part of the sympathetic nervous system.

In addition to the main components of the nervous system—the brain, spinal cord and the nerves of the trunk and limbs—two subsidiary systems exist: the *sympathetic* and *parasympathetic* nervous systems. These two systems have generally opposing effects and are concerned with bodily functions which are not under voluntary nervous control. They control the heart rate, the blood flow to organs and tissues, the secretions of the digestive juices, the movements of the intestinal tract, and sweating.

Among the important functions of the sympathetic nervous system is the control of the caliber (internal diameter) of the arteries, thus influencing the blood flow. The arteries have muscular walls which, when contracted, produce constriction of the vessels (*vasoconstriction*) and a consequent reduction in blood flow and increase in blood pressure. Stimulation of the sympathetic nerves increases vasoconstriction, while paralysis or surgical removal of the nerves produces the opposite effect (*vasodilation*).

When the blood supply to a limb (especially the leg) is poor because the blood vessels are narrowed by spasm (see RAYNAUD'S DISEASE), surgical removal of the sympathetic nerve supply to the limb often results in a great improvement in blood flow. This operation is referred to as a *sympathectomy*. In the case of the leg, it is performed by removing the sympathetic nerve ganglia which supply the legs. These are approached through an incision in the abdominal wall.

Sympathectomy may also be used to treat other forms of vascular disease, including hypertension which does not respond to drugs, and occasionally to relieve symptoms due to excessive sweating.

syncope

A temporary loss of consciousness due to an inadequate flow of blood to the brain; FAINTING.

synovitis

The inner surfaces of a joint are lined by a fine membrane, the *synovial membrane*. Inflammation of this membrane is referred to as synovitis.

Synovitis may be acute or chronic. It usually occurs as a result of disease affecting the joint as a whole. Thus *acute synovitis* occurs in cases of bacterial or viral infection of the joints, after injuries, and in conditions such as HEMOPHILIA in which hemorrhage into joints

SYMPATHECTOMY

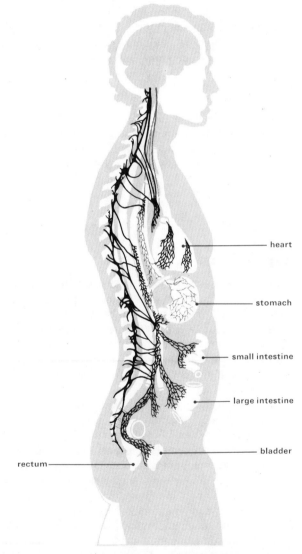

THE AUTONOMIC NERVOUS SYSTEM

The autonomic nervous system has two components—the sympathetic (black) and parasympathetic (gray)—both of which supply the internal organs. Sympathectomy is an operation, usually performed in the neck or the low back, to improve the blood flow to the arms or legs by cutting the sympathetic nerves to the blood vessels.

may occur. *Chronic synovitis* occurs in RHEUMATOID ARTHRITIS and in OSTEOARTHRITIS and in infection of the joints by tuberculosis. The presence of loose fragments of bone or cartilage in a joint may cause acute or chronic synovitis; it occurs in the condition of torn cartilage in the knee (see MENISECTOMY).

Treatment depends on the cause. In synovitis associated with rheumatoid arthritis, for example, generalized treatment of the primary disease is required; in osteoarthritis, drugs are administered for the relief of pain.

In both these conditions, surgical treatment of the joint (including joint replacement operations) may be necessary. Infections are controlled with the administration of antibiotics. Loose fragments of bone or a torn cartilage in the knee will require surgical exploration of the joint.

syphilis

The most serious of the sexually transmitted (venereal) diseases, which may prove fatal if not treated. It is caused by infection with the spirochete bacterium *Treponema pallidum;* the disease is transmitted only by sexual contact or (very rarely) by the transfusion of contaminated blood.

The first sign of syphilis, which appears after a silent incubation period of two to six weeks, is the *chancre*—a hard, painless ulcer on the penis, the female genitalia, or (more rarely) on the lips, tongue or finger. There is some swelling of the lymph nodes nearest to the chancre, which heals slowly in about one month. As the chancre heals, however, syphilis moves into its "secondary stage" with fever, a generalized rash (usually consisting of pale red spots), a sore throat and swelling of lymph nodes throughout the body. Occasionally the infection may inflame the brain coverings (*meningitis*), the membranes that invest the bones (*periostitis*) and the iris of the eyes (*iritis*). Even without treatment this stage will resolve after some weeks, leaving the individual apparently cured; but months or years later "tertiary" syphilitic lesions will appear. These may damage the heart valves or weaken the main blood vessels—causing stretching, swelling and eventually rupture of an artery. The brain and spinal cord may be affected, causing either insanity (*general paralysis of the insane*, or *GPI*) or loss of muscular coordination (*tabes dorsalis*). Indeed, tertiary syphilis may involve any organ and mimic virtually any other chronic disease.

Syphilis can be cured by a full course of treatment with penicillin. Inadequate treatment may only suppress the symptoms, however, and careful medical follow-up is needed to ensure that the infection has been eliminated. Furthermore while penicillin treatment will stop syphilis from progressing it cannot repair damage to the heart valves, nerves, or other organs caused by chronic infection.

An unnoticed syphilitic infection may be suppressed by a short course of antibiotics given as treatment for gonorrhea or any other venereal disease. However, tests on the blood will establish whether or not an individual has syphilis.

Anyone who suspects they may have acquired a venereal disease should be examined and treated by an accredited clinic or specialist.

See also VENEREAL DISEASE.

systemic lupus erythematosus

See LUPUS ERYTHEMATOSUS.

systole

The period when a chamber of the heart contracts and ejects blood. (DIASTOLE is the period when the heart muscle is relaxed and a chamber fills with blood.) During *atrial systole*, blood is pumped from the atria into the ventricles; this period corresponds to ventricular diastole. During *ventricular systole* the right ventricle pumps blood into the lungs where the blood becomes oxygenated while the left ventricle pumps blood into the aorta, and so around the rest of the body.

The term "systolic blood pressure" refers to the pressure in the large arteries during ventricular systole. *Asystole* means cardiac standstill or absence of a heartbeat. If it lasts more than four minutes, deterioration of brain cells begins.

See also BLOOD PRESSURE.

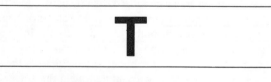

T

tabes dorsalis

A form of tertiary SYPHILIS, affecting men more frequently than women, which appears some years (5 to 20) after the primary infection.

Degeneration occurs in the sensory nerves, which originate in the spinal cord, producing impairment of sensation of temperature and pain and the loss of tendon reflexes. Bouts of acute severe paroxysmal pain ("lightning pains") develop in the legs or arms. Loss of the sense of pain and temperature occurs on the under side of the forearm and arm and spreads over the chest thorax. The abdomen is usually normal, but loss of sensation is again found over the legs.

The patient cannot tell where his legs are when his eyes are closed, and he has to keep his eyes open in order to maintain his balance. He develops a characteristic gait with the feet wide apart, and because he has lost sensation in the soles of his feet he picks them up high when he walks and stamps them down. The same loss of sensation leads to damage of the joints and painless ulcers on the soles of the feet. Sensation from the bladder may be lost, so that the patient suffers from painless retention of urine, and he may be constipated. In some cases there are attacks of acute abdominal pain, with vomiting (tabetic crisis), which may mimic an acute abdominal emergency.

The difficulty in walking gave the disease its alternative name, *locomotor ataxia*.

tachycardia

A marked increase in the rate of the heartbeat, which can be either sudden or gradual in onset. It may arise from some malfunction of the heart, from the action of a drug, from exercise, or from excitement or anger.

talipes

See CLUBFOOT.

tapeworms

Intestinal PARASITES found in virtually every animal species. The two common human tapeworms are acquired from infected pork and beef; a third variety is found in societies which eat infected raw fish. Man may also be parasitized by the larval forms of tapeworms, including some that affect other animals (such as dogs). Infestation of the body with tapeworms is known as *teniasis* (or *taeniasis*).

Infection with the pork tapeworm *Taenia solium* is acquired by eating undercooked "measly" pork, when one or more of the tiny cysticerci (the encysted larval forms of the tapeworm) becomes attached to the small intestine and develops into an adult tapeworm attaining a length of up to 4 meters. A single worm causes few symptoms, but multiple infestation may cause some loss of weight. For the whole of its 30-year life span the worm produces eggs which are excreted with the feces. These eggs are infectious for pigs—and for man. If they are swallowed and partially digested in the stomach, the eggs develop into *oncospheres* (the embryonic stage in which six hooks exist on the head or "scolex" of the tapeworm) which penetrate the intestinal wall and pass in the bloodstream to form cysts in the muscles, brain and other organs. This condition (known as *cysticercosis*) is by far the most dangerous aspect of tapeworm disease, for the cysts in the brain frequently cause epilepsy.

The beef tapeworm, *Taenia saginata*, is common in

TAPEWORM   *Taenia solium*

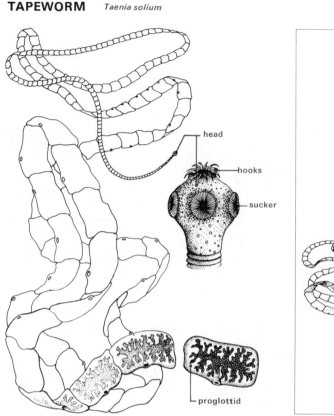

head

hooks

sucker

proglottid

LIFE CYCLE OF
THE TAPEWORM

The adult form of Taenia solium, *the pork tapeworm, is only found in the gut of man, where it may reach a length of 4 m; it attaches itself by the hooks on its head (1). Segments full of eggs (2) are excreted in the feces, and embryos in the soil (3) are eaten by pigs. Encysted larvae (5) reproduce in the pig and develop into adult worms (6) after the human host has eaten infected pork that has not been properly cooked.*

countries where beef is eaten raw. Despite its length (5–6 meters or longer) it rarely causes serious symptoms and the eggs are hardly ever infectious for man, so that cysticercosis is not a problem.

The fish tapeworm, *Diphyllobothrium latum*, is the longest human tapeworm, reaching a length of up to 15 to 18 meters, although the average length is approximately 6 meters (20 feet). Unlike other tapeworms, its presence may lead to serious malnutrition, since the worm competes with its host for vitamin B_{12}; persons infected with the parasites may become profoundly anemic.

Tapeworms may be ejected from the intestines by treatment with special drugs such as quinacrine. The only treatment for cysticercosis is the surgical removal of any cysts causing symptoms.

Compare PINWORMS, ROUNDWORMS.

taste

Although the ancient Greeks recognized nine categories of taste, it is usual today to subdivide them into four—sweet, sour, salty and bitter. The sensation of taste is produced by minute taste buds situated on the surface of the tongue and palate in response to the chemical nature of various substances. Each bud is oval or round and consists of a large number of spindle-shaped cells. Although they appear identical, certain buds (distributed on the tongue in groups) are particularly sensitive to specific tastes. The taste buds at the tip are particularly sensitive to sweet substances, those on the edge to sour (acid) and salt and those on the back of the tongue to bitter substances. At the same time, there is evidence that all taste buds are sensitive in some degree to all four sensations. Chewing the leaves of certain Indian plants destroys the power to taste sweet and bitter substances, while allowing the tongue to recognize those that are salty and sour. This indicates that, although apparently identical, the taste buds have different nerve fibers for the different categories of taste.

Loss or reduction of the ability to taste may be brought about by smoking or the common cold. The once traditional practice of holding the nose while swallowing an unpalatable medicine also indicates that the sense of taste is intimately connected with the sense

TASTE

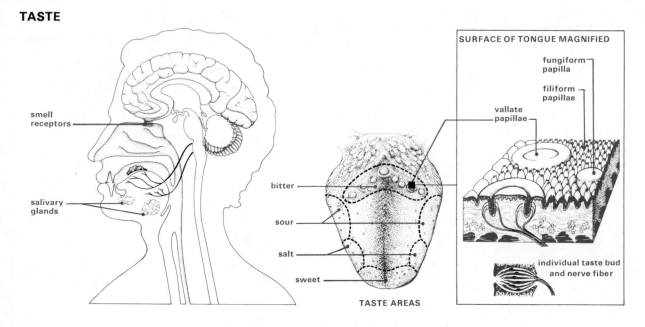

SURFACE OF TONGUE MAGNIFIED

fungiform papilla

filiform papillae

vallate papillae

smell receptors

salivary glands

bitter

sour

salt

sweet

individual taste bud and nerve fiber

TASTE AREAS

The tongue is covered with thousands of taste buds (tiny onion-shaped receptors containing special nerve endings) which respond to substances dissolved in saliva. The buds are found in the fungiform and vallate papillae. All the subtle flavors which we can distinguish are just different combinations of the four basic tastes— sweet, salt, sour and bitter.

of smell. An extremely acute sense of taste to certain substances can be developed—a fact used by wine-tasters or tea-tasters—although this ability tends to lessen after the passage of years. Many tastes are transmitted by the ordinary action of the substance on the tongue, as sensations on the skin are felt. Examples are the "astringent" taste of tannin and the metallic taste produced when a weak electrical current is allowed to pass through the tongue. All tastes produce a reflex flow of saliva, but the awareness of taste also depends to a large extent on such extraneous factors as smell, texture and appearance.

See also SMELL.

tattooing

A method of obtaining a permanent mark or design on the skin by puncturing and the introduction of color. It is of very ancient origin and is found worldwide, except in the darkest-skinned communities and in China. Various methods are used to produce tattooing, the most common being with needles and pigment, though small cuts with special knives are also used.

During the last 20 years tattooing has become increasingly popular among young people in the Western world. In unskilled hands, however, it can be dangerous and has been implicated as a possible cause of some forms of skin cancer. In 1961 the New York City administration severely restricted the practice because of the spread of HEPATITIS caused by contaminated instruments.

Tattooing can be erased only by the removal of the tattooed skin section and the grafting on of new skin.

Tay-Sachs disease

A rare disorder most often found in Ashkenazi Jews, which starts at about the age of six months and affects the nervous system. Victims of the disease, which is inherited as a recessive trait, show retarded physical and mental development, increasing paralysis and blindness, with eventual death by the age of about 18 months to four years.

About one in 30 Ashkenazi Jews carry the gene determining the disease—which is a disorder of fat metabolism—and as carriers can be detected by chromosome tests. They should be screened for the trait before starting a family.

telangiectasia

Small vascular malformations consisting of a group of dilated blood vessels (usually capillaries). They are sometimes seen in the skin in pregnancy, in old age, and in liver disease. The condition may be present at birth, in which case it usually disappears before the age of six.

In most cases the cause is unknown, although telangiectasias may be seen in ROSACEA and certain systemic diseases, such as SCLERODERMA.

temperature

In man and warm-blooded animals the temperature of the body remains almost constant despite the temperature of the surrounding environment. Human beings have a normal body temperature of about 98.6°F (37°C), but the body temperatures of many birds and mammals are somewhat higher. The body temperature of cold-blooded animals (amphibians, invertebrates and fish) varies greatly according to the degree of environmental heat.

Yet even in man the temperature can vary by 1–2°F during the day and is usually highest in the evening. This is probably because of the many movements of the muscles during daytime activity, the energy used being partly dissipated as heat. The intake and digestion of food also slightly increases the temperature of the body.

The temperature can vary in different parts of the body—the skin is about 0.5°F lower than the interior of the body or the natural orifices.

If the body becomes overheated (for example, by exercise) the blood vessels of the skin dilate and sweat is produced. This evaporates and the cooling effect results in the reduction of the body temperature back to normal. When the surrounding atmosphere is very cold the body conserves body heat by contracting the smaller blood vessels especially those near the body surface. In old people and infants the body is less efficient in maintaining a constant temperature and both heat-stroke and extreme loss of heat (HYPOTHERMIA) are more common in these age groups. Hypothermia is especially dangerous in the elderly since its onset may be insidious. An old person living in an unheated house in the winter may lose heat over several days and eventually pass into a fatal coma.

In disease the temperature of the human body may vary from about 90°F (32.2°C) to 110°F (43.3°C) for a time, but there is grave danger to life should it drop and remain below 95°F (35°C) or rise and remain at or above 106°F (41°C). In rare cases, patients have survived a drop in body temperature to below 80°F (26.7°C); indeed, one young patient recovered after a drop in body temperature to 69°F (20.6°C). (Unconsciousness typically occurs when the temperature of the body drops below about 80°F.) Prolonged high fever (hyperpyrexia) can cause irreversible damage to the brain.

The Centigrade scale is normally used in Europe and the U.K.; in the U.S. Fahrenheit is preferred.

tenesmus

A constant desire to evacuate the bowel, although nothing is passed except mucus (occasionally mixed with blood). The condition is spasmodic and extremely distressing. It is likely to be encountered in such disorders of the large intestine as ULCERATIVE COLITIS, DYSENTERY, HEMORRHOIDS or tumor. It can occur when the lower bowel is packed with very hard feces or it may be provoked by fissure of the anus or by a growth. In young children tenesmus may be caused by the presence of worms in the bowel.

Relief of tenesmus depends on treatment of the underlying condition.

tenosynovitis

Inflammation of a tendon sheath—in particular, one of the hand, wrist or ankle.

Tendons are white, fibrous bands of varying lengths which connect muscle to bone. They are very strong. Some tendons consist of round bundles of fibers while others are flat. Most tendons are encased in a sheath similar to the synovial membrane lining joint cavities; this ensures that the tendon glides smoothly over the adjoining bone when contracted.

Tenosynovitis is most commonly found in the wrist and hand and may be caused by bacterial infection following a wound. It may also occur as the result of RHEUMATOID ARTHRITIS or GOUT, or from gonococcal or tubercular infection. The cause may also be obscure and adults of both sexes may be affected. Tuberculous tenosynovitis is most common in the wrist.

Nonspecific tenosynovitis may occur as the result of repeated injuries where frequent and rapid movements of the wrist or ankle are involved. Initial treatment consists of rest and the application of heat. Should this fail, local injections of cortisone may be of value. In extreme cases it may be necessary to excise part of the synovial sheath.

teratogenesis

Literally "giving birth to an abnormality."

The term is used in connection with the production of a physically deformed fetus. This may be caused by the action of certain drugs taken during pregnancy or as the result of a maternal infection during pregnancy, of which the most likely is rubella (German measles).

The drug thalidomide, first used in Germany in 1958, is the best known example of a teratogenic drug. When it was taken by pregnant women (as a tranquilizer), it resulted in the birth of many children with serious physical defects, specifically the absence of limbs. The drug has now been withdrawn. Many drugs have not been adequately tested for teratogenic effects; for this reason, pregnant women are prescribed as few drugs as possible.

If a pregnant woman catches German measles up to the sixth month of pregnancy it may affect the unborn child; it is estimated that in approximately 20% of such cases damage is done to the fetus. Should the mother go to full term and the child is born, the defects caused are varied and serious. They include retarded physical and mental development, brain damage, malformation of the heart, cataract and deafness.

teratoma

This is a true neoplasm (chorionepithelioma) composed of chaotically arranged and bizarre tissues, completely foreign to the type of tissue in which the tumor is found. It occurs most commonly in the testis, and often contains such extraordinary substances as bone, nerve tissue, teeth, gut and, commonly, cysts.

The treatment is removal of the testis and, of course, the tumor, followed by a course of radiotherapy and sometimes an anti-metabolite drug.

testosterone

Testosterone is a male sex hormone—the most important of the group of hormones known as the *androgens*. This group is responsible for the development of internal and external sexual organs, and for the growth and maintenance of the secondary sex characteristics in the male. It is produced in the testicles and in a healthy young man the amount secreted is about 5 mg a day.

Testosterone, in the form of testosterone propionate, is used in the treatment of *hypogonadism*—the failure to develop the secondary sexual characteristic associated with maturity. It is also used to treat PROSTATITIS and certain deficiencies of testicular function.

In females it is sometimes used in the treatment of inoperable breast cancer. Though not a cure, it is of value in arresting the spread of the cancer from soft tissue to the adjoining bone, reducing pain and limiting bone destruction. Testosterone propionate is normally administered in the form of intramuscular injections, but methyltestosterone tablets are given by mouth.

tetanus

An acute infectious disease of the nervous system (also known as *lockjaw*) characterized by spasms of the voluntary muscles and painful convulsions. The cause of the disease is the action of the bacillus *Clostridium tetani* which was first isolated by a Japanese researcher, Kitasato, in 1889.

Spores of the bacillus are commonly found in earth, especially when it is contaminated with manure from horses or cattle. These spores may survive in the earth undisturbed for many years and may enter the body when a wound is contaminated with soil. However, the bacteria cannot multiply in the body in the presence of oxygen, so they grow only in dirty wounds or in dead, bloodless tissues around a deep wound. Once multiplication begins, however, the bacilli produce toxins which destroy the tissue around them, providing ideal conditions for further bacterial growth. The toxins also enter the nerves, spreading up the nerve fibers to reach the spinal cord, where they cause muscle spasms.

The first sign of tetanus is stiffness felt around the site of the wound followed by stiffness of the jaw muscles, irrespective of the location of the wound. The spasms gradually extend to the muscles of the neck and eventually affect the muscles of the chest, back, abdomen and extremities. During such spasms the body may be drawn to the left or right, backward or forward, causing extreme pain and distress to the patient, who remains conscious throughout. In the early stages such convulsions are intermittent, but may be precipitated by any minor disturbance (such as the banging of a door or sudden exposure to bright light). The patient may eventually die from sheer exhaustion due to prolonged spasms.

The treatment of the illness consists of eliminating the infection by cleaning the wound and giving antibiotics, blocking the action of the toxin with specific antitoxins, and reducing the muscular spasms by means of sedatives, such as chlorpromazine or the barbiturates. In severe cases the spasms may be abolished altogether by the administration of muscle-paralyzing drugs such as curare. The patient will then need treatment in an intensive care unit, together with artificial or assisted respiration, until the toxin is finally eliminated from the body.

TRACHEOTOMY may be necessary in order to facilitate breathing in patients treated by paralytic drugs. This form of treatment has cut the mortality rate of severe tetanus from 90% or more to close to 10%.

Tetanus is one of the diseases (including polio and diphtheria) which are entirely preventable by immunization. If children are given tetanus vaccine at the same time as their immunizations against diphtheria and whooping cough they develop lasting immunity against the toxin. This immunity should be boosted with another shot of toxoid as part of the treatment of any dirty or ragged wound.

tetany

An affliction which causes spasms and twitching of muscles, particularly of the arms and hands. The elbows are bent and the fingers squeezed together. Sometimes the lower limbs are similarly affected and sometimes the face. (This condition should not be confused with TETANUS.)

Tetany is due to a fall of the ionic calcium content of

the blood and tissue fluids. It is most common in infants, where it may be associated with RICKETS, excessive vomiting or certain disorders of the kidney. It is also associated with malfunction of the parathyroid gland and with vitamin D deficiency. Tetany can also occur as the result of metabolic disturbances created by *hyperventilation* (one form of which is hysterical overbreathing).

Treatment involves the intravenous administration of calcium, normally as calcium gluconate. Parathormone is administered when tetany results from underactivity of the parathyroid gland.

tetralogy of Fallot

One of the most common congenital multiple defects of the heart. About a fifth of all cases of *cyanotic congenital heart disease* ("blue babies") are in this category. The four defects which make up the tetralogy are (1) interventricular septal defect ("hole in the heart"), (2) transposition of the aorta (the largest artery), (3) narrowing of the pulmonary artery, and (4) enlargement (hypertrophy) of the right ventricle of the heart.

A baby with these heart defects will grow slowly with repeated attacks of breathlessness. The CYANOSIS (blue coloration of the skin and lips) and shortness of breath are worse on exertion. If untreated, the child will develop swollen (clubbed) fingers and be susceptible to attacks of bacterial endocarditis and heart failure. However, surgery is widely and successfully used to improve the circulation through the pulmonary artery and to repair the heart defects, restoring the child to near-normal health. In the majority of children, a complete cure is possible through surgery.

thalassemia

A group of inherited disorders affecting the red blood cells. The "heterozygote" has a form of the disease, *thalassemia minor*, which only produces mild symptoms of hemolytic disease; but the "homozygote" develops *thalassemia major*, a severe disease which is usually fatal in early adult life.

The disease probably had its origin by the shores of the Mediterranean, for it is most common in Sicily, Sardinia and Greece—although it has spread through northern India into Thailand and China.

Affected children may become jaundiced and develop enlargement of the spleen and liver. There is a family history of the disease. Firm diagnosis is made by examination of the blood, which in many cases contains abnormal red cells with a pale rim and a central spot of hemoglobin; an alternative name for the disease is therefore *target cell anemia*. There is no known cure, but palliative treatment is possible.

thermography

Variations of temperature over the surface of the body can be estimated by measuring infrared radiation.

Infrared waves are not visible to the eye, but an infrared camera will show the amount of radiation and therefore the amount of heat given off from a specific area of skin.

The heat given off by the skin is determined by the amount of blood passing through the local circulation and other known factors, so that variations in surface temperature may indicate an underlying abnormality, such as a tumor.

The technique is useful in SCREENING cases of suspected cancer of the breast where an underlying tumor may produce an area of increased temperature in the skin, and in estimating blood flow in limbs affected by circulatory disease.

The diagnostic accuracy of the method in detecting cancer of the breast is not very high, and its clinical use is therefore restricted.

See also BREAST CANCER.

thirst

The instinctive craving for fluid. The sensation of thirst is felt as dryness of the throat and mouth; when there is a deficiency of water in the body, moisture evaporates quickly and immediately from these parts.

In the course of 24 hours the kidneys excrete about $2\frac{1}{2}$ pints of water, while the lungs and skin also lose considerable quantities. To make good this loss, fresh supplies of fluid are required, and thirst is the signal that this has become necessary. In particular, thirst arises from vigorous muscular exercise, owing to the loss of water by the excretion of sweat. Thirst also becomes intense when the body loses a considerable amount of fluid, as in hemorrhage or diarrhea.

Thirst is a common symptom in fever owing to increased body heat and sweating. The thirst which follows the intake of salt or sugar is an indication for the need of the dilution of these substances in the digestive tract and bloodstream. Excessive thirst (polydipsia) is also a feature of DIABETES INSIPIDUS.

thoracotomy

The operation of opening the thorax (chest), the necessary prelude to operation performed on the lungs and heart.

The scope of thoracic surgery has been immensely widened since World War II because of advances in the art of anesthesia, the development of the heart-lung machine, and the discovery of antibiotics. Operations that were technically impossible 40 years ago are now almost matters of routine. It is possible to remove whole lungs or parts of the lung, remove or reconstruct the esophagus, and operate on the arrested heart.

At the same time, the pattern of chest surgery has changed; originally, most chest operations were performed in the treatment of tuberculosis. Emphasis then shifted to the treatment of lung cancer, while now a great deal of time is devoted to heart surgery.

threadworms

Another name for PINWORMS.

thromboangiitis obliterans

A chronic and recurring vascular disease (also known as *Buerger's disease*) which affects the arteries and, to a lesser extent, the veins. A thickening appears in the lining membrane of the affected blood vessel and this progresses until the bore of the vessel becomes progressively reduced and finally obliterated (*obliterative endarteritis*). The disease may take months or years to reach this stage. The cause is unknown but it is definitely worsened by smoking, is much more common in men than in women and is seen more often in certain ethnic groups (young Jewish males are particularly susceptible).

The symptoms are those of a failing blood supply to the limbs, especially the legs, accompanied in some cases by reddened and painful areas over the veins. Symptoms of the failing blood supply are seen in the onset of pain on walking. This characteristically occurs in the calf of the leg after the patient has walked a certain distance, but disappears again rapidly on standing still (a condition known as INTERMITTENT CLAUDICATION). More prolonged pain may occur and there may be ulceration of the skin of the foot or leg; gangrene of the toes or foot may occur if the blood supply becomes seriously impaired.

Treatment is initially conservative (nonsurgical). Tobacco in any form is forbidden since it aggravates the condition. In severe cases, the development of a better circulation through unaffected tributaries of the vessels may be encouraged by a SYMPATHECTOMY operation—which causes dilation of those vessels remaining unobstructed.

Prognosis for life is good but amputation of toes, the foot or even the lower leg is possible if gangrene occurs.

thrombocytopenia

A condition in which there is a deficiency of *thrombocytes* (PLATELETS) in the blood, which gives rise to a number of diseases involving failure of the blood to clot adequately, including thrombocytopenic PURPURA.

Platelets are minute, colorless particles existing in the blood in great numbers, and one cubic millimeter of blood contains about a quarter of a million of them. When a blood vessel is damaged and blood escapes, the platelets fuse together at the site of the injury and so plug the breach. Thrombocytes also release the hormone *serotonin*, which causes the blood vessels to contract and again reduces the flow.

Insufficiency of platelets can result either from their underproduction in the bone marrow or from the destruction of existing platelets. Certain diseases which inhibit the production of white blood cells can also stop the production of platelets. This can happen through radiation, diseases of the bone marrow or leukemia. A deficiency may also arise through a massive transfusion of banked blood, for platelets do not remain viable in banked blood.

Underproduction of platelets may also occur on its own, and not as the result of another disease. In such cases it is known as *idiopathic thrombocytopenia*. This is rare, but is sometimes seen in children and premenopausal women.

Treatment, according to the type of thrombocytopenia involved, is either by drugs (prednisone), removal of the spleen, or by platelets transfusion. The last method is used only in extreme cases owing to the danger of the development of subsequent resistance to further treatment.

thromboembolism

The blockage of a blood vessel by a thrombus that has become detached from its site of origin.

See also EMBOLISM/EMBOLUS, THROMBUS/THROMBOSIS.

thrombophlebitis

Thrombosis (clotting) in veins is divided into two classes, depending on whether or not the wall of the affected vein is inflamed. If it is inflamed the condition is called *thrombophlebitis;* if it is not, the condition is known as *phlebothrombosis*.

In thrombophlebitis the clotting in the vein follows inflammation of its wall. The affected vein is red, tender, painful and hard. The clot sticks to the wall of the vein and there is little danger of it breaking away and producing an embolus. Infection of the vein may be a complication of varicose veins of the leg. It may have no obvious cause, or may be secondary to THROMBOANGIITIS OBLITERANS. Damage to the walls of varicose veins may be produced intentionally by the injection of sclerosing agents as part of a course of treatment, for in this way the varicose veins can be obliterated.

The treatment of thrombophlebitis is initial rest and analgesics (painkillers); elastic support may be comfortable. The affected leg should be used as soon as possible because walking improves the flow of blood through the veins.

See also PHLEBITIS, THROMBUS/THROMBOSIS.

THROMBOPHLEBITIS

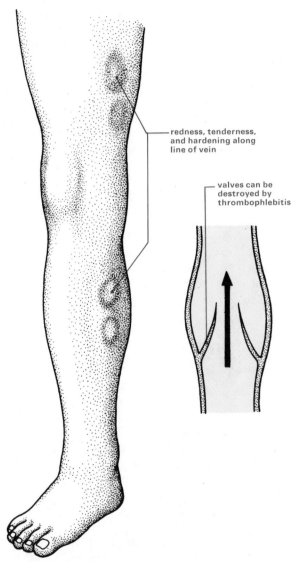

redness, tenderness, and hardening along line of vein

valves can be destroyed by thrombophlebitis

Thrombophlebitis (inflammation of a vein followed by blockage of the vein due to the formation of a blood clot) is usually marked by pain, heat and redness along the course of the involved vein. The illustration shows this process in the long saphenous vein of the leg. The condition is only dangerous if it extends into the deep leg veins from where pieces of blood clot can travel up to the lungs.

thrombophlebitis migrans

This is a condition in which symptoms of THROMBOPHLEBITIS occur in various parts of the body at different times. They may appear in the neck, abdomen, or pelvis as well as in the legs. Small red nodules, which are very tender to the touch, can be seen along the veins immediately under the skin.

This form of thrombophlebitis sometimes arises during the course of an infectious or malignant disease, but can also occur spontaneously for no apparent reason.

thrombus/thrombosis

A *thrombus* is a blood clot; *thrombosis* is the process of formation of a blood clot.

Normally, the inside walls of the blood vessels are smooth; although the blood readily clots when outside the vessels, it remains fluid in normal arteries and veins. If, however, the walls of the vessels are damaged by disease or injury, the blood clots as it comes into contact with the damaged area. This mechanism prevents blood loss in the case of injury, but in disease can lead to the formation of blockages inside the vessels.

Moreover, parts of the clot may break off and travel through the circulation until they are held up and so cause an obstruction to the passage of blood in places remote from the original clot. Pieces of clot which break off in this way are called *emboli*, and the blockage they cause when they become lodged in an artery is an *embolism* (see EMBOLISM/EMBOLUS).

It is possible for arteries to be completely blocked without causing too much disturbance as long as the part of the body affected has a rich blood supply, for the blood needed can still find its way to the tissues by means of bypasses (collateral circulation). If, however, there is no alternative circulation, the tissues normally supplied by the blocked vessel will die. The area of tissue so affected is called an *infarct*, and the process is known as an *infarction*. The effects of a thrombosis are therefore more serious in some parts of the body than others. Examples are (1) the heart, where thrombosis of a coronary artery (*coronary thrombosis*) may lead to the death of part of the heart muscle (*myocardial infarction*); and (2) the brain, where the collateral circulation is poor and a *cerebral thrombosis* leads to loss of function which is manifest by paralysis or weakness of the side of the body opposite to the side of the vascular blockage (see STROKE).

Arterial thrombosis is the end result of atherosclerotic disease of the vessels; but thrombosis of the venous system—commonly seen in the vessels of the lower limbs—may be caused by a number of conditions. Superficial thrombosis of the leg veins is not often of consequence, but thrombosis of the deep veins may be a dangerous condition as emboli may break off and become lodged in other parts of the body, notably the lungs.

Thrombosis of the deep veins occurs principally after childbirth and after surgical operations. It may also occur in women taking oral contraceptive pills and in elderly people confined to bed. If the development of deep vein thrombosis is suspected, anticoagulants are used to minimize the risk of the blood clots breaking off and traveling through the circulatory system.

thrush

A fungal infection of the mouth or throat characterized by the formation of white patches and ulceration of the affected tissues. It is caused by infection with *Candida albicans*, and the condition is known technically as *candidiasis*. See CANDIDA.

thyroid

The thyroid is an endocrine or ductless gland situated in the neck. It has two lobes, one on each side of the larynx, joined by an isthmus. Two *parathyroid glands* lie in each lateral lobe.

The thyroid gland affects the rate of body metabolism, the process by which energy is made available. This is done by the secretion into the blood of two HORMONES, *thyroxine* and *triiodothyronine*, which are produced from tyrosine and inorganic iodine. These hormones stimulate metabolism and increase the consumption of oxygen. They are also essential for normal development and growth.

Deficiency of thyroid hormone brought about by failure of the gland to develop, disease affecting it, or its surgical removal results in HYPOTHYROIDISM. Oversecretion of thyroid hormone results in HYPERTHYROIDISM. The controlling factor in thyroid activity is the *thyroid-stimulating hormone* of the anterior part of the pituitary gland.

Deficiency in the supply of iodine (normally present in the diet in the small quantities needed), an excess of certain foods (such as soya or cabbage), or even an unknown factor may cause the thyroid to enlarge and form a GOITER.

thyroidectomy

Surgical removal of the whole thyroid gland or part of it.

The main indication for the operation is in cases of *thyrotoxicosis* (see HYPERTHYROIDISM), where medical treatment with antithyroid drugs has failed, particularly in patients under 40. It is also indicated in the treatment of goiters, where the size of the tumor is causing trouble. About nine-tenths of the gland is removed in operations for thyrotoxicosis, leaving that part of the gland which is in close relation to the parathyroid glands. In experienced hands the operation is safe, but is sometimes attended by complications ranging from damage to the "recurrent laryngeal nerve," which causes postoperative hoarseness, to tetany due to inadvertent removal of parathyroid glands.

Recurrence of thyrotoxicosis may occur in about 10% of cases; the occurrence of symptoms due to insufficiency of thyroid hormone (HYPOTHYROIDISM) is under 10%. Periodic medical checks are required after thyroidectomy.

The operation is also indicated in the treatment of cancer of the thyroid, but because of the radical operation needed the occurrence of complications may be higher.

See also GOITER, HORMONES.

THYROID AND PARATHYROID

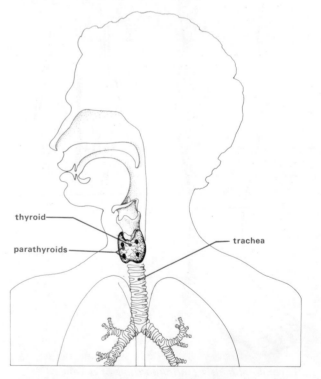

thyroid

parathyroids

trachea

The thyroid gland lies in front of the trachea in the neck and secretes thyroxine, a hormone which controls the rates of many bodily activities. The four pea-sized parathyroid glands embedded within the thyroid secrete another hormone (parathormone) which is essential for maintaining correct levels of calcium and phosphorus in the blood.

thyroiditis

Inflammation of the thyroid gland. It is a relatively rare condition.

Acute inflammation of the thyroid gland may follow severe infections of the upper respiratory tract with streptococci, staphylococci, or pneumococci; subacute infection is thought to be caused by a virus, although definite demonstration of such a virus has not yet been possible. Chronic inflammatory change is found as a manifestation of autoimmunity in lymphadenoid goiter or HASHIMOTO'S DISEASE. The thyroid is enlarged, smooth and rubbery, and may be uncomfortable. Treatment involves the administration of the hormone thyroxine.

In focal thyroiditis similar changes are found. In cases of primary MYXEDEMA in the middle-aged or elderly the thyroid may be found to be very small, with its normal structure lost but small areas left showing the changes of chronic thyroiditis (*diffuse atrophic thyroiditis*).

thyrotoxicosis

A toxic state caused by HYPERTHYROIDISM.

tic

An involuntary movement or twitch of part of the body which is repeated time after time for no apparent reason.

A tic usually represents a movement which would be useful in its proper place, and at one time was made normally because of prevailing conditions. For this reason it is sometimes known as a *habitual spasm*. As an example, a tic of blinking may have come about originally as a result of poor eyesight. This may have been corrected by glasses, but the tic (or habit) of blinking may continue, particularly if the person concerned is of a nervous disposition.

A tic may be a sign of overwork or ill health, and is not usually present during sleep. The movement may be mild, such as blinking, coughing or sniffing, but whole limbs can be affected. The movements are generally sharp and quick, resembling the results of an electric shock. A tic may respond to psychotherapy.

Tic douloureux is spasm of the facial muscles due to paroxysms of pain in the trigeminal nerve; the condition is also known as *trigeminal neuralgia*. It may affect any one of the three parts of the face supplied by this nerve: the forehead and side of the head, the cheek and upper jaw, or the lower jaw. The paroxysms are extraordinarily painful, and even after the attack has subsided the site remains sore and stiff. Normally only one side of the face is affected.

An attack may be precipitated by some minor shock, such as a draft or the eating of very cold food; but in some cases it occurs for no obvious reason. The condition typically occurs in people over the age of 50. Treatment may involve the surgical destruction of the ganglion of the trigeminal nerve.

ticks

Small PARASITES belonging to the spider class (arachnids) which depend on an intake of blood for their growth and development.

Ticks are found in the ground and in undergrowth and attach themselves to the skin of their victim, which may be animal or human. They do this by means of sharp and tenacious teeth and with a probe that sucks the blood into their bodies. Both male and female ticks engorge themselves with blood; the male usually remains unchanged during the process, while the female swells up and resembles a red or purple berry on the skin.

A large number of infections are carried by ticks including ROCKY MOUNTAIN SPOTTED FEVER, African tick typhus, and Queensland tick typhus. They can cause Texas fever in cattle.

Ticks cannot usually transmit infection to man unless they have been on the skin for several hours. In tick-infested areas, therefore, it is a wise precaution to examine the body thoroughly at least twice daily and remove any ticks found. The tick should *not* be rubbed off nor pulled off for fear of further damage to the skin

TICK

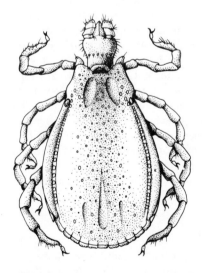

male brown tick *Rhipicephalus appendiculatus*

Ticks (length 5mm) are blood-sucking arthropods which transmit harmful microorganisms to man when they bite. Diseases spread in this manner include tick-borne typhus, relapsing fever, and Q fever.

or tissue. It can either be removed by "drowning" with a heavy oil, such as salad oil or machine oil, or can be killed by carefully applying a lighted cigarette to its body taking care not to burn the person's skin. The use of tick-repellent chemicals on skin and clothing reduces the risk of infection in tick-infested localities.

tinea

A group of common fungus infections of the skin, hair, toenails and fingernails caused by three types of fungus: *Microspora*, *Trichophyton* and *Epidermophyton*. The skin lesions tend to spread outward while the central part heals, thus creating the appearance of a ring. This gives the infection its common name of *ringworm*. The infection is also known as dermatophytosis.

Tinea capitis is ringworm of the scalp. It is found in children under the age of ten and is virtually never present after adolescence. There are a number of round scaly patches on the scalp from which the hair falls out.

Tinea cruris (popularly known as "dhobie itch") is ringworm of the crotch, seen mainly in young men. A red itchy patch of inflammation extends from the crotch down the inner side of the thighs for about two or three inches. It is most common in hot weather, and sweating athletes are particularly vulnerable.

Tinea pedis is the technical name for *athlete's foot*—an extremely common infection, most often occurring in young adults. It is so common that it affects about half the population at one time or another. The skin between the third, fourth and fifth toes becomes sodden and irritating and peels off. The infection may be found on other parts of the feet and may spread to the hands. In some cases the presence of athlete's foot produces skin changes in the hands, although the fungus cannot be demonstrated there. The fungus may also infect the nails (*tinea unguium*); it is one form of ONYCHOMYCOSIS.

Ringworm is spread by direct contact. Treatment is by local application of fungicidal preparations. The development of the antibiotic griseofulvin has made it possible to treat fungus infections orally; the drug is given in appropriate daily doses for about a month, but must be used with caution in patients sensitive to penicillin.

tinnitus

A constant or intermittent hissing, buzzing, or ringing noise in the ear. It may arise from a disorder of the nerves of the ear; it may also occur through blockage of the Eustachian tubes or excessive wax in the ears. Irritation of the auditory nerve may follow large doses of aspirin, quinine, or other drugs. Tinnitus is a common feature of MÉNIÈRE'S DISEASE, in which it is accompanied by gradually increasing deafness.

toilet training

The training of a child to control his bladder or bowel. There are no rigid methods of training, but it is worth keeping in mind a few guiding principles which apply to both bladder and bowel training.

The first is that normal development, maturation, and ability to learn vary enormously from child to child, and a child who is later than others in learning control should not be punished for his failure. Generally, however, the intervals between voiding increase gradually, so that by about the age of $2\frac{1}{2}$ years most children can hold their urine for about five hours.

Babies often empty their bladder or bowel after a meal, and may be conditioned to do so after the age of 2 to $2\frac{1}{2}$ months by placing them on the potty after a meal. It must be remembered that this is conditioning and not voluntary control. The conditioning may break down whenever there is a disturbance in routine, such as during teething. Moreover, if a child is punished for not using the potty he can become conditioned against it. Many children go through a stage of characteristic negativism after the age of one year, during which they rebel against being forced to do anything; over-enthusiastic efforts by anxious parents could result in the opposite effect to what is desired.

Voluntary control does not begin until after a child is about 15 to 18 months old. Often the first indication that a child has reached this stage is that, having passed urine, he can point this out to the mother. This goes on to his being able, on being asked, to say with reasonable accuracy whether or not he wants to void. Finally, he reaches the stage when he can say when he wants to go to the toilet. In the early part of this stage, the child cannot hold his bladder or bowel for very long once the desire to void has set in; if he is not given the opportunity to empty his bladder or bowel when he first announces it, the learning of control may be delayed.

On the other hand, a child soon realizes that a parent may drop everything he or she is doing to attend to his toilet needs, and may use this as an attention-seeking device. It may be difficult to distinguish between natural frequency of wanting to empty the bladder and attention-seeking. If it is due to the latter, the calls should be ignored except at what are thought to be suitable intervals. If it is not likely to be due to attention-seeking, the urine should be examined for evidence of an infection (cloudy urine, containing pus cells, or traces of blood).

In some cases voluntary control may be lost after it has been learned. This may be due to the child deliberately holding back the urine or stool when he is in the middle of an interesting game which he does not want to leave. Accidents may then occur, when he can hold his bladder or bowel no longer; they may be prevented by gently reminding the child who is engrossed in a game to go to the toilet.

See also BEDWETTING (ENURESIS).

tonsillectomy

Surgical removal of the tonsils. The indications for the operation have changed from the past, when it was performed fairly routinely.

Most surgeons are unwilling to operate because difficulties with the tonsils usually resolve themselves with puberty—in girls rather later than in boys—and they confine themselves to operating only in cases of recurrent severe infection involving spread to the ears, or obvious cases of chronic infections which do not respond to medication. They are now inclined to perform adenoidectomy alone, because of middle-ear involvement, and omit tonsillectomy.

In adults it may be necessary to remove the tonsils when they are the seat of a new growth, or have been involved in a QUINSY. The operation is usually performed under general anesthesia for children up to the age of about 12; for teenagers and adults the surgeon may prefer local anesthesia. The most common complication is postoperative bleeding, which requires urgent treatment.

tonsillitis

Infection of the tonsils, which are masses of lymphatic tissue lying on each side of the entrance to the throat at the back of the tongue.

TONSILLECTOMY

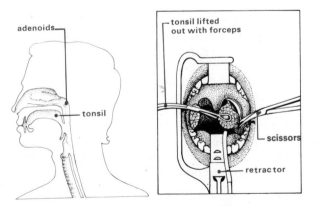

adenoids

tonsil

tonsil lifted out with forceps

scissors

retractor

Tonsillectomy is most often carried out on children who have had frequent attacks of acute tonsillitis. The tonsils are removed under general anesthesia by cutting them off the side wall of the throat with a scalpel and lifting them out with forceps. Very often, the adenoids are removed at the same time.

The infection is very common, particularly in children, and is usually caused by a streptococcus. Very often the infection is self-limiting; but in many cases it spreads to involve the lymph glands which drain the tonsils, and a painful swelling develops behind the angle of the jaw.

Children can become quite ill and run a high temperature during an attack of tonsillitis; if prompt treatment is not obtained, some streptococci produce a toxin which brings out the skin rash of scarlatina (scarlet fever). There may also be abdominal pain and vomiting. Fortunately, however, this is a rare complication today, as prompt and effective treatment eliminates this risk.

The organisms causing tonsillitis are sensitive to antibiotics, and attacks of any severity can usually be controlled with penicillin. Occasionally, infection goes on to abscess formation; an abscess developing in the loose tissue around the tonsils is known as a quinsy. It may need surgical relief.

torsion of the testis

While the fetus is still within the womb the testes are carried in the abdomen; but at birth, or soon afterward, they descend through the muscles of the abdomen into the scrotum. This is normally accomplished within a few weeks, but occasionally one of the testes fails to descend and surgical intervention may be necessary.

In their descent the testes bring with them their duct, the *vas deferens*, and various blood vessels—the whole forming the *spermatic cord*. In torsion of the testis a twisting of the gland compresses the blood vessels in the spermatic cord and so cuts off its blood supply. There is intense pain and tenderness of the testis, often accompanied by nausea and vomiting. Diagnosis may be difficult if the testis is still in the abdomen—as may be the case in infancy. However, torsion of the testis does not happen only during descent of the testes; it can also occur to a mature man as a sudden and devastating event that requires fast medical or surgical intervention if the testis is to be saved.

Occasionally the symptoms may be relieved by untwisting the spermatic cord; more often a surgical operation is needed. Delay may mean permanent damage to or loss of the testis. Whenever torsion has occurred an operation should be carried out on both testes to prevent recurrence.

See ORCHIOPEXY.

torticollis

The medical name for *wryneck*, a condition in which the neck is bent to one side or the other. It may be either chronic or spasmodic.

In *chronic torticollis* the neck is permanently bent due

to shortening of one of the sternomastoid muscles. These are two large muscles, one on each side of the neck, which help to maintain the head and neck in an upright position and act rather like guy ropes. Shortening of the sternomastoid may be the result of injury at birth or later in life, but may also be inherited. It is not usually evident at birth owing to the shortness of the baby's neck, but if discovered will often respond to manipulation. If it does not respond and becomes definitely established, an operation may be required to divide the shortened muscle. Chronic torticollis may also arise from an inflamed gland pressing on the sternomastoid muscle, or from rheumatism.

Spasmodic torticollis is an involuntary twitching of the neck either to the left or right and is often a habit acquired in childhood. It is of nervous origin and can develop into the chronic state. It is extremely difficult to cure but may be relieved by psychiatric treatment.

TORTICOLLIS

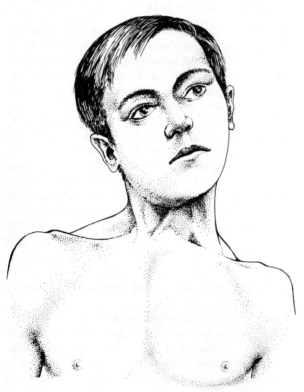

torticollis (congenital wry-neck) in a boy aged 14 years

Congenital torticollis usually affects babies who were breech presentations or difficult deliveries, but its exact cause is unknown. Fortunately, early correction either by repeatedly stretching the neck in the opposite direction or by surgery usually prevents this picture in a teenager.

tourniquet

A band placed tightly around a limb to control severe arterial bleeding. There are several kinds of tourniquets, but basically they consist of a wide band or pad placed around the limb, with an appliance or lever which tightens it enough to stop the flow of blood through a main artery.

Modern medical opinion has discouraged the use of tourniquets except (1) in special operative techniques where blood must be excluded as far as possible from the site of the operation, thus permitting delicate procedures; and (2) for the control of severe bleeding at the end of a limb which has been accidentally amputated and which is not controllable otherwise.

The use of tourniquets is no longer considered acceptable in first-aid work.

toxemia of pregnancy

Another term for PREECLAMPSIA, a rise in blood pressure during pregnancy, with PROTEINURIA, weight gain, and EDEMA, swelling resulting from retained fluid.

toxoplasmosis

An infection with a protozoan parasite, *Toxoplasma gondii*, which is common in both animals and man. Most human infections cause few or no symptoms, but infection during pregnancy can possibly spread to the fetus causing serious damage to the brain or the eyes of the unborn child. This congenital toxoplasmosis occurs in approximately 1 in every 2,000 newborn infants.

Adult toxoplasmosis has assumed new importance in recent years since the disease may be a serious threat in patients whose natural immunity has been lowered by treatment with immunosuppressive drugs after transplantation and in patients given anticancer (cytotoxic) drugs.

Toxoplasmosis often responds to treatment with antimalarial and sulfonamide drugs, but suppression of the disease should be based on public health measures, since the source of human infection is animal excreta and contaminated meat.

tracheitis

Inflammation of the trachea ("windpipe"), the vertical tube extending down from the larynx to immediately above the heart, where it divides into two main *bronchi*, one extending to each lung.

Tracheitis causes pain in the upper part of the chest, accompanied by a dry painful cough. Often it occurs as a complication of a more general respiratory infection, such as influenza or bronchitis. The symptoms may be relieved by inhalation of steam, by cough syrups, or by antibiotics.

See also RESPIRATORY TRACT INFECTION.

tracheotomy

An operation in which the trachea ("windpipe") is opened from the front of the neck and a tube inserted to allow air to reach the lungs. It becomes necessary when the windpipe is obstructed or narrowed as the result of an illness such as diphtheria; or if the larynx has to be excised in the treatment of cancer. Tracheotomy is also necessary whenever the respiration has to be maintained artificially by a mechanical ventilator.

If the opening is made immediately under the chin and above the thyroid gland the operation is called *high tracheotomy*, and below the thyroid *low tracheotomy*. In practice the operation frequently involves cutting through the center of the thyroid gland.

The entry into the windpipe is made by cutting a vertical slit through the skin and fatty tissues of the neck. Tracheotomy tubes are then inserted, an outer tube first which remains in position, and an inner tube which may be removed or coughed out if, for example, it becomes blocked with mucus. The tubes are made of hard rubber or metal and a dressing is inserted between the outer tube and the wound. The entrance to the inner tube is protected by medicated gauze to act as an air filter.

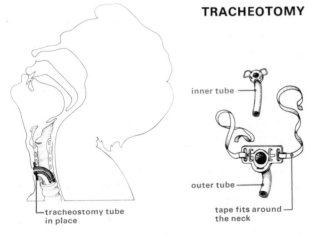

TRACHEOTOMY

inner tube

outer tube

tape fits around the neck

tracheostomy tube in place

A tracheotomy is an opening made in the trachea (windpipe) through which a tube is inserted to create an emergency airway. The main indications for a tracheotomy are: (1) an obstruction in the larynx or upper respiratory tract, (2) an unconscious patient who needs to be attached to an artifical respirator for a considerable period.

Where blockage of the windpipe has taken place, and no other measures give relief, the operation should be performed as soon as possible and before the patient becomes *cyanosed* through lack of oxygen. If delayed until this point the operation may result in sudden cardiac failure and death.

When there is a permanent obstruction the tubes must be left in place. In other instances, such as diphtheria, the tubes are left in for three or four days and then removed, after which the wound will heal.

Patients with a permanent tracheotomy can learn to speak again by regurgitating air from the esophagus— *esophageal speech*.

trachoma

A disease, affecting over 400 million people in the world, which is the chief cause of blindness in tropical and subtropical countries. It is an infection of the conjunctiva by a virus-like microorganism belonging to the group *Bedsonia*.

As the infection spreads slowly through the conjunctival sac, scar tissue forms which distorts the eyelids and renders the cornea liable to ulceration and the formation of dense opacities. The disease is spread by contaminated flies and dirt and is clearly associated with poverty and poor hygiene.

The causative organism is sensitive to antibiotics, and research is being conducted to develop an effective vaccine.

traction

A technique used in orthopedics for treating fractures, straightening the spine, or for treating slipped disks.

When a bone has fractured the resulting inflammation and irritation around the fracture cause the muscles in the area and those attached to the bone to go into spasm. This may result in some overriding of the broken ends of the bone or in their being pulled into an unsatisfactory position. Untreated, the result would be shortening of a limb. Traction is applied by fixing weights and pulleys to the broken limb so that the bones are pulled into the correct alignment. Traction, skillfully applied, can overcome the effects of the muscles which have gone into spasm. Overzealous traction, on the other hand, may pull the fractured ends apart and so delay healing.

Patients with SCOLIOSIS, a type of spinal curvature, may also be treated by traction applied to the head and pelvis or to the spine and pelvis; the steady push and pull of the spine in the desired direction slowly results in some straightening.

Traction is commonly used for treating slipped disks in which the symptoms are thought to be due to pressure of the intervertebral disk on the nerves coming off the spinal cord; traction would then pull the two vertebrae apart on either side of the degenerate disk and allow it to slip back into place. However, there is no definitive proof that this is how symptoms are relieved; a number of experts believe that traction relieves symptoms by enforcing bed rest.

Traction may also be applied by gravity. This is used, for example, in treating upper arm fractures, or congenital dislocation of the hip in children. With upper arm fractures the affected part is held in a wrist sling so that the weight of the upper limb pulls on the humerus (the bone in the upper arm).

Skin traction may also be used. With hip and thigh injuries, elastic devices may be applied around the upper thigh and traction exerted on the elastic by connecting it to weights which run over pulleys at the foot of the bed. Similarly, the weights may be connected to pins or wires inserted into the bone to which traction is to be applied.

transplantation

The surgical replacement of a diseased organ by a healthy one taken from another individual. The donor may be living (usually a close relative) or the organ may be removed from a body shortly after death.

Transplantation began with grafting of the cornea (the transparent layer at the front of the eye) as a treatment for some forms of blindness. When attempts were made to transplant skin, however, it soon became clear that the grafts survived for only a few days: the body's immune defenses *reject* grafts from another individual in the same way that they destroy invading bacteria. The bloodless cornea is the exception to this general rule.

Successful transplantation had to wait for the development of *immunosuppressive drugs*, which temporarily suppress this immune rejection reaction. As these became available, surgeons began the grafting of major organs—including the kidney, liver, heart and lungs. A major transplant operation will usually be considered only in cases of life-threatening illnesses, since the administration of immunosuppressive drugs has potentially dangerous side effects (it lowers the body's defenses against bacteria and viruses; serious infections are thus a risk during this period in transplant patients).

Experience worldwide with over 20,000 transplants, mostly of kidneys, has shown that many factors affect the chances of success. The best results have come when the grafted kidney has been taken from a volunteer who is a close relative (ideally, from the patient's own twin brother or sister). Just as successful blood transfusion depends on matching the blood groups of the donor and recipient, so does successful transplantation depend on close matching of the "tissue types." There are four sets of transplantation *antigens;* among the thousands of possible combinations, the best results come with a match of at least three of the sets. Such matching is most likely to be found within a family, but many transplant centers now use computer banks to select the best match among waiting patients when a kidney becomes available from a patient dying in the hospital. Other factors that affect success are the age of the patient, how many blood transfusions have been given, and the amount of immunosuppressive drugs that are needed. In the early years of transplant surgery another factor was delay between the death of the donor and removal of the organ. But now that the concept of BRAIN DEATH has become widely accepted, this is no longer a major problem.

Kidney transplantation is now a routine in many specialist centers. The operation is successful in about 70% of cases, and many patients are alive and well more than five years after surgery. If the grafted kidney is rejected or ceases to function it may be removed, and second or third transplants are by no means rare. Even so, the operation carries a substantial mortality rate from complications such as infection in the immediate postoperative period—but this is falling steadily in hospital centers with extensive experience in kidney transplants.

Transplantation of other organs has proved disappointing in comparison. Liver, lung and pancreas transplants have been attempted in only a few centers and the mortality rate in the 12 months after operation has been extremely high. The same is true of heart transplantation, with the exception of Professor Norman Shumway's unit in Stanford, California, where the success rate two years after operation is close to 50%.

trauma

A wound, blow or injury, whether physical or psychic.

The response to physical injury is inflammation (followed by healing) or death of the tissue at the site of the injury. Severe physical injury may also produce widespread effects beyond the site of the injury. Shock is an acute failure of the circulation due to a disturbance of the nervous control of the circulatory system or a loss of circulating fluid (such as when massive or prolonged hemorrhage occurs); severe shock may be irreversible, and death is then inevitable.

Special forms of injury include:

1. *Burns*—which may be thermal, electrical, chemical or radiation burns.

2. *High-temperature injuries*—which may be endogenous in origin (very high fevers: hyperpyrexia), or exogenous (as with burns or heatstroke).

3. *Low-temperature injuries*—which may be local (trench foot or immersion foot), due to long-continued

exposure to low but not freezing temperatures; and frostbite, due to exposure to freezing temperatures.

4. *Hypothermia*—the effect of exposure of the whole body to low temperatures.

5. *Crush injuries*—due to sudden prolonged external pressure on the tissue; damage to muscles or death of tissue from compression of blood vessels can lead to the release of a protein from the muscle known as myoglobin, which can lead to shock or kidney failure.

6. *Blast injuries*—due to an airblast which produces high pressure followed by low pressure from all directions, or to an immersion blast in water which produces high pressure followed by low pressure from all directions. These injuries could cause rupture, compression, or laceration of the internal organs.

7. *Radiation injuries*—may produce burns, dermatitis, tissue death, or the radiation may be stored to produce chronic damage. Conditions like leukemia may arise many years after exposure to high doses of radiation.

Psychic trauma is an emotional shock or disturbance that makes a lasting impression—for example, maternal deprivation or a broken home.

traveler's diarrhea

A brief attack (usually lasting one to three days) of DIARRHEA of uncertain cause. When it affects tourists it is also often referred to humorously as *Delhi belly*, *Rangoon runs*, *Tokyo trots*, *Montezuma's revenge*, *Aztec two-step*, and *la turista*.

Besides the diarrhea, there may be nausea, vomiting, rumbling noises in the abdomen and abdominal cramps. This is often accompanied by loss of appetite. The severity varies, but, in all except the unluckiest cases, the attacks are mild.

Treatment consists of rest and a bland diet, starting with perhaps warm sweetened tea, fruit juices and strained broth, progressing to cooked bland cereals, gelatine and soft-boiled eggs. If the diarrhea persists after 12 to 24 hours, antidiarrheal agents such as kaolin may help. Antibiotics are generally avoided since they may adversely affect the intestinal flora and even prolong symptoms.

Most important is the prevention of the condition, especially when traveling to areas where the standard of hygiene is not too high. Drinking water and milk should be boiled, food should be fresh and well cooked, shellfish should be eaten with care, and fruit should always be peeled.

travel sickness

Nausea or vomiting (or both) experienced when traveling in a car, ship, aircraft, train, etc. This is the result of the intermittent and erratic stimulation by the movement of the vehicle of the sensory receptors in the organ of balance in the inner ear.

The organ of balance, or equilibrium, is made up of a continuous system of passages (the semicircular canals) and chambers (the utricle and saccule) filled with a fluid called endolymph and containing sense organs. Movement or a change in position of the head causes movement of the endolymph, which stimulates the receptors. Nerves pass from these receptors to various parts of the nervous system. These connections with the nervous system serve to start off reflex movements which enable the individual to right himself when for some reason he is thrown off balance. However, some of the nerves also connect with the vomiting center in the brain.

Travel sickness may to some extent be a conditioned reflex, so that a person who expects to be sick is more likely to *be* sick; it may also be aggravated by psychological or emotional factors. Keeping oneself occupied is one method of attempting to prevent travel sickness. Tranquilizers or drugs which contain scopolamine or antihistamines may help to prevent travel sickness. They are best taken about an hour before the start of a journey. It must be remembered, however, that they can cause drowsiness; a person who has taken them for a short sea journey, such as on a ferry, should be careful not to drive while the drug still has its effect.

Other measures which help prevent the severity of an attack include adjusting the ventilation to get some fresh air, sitting with the head tilted back as in a dentist's chair, and having small but frequent meals rather than no meals.

tremor

A series of involuntary movements in one or more parts of the body produced by alternate contractions of opposing muscle groups. Tremor may indicate a disturbance in the *extrapyramidal system*—that is, in those parts of the brain and spinal cord involved in motor activities, especially the control and coordination of postural, static, supporting, and locomotor mechanisms. The disturbance may be due to a variety of causes.

Hunger, cold, physical exertion, fatigue, or excitement may produce a transient tremor which is of no special significance. It may also be present as a benign hereditary condition, which becomes apparent during or after adolescence and is found in several successive generations. Other diseases in which a tremor is quite characteristic are Parkinson's disease, hyperthyroidism, Wilson's disease, diseases of the cerebellum and multiple sclerosis. Tremor may be due to the effect of toxins (poisons) on the nervous system, the most common being alcohol; mercury poisoning also produces tremor.

It may also accompany emotional disorders such as anxiety states or hysteria.

The cause of the tremor may to some extent be identified by its characteristics and by the accompanying signs of the underlying condition which produces it. Tremors may be rapid and fine (the type usually seen in thyrotoxicosis) or coarse and slow (as in Parkinson's disease); they may occur at rest (as in Parkinson's disease) or be accentuated when an attempt at a voluntary movement is made (as in cerebellar disease), or they may appear when attempting to maintain the position of the affected part without support.

Treatment depends on the cause of the tremor. When it is due to toxic states, removal of the toxin is the treatment; when due to thyrotoxicosis, control of the hyperthyroid state should remove the tremor. The tremor of Parkinson's disease may respond in part to some drugs; tremor caused by anxiety and emotional disorders usually responds to sedatives, tranquilizers or antianxiety agents, but that due to multiple sclerosis does not respond to drugs. However, the patient can be taught certain postures and maneuvers which may reduce the tremor brought on by a particular movement.

trench mouth

Another name for VINCENT'S ANGINA.

trichomoniasis

Infection with a parasitic protozoan, *Trichomonas vaginalis,* which lives in the vagina and urethra of women and also in the urethra of men (in whom, however, it mostly causes no symptoms). Infection can be transmitted by sexual or other contacts.

Symptoms of an acute infection consist of the sudden onset of an intensely irritating discharge, which may be yellowish, greenish or frothy; the amount of the discharge varies. The vagina feels sore and there is usually pain during sexual intercourse. There may also be the urge to pass urine very frequently, associated with painful urination.

In chronic trichomoniasis, symptoms come and go, usually appearing around menstruation.

The diagnosis is made by examining the discharge under the microscope for the presence of the parasite. Treatment involves the administration of metronidazole (Flagyl) taken orally, or other drugs. Both the patient and her sexual partner (even if he is symptomless) should have the treatment.

Trichophyton

A genus of fungi that attack the hair, skin and nails. The disease they cause is known as *dermatophytosis.*

trigeminal neuralgia

See TIC.

trismus

A disturbance of the motor part of the trigeminal nerve (the Vth cranial nerve), which supplies both motor and sensory nerves to the face, teeth, mouth, nasal cavities, and the muscles of chewing. Irritation of the nerve produces spasm of the muscles around the jaw. Mild trismus results in a fixed grinning appearance known as *risus sardonicus.* In infants, the risus sardonicus may not be very apparent, and the first sign of spasm of the jaw muscles may be difficulty in feeding.

The most common cause of trismus is TETANUS. It may also occur in association with diseases of the mouth, such as dental abscesses, peritonsillar abscesses, or incomplete eruption of the wisdom teeth (third molars). Actinomycosis, which can cause widespread inflammation in the region of the jaw, may also cause trismus. So too may neonatal jaundice and rabies, conditions in which the nerves in other parts of the body are also easily irritated.

Treatment is directed toward the underlying disease. In severe cases intravenous feeds may be necessary. Sedatives and muscle relaxants may partially relieve the muscle spasm.

tropical sprue

A tropical disease of unknown cause, characterized by MALABSORPTION of fats, protein, vitamins, iron and calcium. Its clinical features include muscle wasting, anemia and diarrhea.

Treatment basically involves the initiation of a balanced diet high in protein (but with only normal amounts of fat) and the administration of folic acid, vitamin B_{12} and iron (in the presence of iron-deficiency anemia).

Nontropical sprue is a term used to describe the adult form of CELIAC DISEASE.

truss

A device for retaining in position a hernia which has been reduced into the abdominal cavity. It is most definitely *not* an adequate substitute for surgical repair, and in most cases the use of a truss should be discouraged. A truss is most commonly used for an inguinal hernia. Essentially, it consists of a pad joined to a belt made of various types of material, such as a leather-covered steel spring. The pad is positioned so as to cover the site of the hernia. In infants it is best to use a washable rubber truss.

A truss is usually used when a patient is not fit for surgery or refuses surgery. It is also used for babies with inguinal hernias, who are usually not operated on till they are about three months old.

To be effective, the wearing of a truss requires some degree of intelligence and perseverance on the part of the patient. The truss has to be put on with the patient lying down and the hernia completely within the abdomen; the truss is then applied with some pressure over the hernia site. A truss should fit properly and patients should be properly measured for their truss. The skin underlying the truss should be kept clean and powdered to prevent chafing.

trypanosomiasis

Any of various diseases caused by infection with protozoa of the genus *Trypanosoma*.

See AFRICAN TRYPANOSOMIASIS, CHAGAS' DISEASE (South American trypanosomiasis).

Tsutsugamushi disease

An infection caused by the microorganism *Rickettsia tsutsugamushi*. It is also known as *scrub typhus*, *mite-borne typhus*, or *tropical typhus*. The disease occurs mainly in the Asian-Pacific area bounded by Japan, India and Australia. It is principally a disease of small rodents, acquired by man through the bite of a mite infected with the causative microorganism.

The incubation period lasts from 6 to 21 days, after which there is a sudden onset of fever, chills, headaches and pains in the muscles and joints. At the same time, an ESCHAR develops at the site of the bite; it begins as a firm nodule about 1 cm in diameter, and becomes a blister which ruptures and is covered by a black scab. About a week after the fever starts, a rash appears. There may also be a cough which later becomes a pneumonitis. Other organs in the body may be involved. The heart muscle may become inflamed, the spleen may enlarge, and there may be delirium, stupor or muscle twitching.

Untreated, the fever usually lasts about two weeks, but with the appropriate antibiotics it begins to drop in about two days. The diagnosis has first to be made by examining blood and tissue for the Rickettsia, or by detecting antibodies which the patient produces against the organism.

Preventive measures consist of clearing the bush and spraying infested areas with insecticides to kill the mites, and the use of insect repellents.

tube feeding

The feeding of a patient through a tube which has been passed into the stomach, either by way of a nostril or through an artificial opening made into the stomach through the abdominal wall. Most of the tubes used now are made of plastic and come presterilized.

Tube feeding is required (1) in unconscious persons; (2) in persons who, because of neurological disease, may be conscious but unable to swallow; and (3) in persons in whom the esophagus is partially obstructed so that solids cannot be swallowed.

In a conscious person, the tube is usually introduced with the person sitting up comfortably in bed with the head supported. The nostrils are cleaned with absorbent cotton plugs soaked in a bland antiseptic. As the tube is passed in through a nostril the patient is encouraged to swallow it, if necessary by simultaneously sipping water. A conscious person may be very anxious when the tube is being passed, and may retch so that it becomes extremely difficult for the tube to reach the stomach. A mild sedative given beforehand, or some local anesthetic sprayed on the throat, may minimize the patient's anxiety and discomfort.

Once the tube has reached the stomach, the end protruding out of the nostril is taped to the patient's cheek. Food can then be syringed through the tube. The tube has to be checked frequently to see that it is functioning properly, is unblocked, and that its tip is still in the stomach. Blockage is checked by injecting air into the tube, while the aspiration of gastric juice will confirm that the tip is still in the stomach.

The tube is inserted directly into the stomach by means of a gastrostomy (the formation of an artificial opening into the stomach) when a patient is unable to swallow the tube, or when the obstruction in the esophagus is complete.

tuberculosis

An infection caused by the bacterium *Mycobacterium tuberculosis* (rarely it may be caused by *Mycobacterium bovis*, which normally infects cows).

Practically any organ in the body may be affected by the infection (which may be acute or chronic). The most common site of infection, however, is the lung. At one time, tuberculosis was a common cause of death all over the world, but with control of infection, antituberculosis immunization and chemotherapy, mortality due to tuberculosis has decreased dramatically in most developed countries.

Apart from the few cases in which the disease is spread across the placenta from mother to fetus, tuberculosis is acquired mostly by inhalation or ingestion of infected material in the form of droplets, dust, food and milk. Once the infection has set in, the disease may spread from its primary site—directly to adjacent structures, or it may be carried by the lymphatic system or bloodstream to distant sites.

Symptoms of tuberculosis include malaise (a general feeling of being unwell), lassitude, tiredness, loss of appetite, fever and night sweats. Other symptoms depend on the site affected. For example, with infection of the lungs there may be cough, sometimes with bloodstained sputum. An infection of the intestine (most commonly the small intestine) may produce a malabsorption syndrome, or intestinal obstruction.

There may be a tuberculous meningitis, pericarditis, arthritis, and so on. Very often, the lymph glands draining an infected area enlarge, and it may be the enlarged lymph nodes that draw attention to the presence of an infection.

The infection may often be present for a long time without producing symptoms. Since the lung is the most common site of infection, in areas where tuberculosis is prevalent, persons in close contact with tuberculosis patients are sometimes screened for the disease either by chest x rays or by a MANTOUX TEST.

Diagnosis is made by x rays and examination of various body tissues and fluids for the causative organisms. Treatment consists of a combination of antibiotics, usually for at least six months. Sometimes surgery is necessary. Healing typically results in the formation of a scar at the site of infection. Sometimes organisms remain viable for a long time in the scar and become reactivated at a later date. In most cases the scar itself produces no symptoms; sometimes, however, the scar has some effects. For example, Fallopian tubes which have been infected may become fibrosed and thus produce infertility.

Immunization with BCG is believed to be at least partly effective in preventing tuberculosis in some people. Such an immunization, however, renders the patient permanently positive to tuberculin tests in the future, meaning that they cannot be used for diagnostic purposes.

See also PULMONARY DISEASES.

twins

Two offspring produced in a single pregnancy.

There are two ways in which twins can be produced. Normally only one ovum, or egg, is fertilized. If two ova are fertilized at the same time, the result is a pair of *fraternal* (or *nonidentical*, or *dizygotic*, or *binovular*) twins, who may be as different from each other as any pair of siblings. If only one ovum is fertilized and the resulting embryo divides at a very early stage to produce two embryos, the result is *identical* (or *monozygotic*, or *monovular*) twins. Since the twins would have originally formed from the same ovum and sperm, identical twins would have the same genetic makeup: they would be of the same sex, have the same blood group, same build,

same color of eyes, and even the same pattern of hair whorls.

Twins occur in about 1 in 80 births. The tendency to having dizygotic twins is inherited, especially through the mother's side. Dizygotic twins also appear more

TWINS

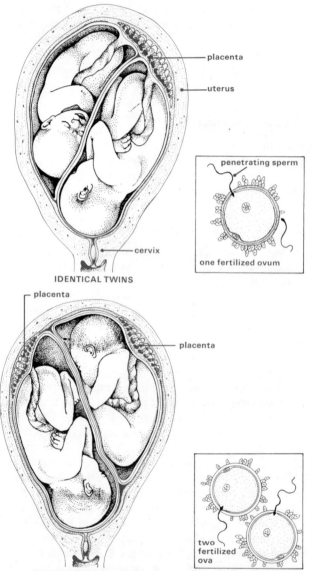

placenta

uterus

penetrating sperm

one fertilized ovum

cervix

IDENTICAL TWINS

placenta

placenta

two fertilized ova

NONIDENTICAL TWINS

Identical twins are the result of a fertilized egg dividing into two identical cells which then separate and develop independently. Since both twins are derived from one sperm and one egg they are genetically identical. Nonidentical twins are no more genetically similar than ordinary brothers and sisters; they develop from two different ova (each fertilized by separate sperms) and have separate placentas.

frequently after the second pregnancy and with advancing maternal age; mothers of 35–40 are three times more likely to have twins than mothers under 20.

Twins have a higher perinatal mortality rate than single children. For a start, life in the uterus is more difficult, and twin pregnancies tend to be associated with more obstetrical complications. Twins are also more prone to fetal growth retardation; this may affect one twin more than the other if the distribution of blood supply to the two embryos is uneven. The difference in growth and development may persist after birth.

There is also a higher rate of mental subnormality, cerebral palsy and of congenital abnormalities in twins. Monozygotic twins may have a higher risk of certain tumors, such as Wilm's tumor, medulloblastoma, retinoblastoma and leukemia.

Less is known about the psychological development of twins, although they can certainly be quite different psychologically; even monozygotic twins reared in the same environment may have quite different psychological makeups. However, if one twin has schizophrenia the other twin—especially if he is an identical twin—has a higher risk of the condition.

Twins should be treated as individuals, each with their unique traits and abilities, and encouraged to develop apart. Otherwise emotional disturbances may develop later, especially if they have to be separated.

Siamese twins or conjoined twins are twins who at the time of birth are physically joined to each other at some part of the body.

typhoid fever

A bacterial infection acquired from food or water contaminated with particles of human sewage containing the causative microorganisms. The bacteria responsible, *Salmonella typhosa*, may be found in dairy produce such as milk and cream as well as in undercooked meats. The disease received its name because of the similarity of its symptoms to TYPHUS.

Typhoid fever used to be one of the most dangerous of the "enteric fevers" affecting adults. It remains a threat to health for people who travel to countries with inadequate sanitation, and there are still a few deaths each year among tourists returning home from certain parts of Europe, Africa and the Far East. The incubation period is from about 5 days to 5 weeks (usually 8–14 days) between the eating of contaminated food and the onset of illness.

Early symptoms include headache, loss of energy, and fever; cough is common and there may be nosebleeds. After 7 to 10 days the fever becomes steady, the abdomen is swollen and the patient may become profoundly weak, confused and delirious. In the second or third week a pink "rose-spot" rash appears; it is at about this time that serious complications may occur, including perforation or hemorrhage in the intestines. In most cases, however, the fever begins to subside at this time and slow recovery follows.

With early diagnosis and antibiotic treatment the course of the illness is cut short; chloramphenicol, co-trimoxazole, or ampicillin are effective in virtually 100% of cases. Even so, a few patients will recover to become symptomless "carriers" who pass typhoid bacteria in their excreta. These carriers are the source of further infections, especially if they are employed in the food industry.

Prevention of typhoid depends on good sanitation, proper hygiene among food handlers and the tracing and treatment of carriers.

Vaccination gives valuable protection to those traveling outside northern Europe and North America: a course of two or three injections is required, but the effect lasts for only one to two years, at the end of which a further booster dose will be needed.

typhus

Any one of three related infectious diseases caused by a species of rickettsia (microorganisms intermediate in size between bacteria and viruses), transmitted to man by human lice.

First described clearly in 1490, typhus went on to kill more soldiers than died in battle in every major European war prior to the late 19th century: between 1918 and 1922 there were 30 million cases with a 10% mortality rate in Russia and Eastern Europe. Also known as *typhus fever*, the disease was prevalent whenever people were crowded together in conditions of poor hygiene.

The microorganisms which cause typhus can multiply in both lice and man. Lice acquire the infection by biting someone with typhus; the microorganisms then multiply inside the louse, eventually killing it—but not before it has had the chance to pass the infection on to another human.

The incubation period between infection and the onset of symptoms is about 14 days. The illness begins abruptly with fever and a severe headache; after three to four days a pinkish rash appears. Typically the high fever is accompanied by confusion and delirium; in untreated cases the mental state may become increasingly stuporous, with eventual coma and death. The mortality rate ranges from 10–50%, varying with the age of the victim and his previous health.

Early treatment with the antibiotic chloramphenicol or one of the tetracyclines is highly effective. A protective vaccine also exists, but prevention is essentially a matter of personal hygiene: the disease can be acquired only from infected lice.

U

ulcer

A defect in the surface of the skin or a mucous membrane exposing tissue normally covered by epithelial cells.

It may develop as the result of several factors, all of which interfere with the proper nourishment of the tissues. These factors include a poor blood supply, poor venous drainage leading to waterlogged tissues, infection, damage by physical agents such as heat and cold, continued pressure, malignant growths and disease of the nervous system leading to loss of sensation and repeated minor trauma. Examples are varicose ulcers, where the venous drainage is inadequate, syphilitic ulcers from infection, frostbite, RODENT ULCERS (which are the result of malignant growths of the skin) and BEDSORES. *Peptic ulcers* form in the stomach and duodenum as the result of loss of the ability of the mucous membranes to withstand the action of hydrochloric acid and pepsin, and occasionally as the

ULCERS

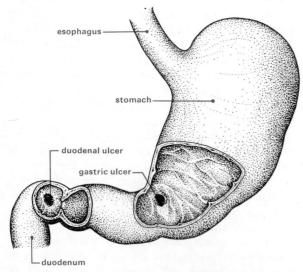

esophagus

stomach

duodenal ulcer

gastric ulcer

duodenum

TWO TYPES OF PEPTIC ULCER

Peptic ulcers are erosions in the lining of the digestive system caused by the action of gastric acid. Many factors—age, sex, occupation, diet, blood group—appear to influence one's likelihood of developing either gastric or duodenal ulcers. Both types of ulcer can usually be managed by drugs and dietary measures, unless complications necessitating surgery (such as hemorrhage or perforation) supervene.

result of a malignant growth (see DUODENAL ULCER and GASTRIC ULCER).

The treatment of an ulcer is by removal of the cause. Patients with varicose ulcers must elevate the leg as much as possible to promote venous drainage, areas liable to develop bedsores must be subjected to as little pressure as possible; malignant growths must be removed.

In some cases plastic surgery is necessary, but treatment cannot hope to succeed unless the circumstances that originally led to ulcer formation are rectified. This is particularly true of varicose ulcers and peptic ulcers, for it is not easy to follow the regimes of treatment often required to heal and then to avoid ulceration, and relapses are frequent.

ulcerative colitis

A nonspecific inflammatory condition of the large bowel (colon) of unknown cause; 75% of cases begin between the ages of 15 and 50. It is slightly more common in women than men, and appears to be more common among Jews.

It has been suggested that the disease has an immunological basis; certainly patients suffering from ulcerative colitis are liable to psychological disturbance.

The lining of the large bowel is ulcerated and liable to bleed, so that the symptoms include incessant bloody diarrhea as well as abdominal discomfort. The loss of protein may be severe enough to produce symptoms of protein malnutrition, and there may be anemia. Complications can occur: the bowel may bleed severely, chronic inflammation may produce a stricture of the intestine, and in some cases the intestine may suddenly distend (toxic dilation)—a condition that requires immediate surgical treatment. The wall of the bowel may perforate, producing PERITONITIS. The risk of developing a malignant growth is significantly greater than it is in the general population.

Diagnosis is based on the patient's medical history, and confirmed by endoscopy of the large bowel and a barium enema. Treatment is difficult; general measures include rest and the correction of any nutritional deficiencies to insure an adequate diet. In severe cases, close collaboration of surgeon and physician is essential, for operative treatment may become needed urgently.

ultrasound

A valuable technique for visualizing internal bodily organs, using inaudible (or ultrasonic) sound waves of a frequency of more than 20,000 cycles per second. These can be formed, like light, into a beam which will reflect from various "interfaces" in the body between structures which have different acoustic properties. The technique (also called *ultrasonography*) can be used to inspect organs or structures which will not show up on an x-ray photograph—for example, blood vessels, or gallstones in position in the gallbladders. It has the added advantage over x rays of producing no radiation hazards, and is therefore extremely useful for monitoring the developing fetus in pregnancy. Another advantage is that the technique is totally painless.

The process is also particularly useful in estimating the position of midline structures in the skull (*echoencephalography*); in echoencephalography the midline structures reflect waves produced by a "transducer" held against the patient's head just above the ear; the time taken for the signal to leave the transducer and arrive back again is proportional to the distance from the transducer to the reflecting structures. Comparison of records taken from the left and right sides of the head will show whether the structures which should lie in the midline are indeed there, or whether they have been displaced to one side or the other.

About 6% of results are misleading, but the technique is very valuable because it does not disturb the patient and can be repeated frequently. In pregnancy the size and shape of the developing fetus can be estimated; moreover, as the beam of ultrasound is reflected from a moving surface a *Doppler shift* of frequency is seen in the reflected signal, so that the beating of the fetal heart can be detected from about the 12th week and the pulse rate counted.

The uses of ultrasound in medicine continue to be the subject of research and the technique is used increasingly in the investigation of blood vessel disease, as well as in the investigation of organs within the abdominal cavity.

unconsciousness

The loss of consciousness, characterized by the inability to respond to sensory stimuli or to have subjective experiences. It may result from a blow on the head, the effects of a disease or disorder (such as the blockage or rupture of a margin artery within the brain) or be induced during general anesthesia.

The degree of unconsciousness may vary from FAINTING to deep COMA.

undescended testis

The development of the testis in the male fetus takes place inside the abdomen near the kidney. It descends into the scrotum before birth, but the descent may be imperfect.

There are three varieties of imperfect descent: (1) retractile testis; (2) incompletely descended testis; and (3) ectopic testis. The retractile testis can be manipulated into the scrotum; it descends completely into the scrotum at puberty and requires no treatment, unless a hernia defect remains.

The incompletely descended testis lies somewhere along the normal path of descent; it may be in the abdomen, in the inguinal canal or at the neck of the scrotum. It cannot be manipulated into the scrotum and it will not descend at puberty. Such cases usually require operative treatment between the ages of 1 and 3. The affected testis is smaller than usual and there is virtually always an associated inguinal hernia.

The ectopic testis has wandered from the normal line of descent and lies somewhere near the inguinal canal, perhaps in the perineum or near the root of the penis. It is usually of normal size, but because of its abnormal position it is particularly liable to damage. Like the incompletely descended testis, it will not produce spermatozoa unless it is surgically replaced in its normal position in the scrotum by the time of puberty. If it proves impossible to replace the testis in the scrotum it should be removed, for ectopic and undescended testes—if left in their abnormal positions—are liable to develop tumors.

uremia

The abnormal accumulation in the body of substances normally excreted by the kidney produces a clinical state called uremia. The name was given to the condition

UNDESCENDED TESTIS

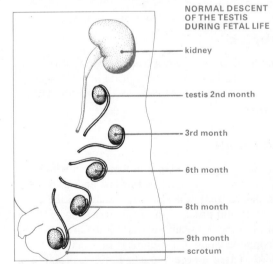

NORMAL DESCENT OF THE TESTIS DURING FETAL LIFE

- kidney
- testis 2nd month
- 3rd month
- 6th month
- 8th month
- 9th month
- scrotum

The downward migration of the testis in the fetus can become arrested at any point, trapping the testis in the abdomen. If it does not descend into the scrotum during early childhood, it should be brought down surgically, preferably before the age of three.

because an excess of the substance *urea* was detected many years ago in cases of kidney failure.

The condition is often of gradual onset. At first the patient becomes tired and is not able to concentrate properly. If the condition progresses, he becomes drowsy and confused. In addition to the lassitude the patient may be out of breath, nauseous and without appetite; he may experience abdominal pain or pain behind the sternum (breastbone). He is more susceptible to chance infection (particularly of the lungs and urinary tract) and may develop diarrhea. Neurological signs may include unsteadiness, weakness and numbness of the legs.

The manifestations of uremia are many, and can include psychological difficulties. On investigation many abnormal substances are found in the blood, and it is clear that kidney function is disturbed.

The nature of the disturbance and the severity of functional loss must be determined, both by examination of the urine and special investigations of the kidneys and urinary tract. If possible the underlying disease is treated; but in some cases the function of the kidneys is so far impaired that the use of an artificial kidney machine is required, and a kidney transplant may have to be considered.

There are many conditions that may damage the function of the kidneys badly enough to produce uremia, some acute, others chronic. Although the precise reasons for the development of clinical uremia are not yet fully understood, it seems clear that it is produced by the retention in the blood of some of the products of protein metabolism.

urethritis

Inflammation of the urethra (the passage that conveys urine from the bladder to the outside of the body).

See NONSPECIFIC URETHRITIS, URINARY TRACT INFECTION.

urethrocele

One form of genital prolapse in females, in which the whole urethra is displaced downward and backward. The displaced urethra is also often dilated. Like other forms of genital prolapse, it arises from damage to or weakness of the ligaments supporting the urethra—the most common cause of the damage or weakness being childbirth. Often it occurs together with a prolapse of the rest of the bladder, the combined condition then being known as a *cystourethrocele*.

The urethrocele may not form until many years after the initial damage. Usually symptoms do not arise till about the menopause when there is some degeneration of the muscles and connective tissue in the pelvis.

Symptoms include a feeling of discomfort or weakness in the vagina, especially after the patient has been standing all day. There may be urinary symptoms, especially stress incontinence, and a tendency to recurrent urinary tract infection.

Treatment involves supporting the prolapse with a pessary, which may relieve symptoms. An operation is required to cure the condition.

urinary frequency

The frequent passage of small amounts of urine.

Control of micturition (urination) in the normal adult is a complex act which is often disturbed in diseases of the central nervous system. Sensory nerves convey pain impulses and a sense of distension to the brain, where these sensations are interpreted. If as a result the person wishes to empty the urinary bladder, impulses travel downward to relax the sphincter muscles and contract the detrusor (expelling) muscles.

Frequency suggests inflammation of the urinary bladder (cystitis). This is most commonly due to bacteria entering the bladder through the urethra. About 50% of married women have a urinary infection at some time in their lives and hence suffer frequency.

Pregnancy distorts the shape of the bladder neck, which is another cause of frequency. PYELONEPHRITIS (bacterial inflammation of the kidney) may also give rise to the symptoms.

urinary tract infection

The urinary tract includes the urethra, bladder, ureters and the kidneys. It is prone to bacterial infection, particularly in women.

The most common organism causing infection is *Escherichia coli* (the "colon bacillus"), which normally flourishes in the large intestine. *E. coli* is often present in the urethra of healthy men and women, and it may be present in the urine without causing symptoms. Usually it causes inflammation when present in the urine in concentrations of more than 100,000 per milliliter; the urine becomes full of white and red blood cells, sometimes to such an extent that the appearance of the urine changes and the presence of blood is obvious. The patient has pain on urination, urinary frequency (especially noticeable at night), and develops a high temperature with shivering attacks (rigors) and complains of severe headache.

Diagnosis is made by examination of the urine for pus cells and red blood cells, and by culture and identification of the infecting organism. Sensitivity tests made on the isolated organism will indicate the appropriate antibiotic to be prescribed.

The incidence of urinary tract infection is fairly high

in children between the ages of 6 months and 4 years, possibly because of the risk of infection from nappies; the incidence then falls until there is a rise among young women of childbearing age, the frequency of infection being about 50 in 1,000. Young men are 10 to 20 times less likely to suffer from urinary infection. The reason for the greater incidence in women is that the urethra is shorter and infection is more likely to spread from the anus and vagina. Moreover, factors which are not fully understood render the pregnant woman especially liable to infection, and many women date a chronic urinary infection back to their first pregnancy.

It is said that infection of one part of the urinary tract means infection of all the structures making up the tract, but treatment with antibiotics will halt the disease even if it has spread from the bladder to the kidneys. Nevertheless, the disease is prone to recur, and in a number of cases infection of the kidney is found without the symptoms produced by bladder infection.

Factors which predispose to chronic urinary tract infection are the presence of stones, anatomical abnormalities and obstructions to the free flow of urine—which become increasingly common with age, with the development of prostatic hypertrophy (enlargement of the prostate gland) in men and uterine prolapses in women. After the age of 60, the incidence of urinary tract infections is approximately equal in both men and women.

Chronic or recurring urinary tract infections require investigation by the urologist, who will try to identify the factors causing repeated infection with a view to definitive treatment; but there are many cases where no abnormality can be found.

In uncomplicated cases of urinary tract infection, *E. coli* are responsible in up to 85% of cases. Other microorganisms which are also able to infect the urinary tract include *Klebsiella* species, *Proteus* species, *Enterobacter aerogenes* and *Pseudomonas aeruginosa*. Less commonly the causative microorganisms may include *Staphylococcus epidermidis, Staphylococcus aureus* and enterococci *(Streptococcus faecalis)*. In many cases these bacteria cause urologic problems only after catheterization of the urinary tract or following operations on the bladder or prostate gland. Indwelling catheters—i.e., those left in position in the bladder for prolonged periods—may set up an irritation that leads to bacterial infection.

URETHRITIS in men may be caused by infection with *Neisseria gonorrhoeae*, the microorganism which causes GONORRHEA. In such cases there may be a purulent (pus-filled) discharge from the tip of the penis. Specific antibiotic treatment usually clears up the infection within a short time.

See also BLADDER PROBLEMS, CYSTITIS, NONSPECIFIC URETHRITIS.

urticaria

A skin eruption not unlike that caused by nettles; raised red-and-white patches on the skin, which cause great irritation, are seen mainly on the trunk and on the face. Also called *hives*. If the swelling extends to the throat (angioneurotic edema) there may be difficulty in breathing. The attack may subside in a few hours or may last several days.

Urticaria is an *allergic* reaction to certain protein foods especially fish or shellfish; to drugs, especially penicillin; and occasionally to insect bites or stings.

As in other allergic disorders, emotional stress and anxiety may be important factors; the condition tends to run in families. In severe cases treatment may be needed urgently, when injections of epinephrine or corticosteroids (such as prednisolone) give dramatic relief. Usually, however, itching may be allayed by antihistamines or by any of the many proprietary "antipruritic" lotions or ointments on the market. Preventive treatment may be given by the administration of *antihistamine* drugs, but the only certain way of eliminating the possibility of further outbreaks is for the factor causing the allergy to be identified and avoided in the future.

URINARY TRACT INFECTION

The urinary system is a common site of bacterial infection. Nearly all cases are "ascending" infections caused by bacteria from the anus entering the urethra and then moving up the urinary tract into the bladder. Women have considerably shorter urethras than men, and are therefore much more likely to be affected.

uterine neoplasms

A growth in the uterus which may be either benign (such as FIBROIDS) or malignant.

Fibroids are overgrowths of the muscle of the uterus; they may be quite small or may grow to weigh several pounds. They may form swellings on the outside of the uterus or within its cavity. Fibroids are found in up to 50% of black women but in only 20% of whites; they often increase in size during pregnancy. These tumors are usually painless and often unsuspected, but they may cause cramping pain, especially at the menstrual period; or they may cause pressure on other internal organs, such as the bladder, and so provoke frequency of passing urine. The most usual symptom, however, is MENORRHAGIA—an increase in the amount and duration of menstrual blood flow. The loss of blood may cause anemia. The only effective treatment of fibroids is surgical removal either of the growth (myomectomy) or of the whole uterus (hysterectomy).

Malignant tumors of the uterus include cancer of its body and cancer of the cervix (the neck of the womb). Cancer of the body of the uterus usually originates in its lining. There may be no symptoms or the growth may cause intermittent and irregular blood loss. For that reason, any unusual uterine bleeding should be investigated without delay. When surgical removal of the uterus is performed early in the disease the outlook is excellent: 75–90% of early cases of this cancer are cured by operation.

Cancer of the cervix is the most common form of cancer in women—and the most preventable, since the condition can be detected in its preliminary stage by examination of a sample of cells taken from the cervix ("Pap smear"). Wherever Pap smears have been used by women as a regular screening test for cancer, the death rate from the disease has fallen precipitously in the last 20 years.

The cancer starts as a small "ulcer" or bleeding point on the cervix, but spread may occur early on to lymph nodes in the pelvis. Treatment is surgical, sometimes backed up with radiotherapy. Again, the prospects for cure are good in cases treated early in the course of the disease.

uterus

The uterus (womb) is a pear-shaped hollow organ situated in the female within the pelvis between the bladder and the rectum. It is about 9 cm long, 5 cm wide and 3 cm thick. Its narrow neck (cervix) opens into the vagina. From each side of the upper portion, one of two Fallopian tubes connects with the ovaries. Underneath it is supported by ligaments attached to the muscular floor of the pelvis. The arrangement is such that the uterus can easily be displaced by pressure from adjacent organs.

In women between the ages of about 13 and 45, the interior lining of the uterus (endometrium) is shed every month (menstruation); a new lining is then grown to prepare for a fertilized ovum. When fertilization occurs the endometrium is no longer expelled, there is no menstruation, and the uterus begins to expand in order to accommodate and nourish the developing embryo.

The muscles which form the outside wall of the uterus have remarkable powers of adaptability and during pregnancy increase from 1 oz. (28 g) in weight to $2\frac{1}{4}$ lbs. (1 kg). After the birth of the child the uterus returns to its normal size within a few weeks and the process of the monthly shedding of the endometrium (menstruation) begins anew.

Owing to its structure and position, the uterus can suffer from downward displacement or PROLAPSE. Another common condition is the growth of benign tumors (FIBROIDS), but these can often be successfully removed.

See also UTERINE NEOPLASMS.

uveitis

Inflammation of the uvea (the pigmented, vascular layer of the eye, including the iris).

See also IRITIS.

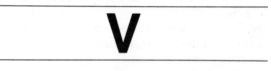

vaccination

See IMMUNIZATION.

vaginal cancer

Primary cancer of the vagina is rare; it accounts for about 1% of all malignant growths of the female reproductive system. It is rarely present before the age of 45, and may be associated with carcinoma of the cervix (neck of the womb) or the vulva. Treatment is surgical with the aid of radiation therapy. The most common form of cancer involving the vagina is that which has spread from adjacent structures such as the rectum, bladder, or uterus.

See also CANCER.

vaginismus

Spasm of the muscles surrounding the vaginal opening, resulting in painful intercourse (DYSPAREUNIA) or preventing penetration of the penis.

It may be due to anxiety, local tenderness, or an unduly small vaginal opening. The anxiety may arise from ignorance of sexual matters, fear of pregnancy, excessive modesty, dislike or distrust of a sexual partner, or dislike of the act of sexual intercourse itself; it may be allayed by psychiatric treatment. Local conditions producing tenderness can be treated as required. In most cases of vaginismus the cause is fairly clear, and the family physician can help a great deal.

vaginitis

Inflammation of the vagina, usually characterized by a vaginal discharge.

The inflammation may be due to a variety of causes, of which infection is the most common—especially that caused by the fungus *Candida albicans* (which produces candidiasis or "thrush"—see CANDIDA) and that by the parasite *Trichomonas vaginalis* (which produces TRICHOMONIASIS). Because the vagina is anatomically related to the cervix, cervical infections (such as that caused by gonorrhea) may also cause vaginitis. In children, vaginitis may occasionally be due to a pinworm infestation.

Foreign bodies are another cause of vaginitis in children. In adults, the types of foreign body most likely to cause vaginitis are pessaries inserted for the treatment of prolapse of the cervix, a tampon left behind after menstruation—either because it has been forgotten or because a second tampon has been put in without removing one already there.

Vaginitis due to a foreign body causes an acute highly offensive discharge which usually responds well to the removal of the foreign body and, if necessary, to a slightly acid douche.

Chemical vaginitis is usually caused by the use of an unsuitable chemical for douching or for contraception. Often the chemical solution is too highly concentrated, or the patient is allergic to it. *Senile vaginitis* is seen in postmenopausal women, or premenopausal women in whom the ovaries have been removed or are not functioning. It is due to deficiency of the ovarian hormone estrogen. The lining of the vagina becomes smooth, thin, shiny and dry, and small hemorrhages may appear. The vagina normally has a slightly acidic secretion which helps protect it against infection; this protection is lost in senile vaginitis, which is treated by administering therapeutic amounts of the hormone to the patient.

vagotomy

The cutting of the two *vagus* nerves. It is often performed as part of the treatment for uncontrolled peptic ulcer, since stimulation by the vagus nerves is one of the main factors in secretion of the digestive juices (hydrochloric acid and pepsin) by the stomach. Patients with duodenal ulcers commonly secrete abnormally large amounts of hydrochloric acid; vagotomy results in a lower acid output and thus reduces the chances of further ulceration.

The vagus nerves begin in the brain stem, travel down the neck close to the jugular vein and then to the abdomen, where branches serve the various digestive organs. In their course, the vagus nerves also provide branches to the heart and lungs.

Vagotomy may be *complete* or *selective*, in which only some of the branches are divided, so reducing the likelihood of unwanted side effects such as diarrhea.

Valsalva's test

Antonio Mario Valsalva (1666–1723) was an Italian physician and Professor of Anatomy at the University of Bologna. He was among the first to recognize the importance of examining diseased organs after death, in an age when autopsies on human bodies were still largely illegal. He also studied the effects of deep breathing on the vascular system.

The *Valsalva test* (or *maneuver*) is the act of breathing out hard while the mouth and nose are held tightly closed, thus raising the pressure inside the chest. The rise in pressure inside the abdomen may help to empty the bowels or bladder. However, the return of blood to the heart is slowed, the heart itself slows, and the blood pressure rises. Straining to empty the rectum may, therefore, cause a dangerous rise in blood pressure in someone with vascular disease and precipitate a stroke or a heart attack.

valvotomy

Literally, "cutting a valve." The valves of the heart normally consist of two or three separate flaps (cusps) which are free to move as the valve opens and closes. As a result of disease (rheumatic fever, for example), the valve becomes inflamed and the cusps may become damaged or scarred and will subsequently stick together. The valve becomes narrowed and no longer functions normally, presenting a considerable obstacle to the free flow of blood (*stenosis* of the valve: *mitral stenosis*, or *aortic stenosis*, depending on which valve is affected).

To overcome the obstruction of the stenosed valve, the valve cusps are divided surgically (valvotomy) to allow freer movement and an unobstructed flow of blood. Alternatively, the diseased valve may be removed and replaced with a plastic substitute (prosthetic valve). The choice of operation depends on the severity of the damage to the valve cusps—although valvotomy is a technically simpler procedure than valve replacement.

varicocele

A network of varicose veins surrounding the testis.

Usually the condition is not a serious one and the patient can be completely reassured. In a few cases an operation may be recommended but in the majority the most that is required is the wearing of a suspensory bandage for comfort.

varicose veins

The blood supplied to the limbs via the arteries is returned to the heart via the veins. While the pressure generated in the arteries by the heartbeat suffices to force blood through the smaller blood vessels to the tissues, no such pressure exists on the venous side of the circulation to return blood to the heart. The venous return is accomplished by a dual mechanism: the veins contain nonreturn valves which allow blood to flow only toward the heart, while the veins themselves are compressed by the contraction of the muscles with each movement of the limb. Blood is thus forced toward the heart and, having passed through the nearest valve, cannot return; further muscle contractions will force it further up the vein.

When this valvular mechanism becomes defective, the veins of the lower part of the leg become swollen by the pressure of the column of blood in the veins higher up the leg. This swelling eventually causes them to become dilated and knotted; they are then described as *varicose*.

In a minority of cases the condition may result from obstruction to the passage of blood up the veins. This may occur when a major leg vein undergoes THROMBOSIS, or when the flow of blood from the leg through the lower part of the abdomen is obstructed by pressure on the veins by a pregnant uterus or a tumor in the pelvis. In the majority of cases, however, the cause is incompetence of the valves in the veins (which may be hereditary).

Varicose veins are a relatively common condition. Many methods of treatment are used, including the use of elastic stockings or bandages to support the veins. The injection of various chemical substances into the veins will cause them to become thrombosed and in due course obliterated by scar tissue. Alternatively, they can be removed surgically (stripping) or tied off at a number of points.

Complications of the condition include the formation of varicose ulcers on the lower leg and a tendency to thrombosis in the dilated vein (superficial THROMBOPHLEBITIS) resulting in a painful, red swelling along the course of the vein.

VARICOSE VEINS

superficial vein

perforating vein

backflow of blood due to incompetent valves

SUPERFICIAL LEG VEINS

NORMAL VALVES

The veins in the legs are arranged into superficial and deep systems, connected by perforating veins. If the valves in the perforating or superficial veins leak, blood flows back down the superficial system causing dilated, tortuous vessels. Varicose veins may be symptomless or cause aching, swelling, eczema and ulceration, as they become distended, enlarged and twisted. Veins almost anywhere in the body can be involved, although those in the legs are most commonly affected.

vasectomy

The operation of cutting and tying the *vasa deferentia* (singular, *vas deferens*), the two ducts passing from the testicles to the seminal vesicles through the inguinal canal.

It is a simple operation rapidly gaining in popularity throughout the world as a means of sterilization of males who no longer want to father children, and can be carried out under general or local anesthesia. In the usual technique, small incisions are made in the scrotum through which the vasa are identified, cut and tied off. It is not the same as castration, for the testes are left undisturbed and functioning.

After the operation a store of sperm is left beyond the block, which means that the man will not be sterile until the live sperms have been ejaculated—a process which may take up to two months, during which another form of contraception is required. At the end of this period consecutive sperm counts are made; two or three negative results are obligatory before the operation can be considered successful. The patient himself will not notice any difference in his sexual activity, for most of the fluid ejaculated at orgasm comes from the prostate gland and seminal vesicles, which are untouched; the secretion of male hormone from the testicles continues without interruption, so that virility and sexual arousal and desire are not affected.

VASECTOMY

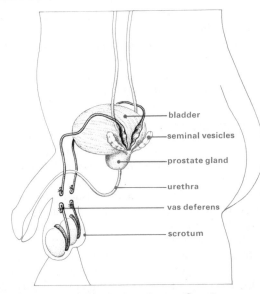

bladder

seminal vesicles

prostate gland

urethra

vas deferens

scrotum

Vasectomy is a method of male sterilization carried out through a small incision in the scrotum. The vasa deferentia are cut and tied back, as pictured above, so that sperm can no longer pass from the testes to the urethra. Very few vasectomies can be reversed successfully.

It is technically possible to reverse the operation, but restoration of the continuity of the vasa deferentia does not always restore fertility.

vasoconstriction

The arteries contain muscle tissue in their walls; contraction of the muscular coat of a blood vessel, reducing its bore and the amount of blood that can flow through it, is referred to as vasoconstriction. It has a valuable physiological function in controlling the flow of blood through a tissue; however, under certain circumstances, an inappropriate constriction of the arterial supply to a tissue can cause serious problems.

The degree of contraction present in the muscular wall of an artery is under involuntary nervous control and is also affected by a number of physiologically active chemicals (HORMONES) circulating in the blood. It can also be increased or decreased by the action of certain drugs.

A common example of the effect of vasoconstriction is the marked variation in blood supply to the hands in hot and cold weather, allowing either extra heat loss (when the temperature is high) or reducing heat loss (when it is cold).

vasodilatation

While VASOCONSTRICTION refers to the contraction of the muscular wall of an artery, reducing its bore and the blood flow through it, *vasodilatation* is the relaxation of the muscular coat. This permits the vessel to increase in bore, thus also increasing the blood flow within it.

As with vasoconstriction, vasodilatation is under involuntary nervous control and is also affected by circulating drugs and physiologically active chemicals (HORMONES) in the blood. Common examples of vasodilatation are seen in the flushing of the skin of the face in response to embarrassment or excitement and the general increase in blood flow in the skin when the body is overheated—allowing more heat to be lost, especially from exposed areas such as the hands.

vegetarianism

The practice of abstaining from all flesh foods of animal origin and living mainly on vegetables. An extreme form of vegetarianism prohibits even the consumption of eggs, milk and dairy products because they come from animals. Upholders of this extreme practice are known (especially in Britain) as *vegans*, to distinguish them from ordinary vegetarians.

Vegetarianism is of extremely ancient origin and was advocated by Pythagoras in the 6th century B.C. During the period of the Roman Empire many religious sects opposed meat eating as a cruel and barbarous practice, as well as being contrary to such beliefs as the "transmigration of souls."

Modern vegetarianism dates from the 18th century, with such famous figures as Benjamin Franklin and Voltaire proclaiming its virtues. The first vegetarian association was formed in Manchester, England, in 1809; it was followed, from 1850, by the founding of similar societies in the United States and Germany. Because the majority of modern vegetarians do not belong to societies or associations, the total number in the United States is difficult to assess. An American Vegetarian Union was formed in 1949 and the American Vegan Society came into being in 1960.

Vegetarians who also eat eggs and dairy produce have no-difficulty in obtaining the required dietary balance (especially of "high quality" proteins), for these foods contain adequate amounts of calcium, protein and B vitamins. Whether or not such a diet is more beneficial and hygienic than a diet containing meat remains a matter of argument. Vegetarian "propagandists" point to the tests made at Yale University and the University of Michigan in 1907 and 1909, respectively, in which it was suggested that vegetarians had far greater endurance and "staying power" than those who include meat in their diets. It is certainly a fact that during World War II, when the Allied blockade severely restricted the import of meat to Norway, the general health of the population improved.

Vegans find it more difficult to maintain an adequate diet, for the minerals and vitamins present in eggs and dairy produce must be replaced from vegetable sources. The diet must include nuts and whole-grain cereals and a wide variety of vegetables and meals must be wisely planned, otherwise there is a risk that mineral deficiency diseases may occur.

Probably the strongest argument for vegetarianism is that such a diet does not lead to the excessive formation of CHOLESTEROL in the blood. As there is a possible connection between this chemical (technically known as a *sterol*) and cardiovascular diseases, a growing number of physicians are of the opinion that a vegetarian diet may lower the incidence of these conditions.

venepuncture

The puncture of a vein with a hollow needle. It is performed for the removal of a sample of blood or the injection or transfusion of drug solutions, blood or other fluids. It is most commonly performed, however, for the removal of blood samples for laboratory testing.

The most accessible veins for the purpose are those on the inner side of the elbow (antecubital fossa), although veins on the hand, wrist and (in small infants) the scalp and neck may be used.

Blood is commonly drawn with a plastic syringe attached to the needle.

Compare VENESECTION.

venereal disease (VD)

Disease transmitted by sexual intercourse.

The organisms responsible vary a great deal, but all depend on the warmth and moisture of the sexual organs for survival—for they die when the temperature drops much below that of body heat. SYPHILIS and GONORRHEA are the best-known venereal diseases, but the range also includes CHANCROID, LYMPHO-GRANULOMA VENEREUM, donovanosis (granuloma venereum, GRANULOMA INGUINALE), NONSPECIFIC URETHRITIS (NSU), REITER'S DISEASE, genital warts, genital herpes (see HERPES SIMPLEX), TRICHOMONIASIS, genital candidiasis (see CANDIDA), MOLLUSCUM CONTAGIOSUM and pediculus pubis (see LICE).

Despite better diagnosis and treatment, venereal diseases have increased during the last 25 years. Changes in public attitudes toward sexual matters, widespread use of contraceptive pills, and the emergence of resistant strains of organisms seem to have contributed to the increase. But the diseases have always tended to spread because of ignorance, reticence and the fact that women may not notice symptoms.

When diagnosed in a man or woman the disease has probably already passed on to the sexual partner; it is therefore important that both should be treated to prevent reinfection. The potential consequences of the major venereal diseases, syphilis and gonorrhea, are so damaging that there is no room for false modesty. Any suspicion of the disease, or of possible exposure to infection, calls for urgent medical attention.

venesection

The "letting of blood" as a therapeutic medical procedure. Also known as *phlebotomy*. It was widely practiced in earlier centuries, but the indications for its use were far from clearly established. It was usually carried out by cutting an arm vein and allowing the blood to run into a basin (venesection literally means the "cutting of a vein").

In modern medicine, it is employed only rarely. In POLYCYTHEMIA there is an overproduction of red blood cells. The simplest way of reducing the red cell count is by the removal of blood, using a needle and a length of plastic tubing, usually 500 cubic centimeters at a time. In HEMOCHROMATOSIS, excessive amounts of iron accumulate in the body and, since iron can only be removed from the body in the form of the hemoglobin pigment in the red blood cells, venesection is the treatment of choice. Blood donation also involves venesection.

Compare VENEPUNCTURE.

venogram

The veins, like most of their surrounding tissues, are readily penetrated by x rays and therefore do not show up on an x-ray film (radiograph). To make them visible they must be injected with material which obstructs the passage of x rays (a *radiopaque contrast medium*). If this is done, the veins will show up as light areas on the film—no blackening has occurred, as no rays can penetrate. Many such materials are available, most of them containing the heavy and radiopaque element iodine.

Liquids containing iodine compounds can be injected at any convenient site into a vein and a series of x-ray pictures taken as the radiopaque material is carried along the vein by the blood flow. Obstruction to the vein can thus be demonstrated. The technique is particularly useful in the diagnosis of THROMBOSIS of the leg veins.

ventricular fibrillation

The normal heartbeat is initiated by an electrical impulse generated in the walls of the upper chambers of the heart (atria). This impulse spreads to the remainder of the heart, producing a coordinated contraction of the muscular walls of first the atria, driving blood into the lower chambers (ventricles), and then of the ventricles themselves, driving blood out into the general circulation.

When a disorder of this regular series of events occurs, the heartbeat becomes irregular and the condition is described as a *cardiac arrhythmia*. (See ARRHYTHMIA.)

The most serious of the arrhythmias is VENTRICULAR FIBRILLATION. In this condition, the ventricles cease to contract regularly and instead show a rapid and uncoordinated contraction of all their muscle fibers without a recognizable rhythmic heartbeat. Since the effect of this is to prevent the heart from performing its normal pumping action, the circulation ceases immediately and—unless immediate measures are taken—sudden death will result. (See DEFIBRILLATION.)

Ventricular fibrillation can occur as a result of damage to the heart or its valves by drugs, infections, or interference with its blood supply via the coronary arteries (*coronary insufficiency*). Its greatest importance, however, is its occurrence as a complication of a *coronary thrombosis* (also known as a *myocardial infarction* or "heart attack")—where it is often the terminal event in sudden death.

Treatment is a matter of extreme urgency. If the situation cannot be remedied within two or three minutes, permanent or fatal damage to the brain from lack of oxygen may occur. Drugs are of limited value; the only effective treatment is to apply electrodes to the chest wall and give a short and controlled direct-current shock to the heart from a machine known as a *defibrillator*. This will lead to restoration of a normal heartbeat in a proportion of cases, although it may fail to do so.

While a defibrillator is being set up, maintenance of the blood circulation by means of closed cardiac massage and mouth-to-mouth artificial respiration is essential. If efficiently performed, it can greatly prolong the normal interval of two to three minutes between cessation of the circulation and BRAIN DEATH and will allow defibrillation to be performed even if the apparatus is not immediately available.

ventricular septal defect

See HOLE IN THE HEART.

verruca

The technical name for a wart.

See WARTS.

vertigo

A condition in which the subject feels dizzy, with a definite sensation of movement, and feels that he is or his surroundings are rotating in space. This last factor is an essential ingredient of true vertigo and distinguishes it from simple dizziness. It is often accompanied by nausea, headache or vomiting.

The loss of balance experienced in vertigo may be caused by motion (as in sea sickness), ear disease such as OTITIS INTERNA (labyrinthitis) or MÉNIÈRE'S DISEASE, damage to the acoustic (VIIIth cranial) nerve, cerebellar disease (the *cerebellum*, a major division of the brain beneath the back part of the cerebrum, is concerned with maintaining balance and coordinating muscular movements), or the effects of some drugs (such as streptomycin).

Sudden vertigo is one of the three characteristic symptoms of Ménière's disease (first discovered in 1861 by Prosper Ménière), the other two being fluctuating loss of hearing and tinnitus (a ringing sensation in the ears). Similar symptoms may sometimes occur, although less violently, after removing wax from the ear with a syringe. Vertigo may also be a symptom of certain stomach and digestive disorders, but in some people it is brought on merely by standing on a height and looking down.

While the attack lasts the patient should lie flat on his back and his collar and clothing around his neck loosened. Sedatives may be administered by a physician if the patient remains conscious. If attacks occur frequently, the patient should consult his doctor to find the cause and permit the appropriate treatment to be given.

Vincent's angina

A noncontagious infection of the gums and throat caused by either of two types of bacteria or a combination of both: a *fusiform bacillus* and a *spirochete*.

Symptoms include painful bleeding gums, excessive production of saliva and fetid breath. In the untreated disease, ulcers form on the gums and sometimes the throat, and the affected tissues may be covered with a gray membrane—the irritation or removal of which typically causes bleeding.

Both types of bacteria are found in healthy mouths, but are normally dormant. In cases of poor oral hygiene, poor general health, prolonged exhaustion, or nutritional deficiencies the infection may suddenly establish itself. (This is the reason why Vincent's angina also has the World War I nickname of *trench mouth*.)

Treatment consists of cleansing the mouth and throat with appropriate antiseptic lotions, rest, and attention to the reestablishment of adequate nutrition and good general health. Antibiotics are not usually required.

viruses

Viruses are the smallest known infectious organisms; with certain exceptions, they are too small to be seen under the ordinary light microscope. They vary in size from 10–300 nanometers (nm) in diameter. The smallest virus is about $\frac{1}{100}$ the size of a bacterium, and about $\frac{1}{750}$ the size of a red blood cell. They are unable to live or multiply outside a host cell since most do not possess the means to synthesize protein.

Structurally, a virus consists of a core of nucleic acid (its genetic material) surrounded by a protein coat. This protein coat is antigenic—that is, it will cause the production of antibodies in the blood of the host; each type of virus has an antigenic property specific for its type. (See ANTIBODY/ANTIGEN.)

Viruses are classified according to the type of nucleic acid they possess and their appearance. The main groups of medically important viruses are the *pox viruses, adenoviruses, herpes viruses, papovaviruses, myxoviruses, rhabdoviruses, enteroviruses, picornaviruses, reoviruses arboviruses* (also known as *togaviruses*), and *arenoviruses*.

Most forms of life (animals, plants or bacteria) are susceptible to virus infection. Viruses affect the cells which they inhabit in several ways. They may kill the cell; they may transform the cell from a normal cell to a cancerous cell; or they may produce a latent infection, in

Viruses, seen here magnified many thousands of times by an electron microscope, have a wide variety of striking, even beautiful, geometric shapes. They are parasitic microorganisms which can only reproduce by taking over the genetic machinery of a host cell (animal, plant or bacterium).

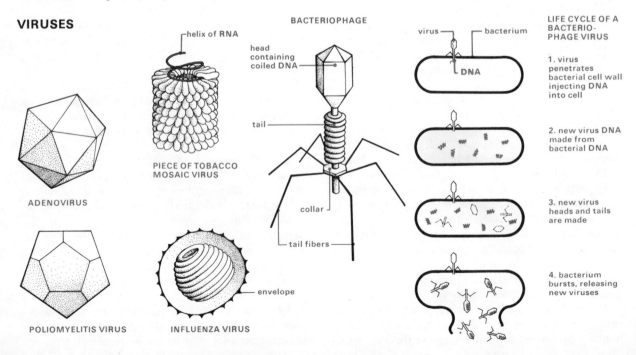

VIRUSES

helix of RNA

PIECE OF TOBACCO MOSAIC VIRUS

ADENOVIRUS

POLIOMYELITIS VIRUS

INFLUENZA VIRUS

envelope

BACTERIOPHAGE

head containing coiled DNA

tail

collar

tail fibers

virus   bacterium

DNA

LIFE CYCLE OF A BACTERIO-PHAGE VIRUS

1. virus penetrates bacterial cell wall injecting DNA into cell

2. new virus DNA made from bacterial DNA

3. new virus heads and tails are made

4. bacterium bursts, releasing new viruses

which the virus remains in the cell in a potentially active state but produces no obvious effects on the functioning of the cell.

Most viruses are inactivated by heat (100°F for 30 minutes, or 212°F for a few seconds), but most are stable at very low temperatures (for example at −95°F). The effect of drying on viruses is variable. Ultraviolet radiation inactivates viruses, and so do oxidizing agents such as formaldehyde, chlorine, iodine and hydrogen peroxide; but chloroform and ether inactivate only those viruses which contain lipid. They are resistant to glycerol, which is sometimes used as a preservative to prevent bacterial contamination of virus suspensions.

Viruses are important causes of human disease. Most virus infections are mild and may go unnoticed by the patient, although the viruses may multiply in the body and be passed on to another susceptible person. In children, the elderly, and those who are debilitated, a viral infection that is normally mild can produce severe effects. Some virus infections (such as smallpox) are severe and have a high mortality rate.

Viruses usually enter the body via the respiratory tract by inhalation, but some enter by ingestion or by inoculation through skin abrasions. The disease produced may be systemic—for example mumps, in which the virus travels through the bloodstream and invades many organs and tissues—or it may be localized and invade only tissues near the site of entry, as in respiratory viral infections.

Unlike some bacteria, viruses do not produce toxins; they produce their effects directly by multiplication in the tissues.

The body attempts to protect itself against viral infections by producing *interferon*, a protein released from infected cells which, when taken up by other cells, renders them refractory to viral infection. The body can also produce antibodies to specific viruses; these antibodies may persist for several years.

Although there are a few drugs which exhibit a degree of antiviral activity, they act only against a few types of viruses. Most viruses are resistant to the antibiotics available. Prevention of viral diseases is accomplished by the avoidance of contact with all infected individuals or by vaccination where the specific vaccines are available.

See also IMMUNIZATION.

vision

The structures concerned with vision are the eyes, optic nerves, and the occipital lobes of the brain.

Light enters the eye through the cornea, the transparent part of the outer covering of the eyeball which overlies the pupil. The pupil is the central aperture of the *iris*, the colored diaphragm which controls the amount of light admitted to the interior of the eye; it is capable of contracting so that the pupil enlarges when the intensity of the light is low. In conditions of high ambient light the pupil is small because the smooth muscle of the iris relaxes. The light reflex (or pupillary reflex) is controlled in the brain stem, and is sometimes affected in disease.

Behind the iris is the *lens* of the eye (also known as the *crystalline lens*), a transparent biconvex structure with the front curved slightly less than the back. Because it is elastic, its shape can be changed by the action of the *ciliary muscle* on the suspensory ligament which supports the lens; in this way the image of objects near the eye can be brought to a focus at the retina (see ACCOMMODATION). With age the elasticity of the lens decreases and the ability of the eye to bring near objects into focus fails; glasses for reading then become useful.

In later life the lens may become obscured by the development of a CATARACT, an opacity which interferes with vision. The image of objects falling on the lens is focused on the *retina*, which consists of receptors sensitive to light; they are of two kinds, called *rods* and *cones*.

There are about 120 million rods and about 6 million cones. Nerve fibers run from them to gather at the optic disk (the "blind spot") where they form the *optic nerve*, which passes from the eyeball to the brain. Behind the

EYE

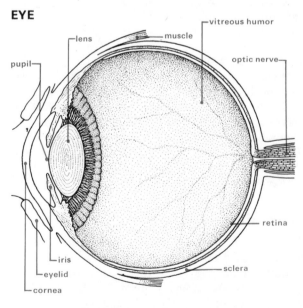

A CROSS SECTION THROUGH THE EYE

The eye is often likened to a camera because it has an adjustable lens and aperture (the pupil) with a light-sensitive film (the retina) behind. The optical images are encoded and transmitted along the optic nerve to the brain, where the simultaneous signals from both eyes are coordinated.

eyes the fibers of the optic nerves in part cross over at the *optic chiasm*, so that images entering the eyes from the right and falling on the temporal or outer side of the left retina and the inner or nasal side of the right retina are conducted to the left side of the brain (and vice versa).

If the shape of the eyeball is abnormal, objects cannot be brought to a sharp focus on the retina—a long eyeball produces short sight, while short eyeballs cannot produce a sharp image of near objects. Both conditions may be remedied by special glasses, as may aberrations of shape of the crystalline lens; if the eyeball is not truly spherical, parts of an image will not be in sharp focus at the retina, producing a defect in vision known as ASTIGMATISM.

Defects in the cones of the retina produce COLOR BLINDNESS, for they are thought to contain the three visual pigments. Rods contain only one pigment (rhodopsin), whose adsorption is greatest for blue-green light. The retina itself may be affected by disease resulting in DETACHED RETINA, hemorrhage or exudation—all of which obscure vision and must be treated medically.

Behind the eye, disease may affect the optic nerve or the crossing of the nerves (optic chiasm) so that there are defects in the field of vision; disease may also interfere with the nerve fibers as they pass through the brain to the occipital cortex at the back of the cerebral hemispheres. Examination of these visual field defects is of great value to the neurologist, who can often (by consideration of the shape and site of the defects) localize brain lesions.

Finally, the movements of the eyeballs must be accurately coordinated. Each eyeball is moved by a complex of six external *ocular muscles* supplied by nerves arising in the brain stem. Interference with the central mechanism of coordination, with the nerves or with the muscles themselves, can result in DOUBLE VISION.

See also BLINDNESS, NIGHT BLINDNESS.

vitamins

A group of unrelated substances, occurring in many foods in small amounts, which are essential for growth, health and life.

Vitamins are generally divided into two broad groups—fat soluble (A, D, E, K) and water soluble (B, C). They were originally named after a letter of the alphabet, but some—such as vitamin B—have since been found to consist of a mixture of several substances. The individual constituents of vitamin B have been given distinctive names: *thiamine* (vitamin B_1), *riboflavin* (B_2), *nicotinic acid, cyanocobalamin* (B_{12}) and so on. The whole group of vitamin B constituents is usually referred to as *vitamin B complex*.

Some vitamins can be synthesized by the body; for example, vitamin D can be synthesized from cholesterol with the action of sunlight on the skin. Others, such as vitamin K, are synthesized by bacteria in the intestine. Still others, such as vitamin C, cannot be synthesized by man and have to be provided in the food we eat.

Each vitamin has a distinctive function, and deficiency of most any vitamin may produce a characteristic group of signs and symptoms. Deficiency may arise (1) because of an inadequate intake of the vitamin or its precursors; (2) because of factors which prevent its absorption or use; or (3) because of factors which increase requirements for the vitamin or promote its excretion from the body.

Excessive amounts of many vitamins (hypervitaminosis) can produce toxic symptoms.

Vitamin A is found mainly in fish-liver oils, liver, egg yolk, butter and cream; its precursors are found in green leafy and yellow vegetables. Vitamin A deficiency produces NIGHT BLINDNESS (nyctalopia), eye changes and thickening of the cells which cover internal and body surfaces such as the skin and the lining of the gastrointestinal and urinary tracts. There is also susceptibility to infections. *Hypervitaminosis A* may be acute, and causes increased pressure in the brain producing drowsiness, irritability, headaches and vomiting. Chronic vitamin A toxicity produces loss of hair, rough skin, cracked skin and lips, and later severe headaches, generalized weakness, bony ·changes and pain in the joints.

Vitamin D comes from the same sources as vitamin A. Its deficiency results in rickets or osteomalacia, while *hypervitaminosis D* causes loss of appetite, nausea, vomiting, thirst, the passage of large quantities of urine, weakness, nervousness, itch, impairment of kidney function and calcification in various tissues.

Vitamin E is found in vegetable oils, wheat germ, leafy vegetables, egg yolk and legumes (peas, beans, etc.). Its role is to maintain the stability of cell membranes; deficiency can lead to early breakdown of red blood cells.

A deficiency of vitamin K causes bleeding, while excessive amounts cause breakdown of red blood cells.

Vitamin B_1 is found in dried yeasts, whole grain, meat, legumes (peas, beans, etc.) and potatoes; deficiency produces BERIBERI.

Vitamin B_2 is found in milk, liver, meat and eggs; deficiency produces inflammation and ulceration of the skin, mouth, eyes and genital areas.

Niacin, or nicotinic acid, is found in the same foods which contain vitamin B_1; deficiency produces pellagra.

Vitamin B_6 comprises a group of related compounds which are involved in the metabolism of many tissue systems; deficiency does not usually produce characteristic symptoms, although a number of vague symptoms may occur which can be relieved by treatment with vitamin B_6.

Vitamin C (ascorbic acid) is found in citrus foods and green vegetables; deficiency causes SCURVY, once a common disease among seafarers.

Folic acid is a B vitamin found in many animal and plant tissues. Deficiency is associated with malabsorption of food from the small intestine and megaloblastic anemia. Similarly, deficiency of vitamin B_{12} (which is found in meat and dairy products) may produce megaloblastic anemia.

vitiligo

A condition in which light-coloured blotchy patches appear on the skin or hair as a result of the localized absence of the pigment *melanin*, the presence of which gives the skin its characteristic color.

vomiting

The forcible ejection through the mouth of the contents of the stomach, caused by a reflex controlled by a vomiting center in the brain. Retching is vomiting without the production of stomach contents.

The vomiting reflex can be set in motion by many different stimuli. Direct stimulation of the vomiting center occurs in meningitis, migraine, and the state of increased pressure within the skull caused by tumors or hemorrhage. This type of vomiting is not accompanied by nausea; it may also be caused by various drugs.

Many people vomit as the result of emotional shock—for example, at the sight of a bad road accident, or the perception of a disgusting smell; others vomit when unduly excited or anxious. Travel sickness is a problem for a number of people, particularly the young. It is caused by stimulation of the vomiting center by impulses arising in the inner ear.

The most common cause of vomiting is intestinal disturbance, when irritation brought about by over-distension or inflammation sets up the reflex through the vagus nerve—which serves both to carry stimuli to the vomiting center and to transmit the outgoing nerve impulses necessary for the accomplishment of the act.

The vomiting which often occurs during pregnancy may be due to changes in hormone balance, but the cause is not definitely known.

Vomiting in children may herald the onset of an infectious fever, while in babies it is often the result of injudicious feeding or the swallowing of too much air.

So many disturbances cause vomiting that it is not possible to generalize about the most effective treatment, which must depend on the treatment of the underlying condition. One danger of vomiting to excess, particularly in young children, is loss of water and salts from the body with consequent dehydration and imbalance of electrolytes. A more immediate danger is inhalation of vomit, which may occur in unconscious or semiconscious persons.

von Recklinghausen's disease

A hereditary condition (also known as *neurofibromatosis*) in which numerous "neurofibromas" are found all over the body. These are benign tumors that arise in the skin or in the fibrous tissue surrounding peripheral and cranial nerves. The neurofibromas may occur on any nerve. If superficial, they may be seen as nodules under the skin; if they develop around deeper nerves, they may not be noticed until they produce symptoms by pressing on adjacent structures.

The symptoms of the disease depend largely on the severity of nerve involvement. In many cases, where the peripheral nerves are affected, there may be no symptoms at all (except perhaps pain on pressure over the course of the affected nerve or nerves). However, if the cranial nerves or the roots of the spinal nerves are involved, serious disability may result—depending on the function of the damaged nerves. Associated tumors of the brain (although relatively uncommon) can be particularly serious; surgical removal of accessible tumors is usually attempted.

Aside from surgical intervention (where appropriate), no specific treatment currently exists for von Recklinghausen's disease. It is very rarely fatal; the major complications arise in those patients who develop a malignant degeneration of the affected tissues.

vulvitis

Inflammation of the vulva, the female external sexual organs excluding the vagina. The vulva consists of the labia majora, labia minora, clitoris, the urethral meatus and various glands. It may become inflamed as the result of many types of skin disorders.

Infections which may be involved include the herpes simplex virus, other viruses, and Trichomonas. Infections by fungus and yeast organisms are often associated with pregnancy and diabetes. They lead to a beefy red appearance and severe itching. This type of infection can usually be controlled quickly and effectively with local applications of nystatin.

It is also essential to control the underlying disease in cases of diabetes. *Molluscum contagiosum*, a viral disease of the skin, is noted in the vulval area and can be transmitted during sexual intercourse.

In general, dermatological problems such as psoriasis, seborrheic dermatitis and folliculitis often involve the vulva. Friction, allergies, or irritation can lead to "eczematoid dermatitis," which responds well to local hydrocortisone and antihistamines. INTERTRIGO may involve the labial folds. It is not uncommon for vulvitis to be initiated by vaginitis spreading to the vulva by the agency of an extensive discharge, with resultant severe vulvar edema and itching. Treatment is directed at the underlying cause.

warts

Small solid benign tumors that arise from the surface of the skin as a result of a virus infection.

Warts (or *verrucas*) are extremely common and usually completely harmless, although they may be unsightly and irritating. A wart appears when the activity of the virus causes hypertrophy of the papillae of the skin. This results in the growth of a bundle of fibers from the skin's surface, capped by the horny cells that cover the cuticle. The mass of the wart is surrounded by a ring of thickened cuticle and the fibers can be seen particularly well when the wart has been growing for some time and has become abraded. The color of the wart is usually darker than that of the background skin, but this is because dirt becomes lodged in the minute crevices between the fibers.

Warts are common in children, probably because of a lack of immunity to the causative virus. They often appear more thickly on areas such as the knuckles, the insides of the knees and the face—where the skin is more likely to be irritated. Adolescents and young adults often suffer from epidemics in schools and other institutions, such as military camps, where physical education and swimming may be conducted in bare feet. The wart transmitted in these cases, the *plantar wart* on the soles of the feet, can be painful because of the pressure of the body's weight during walking. Older people suffer from *senile warts* and there is a type of *soft wart* on the eyelids, ears and neck which can occur among people working with hydrocarbons.

Treatment of warts is usually accomplished successfully, where it is thought necessary, by the simple expedient of removing them by application of a freezing agent such as liquid nitrogen or carbon dioxide snow. Plantar warts unsuitable for this treatment may need surgical excision. Chemical agents for the removal of warts are now little used: their effects are slow and repeated applications are necessary.

Wasserman reaction

A serological test for syphilis, which is positive five to seven weeks from the date of infection. However, a positive reaction does not necessarily indicate the presence of syphilis, since false positives may occur with some autoimmune diseases.

weaning

Teaching a baby to eat foods other than milk. In the past 30 years some nutritionists have argued that weaning can be started in the first month of life; others have urged that it should be delayed until the age of six months. This lack of any consistent expert advice is evidence that a baby will come to little harm whichever policy is followed.

Although the early introduction of solid foods is well tolerated, it is probably not necessary for the nutritional needs of the child. So long as a baby seems content and gains weight satisfactorily on a milk diet there need be no hurry to wean him.

wheeze

A noise produced in respiratory diseases when the walls of the larger airways are in apposition and behaving like the reed of a toy trumpet.

Wheeze is frequently observed in patients with airway obstruction and is often worse in the morning, during and after exercise, and following a chest infection. A particularly high-pitched wheezing is characteristic of acute asthma.

Although wheezing is diagnostic of chest disease and is one of the signs looked for by the doctor, it is also heard in normal people during a sudden violent expiratory effort.

See also PULMONARY DISEASES.

whiplash injury

If an automobile is suddenly hit from behind, the head and neck, which are more mobile than the trunk, move violently forward and backward like the lash of a whip. The movement can damage the neck, or in violent accidents the spinal cord or even the brain.

A very common complaint even after minor collisions is stiffness of the neck. This usually wears off, but the injury can be severe enough to require the wearing of a collar to limit movement of the cervical spine until recovery is complete. Unfortunately, the effects of whiplash injury may take a long time to show themselves, and the development of "cervical disk syndrome" can sometimes be traced back to an accident that occurred some years before.

Headrests (or more properly, head restraints) fitted to car seats protect against these injuries by preventing the backward whiplash movement of the neck.

whitlow

See FELON.

whooping cough

An infectious disease of the mucous membranes lining the air passages. Also called *pertussis*. It mainly affects children, who achieve lifelong immunity after infection. Thanks to improved health care and vaccination, it is no longer the menace that it was.

Whooping cough gets its popular name from the fact that the irritation of the upper respiratory passages causes convulsive bouts of coughing, followed by a peculiar indrawing of the breath. Children, particularly those under the age of one year, were once greatly at risk from whooping cough. In 1906 the causative organism, *Bordetella pertussis*, was isolated for the first time and in the last three or four decades vaccines of greater and greater efficacy have been prepared. The effect has been to make whooping cough a comparatively rare disease. Some cases of brain damage to vaccinated children have been reported, but this risk is smaller than the risk of similar damage caused by the disease itself.

In cases where vaccination has not been performed, three stages of the disease may be expected to occur. The initial "catarrhal" stage is followed by the "spasmodic" stage—in which all the classical symptoms appear—and by the stage of decline. During the spasmodic stage the bouts of coughing and "whooping" last about 30 to 45 seconds and can be extremely distressing and frightening to a child.

The spasmodic stage may last four to seven weeks and in rare cases may leave behind side effects such as EMPHYSEMA or a liability to attacks of ASTHMA. Whooping cough is highly contagious. Where a case occurs it is wise to isolate the sufferer from other children, or even adults, who have not previously had the disease (or have not been vaccinated). The patient should be kept warm and restricted to bed until the symptoms become less severe. Spasms of coughing may be relieved by the administration of drugs such as phenobarbital.

Vaccination should be performed at as early an age as possible, with a reinforcing dose at a year to 18 months.

X

xeroderma

A disorder in which the skin is very rough and dry.

The most common form is also known as *ichthyosis*

simplex, in which large corrugated papery scales form on the skin (which is deficient in sebaceous glands and sometimes also in sweat glands). *Xeroderma pigmentosum* is a rare disease, usually appearing in childhood, in which the skin atrophies (wastes away) and contracts. It is associated with overexposure to harsh sunlight, but there is also a familial tendency. Sufferers have photophobia (abnormal sensitivity of the eyes to light) and the warty and "keratolytic" lesions of the disease quickly become malignant. The skin has the appearance of senility even in young patients.

X rays

X rays, discovered in 1895 by the German physicist Wilhelm Konrad Roentgen (1845–1923), have become one of the best-known aids to both diagnosis and treatment.

A standard radiograph (or "x ray picture") is produced by placing the hand, for example, on a sheet of x ray film enclosed in a light-proof envelope and exposing it to radiation from an x ray tube. The bones, being resistant to the passage of x rays (*radiopaque*), will appear on the film as a white unexposed area, while the soft tissues, offering no resistance (*radiolucent*), allow the film underlying them to be exposed and blackened by the rays. The result, in photographic terms, is a "negative" picture of the bones of the hand.

Since most soft tissues are radiolucent, their visualization requires special radiographic techniques; although the lungs, since they are air-filled, are so much more radiolucent than other tissues that the lung fields can be easily studied on a simple chest x ray. A technique with wide applications, however, is to inject or give by mouth or otherwise introduce into the body a fluid contrast material which is opaque to x rays. The upper part of the intestinal tract can thus be visualized on x rays if the patient first swallows a suspension of barium sulfate (*barium meal*); to visualize the large intestine on an x ray, a similar suspension can be given as an enema (*barium enema*).

Certain iodine-containing compounds can be injected into a blood vessel to allow x-ray visualization of the heart, arteries and veins (*arteriogram, venogram*). Similar material, on injection into the circulation, is rapidly excreted by the kidneys, allowing the kidneys to be visualized (*intravenous pyelogram*); by the same means the liver, gallbladder and bile ducts can be visualized (*cholecystogram*). Injection of iodine-containing material into the cerebrospinal fluid (around the brain and spinal cord) allows these structures to be seen on an x-ray (*myelogram*).

A new technique for soft tissue visualization is *tomography*. Movement of the x-ray tube during the exposure allows a plane of tissues to be examined in more detail, since there is no interference by tissues which lie above or beneath. This technique will reveal soft tissue structures not identifiable on a standard x-ray. A more recent development still is *computerized axial tomography (CAT scan)*. Here multiple tissue planes are viewed by tomography and the results are analyzed by an attached computer to build up a detailed picture of the soft tissue structures. The computer coordinates, integrates, and interprets a vast amount of data in clear, crisp images of high resolution that clearly demonstrate abnormalities of a size imperceptible to earlier machines. The CAT Scan is applicable to the diagnosis of tumors and other lesions within the brain, liver, and other organs not easily visualized on x rays by other means.

X rays are also widely used in the treatment of cancer.

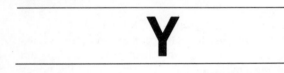

yaws

An infectious disease occurring in the hot moist tropics—especially in Africa, the West Indies and some parts of the Far East.

It is caused by a spirochete known as *Treponema pertenue*. The disease is also known as *frambesia* (from a French word meaning raspberry), because of the resemblance of the lesions to squashed raspberries. The first manifestation of yaws is an initial lesion of the skin, which is known as the mother yaw (or mamanpian). After this lesion has appeared, probably as a result of the transmission of the spirochete to the skin by various species of flies, or by direct contact with a sufferer, other lesions follow over the surface of the body. If the disease is left untreated more damaging lesions can occur, eroding both skin and bones.

The incubation period for yaws is two to four weeks, during which time the patient may experience a general feeling of being unwell (malaise) as well as pains, fever and a severe itching of the skin. A scaly eruption on the body and legs turns into the characteristic lesions with the appearance of lumps. Some of them may develop to be several inches in diameter and when the general level of health is low they may break down and form ulcers.

In most cases the lesions shrink slowly and eventually disappear after a few weeks or months. Yaws is one of the more important debilitating diseases of the tropics, especially in people who are malnourished or otherwise not in good health. It can be an especially severe disease when it occurs in combination with syphilis or tuberculosis. Since the introduction of antibiotics, however, its effect on the economic and social life of the people of the tropics has diminished; penicillin has dramatic effects on the lesions by killing the infecting microorganisms. Prevention is by normal hygienic safeguards; spread of the disease can be checked by isolating sufferers.

yellow fever

An acute viral infection of the liver, kidneys and heart muscle transmitted by a female mosquito of the genus *Aedes*. It occurs in tropical Africa and parts of America lying between Brazil and the southern United States.

In the last century yellow fever killed so many workers engaged in constructing the Panama Canal that the French Panama Canal Company became bankrupt. During the Spanish–American war in 1900 a team of Army doctors—including Walter Reed—showed that the disease was transmitted by a species of mosquito known as *Aedes aegypti*. An efficient vaccine was eventually produced, giving up to ten years protection.

There is no known specific treatment for yellow fever. From about 3 to 14 days after being bitten by an infected mosquito the patient develops a headache, fever, and pains in the muscles. In a severe attack the temperature rises, the face becomes flushed and the mind confused. After two days the fever abates and confusion clears; but within 48 hours delirium may return, the pulse becomes slow and weak and the patient ceases to pass urine and becomes yellow as the infection spreads in the liver, kidneys and heart muscles. About one in five of those who develop jaundice die.

The control of yellow fever depends on strict control of the *Aedes aegypti*, which is a domestic mosquito breeding in pools of stagnant water and the water in the bottoms of old pots and pans and oil drums left near houses.

All travelers to places where the disease exists must be immunized at least ten days before they travel.

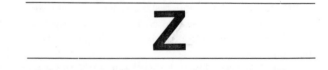

zoonosis

Any disease shared by man and other vertebrate animals.

More than 150 zoonoses, carried by a variety of animals, are known; but modern medicine and veterinary science have been able to control many of them, or to ameliorate their effects. Even so, some of them still present a very real threat to human and animal life.

Examples of zoonoses are ANTHRAX, BRUCELLOSIS, PSITTACOSIS and RABIES.